Problem Solving in Clinical Medicine

From Data to Diagnosis

SECOND EDITION

Problem Solving in Clinical Medicine

From Data to Diagnosis

SECOND EDITION

Paul Cutler, M.D.

Clinical Professor of Medicine
The Jefferson Medical College
Philadelphia, Pennsylvania

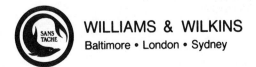

WILLIAMS & WILKINS
Baltimore • London • Sydney

Editor: James Sangston
Associate Editor: Victoria M. Vaughn
Copy Editor: Deborah K. Tourtlotte
Design: Bert Smith
Illustration Planning: Joseph P. Cummings
Production: Raymond E. Reter

First Edition, 1979
  Reprinted 1980

Library of Congress Cataloging in Publication Data

Cutler, Paul, 1920–
   Problem solving in clinical medicine.

   Includes bibliographies and index.
   1. Diagnosis. 2. Medical logic. 3. Problem solving. 4. Medicine, Clinical. I. Title.
[DNLM: 1. Diagnosis. 2. Internal Medicine. 3. Problem Solving. WB 141 C989p]
RC71.3.C88 1985   616.07'5   84-11946 ISBN 0-683-02252-0

Composed and printed at the
Waverly Press, Inc.

to Helene

who is *still* always with me

Preface to Second Edition

An author usually writes a second edition because 4 years have elapsed since the first, because small changes have occurred which render the book's contents obsolete in a few areas, and because competition with publishers of similar books makes a new edition economically advisable.

Such is not the case here. Except for books written primarily for educators, I know of no comparable text that teaches and exemplifies medical problem solving at the elementary level compatible with student comprehension.

Since 1979, problem solving, problem-based learning, probability theory, and decision analysis have become key concepts in educational circles, and they have started to flood the medical literature, to creep slightly into standard textbooks, and even to enter into formalized undergraduate courses in a few schools.

The blind men from beyond Ghor have begun to confer with each other, and a more holistic and accurate concept of both the elephant and the profession of medicine is under construction.

Much ongoing research aims to determine how the mind works, how patient information is processed, and how the clinician solves problems and makes decisions. The transactions of the young Society for Medical Decision Making are testimony to the progress being made in these areas.

Patients and their families, hospital and public policy, and administrators, politicians, attorneys, and clergy—all demand that students learn and physicians practice medicine with ever increasing new concerns in mind. Simply providing the best possible care is not enough. Consideration must be given to accountability, cost containment, health care rationing, and the various legal, moral, and ethical issues that are implicated by these new slants.

And at long last the concrete curricula of ivied and ivory towers are being eroded by the realization that students learn better by teaching themselves than by rote memorization and regurgitation of didactic lectures. Not since the days of Flexner have curricula been under such scrutiny, criticism, reevaluation, and revision. Students must be inspired to think, to read, to learn, to solve, to decide—not to memorize. Demonstrating the intellectual beauty of problem solving should do much to restore the enthusiasm and scholarly attitude of medical students who are being drowned by thousands of facts which they will mostly never use again.

Greater stress is being laid on protocols, flow charts, algorithms, and decision trees. Nevertheless, the fact remains that problem solving begins with and depends primarily on the taking of the history and on the processing of patient data—two skills in which students are notoriously weak.

Any book that attempts to teach students of the 80's to deal with patient problems must include: the concept of imperfect information; the consideration of informed consent and cost of medical care; the intelligent selection of tests and treatment; the availability of new but expensive procedures that may short-cut, although sometimes complicate, the diagnostic process; attempts to make computer programs that simulate natural intelligence; and efforts to construct mathematical models that add precision to intuitive and judgmental decisions.

To accomplish these objectives, the section on the problem-solving process was rewritten, revised, and expanded. Chapters on data processing, data relevance, decision making, the impact of new diagnostic tools, and the ordering and interpretation of tests were added. All case studies and their associated "Suggested Readings" lists were updated. An introductory chapter instructs the student or teacher how, where, and when to best use this book. Numerous exercises and self-evaluation procedures have been interspersed throughout the text; the answers follow.

It is hoped that this book will increasingly serve as a model for teaching students how to to think—to learn—then think again.

May I express even greater gratitude than before to my wife and friend, Helene, not only for her encouragement and forebearance (perfunctory functions of most spouses), but for her exceptional typing, proofreading, and editing—and for the remarkable ways in which her Betz cells have filled the void created by those which may have disappeared from my own cortex.

PAUL CUTLER, M.D.
Philadelphia, Pennsylvania

Preface to First Edition

Just as King Savatthi's blind men described the elephant—student, teacher, practitioner, and patient each sees medicine in his own way. The student asks, "How much must I learn? What's important, and how do I put it all together to solve the patient's problems?" The teacher answers, "Learn it all! $a+b+c=x$. Proceed in an orderly complete fashion." The practitioner is concerned with shortcuts, speed, experience, and clinical judgment. The patient wants to know, "What's wrong, can you cure me, and how much will it cost?"

And each is right.

And each is wrong.

Having observed medicine for 38 years from all four viewpoints—as student, teacher, practitioner, and patient—not like the blind men, but in a holistic and overlapping manner—I have noted that the effectiveness of many students and physicians is impaired because they have never really learned or acquired certain vital skills and categories of information. These include:

1. Collection and interpretation of data
2. Pathophysiology of disease
3. Processing of data into what is relevant
4. Many presentations of a disease
5. Many diseases causing a presentation
6. Appreciation of what is common and likely
7. Solution of problems.

In addition to being covered in many good books, the first two items are now taught intensively at most medical schools. Physical Diagnosis and Introduction to Clinical Medicine take care of data collection (1); the pathophysiology of disease (2) is taught in an integrated modular fashion or in traditional separate subjects, depending on the curricular structure of each school. Yet few schools, and almost no books, teach the student how to process or synthesize acquired data into diagnoses or problem lists— a skill requiring knowledge of items 3 to 7. This book is concerned mainly with these last five items; principal emphasis, however, is on problem solving, since mastery of its intricacies differentiates the outstanding from the mediocre student or physician.

Sometimes data synthesis and problem solving are half-heartedly included in Physical Diagnosis or Introduction to Clinical Medicine. More often they are left for the third-year medicine clerkship, where it is hoped the student will somehow acquire those skills by himself, from the busy intern or resident, at the foot of the attending physician, by observation or by osmosis—but rarely is time allotted for the formal teaching of this material.

Modern curricula are accelerated. The student usually sees patients in his first year, and on completion of his third year he has seen, felt, heard, and learned more than the previous generation had experienced after 5 to 10 years in practice. Everything is taught earlier. Why not problem solving?

Sometime between the second and fifth years of medical education, the student must learn to think, to solve, to relate, and to manage. Some do. Many do not. A few never do!

To illustrate: I used to know a physician who had quick indiscriminate recall of thousands of facts. He attended all conferences, read numerous journals, and took assiduous notes. Yet he did not know how to handle facts and could not solve patient problems. He had no judgment, no common sense, and was a failure so far as patient care was concerned. If he saw someone who was sick, he could list 10 possible diseases, but he could not tell what was *most likely* to be wrong. Patients were usually frightened away by his imposing differential diagnoses. Once at 2 AM he saw a 65-year-old woman who had epigastric discomfort and vomiting due to a dietary indiscretion. As possible causes of her illness he listed everything from acute gastritis, perforated ulcer, and cancer of the stomach to coronary thrombosis and dissecting aneurysm—all unlikely except for the first. By 8 AM she had placed herself under the care of another physician who recognized that she needed only a tranquilizer and reassurance. The first physician had never learned problem solving—either in school or 20 years after.

Should the medical student be expected to know disease probabilities, odds, and likelihoods? How does he deal with the absence of a crucial clue or the presence of one that does not fit? Can he learn to categorize symptoms or groups of symptoms which overlap into many diseases? Should he be able to cope with the varied presentations of a single disease? Which clues form a plausible cluster? Can he deal with the specificity and sensitivity of clues in the history, physical examination, and laboratory profile? What about the orderly selection of appropriate diagnostic studies? Are we dealing with one disease or are there several? Indeed, is it possible to teach the student to think in these terms and can we give him guidelines for solving problems?

I believe so.

This book purports to teach the student to reason in a logical, rational manner. After a general discussion of preliminary key issues, it goes on to describe and give examples of more than 25 methods of problem solving called upon daily by the clinician. As a rule these techniques are used almost subconsciously in a manner which the capable physician does not conceptualize and may not even be aware of.

After a second section on data synthesis, 65 common patient presentations in Section Three demonstrate the use of previously discussed techniques. Different methods are used in each case, depending upon the nature of the problem and the approach of each contributing author. Section Four contains specialized aspects of problem solving.

Some of this material is derived from scattered references. Much is the distillate of 30 years' experience in private practice, primitive medicine in central Asia, and academia. I regret not being able to give due credit for the numerous "pearls, nuggets, and aphorisms" incorporated into my own knowledge base from long-forgotten sources, but who can remember where he learned or read all that he knows?

Sincere thanks to my more identifiable sources of assistance: the contributors; the students who taught me what they needed to know; those of the Williams & Wilkins Co. who gave guidance and planning; Leon Cander, M.D., the chairman of medicine who gave me his friendship and the freedom, advice, and support needed to develop new ways to teach students to think and learn; Terry Mikiten, Ph.D. for his early suggestions regarding clarity and content; Lee B. Lusted, M.D., Edmond A. Murphy, M.D., and Alvan R. Feinstein, M.D., whose writings were inspirational; my wife, Helene, for her encouragement, critiques, manuscript typing, proofreading, and editing; and, last, my father, Meyer Melechovitch Kotlyarenko, but for whose emigration 75 years ago this book might have been written in Russian or not at all.

PAUL CUTLER, M.D.
San Antonio, Texas

Contributors

H. Leonard Bentch, M.D.
Clinical Associate Professor of Medicine
The University of Texas
Health Science Center
at San Antonio

Charles L. Bowden, M.D.
Professor of Psychiatry
The University of Texas
Health Science Center
at San Antonio

Timothy N. Caris, M.D.
Professor of Medicine
The University of Texas
Health Science Center
at San Antonio

Charles A. Coltman, Jr., M.D.
Professor of Medicine
The University of Texas
Health Science Center
at San Antonio

Michael H. Crawford, M.D.
Professor of Medicine
The University of Texas
Health Science Center
at San Antonio

Paul Cutler, M.D.
Clinical Professor of Medicine
Jefferson Medical College
Philadelphia

Herschel L. Douglas, M.D.
Professor of Family Practice
and Dean
Quillen-Dishner College of Medicine
Johnson City

Marvin Forland, M.D.
Professor of Medicine
The University of Texas
Health Science Center
at San Antonio

Samuel J. Friedberg, M.D.
Professor of Medicine
The University of Texas
Health Science Center
at San Antonio

James N. George, M.D.
Professor of Medicine
The University of Texas
Health Science Center
at San Antonio

Ralph S. Goldsmith, M.D.
Professor of Medicine
University of California
School of Medicine
San Francisco

Gary D. Harris, M.D.
Associate Professor of Medicine
The University of Texas
Health Science Center
at San Antonio

David W. Hawkins, Pharm.D.
Associate Professor of Family Medicine
East Carolina University
School of Medicine
Greenville

James D. Heckman, M.D.
Associate Professor of Orthopaedic Surgery
The University of Texas
Health Science Center
at San Antonio

Lawrence D. Horwitz, M.D.
Professor of Medicine
University of Colorado Medical Center
Denver

Robert W. Huff, M.D.
Professor of Obstetrics and Gynecology
The University of Texas
Health Science Center
at San Antonio

Waldemar G. Johanson, Jr., M.D.
Professor of Medicine
The University of Texas
Health Science Center
at San Antonio

David A. Kronick, Ph.D.
Professor of Medical Bibliography
The University of Texas
Health Science Center
at San Antonio

David J. Kudzma, M.D.
Clinical Associate Professor of Medicine
University of Miami
School of Medicine
Miami

Shirley P. Levine, M.D.
Associate Professor of Medicine
The University of Texas
Health Science Center
at San Antonio

Meyer D. Lifschitz, M.D.
Professor of Medicine
The University of Texas
Health Science Center
at San Antonio

Roger M. Lyons, M.D.
Clinical Associate Professor of Medicine
The University of Texas
Health Science Center
at San Antonio

Arthur S. McFee, M.D., Ph.D.
Professor of Surgery
The University of Texas
Health Science Center
at San Antonio

Carlos A. Moreno, M.D.
Assistant Professor of Family Practice
The University of Texas
Health Science Center
at San Antonio

Arvo Neidre, M.D.
Clinical Assistant Professor of Orthopaedic
    Surgery
The University of Texas
Health Science Center
at San Antonio

Carlos Pestana, M.D., Ph.D.
Professor of Surgery
The University of Texas
Health Science Center
at San Antonio

Alexander W. Pierce, Jr., M.D.
Professor of Pediatrics
The University of Texas
Health Science Center
at San Antonio

Henry J. Reineck, M.D.
Associate Professor of Medicine
The University of Texas
Health Science Center
at San Antonio

David A. Sears, M.D.
Professor of Medicine
Baylor College of Medicine
Houston

Paul C. Weinberg, M.D.
Professor of Family Practice
The University of Texas
Health Science Center
at San Antonio

Ernest Urban, M.B.B.S.
Associate Professor of Medicine
The University of Texas
Health Science Center
at San Antonio

Elliot Weser, M.D.
Professor of Medicine
The University of Texas
Health Science Center
at San Antonio

Contents

Preface 2   vii
Preface 1   ix
Contributors   xi

Introduction: How To Use This Book

Aims of This Book   xxi
What It Teaches   xxi
Section by Section   xxii
Self-Evaluation   xxiii
Objectives   xxiii
Need to Teach Problem Solving   xxv
Where, When, and How It's Taught   xxvi
Problem-Based Learning   xxvi
On the Subject of Supplementary Reading   xxvii
A Recommended Way   xxix
Some Final Comments   xxxi

Section One   The Problem-Solving Process

Chapter 1   Problem Solving: What It Is

Three Questions   2
What the Physician Does   2
What the Student Must Do   3
Faculty Faults   6
Confessions of a Problem Solver   7
Patient Management   7
Necessary Student Skills   10
The Three Questions Revisited   10

Chapter 2   Data Collection, Data Processing, Problem Lists

Data Collection   12
History Taking   13
Physical Examination   21
Paraclinical Studies   27
Data Processing   30

Problem Lists   34
Self-Evaluation Exercises   37

Chapter 3   Clues: The Building Blocks **40**

Chapter 4   From Odds to Ends

Application of Logic   50
Depth of Study   53
Shortcuts   55
Coming to Terms   56
The Decision-Making Process   58
The Science of Diagnosis   59
Tactics and Strategies   60
Why Clinical Pictures Differ   62
Conclusions   63

Chapter 5   Digits, Decimals, and Doctors

Who Needs Math Anyway?   65
Boole à Bayes   67
Making Sense of Numbers   72
Pas de Deux   77
The Ways of Bayes   81
The Nays of Bayes   88
Adding by Multiplication   89
Some Final Reflections   93
Self-Evaluation Exercises   93

Chapter 6   How to Use Tests **98**

Why We Use Tests   99
Know Your Lab   100
What Normal Is   103
Correct Test Usage   105
Misuse of Tests   108
Alteration of Testing Formats   110
Strategies for Testing   112

Chapter 7   The Impact of New Technology **118**

Complex Considerations   119
Ultrasound   120
Computed Tomography   121
Nuclear Imaging   122
Biopsies   122
Newer Radiologic Modalities   123
Are We Better Off?   124

Chapter 8   Making Medical Decisions

On Zen, Zoos, Zealots, and Zeitgeist   127

What Decision Theory Is **129**
Where the Numbers Come From **137**
Risks, Costs, Benefits **139**
A Case in Point **141**
Uses, Pros, and Cons **144**

Chapter 9   Problem-Solving Methods **148**

Section Two   Data Management: Synthesis and Analysis

Introduction to Section Two **172**
Chapter 10   From Patient to Paper

Patient Interview **174**
Written Record—Author's Version **178**
Mistakes Students Make **181**
The First Few Minutes **183**

Chapter 11   From Data Base to Problem List

Some Aids First **187**
Sample Data Base 1 . . . .   **188**
Sample Data Base 2 . . . .   **193**

Chapter 12   The Case Presentation

The Medes and Persians **199**
Abbreviated Data Base (A) **201**
Abbreviated Data Base (B) **202**
Abbreviated Data Base (C) **203**
Abbreviated Data Base (D) **203**

Chapter 13   Data Resolution Skills

Selecting Data Subsets **205**
Performing Relevance Exercises **209**
Decoding Problem Sets **217**

Section Three   Problem Solving in Action

Introduction to Section Three **222**
Chapter 14   Hematologic Problems

Introduction **225**
Case 1   Weakness and Joint Pains **227**
Case 2   Bleeding Gums and Bruising **232**
Case 3   Lethargy and Confusion **236**
Case 4   Backache, Weakness, Nosebleeds **241**
Case 5   Cough, Fever, then Fatigue **245**
Case 6   Elevated Hematocrit **250**

Case 7   Jaundice, Weakness, Pallor   256
Case 8   Neck Lumps   260

Chapter 15   Endocrine Problems

Introduction   266
Case 9   A Thyroid Nodule   269
Case 10   Glycosuria   273
Case 11   Weakness, Anxiety, Sweating   278
Case 12   Obesity and Hirsutism   282
Case 13   Nervousness and Weight Loss   286
Case 14   Polyuria and Polydipsia   290

Chapter 16   Cardiovascular Problems

Introduction   295
Case 15   Abnormal ECG   298
Case 16   Dyspnea on Exertion   302
Case 17   Severe Substernal Tightness   306
Case 18   Systolic Murmur   310
Case 19   Palpitations   315
Case 20   Swollen Legs   318
Case 21   Sharp Chest Pains   323

Chapter 17   Pulmonary Problems

Introduction   327
Case 22   X-ray Abnormality   329
Case 23   Wheeze and Dyspnea   335
Case 24   Coughing of Blood   340
Case 25   Cough, Fever, Chill   344
Case 26   Sudden Shortness of Breath   349
Case 27   Chronic Cough and Expectoration   353
Case 28   Worsening Shortness of Breath   358

Chapter 18   Gastrointestinal Problems

Introduction   363
Case 29   Difficulty in Swallowing   365
Case 30   Vomiting of Blood   369
Case 31   Indigestion   372
Case 32   Sudden Upper Abdominal Pain   377
Case 33   Diarrhea and Weight Loss   382
Case 34   Lower Abdominal Pain   387
Case 35   Black Stools   392
Case 36   Jaundice and Pain   397
Case 37   Cramps and Nausea   403
Case 38   Fever and Confusion with Cirrhosis   408

Chapter 19   Renal Problems

Introduction **413**
Case 39   Bloody Urine **415**
Case 40   Frequent and Painful Urination **422**
Case 41   Sharp Flank Pain **427**
Case 42   Swelling of Face and Legs **432**
Case 43   Unconsciousness **437**
Case 44   Nausea, Weakness, Confusion **442**

Chapter 20   Electrolyte Problems

Introduction **447**
Case 45   Fatigue and Abnormal ECG **449**
Case 46   Hypercalcemia **454**
Case 47   Weakness and Disorientation **459**

Chapter 21   Gynecologic Problems

Introduction **465**
Case 48   A Missed Menstrual Period **467**
Case 49   Acute Pelvic Pain **471**
Case 50   Abnormal Vaginal Bleeding **474**

Chapter 22   Musculoskeletal Problems

Introduction **479**
Case 51   Painful Swollen Joint **481**
Case 52   Shoulder Pain **485**
Case 53   Painful Stiff Joints **490**
Case 54   Backache **495**

Chapter 23   Neurologic Problems

Introduction **500**
Case 55   Headache **502**
Case 56   Convulsions **507**
Case 57   Dizziness **512**
Case 58   Paralysis **516**

Chapter 24   Multisystem Problems

Introduction **522**
Case 59   Weakness, Weight Loss, Anorexia **523**
Case 60   Swelling of the Abdomen **527**
Case 61   High Blood Pressure **531**
Case 62   Sudden Coma **536**
Case 63   Fainting Spells **540**
Case 64   Strange Behavior **545**
Case 65   Prolonged Fever **550**

Section Four   Special Aspects of Problem Solving

Introduction to Section Four 558

Chapter 25   Information Retrieval 559

Chapter 26   Triage, Screening, Urgent Care 565

Chapter 27   Doctor- and Drug-Induced Diseases 570

**Chapter 28   Special Aspects of Problem Solving in the
Psychiatric Patient** 577

**Chapter 29   Special Aspects of Problem Solving in the
Pediatric Patient** 584

**Chapter 30   Special Aspects of Problem Solving in the
Geriatric Patient** 588

Index 595

Introduction: How To Use This Book

Feedback from teachers and students has indicated a need to explain ways to use this book. Simply reading it is not enough.

Since curriculum structures differ, and since the styles of intertwining Physical Diagnosis, Introduction to Clinical Medicine, and the medicine clerkship vary, it may be difficult to decide just where and even whether *problem solving* should be taught and this book used. A few schools cover this subject in an expanded Physical Diagnosis course; in others it is interdigitated with Introduction to Clinical Medicine; elsewhere it is included in the third-year clerkships. Some teach problem solving during an interphase period between the end of the second year and the beginning of the traditional third-year clinical rotations. Others suggest that students independently read books on problem solving as an optional or recommended exercise. A few are more daring and give separate specially designed courses or electives on the subject. These cut across traditional course boundaries. But most schools ignore the issue and expect students to acquire clinical reasoning skills "naturally."

Experiences in the past 5 years have suggested ways in which users of this particular book may benefit more. These users include course directors who employ the book as a guide, course directors who want their students to use it, and students who want to get their money's worth and thereby profit the most. These methods will be explained later in this introductory section.

Aims of This Book

Essentially, this book attempts to bridge the chasm between basic science and the bedside, between pathophysiology and the patient, between knowledge and the application of knowledge—but mainly the gap between the collection of data and their synthesis into defined problems. *Diagnosis* is the name of this game.

Consequently, the contents are directed at second-year students who are studying Pathophysiology and Introduction to Clinical Medicine, at third- and fourth-year students who are beginning to apply their newly acquired skills at the bedside, and at some graduate students or practicing physicians for whom this book may serve as a continuing education exercise. Specialists may detect models applicable to their own fields. The physician's assistant or nurse-practitioner who is learning to deal with problem solving may also benefit.

What It Teaches

We propose to teach methods, ideas, and skills through the medium of a core of commonly encountered patient presentations. While the reader may learn a multitude of facts as a spinoff from this technique, the principal goal is to teach the reader how to process acquired data into relevant or irrelevant information (separate the wheat from the chaff); how to properly group related bits of data; and, most of all, how to apply logic in order to solve patient-problem presentations.

Let us assume that the reader already knows how to gather data (history and physical examination), that he already knows about disease processes and how they cause symptoms (pathophysiology), and that he has had some exposure to basic diagnostic techniques, such as thoracentesis, lumbar puncture, clinical laboratory studies, radiology, and electrocardiography. Having satisfied ourselves in these regards, then, the essence of the book will be problem solving: the transformation of a data base into a problem list. Put more basically, the book will try *to teach the student how to find out what is wrong with the patient.* This is the stuff that medicine is made of.

It is our intention not to supplant but to supplement the existing numerous excellent textbooks of physical diagnosis and medicine. The former teach students how to elicit information; the latter offer huge stores of facts that are categorized by disease headings. Those books teach students "what are the effects of a cause." We concentrate here on "what are the causes of an effect." Expressed differently, traditional textbooks teach: "Given a disease, what are the clinical features?" We prefer: "Given a clinical picture, what are the disease probabilities?"

Section by Section

The table of contents gives more detailed and precise definition of the material to be presented.

Section One is devoted to the principles and mechanisms of problem solving; it dwells heavily on the logic, mathematics, skills, techniques, probabilities, and decisions that are applied in the problem-solving process.

Section Two consists of physician-patient interviews which are constructed so as to allow the reader to enter the physician's mind during the gathering of data and to learn why he pursues certain pathways in his quest for solutions. This section on data synthesis and analysis also includes a chapter

in which the reader is taught to transform his acquired data into an orderly well-written record. Several complete patient write-ups are detailed and problem lists are synthesized, then assessed and completely analyzed. Separate portions are devoted to teaching data evaluation and data processing. Also included is a chapter which demonstrates how to miniaturize a long case for presentation on rounds. The reader is then informed of errors commonly made by students in the performance of these various data management skills.

Section Three is composed of a carefully selected collection of cases which illustrate *problem solving in action.* Each case is arranged in "data-logic-data-logic" sequence so as to set forth a detailed analysis of the relevant points or clues in the history, physical examination, and paraclinical data. This format fosters a "think along with me" relationship between the author and the reader. Woven into the case studies are how these clues relate or do not relate to solving the problem; whether these clues tend to confirm or negate tentative diagnostic hypotheses; and a step-by-step approach to the selection and interpretation of additional information which may be of value in each instance.

The problem-solving techniques vary from case to case. At the conclusion of each "logic session" the techniques used are identified and explained in the "Comment." The various patient discussions are arranged in groups which parallel the modular type of curriculum. Each deals with a particular body system. The selection of case material is designed to cover the bulk of common clinical presentations—a "core of medicine," so to speak. Occasionally a not-so-common clinical entity is presented because it may serve as an excellent teaching model.

Section Four is a *mélange* of subjects that are related to problem solving as applied to different population subsets and that are considered important enough to be called to the reader's attention. Particularly worthy of note are the chapters on how to seek out information about a special subject in the library, how to solve problems in the unique environments of emergencies and emergency rooms, and how to deal diagnostically with complications caused by drugs and doctors.

Self-Evaluation

Since student participation makes for more effective learning, active reader involvement is accomplished by exercises and problems offered via a variety of techniques that become evident as the book unfolds.

The answers and their explanations trail each group of exercises.

Chapters 2, 3, and 5 in Section One include self-evaluation exercises. Additional exercises testing the reader's mastery of Chapters 8 and 9 are found in association with selected individual cases in Section Three. For example, Case 22 on the subject of the asymptomatic pulmonary nodule is followed by a section that tests your judgment on diagnostic protocols. Case 39 is about hematuria; it is followed by a series of exercises that are applications of, and tests for the comprehension of, the decision-making and problem-solving processes taught in Chapters 8 and 9. Case 56, on the subject of convulsions, is followed by an exercise that tests your clinical judgment. Note again that answers and explanations follow.

Chapter 13 of Section Two consists entirely of tasks that gauge the reader's comprehension of the rest of the section. This chapter deals with data processing, the selection of data subsets, determining the relevance and relationship of clues, and decoding problem sets.

Chapter 14 is concerned with hematologic problems. This entire chapter of eight cases is followed by self-evaluation exercises that test the reader's comprehension of some cases in this chapter. But none of the other modular chapters is followed by a similar exercise covering the entire chapter. The course instructor is free to model exercises for each chapter and to construct case vignettes to test the student's comprehension in whichever style is desired.

However, almost *every* case *is* followed by an examination containing three, four, or five questions with the answers close behind. These serve to both test and teach.

Objectives

Primarily, this book teaches the reader to:

* *elicit and process patient data*
* *utilize problem-solving techniques*
* *establish diagnostic strategies*
* *deal with common presentations.*

But each of these principal objectives can be subdivided into less encompassing ones with overlapping components.

Assume the reader has digested the book, worked through the various case histories and logic sessions, read the suggested problem-based instructional material, and participated in the exercises and self-evaluation portions. He should then be able to:

1. elicit patient information in an intelligent purposeful order
2. process, evaluate, and cluster patient information according to relevance, significance, and relatedness
3. formulate single, multiple, or competing hypotheses which suggest possible diagnoses
4. confirm or reject hypotheses with additional carefully selected and acquired bits of patient information
5. utilize various problem-solving techniques and be consciously aware of their use
6. create diagnostic game plans and structure decision scenarios that are reasonable, orderly, precise, and considerate of cost-benefit-risk-time factors
7. gather additional information about the patient in accordance with a problem-based student-motivated format
8. decide what additional data are needed and what further tests to order, bearing in mind the concept of imperfect information
9. transcribe patient information into an

orderly well-written data base that includes the history, physical examination, and basic paraclinical procedures

10. relate clues in the patient's data base to the underlying pathophysiology

11. construct a complete problem list from the available patient information and be able to assess each problem

12. solve patient presentations and confirm diagnoses rapidly, like the seasoned clinician who uses shortcuts, tangents, selected data subsets, and high-yield tests

13. develop a more intellectual approach to problem solving by knowing what diseases are most common and therefore most likely to be present, by knowing the various presentations of a single disease, and by realizing that several diseases may coexist in one patient

14. understand and deal with the taxonomy of quantitation. The reader must appreciate the meaning of such poorly quantified phrases as "usually," "almost always," and "most of the time"

15. identify a "core curriculum" and deal diagnostically with a large majority of clinical presentations; almost all that the practicing physician sees can be pared down to a reasonably limited number of presentations and diseases

16. judge who needs a complete workup and who can be managed quickly with a small data base; not everybody needs a lengthy study, since most patients see the physician with simple problems that can be solved with a few questions, a brief examination, and no laboratory work

17. miniaturize a case for presentation to others.

Why should it be necessary to teach material with such objectives? It's simply because these are the steps or processes that the physician or student must use in many patient encounters. These skills do not come easily to beginners.

A Living Example. You see a 42-year-old woman who complains of painless swollen legs for 2 weeks. Immediately you consider several possibilities and begin to seek special bits of information which you hope will yield positive or pertinent negative information; these will tend to diagnose or exclude the various hypotheses—renal, cardiac, hepatic, lymphatic, or venous disease.

First, you wonder if the edema or swelling is actually there, so you look and feel. It is. Then ask a few questions. Has it happened before? Is there edema elsewhere? Has there been shortness of breath on exertion? Any cough? How many pillows? Any heart trouble? Murmurs? Kidney trouble? So far no help. All answers are negative.

A possible lead is revealed: she takes aspirin intermittently for some kind of arthritis which recurrently affects many joints. You look at her hands and wrists; some of the joints are swollen and stiff. Is this clue helpful?

Further information: she doesn't drink alcohol, never had jaundice or hepatitis, menses are normal, no abnormal vaginal bleeding or discharge, has not been immobile, no long trips, slight weakness, no weight loss, good appetite. But she has had untreated mild hypertension for 5 years; no diabetes, but her mother did have it. Strong points against some possibilities. Weak suggestions for others. The competing hypotheses are lining up according to their respective probabilities.

Heart and liver disease are unlikely. There is no suspicion of malignancy or any other predisposing cause for lymphatic or venous obstruction.

A quick examination of the heart, lungs, liver, and abdomen is normal. Except for pallor, so is general inspection. The blood pressure is 150/96 in both arms and the fundi are normal. No lymph nodes are found. Pelvic and rectal examinations are normal. Homans' sign is negative and there is no calf tenderness. A quick dipstick test shows 4+ albuminuria. The blood count reveals a mild anemia. Blood glucose is 165 mg/dl.

The hypotheses change their order of likelihood. She has kidney disease and a possible nephrotic syndrome. Cirrhosis, heart failure, pelvic disease, and venous disease are now most unlikely. Some form of arthritis, hypertension, and possible diabetes are present. What is the interrelationship, if any?

More facts are needed from the information bank—i.e. textbooks and review articles. So you read about the nephrotic syndrome and its causes. Can arthritis relate to her renal disease? Is early diabetes mellitus a factor? Read further about rheumatoid arthritis, analgesic nephropathy, diabetic nephropathy amyloidosis, and systemic lupus erythematosus. Research the latest literature on whether mild hypertension should be treated. Is the hypertension a cause or a result of her kidney disease? Learn about immunologic markers for autoimmune diseases. Decide what additional diagnostic procedures are indicated.

Further data—low serum albumin and 8 g of albumin/24-hour urine collection—allow you to cluster the triad of the nephrotic syndrome. Its cause is still uncertain. But you can now write a data base and problem list, decide on further studies, understand most of the pathophysiology, and present the case to others.

In developing this case, you have benefited from almost all of the 17 learning objectives listed. Reread them and the case, and see that this is so.

Need to Teach Problem Solving

Why bother teaching this particular skill? To a few students it comes naturally, but to most it doesn't, and those students have difficulty handling the large amounts of patient data with which they are deluged. Unfortunately, there are no *good* educational studies to prove that teaching the problem-solving process turns students into better problem solvers. Though many prominent educators have made valiant efforts at such

proof, there are those who say the experiments are untested, uncontrolled, and of dubious value. Yet most feel that students are best equipped to approach medical diagnosis in a logical manner when they are familiar with a wide variety of problem-solving tools.

But are double-blind controlled studies really needed? We don't need them to recognize the superiority of airplanes over wagons, television over radio, or computers over ledgers. Can there be any reasonable doubt that the student who learns to think and solve will make the better doctor?

Considerable time in the medical curriculum is allotted to teaching students how to acquire a data base. But problem solving (the synthesis of data into a diagnosis) is often considered nonteachable or difficult to teach, and is ignored, neglected, or recognized as important but no time allowed for it in the curriculum. Only sometimes is it taught as a separate discipline. This is unfortunate since problem-solving skills are eminently teachable and learnable; and *the idea that the art of clinical medicine is intuitive and results only from experience is a counterproductive myth.*

Symptoms of Curricular Diseases. Numerous curricular failings have kept problem solving from its rightful place. These include too many curriculum hours, excessive didactic teaching, too many lectures and too little problem solving, no student responsibility for learning or thinking, capitulation to students who want only predigested facts, unwilling or incapable teachers, and resistance to change (1).

Interdepartmental squabbling, hedonistic students, reverence for sacred cows, and passive faculty have led to patchwork curricula that are not in the best interests of the student's education. "There is excessive reliance on the lecture as the main vehicle of student learning, thus tending to induce passivity among learners; this may be associated with detrimental reliance on the note service, poor class attendance, inadequate development of critical thinking, and sloppy lifelong habits" (2). An R2D2 of silicon and copper could score high on examinations in an educational program of this type.

Where, When, and How It's Taught

Clinical reasoning and problem-solving skills are taught at different times in diverse ways at a variety of schools. From Beersheva in the Negev Desert to the hallowed halls of Harvard, some educators have recognized the need and have provided time for the teaching of this discipline.

There is no uniform method or style for teaching the student to solve problems, and there need not be. It can be compulsory or elective and may be taught in the second, third, or fourth year. A required course in decision making is given to preclinical students at Ben Gurion University; in it, students are taught to construct algorithms, solve problems, and make decisions according to the latest concepts of decision analysis (3) (Chapter 8). In Pittsburgh, a second-year elective gives students selected reading on problem solving, Socratic sessions, and interactions with Internist I, a computer program that is a readily accessible repository for accumulated medical knowledge; patient encounters are videotaped and later analyzed (4).

In recent years much has been done with the PMP (patient management problem), though the effectiveness of such a learning tool has been extensively studied and debated. In this procedure the student is presented with an opening clinical scene and is then confronted with five different menus from which he may request information referable to the history, physical examination, studies, differential diagnosis, and treatment. The latent image process provides instant feedback and a basis for student self-evaluation. But in this method students are cued to answers by the choices given and free inquiry cannot take place. In addition, it has been shown that this method does not correlate well with performance on MCQs (multiple choice questions) or with performance at the bedside in live situations.

Other methods of teaching students to solve problems employ encounters with real patients, simulated patients (actors), paper patients, and computer patients. Each has its merits and constraints. In any event, small-group discussions with tutors and properly conducted bedside teaching are still very effective adjunct tools.

Problem-Based Learning (PBL)

A new technique that teaches clinical reasoning and problem-solving skills has become stylish in a number of schools. Though simple, this valuable method represents a major breakthrough in the field of education (5).

Medical students facing a problem are responsible for their own education in a way that develops a systematic approach, fosters retention of information, and facilitates transfer of this information to today's and tomorrow's clinical tasks.

PBL is a process whereby students learn by using a problem as a stimulus to discover what added information they must acquire in order to move toward a solution (5, 6). The amount of inquiry needed depends on the cognitive level from which the inquiry begins. A first-year student must learn the pertinent anatomy, physiology, and biochemistry, in addition to the clinical features. The third-year student may have to review his basic science, but he can then proceed to gather information primarily at a more advanced level. The clinician, whose knowledge base is larger and more solid, may need very little additional information and may only have to find out what's new.

Many physicians and students have used PBL for years without conceptualizing it. Faced with situations in which there were wide gaps in my knowledge base, I learned about my own patients in a PBL mode. For there, surrounding me at my desk, were my physiology notes, anatomy textbook, cardiology notes and text, notes from a recent seminar, a reference or two—whatever was needed to fill the blanks and provide the answers. No doubt any good practitioner does this whenever he comes upon a problem that is difficult to solve. Read about it. Learn about it. Then return to the patient with new information and apply the necessary measures to reach a solution.

How It's Done. First the student is introduced to a patient problem by tape, paper, or interview. Teacher and student discuss the issues and outline the subjects in *all related disciplines* that need to be learned in order to understand and manage the clinical problem (6). The list should cover a wide span of subjects—not only the medical aspects, but the social, environmental, and behavioral issues as well. The teacher may guide the student in selecting the reference sources and may even supply study materials. These can include videotapes, journals, textbooks, abstracts, slide programs, mannikins, PMPs, prepackaged PBLMs (problem-based learning modules) (7), and so forth.

After learning the related materials, students meet with instructors for group interaction and further planning. And on it goes.

For Example. Suppose the patient to be studied is a 38-year-old woman who complains of palpitations and episodes of rapid heartbeating. Subjects to be learned include the conduction mechanisms and electrophysiology of the heart and common disturbances of rhythm, including their characteristics, manifestations, causes, diagnoses, and treatments. Also to be considered are the effects of this disturbance on her social activities, her job, her family, and her psyche.

Why It's Good. There can be little question that PBL optimizes the learning process (8). It exposes the student to the disciplines of independent learning and clinical reasoning and promotes interest, motivation, satisfaction, and achievement. The student is encouraged to cross course boundaries and to keep his own notes or a filing system, thereby encoding specific plans for similar problems to be faced in the future. Hopefully, lifelong habits will be established.

Differences of opinion center about whether an entire curriculum should be structured about PBL, whether PBL should be used an as aid to inspire learning during a more traditional curriculum, or whether it is only a meteoric educational fad that will soon vanish. I recommend the middle option—that it be used *after* the student has learned traditional basic sciences, as he begins to face clinical problems, *and forever after.*

On the Subject of Supplementary Reading

Over the years, I have come to realize how little supplementary reading is actually done. It seems almost a waste of space and energy to publish a list of *extra* reading; most learners are content to read the body of the text or, better yet, a conclusion or summary of each chapter. Articles published in learned journals may be followed by as many as 200 references which are of value for only the rare reader. The list of references may be almost as long as the article.

One may therefore hesitate to append such a list, especially when dealing with medical students who are inundated with work from all departments. Accordingly, the "Suggested Readings" list at the end of each case discussion in Section Three has been carefully conceived, constructed, and annotated. With the understanding that the depth of reading must vary with the educational stage of the reader, a general method for adjunct reading about each case follows.

Assume that the student has completed basic sciences, physical diagnosis, and pathophysiology and is either in the middle of Introduction to Clinical Medicine or has already studied it. When going through a case study, he may have to review some of the mentioned material that he has either forgotten or never really learned. This may include items such as a third heart sound, a classification for rales, the symptoms and signs of pancreatitis, the puddle sign, values for a normal blood count, how to calculate the mean corpuscular volume or creatinine clearance, where the dorsalis pedis is felt, which diseases cause clubbing, what the forced vital capacity is, and so on.

At the very least, this student should also read the basic material referable to the case in a major textbook. This may be a textbook of medicine, surgery, obstetrics, or whatever subject is applicable; it may involve only four or five pages of reading. If the case being studied is a patient with the nephrotic syndrome, the least amount of reading should include didactic material on the definition, diagnosis, causes, and treatment of this entity. A review of myocardial infarction and its pathophysiology, clinical picture, complications, and treatment may mandate a few more pages.

While most schools using *Problem Solving in Clinical Medicine* do so in the second year, some recommend its use in the third-year medicine clerkship. Others use it during a transitional period preceding the third year. In these latter instances, students should have to review less but read more extensively. Since the S_3, clubbing, mean corpuscular volume, and forced vital capacity have already been learned, more reading should be required. A standard textbook is not enough. Here the student should be encouraged also to read related portions in a subspecialty book and to read one or two recent review articles on the subject. Better yet, he should also read the article in the latest issue of America's Best Journal, photocopied and given to him by his resident. More advanced learners, including practicing physicians who are continuous learners, may merely corroborate and solidify their own cognition and skills. The physician whose area of practice is limited may find himself at the same level as second- or third-year students when the subject material is outside of his field. He may both review and read, and it may be enjoyable for him to know what his colleagues in other fields have to deal with.

The amount of "required" extra reading will, of course, vary from school to school and from teacher to teacher. It wil depend on what the course planners and educational directors feel is adequate and appropriate for their students at this level at that school. But in order to make sure that the student does

his supplementary or required reading, material from the reading *must be included in his examinations.* Unfortunately, most students read only what they must in order to pass, and the teacher must deal with this reality.

Case-Based Learning. Suppose we consider Case 33 (page 382), a patient with diarrhea and weight loss who turns out to have celiac sprue or gluten enteropathy. In going through the data and logic needed to solve this problem, numerous points are made and issues are raised which may need further reading for clarification.

To get the most out of this case, in addition to reading the case study, the student should read enough to know all about:

1. the causes of chronic diarrhea
2. the types of stools seen in such diseases
3. chronic ulcerative colitis, regional enteritis, tuberculous enteritis, amebiasis, and other parasitic diseases of the colon
4. carcinoma of the colon
5. endocrine-induced diarrhea
6. the malabsorption syndrome and the pathophysiology of each and all of its manifestations; this should include the nature of the stool, causes for vitamin deficiencies, weight loss, lower serum protein, fat, protein, and carbohydrate metabolic disturbances, clotting defects, anemia, associated electrolyte disorders, etc.
7. the normal physiology of digestion and absorption
8. the roles of the liver, bile salts, pancreas, and small intestine in creating disturbances of digestion or absorption
9. causes for the malabsorption syndrome and the clinical and radiologic manifestations of each cause
10. sigmoidoscopic findings and radiographic features of the diseases mentioned in item 1
11. methods to qualitatively and quantitatively examine the stool

12. diagnostic tests to determine what is being poorly absorbed
13. the role of and findings in peroral jejunal biopsy
14. celiac sprue and its special pathophysiology.

Included in this case is a veritable mountain of information, provided the case is properly studied and extra reading is done. *Don't forget!* You must know exactly how to do a *d*-xylose test, and you must know what a blind loop syndrome is. If you don't, then *look it up*. The reader who follows these recommendations for this case alone will have mastered a sizable percentage of all medical knowledge. Add this to the next case and then the next, and soon the learner will have a most respectable knowledge base. Students working with patients during clerkships would benefit by studying all about each patient in the same way.

The first case in each module of disease (Chapters 14 to 24) has a section on problem-based learning preceding each "Suggested Readings" list. Other case studies in each module should be treated in the same way: Decide what subject materials should be learned, and read about them.

To further aid the reader in looking up information about a patient's disease, an entire chapter in Section Four (Chapter 25) covers the subject of information retrieval. Students must know how to effectively utilize information storage systems, such as libraries and their ancillary facilities. Other than standard textbooks, the *Index Medicus* is your best friend in this regard. In selected instances, computerized data banks may be of great help.

A Recommended Way

It may be presumptuous to offer advice on how to teach and learn problem solving, and in particular how to use this book to achieve such ends. This recipe is a result of trial, error, and experimentation with various techniques, plus pinches of what's done at some other schools.

Teach it as you would any other skill. First give didactic information, next some demonstrations, then homework, reading, and practice; follow this by student performance under supervision and then evaluation.

A student can cover the entire subject and book by himself. My preference is that it be taught as part of a larger course or as a separate entity somewhere between the latter part of the second year and the early part of the third.

First, the principles of problem solving as detailed in *Section One* may be learned by reading, by analyzing the didactic presentations, and by performing exercises given in the text. The student must acquire the ability to deal with the concepts of hypothesis generation, Bayes' theorems, sensitivity, specificity, and predictive values. This will prepare him for much of the medical literature that will be published in the next 10 years. Exercises in the text will allow the student to calculate predictive values and to construct algorithms, flow charts, and decision paths. Additional exercises may be composed by the instructor.

Section Two can also be covered with only little classroom activity. Data processing can be learned by reading the section and understanding the transition from data collection to data transcription. Exercises will teach the student who is presented with a chief complaint to prepare selected data subsets, determine data relevance, do writeups, and present cases. The instructor may give the students several taped interviews and have them rearrange the data and write the history in correct format. Or the same may be done with live patients. Give at least two exercises that require the students to write complete data bases, problem lists, assessments, and diagnostic plans. These can be presented and critiqued in class or in small-group sessions. Students may also benefit by observing live or videotaped physician-patient interviews. The order of, reasons for, and results of questions and directions of lines of inquiry can be discussed.

The 65 cases in *Section Three* should be read, studied, and broadened by "case-based learning" as described earlier. Note and analyze the problem-solving techniques that are used and that are explained in the editor's *"Comment."*

A classroom or small study section's critique of the problem-solving scenario used by the author of each case may be a useful teaching tool. Students may suggest better or more efficient ways to solve the problem.

Most of the case studies are followed by mini-cases or case vignettes. These are contained in the questions and answers at the end of each case discussion, and they serve both to expand on the informational value of the cases and to test the reader's medical logic.

In addition, students may be given carefully constructed take-home exercises that are related to a case studied in the textbook. Such homework can consist of abstracts or mini-cases that are prepared by the course instructor. From these case abstracts, the student may be required to prepare high-yield information request lists or to furnish answers to specific instructor-generated questions.

More specifically, suppose the students are asked to study Case 16 on the subject of "dyspnea on exertion" and to read all about this presentation according to the concept of problem-based or case-based learning. The instructor then gives the students several brief case vignettes that resemble the original case but lead along different branches of the diagnostic tree and terminate in, say, pulmonary fibrosis, chronic obstructive pulmonary disease, pleural effusion, left ventricular aneurysm, mitral stenosis, or severe anemia.

For example: "Give all the pertinent information you would seek in a 40-year-old woman who has progressively worsening dyspnea on exertion." Or: "What information do you seek in a 60-year-old man who smokes heavily, has a chronic cough, and has recently developed dyspnea on exertion?" Or: "What do you look for in the history, physical examination, and ancillary studies in a 56-year-old man with known coronary heart disease who is beginning to complain of shortness of breath on walking a block or two?" Further: "Zero in on the questions, findings, and studies for a 38-year-old woman who complains of palpitations, worsening dyspnea on mild exertion, and recent orthopnea and night cough." And last: "What data do you seek in a 46-year-old man who appears to be extremely pale and who complains only of dyspnea on exertion?"

Consider the latter examples, and have the students determine the additional information to be rooted out if the expected diagnosis were specifically sarcoidosis, asbestosis, lung cancer, bronchiectasis, recent myocardial infarction, aortic regurgitation with left ventricular failure, pernicious anemia, hookworm infestation, or any one of many possibilities.

In regard to each mini-case study, the students may be given several important questions for which answers must be furnished. (*a*) What if the patient were not a smoker? (*b*) What if pleuritic pain were present? (*c*) Suppose the patient complained of a swollen achy left leg too! (*d*) If the chest x-ray were normal, what would you do next? (*e*) How do you relate the anemia to dyspnea? (*f*) Explain the possible coexistence of heart and lung disease in this patient! And so forth.

These matters should subsequently be discussed in class or in small group-instructor sessions. In such ways, the instructor can evaluate the student's acquired ability to solve problems rather than his ability to parrot material he has read. These discussions generate additional thought, questions, and answers. And since active participation by all students is the desired goal, the instructor must not permit a few vocal students to dominate the exercise.

These methods of teaching and learning are excellent ways for the student to review pathophysiology and "put it all together." The student learns to reason—first by observing, and then by doing. Questions are designed to make the student think.

In short there are limitless ways in which the 65 cases can be used to encourage the student to read, to reason, to participate, and to learn. All tend to make medical school education a more stimulating, more enjoyable, and more intellectual process—for both the student and the teacher.

Section Four can be adapted to classroom teaching and discussion in countless ways. Students may be required to research an assigned subject according to the chapter on data retrieval. Discussions can revolve around determining if and when a presenting symptom is urgent. Separate sessions can be devoted to special aspects of solving problems in neuropsychiatric, pediatric, alcoholic, underprivileged, and geriatric subsets of the population.

A "Suggested Readings" list is appended to each chapter in this section since some of the subjects may not be covered in adequate depth for students who wish to know more.

Some Final Comments

Several medical schools have initiated "experimental" curricula that are based on problem-oriented study and that depart from the traditional discipline-based, teacher-centered program. Instead, emphasis is placed on the interdisciplinary piecemeal study of courses as they relate to a particular patient problem. Formal lectures are given only when necessary, self-learning is emphasized, and small group-teacher interactions are employed. The goal is to produce young physicians who are not repositories of facts but are problem solvers, decision makers, and ongoing learners.

Along these lines, I have often wondered why short textbooks of medicine (300 to 600 pages) or, for that matter, short textbooks on any major discipline are so popular with second- and third-year medical students. I must conclude that students are taught too many facts. For example, it is not necessary that a second-year student learn all there is to know about infective endocarditis in a 1- or 2-hour lecture. At this educational level, 10 minutes can relay the fundamental pathophysiology and the five or six clinical points that must be remembered. One page of reading is enough.

After 40 years in medicine, *I* do not know *all* about infective endocarditis. But I do know the predisposing causes, the pathophysiologic mechanisms, and the fact that fever, splenomegaly, murmurs, anemia, microscopic hematuria, and embolic phenomena should be sought. Isn't that really enough? Once the disease is suspected or proven by blood culture, I (or a student) can then consult a 2000-page textbook and the *Index Medicus* for more detailed information. This latter step is needed if the diagnosis is still in doubt, if the patient is to be presented for discussion, or if further information about complications and treatment is needed.

Listen to many in-depth lectures that students hear and inspect the amount of reading they are asked to do. Then look at the examination given on the subject in question. Note that many questions involve minutiae delivered in lectures and require only regurgitation of facts; few questions, if any, demand thought, logic, and reason; few questions, if any, are derived from either recommended or "compulsory" reading. Under such a system, students soon learn that it's not necessary to read or think. Just memorize the lectures!

Let's face the fact that students who score high on an examination because of memorization of minutiae will do poorly if examined on the same subject material 6 months later. Rather than force the student to perfect short-term memory, it is better to transform him into a reader, a learner, a thinker, and a solver.

The course outline recommended in the preceding section is designed to be a prescription for the cure of many curricular maladies. The ingredients are: fewer lectures, more self-teaching, and more small-group discussions of patient problems. Students should be encouraged to learn and think! This is what I have tried to accomplish in the four sections of this book. (*P. C.*)

References

1. Eichna LW: A medical school curriculum for the 1980s. *N Engl J Med* 308:18–21, 1983.
2. Gonnella JS: Problems and strengths of the medical college curriculum. In *Jefferson Medical College An-*

nual Report, 1980–1981. Philadelphia, Jefferson Medical College, 1981.

3. Margolis CZ, Barnoon S, Barak N: A required course in decision-making for preclinical medical students. *J Med Educ* 57:184–190, 1982.

4. Miller RA, Schaffner KF: The logic of problem solving in clinical diagnosis: a course for second year medical students. *J Med Educ* 57:63–65, 1982.

5. Barrows HS, Tamblyn RM: *Problem Based Learn-
ing: An Approach to Medical Education.* New York, Springer, 1980.

6. Neame RLB: How to construct a problem-based course. *Med Teacher* 3:94–99, 1981.

7. Distelhorst LH, Barrows HS: A new tool for problem-based, self-directed learning. *J Med Educ* 57:486–488, 1982.

8. Schmidt HG: Problem-based learning; rationale and description. *J Med Educ* 17:11–16, 1983.

Section One

The Problem-Solving Process

Chapter 1. Problem Solving: What It Is

Chapter 2. Data Collection, Data Processing, Problem Lists

Chapter 3. Clues: The Building Blocks

Chapter 4. From Odds to Ends

Chapter 5. Digits, Decimals, and Doctors

Chapter 6. How to Use Tests

Chapter 7. The Impact of New Technology

Chapter 8. Making Medical Decisions

Chapter 9. Problem-Solving Methods

Chapter 1

Problem Solving: What It Is

PAUL CUTLER, M.D.

KEY WORDS

1. experience
2. judgment
3. logic
4. hypothesis
5. diagnosis
6. patient presentation
7. precision
8. acronyms
9. patient management process
10. data base
11. problem list
12. problem solving
13. medical information base
14. assessment
15. problem-oriented medical record
16. data management
17. student skills

Three Questions

Year after year, students ask the same three questions:

1. How much do we have to learn now?
2. How can we shorten patient workups?
3. How do we pull it all together?

First, the student* wants to know how much of the vast body of information being taught him is relevant, important, and necessary in his present stage of development. Next, he is seeking shortcuts to the tradi-

---

* In referring to a student, "he" will be used for simplicity even though "she" becomes more applicable each year.

tional 3- to 6-hour data-gathering process. And last, he wants to learn how to apply logic, judgment, and synthesis so he may interlace a patient's data base with his own knowledge of disease and thereby find out what is wrong with the patient.

Medical students need to know, yet medical educators fail to teach, the answers to these three questions. The answers do not lie in clichés like: "it's all important—learn it now"; "it gets easier and shorter when you get experience"; or "you'll acquire the knack in time."

There is indeed a basic core of information the second- and third-year medical student must learn immediately and enlarge later, but it is ill-defined. And since he deals with patients early, he must quickly acquire the answers to all three questions. He cannot wait for experience, which comes slowly, or for judgment, which may not come at all. For *experience* can be a matter of doing the wrong thing a hundred times, and *judgment* may be based upon such experience.

What the Physician Does

The capable physician practiced quality medicine and successfully managed patients long before the concepts of clinical judgment (1), problem-oriented medical records (2), probability theory, and decision analysis became well known. All the physician did was take a history, do a physical examination, and order a few basic tests. During the data-gathering process he filtered clues through his information base. He formed then rejected or accepted diagnoses based mainly on his own knowledge, logic, judgment, and experience. Tentative diagnoses were confirmed or negated by additional studies. He may have put two crucial symptoms together and immediately confirmed a single physical finding to establish the diagnosis. He may even have solved the problem with his first question or glance. Therapy optimally followed diagnosis, though it might have begun anywhere during the diagnostic process depending upon the urgency of the situation.

The logic that he used is the traditional logic used by problem solvers in all fields. It is the science of correct reasoning, a system of formal principles of deduction or inference, a discipline with strict criteria of validity in thought, correct predication, and tenets of reason—much like the arguments and concepts propounded by Socrates and Aristotle.

Medical problem solvers utilize such logic in addition to less formal principles of reasoning. In so doing, the problem solver must intermesh his own information base with the patient's data base. This can be done by persons of reasonable intelligence who have never studied formal logic.

Today's good clinician may solve problems quickly and easily, albeit in an almost subconscious manner, by using a highly developed system of logic and numerous problem-solving techniques which he himself has not clearly conceptualized. However, the educator *has*. Studies have shown that the physician forms early hypotheses, tracks a key clue, forms a cluster, spots a triad or tetrad, considers a differential diagnosis right away, pursues only one subset of the data base, and rapidly zeroes in on a diagnosis.

Elstein et al (3) have shown that "rather than follow a set order of constraining questions, the experienced physician appears to leap directly to a small array of provisional hypotheses very early in his encounter with the patient." Thus, the logic of good physicians is applied by generation, testing, and acceptance or rejection of diagnostic hy-

potheses throughout the data collection process. The number of hypotheses formed will vary with the educational level of the problem solver, his experience, and whether his specialty matches the nature of the case.

At any step in gathering data, the experienced physician, both today and then, having put together a few clues, may go off on a Sherlockian tangent to reach a rapid conclusion. Then again, he may find that his algorithmic departure at some branching point has led him down the wrong path. So he returns to the branching point and continues in another direction. This technique does not negate the need for thoroughness. The rest of the history and physical examination can be filled in even after conclusions have been reached.

It is important for the physician and student to know that, even though the main problem is neatly and quickly solved with a few bits of information, a complete data base must usually still be fleshed out. The purpose is not only to make sure the original impressions are correct and to discover the possible coexistence of other diseases, but to stumble on clues which don't fit your impression, perhaps to rerank the order of likelihoods, and, last, to establish a baseline of normality for future comparison.

Nobody wants to be locked into a wrong hypothesis.

Even though the physician is unaware of it, much of his logic is not intuitive but is based on syllogisms, strategies, and information which have been programmed into the silicon chips of his short-term, long-term, and submerged memory. By pressing the correct punch-key, the internal logic and natural intelligence of this system are activated; what is displayed on the print-out is euphemistically called "medical intuition." The concept that intuition is more science than art will be explored in Chapter 5.

What the Student Must Do

Who could not have some compassion for the medical student in his early patient encounters, overwhelmed by a flood of data he can't quite handle? He can't decide what's important, what's relevant, which clues to cluster, which don't relate, which course of inquiry to pursue next, and how reliable, sensitive, and specific certain clues are. He doesn't fully understand the overlap of clues into many diseases, the probabilities, odds, and likelihoods. For these are but a few of the special skills needed to synthesize a data base into solutions and solve a problem.

Students should be trained to form diagnostic hypotheses early so that their performances will more closely resemble that of the expert physician. These hypotheses are often generated during history taking, and the student should branch into appropriate questions, look for confirmatory physical signs, and select diagnostic methods for testing or refuting his tentative impressions.

Traditionally, students have been taught to gather a data base and solve a problem in separate, inviolate, orderly blocks. First, do a complete history. Second, do a complete physical examination. Then order routine laboratory tests, x-ray, and ECG. When these are completed, pick out the important clues from each of the three sources, then put them together so they fit a known diagnostic pattern as closely as possible. But this is not usually the way it is done "in real life" by practicing physicians. In fact, the teacher who sees patients does not do as he teaches. He begins to solve problems with his first question.

The main concept to learn, then, is that problem solving is a lively, seemingly disordered though highly intellectual process, rather than a rigid structured one. It cannot readily be done by following printed forms, flow charts, and computer print-outs. Admittedly there are some who disagree.

Like an embryo, the diagnosis is conceived, germinates, develops, and may even be delivered during the dynamic taking of a history. This is undoubtedly the most important part of the doctor-patient interaction, and the entire drama of problem solving may unfold without leaving the stage-set of two chairs and a desk. The history taker should proceed in a conversational style,

conducting his investigation in whatever direction he must in order to arrive at either useful information, new pathways of inquiry, or perhaps even a dead end.

The Time Factor. As for the length of time needed to gather data and solve a problem, the answer is not simple. Since second- and third-year medical students spend 3 to 6 hours with each new patient, fourth-year students 2 hours, the intern and resident 1 hour, and the practicing physician perhaps less, something must have transpired during their interim development and maturation (Fig. 1.1). This estimated time-training parabolic curve has been nicely corroborated by a recent clinical study (4). Certainly it is not that the finished physician simply does everything faster and thus telescopes all his data gathering into less time. Rather, he has been mastering the skill of problem solving by quickly grouping clues, intelligently selecting key questions, examining where indicated, going off on appropriate tangents, and taking the correct turns at branching points. Thus he reaches conclusions more rapidly. He may begin this process on meeting the patient and shaking his hand, even before starting the history, and be well along toward solving the problem on first hearing the chief complaint (5).

Like It Is. In almost all cases, the physi-

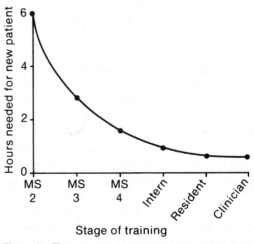

Fig. 1.1. Time spent with new patient in relation to level of experience.

cian generates his hypotheses (diagnostic possibilities) in the first minute or two of the patient interview. The student should do likewise. Each hypothesis may be as general as "gastrointestinal disease" or as specific as "carcinoma of the descending colon."

Your patient complains of weight loss and poor appetite, so you think of cancer and depression and ask questions accordingly. Another patient has hoarseness for 3 days; this conjures up a set of hypotheses and subsequent questions different from those to be pursued if the hoarseness had been present for 3 *weeks*. If the presenting symptom were simply abdominal cramps, a gastrointestinal problem would be possible. But if, in addition, rectal bleeding and worsening constipation were present, your supposition and line of inquiry would be more specific.

Suppose you see a patient with fever and weakness who looks pale and says he has not felt really well since a tooth extraction 4 weeks ago. Immediately you think of infective endocarditis, though you have not ruled out a blood disorder or tuberculosis, both of which may be unrelated to the tooth extraction. So you test and verify or reject your principal working hypothesis by seeking specific bits of information.

The patient never had a murmur that he knows of, never had acute rheumatic fever, and does not have any murmur now. Though you have searched carefully, there are no visible embolic phenomena nor is the spleen palpable. You are beginning to have doubts. The urinalysis shows no red blood cells, and the complete blood count shows evidence of myelogenous leukemia. Several blood cultures are negative. Thus you can reject the original hypothesis and accept a secondary one. But, since disseminated tuberculosis can cause a leukemoid blood picture, you are still not sure and must therefore test and reject or accept one of the two secondary hypotheses. And so it goes.

Protecting Your Flank. Students should be urged to form tentative hypotheses rapidly, explore these hypotheses quickly, and either accept or reject them based on further questioning and examination—just as Sher-

lock Holmes solves his mysteries with one or two bits of incontrovertible evidence. The student must attempt to do this even though he lacks the knowledge, judgment, and experience of the physician. Having done so, he must always check and double-check to make sure he is right by ruling out all other possibilities and defending his conclusions against any possible assault. He does this by subsequently gathering all evidence in the traditionally complete manner, hoping to reach the same solution to the mystery. The expert physician does likewise.

How Much to Learn. The question of how much the second- and third-year medical student should know is difficult to answer. He cannot be expected to know everything. He has 1 or 2 years more of medical school, postgraduate training, and a lifetime of continuing education for that. If he absorbs a carefully predetermined basic fund of knowledge, develops an organized method of problem solving, and knows how and where to seek additional information, that should be enough.

It is more important for the student to learn techniques, attitudes, and concepts than a huge quantity of facts. He will remember ideas long after he has forgotten the contents of the brachial plexus, the biochemistry of the Cori cycle, or the manifestations of the Laurence-Moon-Biedl syndrome. The memorization of thousands of facts is unrealistic and not a sensible goal. It is better to learn correct behavior—which includes thoroughness, efficiency, reliability, analysis and synthesis, the ability to define a data base, and how to identify and solve problems.

How Much to Teach. A discussion of what the student should know brings another question to mind: What shall we teach? Why spend 5 hours teaching a student about a disease he will see once in a lifetime, and 1 hour or less on a problem he will see every day? Here we who educate are responsible. We may concentrate on a rare disease since it is our special field of research or interest, or it is in vogue in the current journals. Yet we sometimes neglect common basic problems since they are dull, mundane, and seemingly too simple to bother teaching.

After medical school and 4 years of postgraduate training in internal medicine, I found myself unable to handle most of the problems first seen in my practice. While I could easily treat a myocardial infarction complicated by arrhythmias, cardiac failure, and diabetic ketoacidosis, or even diagnose Whipple's disease (if one had come along during that decade), I had not the vaguest idea what to do with the office patient who complained of itching skin, backache, or headache, or who had newly discovered diabetes or hypertension. I suspect that this unfortunate situation still exists. That's too bad, because well over 95% of what the physician most commonly treats can be included in a very short list.

Educators must taken the blame too for making their teaching disease-oriented rather than patient-problem-oriented. It is trite to say that a patient does not come into your office with a disease label on him. But it is true. We learn about diseases, but not enough about the patient who presents with a symptom or constellation of symptoms and how to go about solving his problem. The student must turn his brain storage space around and think in reverse. He must determine what diseases can cause this particular clinical presentation, in addition to what clinical presentations a disease can cause. In the early stages of student maturation, it is easier to learn the various presentations and the clinical picture of a disease; these can be found in any textbook of medicine. All the student has to do is look up the disease in the index. But it is more difficult and more important to know the opposite: the various diseases which can all present in the same way. For instance, cancer of the stomach causes weakness, weight loss, and anorexia. But patients with diseases in any one of seven different systems can have the same cluster of symptoms. It is simple to learn how lung cancer may manifest itself, but there are very few good sources that discuss the diseases which present with cough, expectoration, and hemoptysis.

Faculty Faults

Teachers and course planners should revise teaching in other respects too. I can remember one lecture on carcinoma of the pancreas given to second-year students. First it was stated that 25,000 cases occur each year in the United States. Quick calculations tell us that a primary care physician will see one new case every 5 to 10 years—a rare incidence. All a second-year student need know about this disease can be taught in 10 minutes. Yet most of the lecture centered about its surgical, chemical, and radiation therapy. The same course devoted 1 hour to hypertension and 1 hour to diabetes mellitus. Such misuse of curriculum time needs no further explanation. Such misuse of a precious lecture hour needs no further comment either.

It has been facetiously stated that textbooks should be arranged with the most common entities in the front and the most rare diseases in the back. Students should memorize the front, be aware of the middle, and be curious about the back. While books need not be written so, such priorities must be symbolically respected.

This chapter was not initially designed to cover faculty failures, but a few more shortcomings will be mentioned insofar as they result in student problem-solving weaknesses. In a school where there is no shortage of good teachers there is no excuse for a lecturer who is not well prepared, has poor delivery, cannot be heard or understood, or whose slides are upside down or contain misspelled words. We cannot expect thought, precision, and organization from students if their teachers do not exemplify these qualities.

Too often teachers do not insist on precision, nor do they probe a little beneath the surface. If a student uses sloppy imprecise language, he needs correction. The instructor should not be satisfied with statements like *"essentially* within normal limits," "a *somewhat* enlarged liver," or "an enlarged, displaced apex beat." The student must explain exactly what these phrases mean.

When he rattles off a list of negative facts, he should be able to state why these negative findings were mentioned, since they were obviously considered to be pertinent negatives. But if he is only parroting the intern's language, he may not know why. Ask. Also, he should know the meaning of the abbreviations he uses—e.g. CREST, GGT, COPD, PERLA, etc. It's shocking how often he does not!

It is surprising too how often a student will say that pupillary reactions are normal to L, C, and A, that the liver size is normal, or that the trachea is in the midline. Yet ask him how he made that determination, and he shows how bad his examining skills are. The instructor doesn't know this unless he probes.

Confessions of a Problem Solver

You need not be thought a medical Savonarola if you admit that problem solving is usually easy and simple! Most patient problems are easy to solve, since most patients have common diseases that present simply.

Nausea, vomiting, and diarrhea for 24 hours equals acute gastroenteritis; sore throat with stuffy nose equals head cold; sore, tender, swollen finger equals infection. No difficulties here! Many patients are revisits with already known diagnoses. Perhaps a little more problem solving is required in the patient with newly discovered diabetes mellitus or essential hypertension. While ambulatory patients do not commonly need the application of extensive problem-solving principles, complicated and acutely ill hospitalized patients usually do.

It may be startling to hear that it is not always necessary to make a precise diagnosis. If an acute, predictably self-limited disease strikes a healthy person and the treatment is the same no matter what, why perform tests? Must we differentiate between viral and bacterial gastroenteritis? Must we distinguish between a severe head cold and influenza?

Consider the patient with advanced in-operable coronary heart disease who develops weakness and weight loss. A detailed search for occult cancer would probably be considered bad judgment and poor management. It is also true that a patient with far-advanced cancer who develops angina pectoris does not need coronary artery disease studies.

The question of how certain a diagnosis must be before proceeding with treatment will be discussed in Chapter 5.

Patient Management

Total management of the patient includes diagnosis, treatment, and education. If you see a head cold, you prescribe aspirin and nosedrops. If the problems are more complicated or more difficult to solve, you may go through a detailed stepwise approach. These steps—the patient management process—can be listed as follows:

1. Collect data base.
2. Select and group clues.
3. Form initial problem list.
4. Assess problem list.
5. Devise additional studies and treatment plan.
6. Form final problem list.
7. Assess or modify therapy.
8. Add to data base and recycle.

These eight steps may be more meaningfully arranged in a circular diagram (Fig. 1.2). Note how the physician must continuously apply his knowledge and thought processes to bridge every part of it. First, each of the eight steps concerned with patient management will be described. Then the initial three—data collection, data processing (selection and grouping of clues), and the formation of the problem list—will be discussed in detail, since these are the principal parts of the problem-solving process. Attention will then be focused on the application of logic in medicine, who needs a complete study, the feasibility of shortcuts, the selection of clues, and decision making—important aspects of problem solving.

Examine Figure 1.2 carefully before pro-

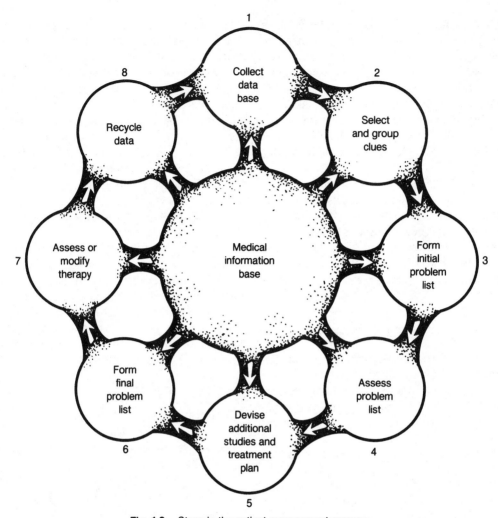

Fig. 1.2.   Steps in the patient management process.

ceeding. It is the foundation of the intelligent practice of medicine. The medical information base is the physician's fund of knowledge, whether it be internally or externally retrievable. The data base is information acquired by the physician from the patient. Note how the free flow of thought and logic from the physician's brain relates his information base to the patient's data base and makes the wheel go around from step to step as he solves the problems and treats the patient.

The medical information base is of paramount importance and is central to the entire patient management process. This base refers to the physician's knowledge of symptoms and signs, skills in eliciting them, and knowledge of pathophysiology and disease. Unless he has a good understanding of disease, he cannot satisfactorily complete the entire cycle. Also preeminent in the problem-solving process is "logic," indicated in the figure by the *shaded areas* and *arrows.* Logic invokes the thought processes, decisions, probabilities, unlikelihoods, and judgments which pervade and envelop every part of the diagram. This allows the physician to utilize his information base on each portion of the circle and to proceed from one item to the next.

Certain skills and information are necessary in order to acquire a data base (*step 1*).

For instance, you must know how to take a good history, the format thereof, the techniques of doing a physical examination, how to recognize abnormalities, and how to request and interpret laboratory data.

The physician must have the ability to select certain pertinent clues from the data base, be they points in the history, physical examination, or laboratory profile. He must then group these clues and label them as problems if possible (*step 2*). This is data processing. It requires the ability to pick out important clues, to know what is abnormal, and to process all the data properly, separating the relevant from the irrelevant. This too requires skill, a good medical information base, and the application of logic.

Having selected and grouped the clues, an initial problem list is formulated (*step 3*). There may be one or many problems.

It seems appropriate here to engage in semantics, since the word *problem* is being used in two different contexts. The phrases *problem solving* and *problem list* should not be confused with each other. A patient sees a physician because something is wrong and the patient has one or more symptoms. Problem solving is the process of transforming the patient's data base into known diagnoses—finding out what is wrong. The things that are wrong with the patient comprise the problem list. Some might prefer to call it a *solution list* or *list of diagnoses*.

But these latter two designations are not strictly correct. Some of the items entered into the problem list may be isolated symptoms, physical findings, or laboratory abnormalities which may not be part of the principal diagnosis. For example, the main problem on the list may be acute myocardial infarction. But, in the course of data collection, a history of chronic backache and albuminuria was noted. The initial problem list then would be:

1. acute myocardial infarction
2. chronic low backache
3. albuminuria

Problem 1 is a definite diagnosis and needs prompt attention. Problems 2 and 3 remain to be resolved.

All the problems must be raised to as high a level of resolution as possible by getting further data. Some problems may never be solved. Ideally and eventually, though, the problem list should be composed only of diagnoses.

Assessment of the problem list is now indicated (*step 4*). The physician must analyze his problem list and review the clues in this patient that led him to designate a specific problem. He must ask himself many questions. Are there any clinical features of a solved problem which are lacking? Are there features present which point away from this particular diagnosis? Are additional studies needed to raise the problem to its highest level of resolution, i.e. make a definite diagnosis? What other possibilities might explain the problem? Is there a differential diagnosis? What bits of seemingly pertinent data do not fit the main problem, and could there be other problems present that have not yet been resolved? Is urgent treatment indicated?

After assessing the initial problem list, you must devise and begin an additional study plan and a plan of treatment (*step 5*). Further studies may be needed to establish a definite diagnosis, to eliminate other possibilities in the differential diagnosis involving a particular problem, and to determine the cause of secondary or coincidentally discovered unresolved problems. Treatment may be devised and implemented at, before, or after this stage, depending upon the urgency of the situation. This is where treatment usually begins. So does patient education. But if circulatory or respiratory failure exists, treatment must start the instant you see the patient, even before a diagnosis, problem list, or data base is formed. If there is no emergency, it might be better to wait for further studies before starting treatment, e.g. in the case of fever of undetermined origin or an enlarged spleen.

With the passing of additional time, further observation, and more studies, you should formulate a final problem list (*step 6*). It ought to be definitive and again must represent the resolution of problems to as high a level as possible.

Therapy may be reassessed, continued, or modified, depending on any change in the problem list or the results of treatment so far (*step 7*).

The last step (*step 8*) represents the expansion of the data base by recycling into it all of the additional information harvested from steps 4 to 7. As the management of the patient continues, the data base keeps expanding with the results of additional studies, response to treatment, new physical findings, progress notes, and originally overlooked historical data. And so the cycle keeps repeating itself as long as the patient requires care.

Note that at each stage of the cycle, and in proceeding from one stage to the next, the physician's logic is at work extending his information base into all aspects and directions—the spokes, the hub, and the wheel of the patient management process.

I do not mean to imply that one has to adhere rigidly to this eight-step cycle in all patients. As hinted earlier, and as will be explained later in greater detail, shortcuts may be taken and portions of the diagram omitted in certain instances. For example, you can proceed from step 1 directly to step 6 if the situation warrants it. Or, while performing step 1, you can order additional studies or start treatment immediately (step 5) if this bypass seems appropriate to the case. Then, you may inherit a new patient at step 7 and decide to skip back to step 4, or even restart at step 1, should you conclude that the previous physican was on the wrong track.

Be aware that the problem-oriented medical record and the problem list format have not found universal acceptance. Many still prefer the use of the differential diagnosis. This issue will be further explained in Chapter 2.

Necessary Student Skills

To simulate the clinician who solves problems the student must acquire and master many skills. Each of these will be detailed in subsequent chapters.

First is the ability to relate well to the patient. Good interpersonal skills are essential to eliciting patient data. Next is the ability to take a history or obtain verbal information from the patient. Third, the student must be adroit in performing a physical examination. Then, having acquired an initial patient data base, the student must evaluate and process the information, putting it together so that it makes sense. Also needed is the talent to write a problem list, raising each problem to as high a level of resolution possible with the information on hand at that moment.

It is interesting to note how many of the skills just noted are identical to those needed to take good lecture notes. The student who takes his own notes has acquired data-processing skills in doing so because he has learned how to select important information from a lecture. This same process is used by the student who takes a history from a patient; he too must process data in the same way that notes are derived from a lecture. However, the student who has relied on a note service has allowed these skills to atrophy.

Additional reasoning skills include the assessment of a problem list and a determination of what further data can be helpful. Remember that obtaining patient information is not the same action as writing the material into the chart so that it is orderly, legible, and understandable—another skill. And in order to get more medical information about the patient's problems, the student must have information-search skills. Oral and written communication skills are necessary so that the student can present succinct summaries of his patients to others. And last, the student must have the ability to assess the quality of his own work by setting his own standards, by comparing his work to that of others, and by enlisting the help and criticism of those with whom he labors.

The Three Questions Revisited

The first page of this chapter listed three questions that students repeatedly ask. The answers are not simple. Learn enough to manage patient problems at your level of sophistication. This means knowing a basic core of disease processes, their symptoms and signs, common clinical presentations, what may be causing them, and what clues are helpful in deciding on the cause. To shorten patient workups and to pull all the data together, the student must learn data evaluation, data processing, data clustering, and problem-solving shortcuts. These subjects will be covered in chapters which follow.

References

1. Feinstein AR: *Clinical Judgment*, Baltimore, Williams & Wilkins, 1967.
2. Weed LL: *Medical Records, Medical Education and Patient Care*. Cleveland, The Press of Case Western Reserve University, 1969.
3. Elstein AS, Shulman LS, Sprafka SA: *Medical Problem Solving: An Analysis of Clinical Reasoning*. Cambridge, MA, Harvard University Press, 1978.
4. Sivertson SE, Stone HL: Efficiency in examining adult patients on preceptorship. *J Med Educ* 58:657–659, 1983.
5. Benbassat M, Schiffman A: An approach to teaching introduction to clinical medicine. *Ann Intern Med* 84:477–481, 1976.

Chapter 2

Data Collection, Data Processing, Problem Lists

PAUL CUTLER, M.D.

The principal steps in problem solving are the collection of patient data, the processing of these data, and then the formation of a problem list (or a differential diagnosis). It is difficult to separate these three into sequential steps since they usually proceed simultaneously.

Information about the patient is processed piecemeal as soon as it is obtained. The gait, clothing, general appearance, handshake, age, and gender are entered into the data processor even before a single word is spoken. Already impressions are formed and hypotheses considered. Add the chief complaint and the way it is elicited and articulated, and then, as you wind your way through the history of the present illness, you are well on the road toward the diagnosis. Interpret each bit of information as being relevant or irrelevant, important or unimportant, and relegate it to short-term memory or discard it in light of the information and impressions that came before.

Clinical reasoning begins with the medical history and continues throughout the collection of patient data. In fact, it is clinical reasoning and problem solving that direct the flow of traffic through the circuitry of data acquisition during the doctor-patient encounter.

Data Collection

This represents all information obtained from and about the patient. Only a few points will be made here, since this subject is amply covered in many good textbooks where the rigid formats and formal outlines of the patient data base may be obtained.

Included in this data base are: (*a*) the history; (*b*) the physical examination; (*c*) laboratory tests which include blood chemistries, complete blood count, and urinalysis; and (*d*) chest x-ray and electrocardiogram.

What is the relative importance of each? Certainly a diagnosis can be strongly suspected or definitely made during any one of the data-gathering processes. Sometimes a chest x-ray is the determining factor, as in the patient with low-grade fever and fatigue who has an infiltrate in the right apex. At times a single physical finding may be the concluding factor, as in the 56-year-old man who complains of weakness and weight loss and in whom a hard nodular prostate gland is found. An elevated serum amylase may be the key point in the diagnosis and therapy of the patient with severe pain, tenderness, and rigidity in the upper abdomen.

But in the great majority of cases the *history is the most important* and most revealing portion of the data base. By dialogue alone you can usually be reasonably certain of what is wrong. If it were possible to quantitate the relative importance of each portion of the data base in arriving at a problem list, it would probably be in the range of: history 70%, physical examination 20%, and laboratory tests and other procedures 10%.

History Taking

A Neglected Skill. Unfortunately, history taking has always been, and probably still is, the student's and physician's least perfected and most neglected skill. There are few poor historians but many poor history takers. Too often we ask a few questions, do a cursory examination, then order a huge array of studies, hoping to find the answer there. These studies may be inaccurately done, poorly interpreted, and misleading—so that time and dollars are wasted. The consultant who is asked to solve the problem usually does so by asking an additional question or by finding something that was overlooked on the original physical examination, not by ordering a little-known test.

A Difficult Art. Nowhere in the practice of medicine are interpersonal skills needed more than in taking a history. This is not to say that much less care is required in the performance of the physical examination, the ordering of tests, and the explanation of diagnoses and treatment.

When patients give reasons why they change doctors, over half do so because the doctor is cold, abrupt, and impersonal. Most of the others switch because the doctor is evasive and gives "inadequate treatment."

Common criticisms of a doctor's demeanor include statements that the doctor is arrogant, bored, impatient, or aloof, seems rushed, explains too little, or confuses the patient.

On the other hand, patients seem satisfied with doctors who are relaxed, take time, explain things and answer questions, have patience, are cordial, and seem interested in them.

What It Takes. While it takes only months to learn about laboratory procedures and perhaps a year to acquire examining skills, many years are required to master the art and science of history taking. As a student, you begin by learning how to approach a patient with sympathy, politeness, humility, and a smile. Extend your hand, introduce yourself, and tell the patient why you are there. And then begin with a kind introductory comment. Be informal and conversational but never familiar. You should not have to follow printed forms.

Above all, encourage the patient to talk, and do not dominate the conversation. Don't forget that the patient is trying to tell you what's wrong with him. Therefore, a good history taker must be a good listener.

Do and Don't. There are many do's and don't's. Don't smoke. Don't sit on the bed. Don't give false reassurance, but do give reassurance when it is justified and helpful. Don't address the patient by first name, "granny," or "dad." Do say "Mrs. Smith" or "Mr. Jones." Speak low and provide privacy. Act with dignity and show respect to the patient. Take notes, but tell the patient what you are doing, and don't keep your head buried in the chart. Maintain frequent eye contact. Make sure the patient understands and hears you and that his memory is good; use the vernacular if necessary, but don't use medical jargon. And be certain you understand what the patient means when he refers to such symptoms as dizziness, blackout, or gas.

At the beginning use mainly open-ended questions that allow and encourage the patient to talk. For example, "tell me more," "what about that?," "and then?," "yes?," and "you had pain?" are all invitations for the patient to continue. Specific closed-ended questions come later. For example, "did the pain make you vomit?" and "what was the color of your stools?" require simple answers. But try not to suggest the answers with your questions, and do not behave like an attorney cross-examining a witness.

Unspoken Language. Silence can be golden or awkward depending on its use. It may indicate interest and spur dialogue if it is accompanied by a nod, a postural shift forward, eye contact, a "yes", or "uh-huh." On the other hand, if the interviewer looks elsewhere, sighs heavily, or looks evaluatively at the patient, the silence can be counterproductive.

Body language is almost as important as what you say. A head scratch, a tongue in the cheek, a shake of the head, or a sudden widening of the eyes can be disconcerting, whereas a smile, a sympathetic expression, or properly timed nods may be encouraging. The same expression used differently can mean vastly different things to the patient. Consider the use of: "oh?"; "oh!"; "oh, oh!"; and "oh-HO!"

Getting at the Truth. Some difficulties inevitably arise in trying to get at the facts. Truth is often colored by the patient's personality and attitudes; he may minimize, exaggerate, or hide the truth or be fearful, angry, quiet, or shy. There may be reluctance to be honest because of alcoholism, drug addiction, excessive eating, malingering, sexual difficulty, venereal disease, marital problems, criminal record, unstable job history, contact with a previous physician, or lack of adherence to a previous treatment program.

Don't forget that you are interviewing a patient who is not only sick but is experiencing all of life's events, such as disability, divorce, separation, retirement, parenthood, terminal illness, suffering, despondency, and perhaps responsibility. Some issues may be incompletely or inaccurately addressed if family members are present.

Since the purpose of getting a history is to elicit accurate bits of information that contribute to the problem-solving process, all the factors that may inhibit or expedite this process must be considered.

Rigid and Flexible Formats. While we teach students to be rote in gathering data, physicians are fluid and freewheeling when they take histories. Why is there such a difference, and where does the change take place?

Of necessity, students who are just beginning to take histories must learn the time-honored, well-defined plan and sequence of questions. First come the identification data, next is the chief complaint, then the history of present illness, the family history, systems review, and so forth. Beginners need a format (1).

But the sooner the student learns to take histories like the physician, the better. The physician uses a flexible approach and a conversational style. He seems to change order, bypassing some questions and asking others which are not in the traditional sequence. But this is always done for good reasons. He has formed one or more early provisional hypotheses and is asking questions with high sensitivity (to exclude a hypothesis if negative and to build a pattern of support for a hypothesis if positive) and questions with high specificity (to confirm a hypothesis if positive and to build evidence for rejection of a hypothesis if negative).

For example, if the patient complains of angina-like chest pain, the physician may quickly select sensitive questions that would guide him in solving this problem. He would at once want to know if the patient has hypertension or diabetes; thus he has immediately invaded the past medical history and would do likewise to the family history by asking if the patient's father had coronary disease. He might then selectively inquire about cigarette smoking and not wait until the patient profile is reached. The responses would support a diagnosis of coronary disease if positive and be against that diagnosis if negative. A question with high specificity might be "tell me about the chest pain; when does it come and what does it feel like?" If it comes on exertion, feels like a constricting vise, and radiates down the inner aspect of the left arm—a pain which is specific for coronary heart disease—the diagnosis of angina is confirmed by history alone. The matter of sensitivity and specificity will be expanded in detail in Chapter 5.

Another example of seemingly disordered inquiry might occur with a patient who sees the physician for recently discovered hypertension. Early questions would relate to a family history, the presence of kidney disease, symptoms resulting from complications of hypertension, such as visual disturbances and dyspnea on exertion, and whether oral contraceptives that can cause hypertension are being taken.

If the patient with angina said that he had diabetes too, the physician might tangentially at this point ask all about the diabetes. This would include its onset, a family history, its course, its current state of control, information about diet, exercise, and medication, and questions that might alert him to any other possible diabetic complications. After this avenue had been explored, the physician would return to his original line of conversation.

The elderly patient complaining of weight loss, weakness, and loss of appetite would rapidly be asked about depression and symptoms referable to malignancies anywhere. And so there really is a rhyme and reason to the questions doctors ask of patients. It might be labeled a *hypothesis-verifying method of inquiry* rather than a rigid classical one.

Obviously there is a difference between the way history taking is taught and the way history taking is done. The good clinician does not do as he teaches. He solves problems by employing a variety of subconscious techniques which he has not conceptualized. He does not follow a constrained list or order. But by subtly guided conversation he initially forms a cluster of clues and generates early hypotheses which he then proceeds to refine, prove, or disprove by pursuing selected subsets of the data base, i.e. using both inquiry strategies and examining skills almost simultaneously. The collection of data is a discriminatory activity, like the

picking of flowers and unlike the action of a lawnmower (2).

The more the student understands about disease processes and the greater his knowledge base, the more readily he can detour from traditional pathways, and the quicker he can get to the root and heart of the issues. This he does by determining a sensible, more fruitful, and more productive series of questions. Actually, the traditional and ad hoc methods of inquiry should be complementary and synchronous.

Two Minutes In. Studies have shown that initial hypotheses are formed very early during the patient interview. The time needed to form hypotheses and the number of hypotheses formed will vary with the maturity of the history taker and his specialty vis-à-vis the type of disease process encountered. For example, beginners take longer and form more hypotheses than experienced clinicians. If the problem resides in the gastrointestinal tract, the gastroenterologist forms fewer and earlier hypotheses than would a cardiologist facing the same problem. Very often the correct hypothesis is reached by the time the physician is only 2 minutes into the history.

But even before *initial hypotheses* can be generated, *initial concepts* must be formed. An initial concept is based on the age, gender, chief complaint, and one or two additional bits of information. Here are two examples of initial concepts: "28-year-old woman with recurrent polyarthritis"; "64-year-old man with 6 months of worsening cough, expectoration, and dyspnea on exertion."

The first initial concept would generate initial hypotheses of acute rheumatic fever, rheumatoid arthritis, and systemic lupus erythematosus; the second would warrant the consideration of chronic obstructive pulmonary disease, lung cancer, tuberculosis, and other diffuse parenchymal diseases.

Initial hypotheses can vary from items such as "trouble in the gastrointestinal tract" to items as specific as Whipple's disease. Impressions can include diseases, syndromes, and pathophysiologic states. The diseases may vary in precision and sophistication from heart disease to Wolff-Parkinson-White syndrome with paroxysmal atrial tachycardia. Pathophysiologic states include such designations as chronic renal failure, inappropriate antidiuretic hormone secretion, hypokalemic alkalosis, or malabsorption syndrome. The initial hypothesis list is usually multiple, containing from two to seven entries.

To Exclude or Confirm. Having formed initial hypotheses, the history taker then moves into areas of the interview in which he will gather information tending to exclude most possibilities and confirm one. This is called the *hypothetico-deductive method.* To use it, the interview must be highly directed and hypothesis-driven, so that shortcuts can be taken and hours not be spent gathering high-volume, low-value information. Hypothesis evaluation is accomplished by requesting and assessing new information in the light of the tentative hypotheses. It depends in large measure on the physician's knowledge base, template-matching ability, and exploration, confirmation, elimination, and case-building strategies. The interviewer searches for clues that are usually present if a hypothesis is correct; if these are present or positive, the hypothesis is more likely to be correct. If these clues are absent, then the hypothesis is likely to be incorrect, especially if these clues have a high incidence of positivity (sensitivity) in this disease.

Suppose a historical clue is *always* present in a certain disease; if it is not present in the patient under investigation, the disease is ruled out. For example, edema is always present in the nephrotic syndrome; *its absence excludes* this hypothesis. On the other hand, a history of greasy, foul, floating stools is specific for the malabsorption syndrome; *its presence confirms* such a clinical impression.

Strengthening Your Impressions. As the history is expanded with more conversation and questions, the physician is sorting, extracting, subtracting, and adding bits of information into meaningful groups. He may enlarge on all aspects of a positive response,

e.g. when, where, how, and why an abdominal pain is manifested, what brings it on, and what relieves it. Negative responses are evaluated in the light of how strongly they militate against a hypothesis. Those hypotheses being considered undergo probability revision and reranking as the dynamic search for helpful information proceeds.

Searching questions are those which establish, shape, refine, support, strengthen, or rule out hypotheses. *Scanning* questions, on the other hand, are merely fishing expeditions whereby the questioner is looking for new clues and new leads if he is temporarily stumped and needs time to think. For example, he can embark on a review of systems looking for a new lead. Search questions are usually more valuable than scan questions, though the good interviewer will use both types, switching back and forth (3).

The term *"rule out"* is frequently used in medical circles. It means that a diagnosis or hypothesis has been eliminated from the list of possibilities by requesting data which, if negative or absent, more or less excludes the hypothesis under consideration. For example, the absence of a wet street and sidewalk would rule out the hypothesis that it is raining. Similarly, the existence of congestive heart failure can be ruled out by the absence of dyspnea on exertion, orthopnea, basal rales, enlarged heart, and edema.

Imagine a 38-year-old woman who consults you because of a swollen abdomen. The question of whether she may be pregnant arises. You conclude that she is not pregnant on the basis of many bits of historical evidence, but each bit has only comparative strength and must be carefully weighed: (*a*) she is not married; (*b*) she is not concerned about pregnancy; (*c*) she says she has not had sexual relations; (*d*) she has never been pregnant before; (*e*) she had a pelvic operation 1 year ago; (*f*) she has irregular menses; (*g*) she uses oral contraceptives; (*h*) she says her breasts have not enlarged; (*i*) she has anorexia and has lost weight but has no nausea or vomiting. You can see how some of these statements might raise an eyebrow, while others would make you reasonably certain she is not pregnant. Each item requires thought, consideration of psychosocial and pathophysiologic factors, and the application of logic. And each item tends to rule out pregnancy with varying degrees of certainty.

On the Question of Questions. The following script portrays a simulated doctor-patient interview. During the dialogue, *the physician's thoughts and actions are denoted in parenthetical italics.* This allows you to understand his logic, the reasons for questions, and how he deviates from the orderly data-gathering process. Occasionally the patient's thoughts will be similarly stated. It should come as no surprise to students that the patient is simultaneously evaluating the doctor.

Mrs. Jones is a 60-year-old homemaker.

DOCTOR: Hello, Mrs. Jones. I haven't seen you in several years. What brings you here?

PATIENT: I've been short of breath, doctor.

DOCTOR: *(She looks apprehensive—I'll ask her an open-ended question.)* Short of breath? Tell me about it.

PATIENT: I've had some difficulty in breathing for the past 3 or 4 weeks. Mainly it's when I walk fast or carry bundles home from the supermarket. Even the one flight up to my apartment makes me short of breath. It seems to be getting worse, too.

DOCTOR: *(Hm-m-m! Sixty-year-old woman with recent onset of worsening dyspnea on exertion—sounds like an organic problem since it occurs only on exertion— the gradual worsening and vague onset suggest an organic process of slow progression— perhaps left ventricular failure or a chronic lung disease—she doesn't look pale so anemia can't be a causative or contributing factor—better make sure it's not simple hyperventilation though it doesn't sound like it.)* Do you get short of breath if you sit around or do nothing?

PATIENT: No, I feel OK then. It's only when I exert myself.

DOCTOR: *(Probably an organic process, but I'll ask one or two more questions to rule out a functional disorder.)* When you get short of breath, do you also yawn, feel giddy, or have tingling of the fingers?

PATIENT: No. None of those. *(What can he be thinking of?)*

DOCTOR: Are you having any emotional problems at home, perhaps your husband or children?

PATIENT: No, doctor, everything else is fine. My husband is in good health; my children are married and happy and so am I. *(It sounds like this doctor doesn't believe me; he doesn't think I'm sick!)*

DOCTOR: *(I guess we can forget about psychogenic factors and the hyperventilation syndrome and concentrate on the heart and lungs—she doesn't look pleased with me!)* That's good. Has this ever happened before?

PATIENT: No, doctor.

DOCTOR: *(That one didn't help much. Anyway, I was just scanning.)* Do you have any other symptoms? *(scanning again)*

PATIENT: Well, I do get tired very easily.

DOCTOR: At the same time as you get short of breath?

PATIENT: Yes.

DOCTOR: *(Dyspnea and fatigue on exertion—sounds definitely organic. Let's search.)* Do you have any chest pain or cough, and do you bring up phlegm?

PATIENT: No chest pain or phlegm, but I do cough a little when I lie down at night.

DOCTOR: At night?

PATIENT: Yes. I find I'm not comfortable unless I sleep on three pillows.

DOCTOR: Is that unusual for you?

PATIENT: Well, I always slept on one pillow, but lately I've found it necessary to use three.

DOCTOR: *(Oh, oh—orthopnea?)* Why?

PATIENT: Because if I don't, I wake up short of breath.

DOCTOR: *(Must be early left ventricular failure, though I don't know its cause yet; maybe it's her hypertension. Lung disease is unlikely, but a pleural effusion or chronic fibrotic process could present in this way.)* Mrs. Jones, I saw you 3 years ago for high blood pressure and gave you a prescription and diet. What happened?

PATIENT: We moved to Florida and my

blood pressure was normal the one time I checked it there, so I stopped the medication. And I haven't seen a doctor since then.

DOCTOR: Let's take a look at you. (*On examination*, the doctor finds blood pressure 220/110 mm Hg in both arms; pulse 98/minute; grade 2 hypertensive retinopathy; normal lungs except for fine moist end-inspiratory rales; a diffusely forceful apex beat in the sixth left intercostal space 12 cm from the midsternal line; a grade 2/6 pansystolic murmur at the apex, a grade 2/6 systolic ejection murmur at the base, and a loud second heart sound.)

DOCTOR: Mrs. Jones, I think your heart is not functioning as well as it should because of untreated high blood pressure. Let's go over you very carefully so we can be sure of the extent of the problem and its cause. Then we can begin treatment.

Note that the interview was conversational and flexible, and that mainly open-ended questions were asked. The physician formed an initial concept and then some provisional hypotheses. Using an exclude-and-confirm technique, he eliminated some possibilities while promoting one. The examination did the rest. He might have performed parts of the physical examination during the interview, though his instincts told him to proceed a little more slowly with this patient. You might even validly criticize the doctor for having landed too soon and lingered too long on psychogenic aspects.

Complete Histories. While espousing the philosophy of shortcuts in history taking in other parts of this book, I do not imply that complete detailed histories are archaic. They must be done even though you may have decided on the major problems early in the anamnesis. In so doing you confirm or reject these problems, uncover new ones, or find isolated historical facts which fit nowhere. Moreover, you may realize that what was thought to be a simple problem is really complex or involves more systems than had been suspected.

Who Takes the History. Today many other people gather data for the busy physi-

cian. It may be heresy, but I firmly believe that only the physician* should take the patient's history. What an old-fashioned idea! It should not be done by an untrained person or by the patient filling out a form or punching information into a computer. For it is primarily in taking the history that the physician establishes rapport and begins to understand the patient's personality. The patient drops clues that the discerning physician detects. He notices a patient's reaction to a question, the words he chooses, and what he emphasizes. By the expression on the patient's face he may suspect that a negative answer may not actually be true and probe further. The physician is best qualified to change the focus or direction of questions, to deduce simultaneously, to elaborate, and to discern fine shades of meaning. It is here where depression, anxiety, fear, exaggeration, and denial are detected, facial nuances can be weighed, and problem solving begins. Furthermore, he may discover that the presenting symptom is not really the patient's main concern. What computer or form can do all these things?

Any simplistic approach which attempts to add clues together in a machine that prints out the answers is probably naive. Such an approach completely ignores the critical value of the human intellect and is not a substitute for human thinking and patient-physician interaction.

Oblique Questions. For example, the physician may sometimes have to resort to oblique rather than direct questions. If he inquires about chest pain on walking, the answer may be negative. But if he then asks "how often to you stop to look in shop windows when you go out walking?" he may get valuable information. Similarly, "have you noticed that your hands are weaker than they used to be?" might better be asked "can you still pour a full teapot with one hand?"

---

* The use of the word "physician" in many portions of the text is meant to include the physician's assistant or nurse-practitioner who may be trained to gather certain types of data and aid in problem solving.

And "have you given up your bedtime cup of tea?" may give more positive information than "do you get up at night to urinate?"

On Being Critical. Be most critical in history taking. Do not accept vague or suspicious statements as gospel truth. If your patient is "allergic to penicillin," ask in what way. The symptoms following the antibiotic may have been completely unrelated to allergy. "Sinus trouble" is another vague symptom which warrants further questions.

A 60-year-old man tells you he had a "heart attack" at age 29. It almost certainly is not so. Ask more questions. How long was he in bed? What was the pain like? What was the treatment? Did he go back to work promptly? Has he had trouble since then?

If the patient states he has gained or lost weight, make sure this is actually so by inspecting his skin, noting the fit of his clothes, and talking to his family. A gain in weight may be simple obesity because the patient is eating more. A loss of weight usually signifies serious disease unless a diet has been imposed. If weight loss is verified, a detailed and usually costly investigation is indicated. "Swollen legs" and "swollen abdomen" must also be verified. The former may be a plethora of connective tissue or fat around the ankles which the patient has had all through life. The latter can be simple obesity or constipation with gas.

A change in symptoms is important. When a cough suddenly gets worse, sputum changes color, angina intensifies, or black stools begin to accompany chronic indigestion, the patient's clinical state has changed. Be alert for a complication.

Students often fail to find out why a patient consults a physician at a particular time. While cough and expectoration, headaches, or indigestion may have existed for years, there is usually a precipitating event that occasions the consultation. What was the straw that broke the camel's back? While it may be a new, more frightening symptom, it can be as simple as a television commercial, a warning piece of literature, or the spouse's insistence.

Independent History Taking. In order to

escape the biases of students, interns, or physicians who have previously questioned and examined the patient, it is necessary to do it yourself. If you look at the chart and read someone else's logic, you may find yourself following in his footsteps and making the same mistakes. Take the history before being influenced by others; review the chart after you yourself have acquired the data base (4).

The clinical clerk may see a patient after the emergency room physician has already made an alleged diagnosis. Or in later years the consultant sees a patient whom the attending physician has already diagnosed or at least investigated. The approach is the same. While some information is already available, you must wipe the slate clean and start afresh. Take your own history; do your own examination; check the paraclinical studies yourself. While respecting the previous physician's opinions, take nothing for granted. Be doubting; be skeptical; be critical; be unbiased; and your yield will be high.

Is This Symptom Normal? When is a symptom abnormal, and when is it merely something that often occurs in normal individuals? Everybody gets dyspneic on running. But what degree of dyspnea is normal after intercourse, on walking fast, or on going up two flights of stairs? Such quantitation must also be applied to headaches, insomnia, and menstrual cramps, all of which if frequent or severe may be abnormal but otherwise can be normal. Almost everybody has an occasional cough, wakes up now and then with a stuffy nose, raises some phlegm, or sometimes has ringing in the ears. And many people have constipation or diarrhea from time to time, or have "gas," or complain that they bruise easily. Drawing the line between disease and health may be difficult.

It may be helpful to know that many symptoms go unreported. If you were retrospectively to survey hundreds of healthy people, almost all would tell you of headaches and periodic changes in energy. Many would be reminded of backaches, gastric dysfunction, and abdominal pains; some would have had any complaint you could mention. These symptoms did not prompt a visit to the doctor. The incidences of symptoms as experienced by the patient and as seen by the doctor are not identical; the relationship is very complex and varies with the person, his pain threshold, attitudes, finances, social class, and physician consciousness. Many of these seemingly irrelevant symptoms come to light during a systems review and may be difficult to evaluate.

Sources for History. Gathering historical data from sources other than the patient must be mentioned. The facts elicited from the patient may be fuzzy, incomplete, or even false. Patients forget, sometimes do not understand, or never knew what was diagnosed or removed in the past. A relative, neighbor, or co-worker may be most helpful. On day 1, the patient may be too ill to give an accurate history. A telephone call or letter to a former physician or to the record room of a previous hospital or a search of military records may be of tremendous value. The necessary information is often tucked away in an old medical report. Much money and time can be saved. Too often a multitude of studies will be ordered where one telephone call would have sufficed. Do not substitute tests for talk. Talk is cheap—tests are not; both can be effective.

Only the History Can Help. Often a history is the only means of establishing a diagnosis. Migraine is recognized purely by history. There are no physical findings or studies to confirm it. Paroxysmal atrial tachycardia is often strongly suspected by history alone, since the attack may be gone by the time the physician is able to listen or record; the interval ECG is usually normal, and Holter recordings are tedious, expensive, and often fruitless. The same can be said for angina pectoris where, short of a coronary angiogram or treadmill test, all else may be normal but the history unmistakable.

A carefully investigated chief complaint may provide you with the answer without seeking any additional information. Kipling's six honest serving-men—*What*, and *Why*, and *When*, and *How*, and *Where*, and *Who*—teach you all you want to know about chief complaints or symptoms.

Six Senses. Today there is too great a tendency to study all the body effluvia, invade all the orifices, create some artificial ones to invade, and use a profusion of new electronic and computerized gadgetry. Learn rather to use your five senses, depend even more on the sixth—common sense— and prove Voltaire was wrong when he said, "common sense is not common!"

Functional vs Organic. As in the script presented above, the distinction between functional and organic disease is often crucial. Functional problems lie in the psychosomatic sphere, whereas organic problems can be attributed to known or postulated biologic, metabolic, microbial, or physicochemical disturbances. Each of the two must be managed differently, though they often coexist. This subject will be detailed in Chapter 28.

But for now it is important to learn how to distinguish between a psychosomatic disorder and an organic disease during the process of taking the history. This may well be the single *most important diagnostic skill* in all of medicine.

No matter how talented, the physician inevitably makes mistakes in this area. The 38-year-old obviously neurotic woman complaining of abdominal "cramps and gas" may turn out to have carcinoma of the colon, not a "nervous bowel." The person with headaches for years may develop a new type of headache—this time a brain tumor. Do not label a patient psychoneurotic for life, since he too must someday die of an organic disease. Each new complaint must be regarded seriously. Generally speaking, though, the more complaints, the more surgery, the more doctors, and the more hospitalizations—in a healthy-appearing person—the less disease there is.

Symptoms in psychoneurotic patients occur in all organs but seem to relate mainly to the head, special senses, heart, gastrointestinal tract, and sexual organs. Common complaints are weakness, headaches, light headedness, abnormalities of sight and sound, indigestion, gas, heartburn, cramps, difficulty in breathing, palpitations, and bizarre sensations around the sexual organs. Each of these symptoms obviously can have an organic basis too. It may take a lot of conversation, examination, and tests to be sure. And even then you may not be certain.

To evaluate one of these symptoms you must judge the patient's entire profile. Is there a cause for anxiety or conversion? Are there any associated symptoms which point to organicity? If the answers to *all* questions are positive, it is unlikely that so many symptoms could exist on an organic basis in a single patient. Good doctor-patient verbal interaction is most important when trying to distinguish between functional and organic disease.

Physical Examination

The Two Types. After having completed the history, or even a subset of the history, the physician already has a good idea of what may be wrong with the patient. In proceeding to the physical examination he knows what he should be looking for. In fact, he may already have done some parts of the examination during the taking of the history. Thus he does two types of physical examinations simultaneously. One is a specific or ad hoc examination in which he is looking for findings which will confirm or rule out his impressions. The other is a nonspecific or complete examination in which he is being thorough; here he may stumble upon unexpected clues and additional problems.

Pitfalls. In doing *complete physical examinations* there are no substitutes for orderliness, thoroughness, and attention to one thing at a time. Often the solution is to be found in the fundi, the supraclavicular nodes, the spleen, the rectum, testes, or pelvis—much neglected or poorly examined areas. Most errors here are due to lack of thoroughness, not lack of knowledge. The general inspection of the patient is the part of the physical examination that is often inadequately done, and it is where important

findings are missed. This inspection should be done at the beginning. All you do is look—do not touch or listen. Take a few minutes to do it and do it systematically. Program yourself to look successively for jaundice, anemia, cyanosis, plethora, rashes, and a wide variety of findings often overlooked because there is no specific place in the rest of the physical examination for them.

Other items to be successively evaluated during the inspection period are the body build, endocrine or genetic habitus, state of nutrition and hydration, body deformities, correlation of apparent and actual ages, and so forth.

Who has not done a complete physical examination and overlooked the fact that the patient was pale or even slightly jaundiced because it wasn't looked for? These are noted mainly on general inspection since once you get to the rest of the body, these items are already out of mind. Two days later you note the laboratory abnormalities and return to the patient for a more careful look.

Endocrine or genetic disorders (myxedema, acromegaly, hyperthyroidism, Cushing's syndrome, Turner's syndrome) can often be diagnosed at a glance, but only if you are looking for them. Otherwise they may be missed. The patient who is gradually developing hypothyroidism under your very nose may remain undiagnosed until she is seen by another doctor who opens his unbiased eyes wider than yours. (Refer to "How Inspection Helps," Chapter 4.)

Smelling should be included in general inspection. Put your nose to the patient's mouth as he exhales. Do not be timid. You may diagnose hepatic failure, renal failure, alcoholism, diabetic ketoacidosis, or pulmonary suppuration with just a sniff.

Palpation too is an underutilized and poorly understood skill. The amount of information that can be obtained by simply touching and feeling is amazing, and students are often unaware of such multiple utilities. For example, light palpation with the fingertips can detect texture, moisture, crepitus, tenderness, fluctuation, and masses. Slightly firmer palpation with the distal phalanges elicits deep tenderness, rigidity, ballottement, thrust, and pulsation and may further delineate and characterize masses. Certain parts of the hand are best for eliciting other findings. For example, the dorsum of the hand is best for temperature sensation, and the hypothenar eminences and palmar aspect of the metacarpophalangeal joints are best for vibratory sensation; this includes the detection of tactile fremitus, vascular thrills, and friction rubs.

While on the subject of palpation, it must be stated that the heart is "underpalpated" and perhaps "overauscultated." Examiners will often be satisfied with only the detection of the apex beat. But there are many areas of the precordium to be palpated. These include the upper sternum, the aortic valve area, the pulmonic valve area, the presternal area, the area over the sliver of left ventricle, the ectopic area, and the epigastrium, as well as the apex beat. And don't forget to palpate the liver, since systolic or presystolic liver pulsation may be related to tricuspid valve disease.

The cavil to pay attention to one thing at a time sounds simple, but it isn't. It means that the examiner must program his mind to look for only one thing to the exclusion of all others. The mouth is not examined by an overall scan and a glance at the tongue. Instead there are at least ten parts to be individually inspected, one at a time. If you were to hear a symphony and were then asked if you had heard the oboe in the background, you probably would answer "no." But if you were told in advance to listen for the oboe, most of you would hear it. Therefore, in doing your examination, always listen for the oboe.

Other Common Errors. Numerous other errors are often made in performing the physical examination. These can be classified as errors of (*a*) technique, (*b*) omission, (*c*) detection, (*d*) interpretation, and (*e*) recording (5).

Failures in technique include faulty examining equipment and improper methods of examination of the trachea and thyroid, neck vein waves, jugular venous pressure, low- and high-frequency murmurs, diaphragmatic movements, spleen and liver size, abdominal bruits, popliteal pulses, and testes.

Errors of omission are common in the inspection of various parts of the eye and the nasal cavity; auscultation of the neck vessels; palpation of the point of maximal impulse; auscultation of the lateral chest and apices; cardiac auscultation in various positions; palpation of the spleen in the right lateral decubitus position; palpation of the prostate, ovaries, and kidneys; rectal and pelvic examination; plus numerous parts of what ordinarily constitutes a complete neurologic examination.

Errors of detection include failure to detect abnormalities which are present or reporting a sign that is not present. Typically these include thyroid nodules, tracheal deviation, bruits, scleral icterus, breath odors, chest lag, crepitus, bronchial breathing, faint aortic and mitral diastolic murmurs, third and fourth heart sounds, fine rales, minimal splenomegaly, small hernias, prostatic nodules, aortic aneurysms, and small abdominal masses.

Errors in the interpretation of abnormal physical findings concern tracheal deviation, venous pulses, jugular pressure, dullness, bronchial breathing, systolic murmurs, whispered voice, aortic dilatation vs aneurysm, venous flow patterns, liver size, and eye signs.

Errors in recording include failure to record an abnormal finding, illegible handwriting, obscure abbreviations, improper terminology, and bad grammar. Descriptions of heart murmurs are often poor.

Excusable Errors. Wiener and Nathanson's (5) excellent study was accomplished by the direct observation of students and should serve as a guide to others who teach examination skills. However, some of the above are not really errors. There can be legitimate disagreement between equally competent observers. This is common, for instance, in cases of hearing a murmur, an

S_3 or S_4, or the palpation of a splenic tip. Observer variations can occur in history taking too. The second history may differ in many respects from the first. The patient may be more alert, he may already be cued to questions, his memory may be improved, or his rapport with the second physician may be better. Interpretations of biopsies and cancer cell smears may differ, and electrocardiographers frequently disagree too.

Are Educators to Blame? Teachers must take most of the blame for many of the examining errors that students make. Our much vaunted American medical education system is failing in its responsibilities to prepare physicians in the most fundamental of all medical skills (6).

Few students have ever been monitored while actually doing a history or physical examination—or at best they have been monitored only once or twice. Nor do their clinical instructors show them how it is done. Most students complete all their training and go into practice without once having been observed for acquired examination skills, even during internship and residency. Two often we succeed in producing a physician who is ill-equipped for patient management and problem solving and who can only suggest more diagnostic tests. The American Board of Internal Medicine has attempted to correct this by demanding that attending physicians observe and evaluate housestaff performing these skills. But often there is a disparity between the requirement and its observance.

Knowing What Is Normal. You can't be sure that a physical finding is abnormal unless you know what normal is. This would seem to go without saying, but I am constantly amazed by students and housestaff who present physical findings without knowing for sure whether they are abnormal. Indeed, how can you determine if a physical finding is relevant or irrelevant unless you first know whether it is abnormal?

Take the size of the normal testicle. It has three dimensions and a volume which is the product of these dimensions. yet how many examiners know that the volume of an average-sized normal testicle is greater than 15 cm^3? You must know this to suspect testicular atrophy and hypogonadism from any cause. Careful measurements must be made; just a feel is not sufficient.

Similarly, you must know the sizes and shapes of normal livers, the distance the diaphragm normally moves with deep inspiration, the normal arterial-venous ratio in the fundus, and so on. Limits of normal variation must also be known. For example, the systolic blood pressure normally does not change more than 10 mm Hg on shifting from the supine to the erect position or on breathing in and out, and it will not vary more than 10 mm Hg from one arm to the other.

There are numerous other considerations. For instance, the absence of dorsalis pedis pulses may be normal in a small percentage of people. An innocent murmur may have been present since childhood and be unrelated to the patient's vague symptoms. An alleged mass in the right upper quadrant may be an anomalous Riedel's lobe or a misplaced kidney. You suspect Marfans syndrome and look for evidence of a highly arched palate. But since you do not know the normal palatal arch, you cannot be sure. How much hair on the face is abnormal in women? Are those stretch marks due to obesity or pregnancies, or is it Cushing's disease? How much pigmentation is normal in the mouths and eyes of nonwhites? Is this lymph node really enlarged? Each of these may be critical in deciding whether a finding is a clue or is normal.

In some instances, it is difficult to distinguish between normal and abnormal. Consider the patient with a few palpable cervical lymph nodes which range between 1 and 2 cm in length. Important diagnostic decisions hinge on whether or not these nodes are normal.

The Clinical Measurement. Accuracy does not always result when a measurement is made, and measurements do not always result in predictable precision. In a simple well-designed experiment, groups of medical students were asked to determine a blood pressure, measure papules that simulated purified protein derivative reactions, and measure heart and kidney size on radiographs. Errors and variability were prominent. There was a 52 mm Hg range of blood pressure values, a wide range of skin lesion size, and wide ranges in heart and kidney size. Some errors were procedural, but others were technical. The variability of clinical measurements demonstrates the need to learn how to deal with what is obviously imperfect information when making diagnostic decisions (7).

Recent clinical investigations have shown the inaccuracies of measuring liver size, diaphragmatic motion, and the presence of ascites by traditional physical diagnostic maneuvers. In comparing measurements made by groups of clinicians to the results of x-ray, isotope scans, and ultrasound, it was shown that the clinicians were frequently wrong. Percussion for liver size had an overall accuracy of 50%, information that could have been gotten from the flip of a coin. The results of percussion for diaphragmatic excursion correlated so poorly that the authors of this study recommended it no longer be done as part of a routine physical examination (8). In a series of patients with *questionable* ascites, the various physical maneuvers had an overall accuracy of only 58% when compared with ultrasound studies which were regarded as 100% accurate. Bulging flanks, flank dullness, shifting dullness, fluid wave, and puddle sign were each evaluated for sensitivity and specificity, and the overall accuracy was then calculated. The three observers used showed very little interobserver variation (9).

It would seem that all our physical examination skills need careful reappraisals of this sort. Hopefully, such studies will not result in more diagnostic procedures being done but will instead stimulate the more critical evaluation of data.

To Do and Not to Do. Once the examiner has mastered a certain number of specific skills, the physical examination portion of the data-gathering process is easy and should require only 10 or 15 minutes. Again, the key to the examination is orderliness, thoroughness, and doing one thing at a time. Too often the examiner falls into the slovenly habit of doing an abbreviated helter-skelter physical examination, which includes a look at the tongue, a tap on the chest, a listen to the heart, and a pat on the abdomen. Even if the patient comes in complaining only of lumps in the neck and axillae, it is not enough to simply examine the lumps and know immediately that he has leukemia or lymphoma, which may well be the case. Completeness is indicated since other manifestations of the disease, as well as other diseases, may be uncovered.

Orderliness is important lest one unintentionally omit an important aspect of the examination, such as the fundi or the rectum. Attention to one thing at a time is crucial since the brain can appreciate only one thing at a time. In examining the eyes, there are approximately 15 items that must be checked. A single glance does not take them all in. In listening to the heart, do not listen for 15 seconds then stop. Instead, concentrate first on S_1 at the apex, then S_2 at the base, systole, diastole, individual valve areas, and so forth. Allow the ears and brain to focus on one item at a time, blocking out all other sounds. If this is not done, much of importance can be missed. The cost or complexity of the stethoscope is of less consequence than the caliber of the brain interpreting the sound reaching the ear.

One Skill Dissected. On the surface, it might seem that a single examining skill would be simple. But most are not; they require many separate actions in order to be properly executed. Take, for example, the location and description of the cardiac apex beat. *First*, try to locate the apex beat by inspection; perhaps only 25% are visible. *Second*, place the palm of the right hand over the precordium and feel the apex beat; perhaps only 50% are palpable. If you cannot feel it, have the patient gently exercise and then lean forward; this maneuver may make the apex beat more palpable. *Third*, place your index finger where the apex beat was felt and mark the location. *Fourth*, locate the sternal angle and the second rib on the left. *Fifth*, count downward one rib at a time until you reach the interspace where you felt the apex beat. *Sixth*, measure the distance tangentially and horizontally from the midsternal line to the apex beat. You have now located the apex beat. *Seventh*, again feel the apex beat, noting its strength, shape, duration, and diameter, and whether there are associated impulses preceding or following it.

You are now ready to describe the normal apex beat. "The apex beat is in the fifth left intercostal space, 8 cm tangentially from the midsternal line. It is of normal force, lasts less than 0.1 second, occupies an area with a 2-cm diameter, has a normal shape, and is not associated with any other impulses."

Almost every examining skill can be broken down into its component parts in a similar manner. This enables the student to learn, do, and report his examination with accuracy and precision. Any student describing the apex beat as was just done would be regarded by his listeners with awe and respect.

Many Skills per System. While it is not the purpose of this book to cover the field of physical diagnosis, it should be pointed out that each organ system has many examining skills associated with it. If a complete examination is indicated, it is not enough to examine only one or two parts. For example, an examination of the eyes includes: inspection for symmetry, protrusion, and position; the eyelids, eyebrow, conjunctiva (with lid eversion), cornea, sclera, pupils, and lacrimal apparatus; all three pupillary reactions; tonometry, visual acuity, visual fields, and extraocular motions; and, last, ophthalmoscopy. Most of these skills can be broken down into many parts.

The same can be said for the examinations of the ears, mouth, neck, heart, lungs, abdomen, genitalia, and so forth. To master each skill, read about it, watch it being done, study it, practice it, then have a senior person check your performance to make sure you are doing it correctly. Once mastered, you should know it forever.

On Light, Clothes, and Position. Other aspects of the physical examination almost too basic and simple to preach—yet often ignored—include the presence of proper light, having all necessary instruments, the comfort of patient and examiner, informing the patient of certain sensitive areas to be examined, gentleness, and the patient's being disrobed and properly draped. You cannot possibly examine a female's heart while her brassiere is on, nor her abdomen through a girdle. Yet how often it is done! Frequently jaundice or anemia is missed because the light is poor. And while you should do your examination in an order permitting a minimal number of changes of position for the patient, it is difficult to hear faint aortic regurgitation in a reclining patient, nor can diaphragmatic motion be properly assessed unless the patient sits up, and perhaps not even then.

The Proper Positions. The novice examiner often has difficulty deciding on the proper sequence of examination vis-à-vis patient-doctor positioning. A good routine should be established. This will depend on whether the patient is ambulatory, in bed but mobile, or in bed and too sick to move about. In general, the patient has three positions during the examination—lying, sitting, and standing. The examiner stands either in front, behind, or to the right of the patient; he should aim for a minimum number of changes of patient position and spare the patient the inconvenience and discomfort of a helter-skelter disordered examination.

Since almost all patients can sit, the ambulatory patient should sit over the side of an examining table, and the hospitalized patient should sit over the side of the bed. With the patient in this position, the examiner can now complete the general inspection, obtain the vital signs, and study the head and neck, eyes, ears, nose, mouth, throat, back and front of the chest, heart, breasts, and axillae. The patient then lies down, and the heart, breasts, and axillae are reexamined. In this position, the abdomen, external genitalia, rectum, extremities, and peripheral circulation are reviewed.

A few selected parts of the examination can then be done in the standing position. These include a search for hernias and inspection of the leg veins.

As for the neurologic examination, the cranial nerves, reflexes, motor power, and sensation could have been tested while the patient was sitting. Cerebellar function is tested while sitting and standing. The pelvic examination occupies a position by itself, probably best at the end of the examination; the rectum can be examined at the same time in the female. The musculoskeletal system is examined in the sitting and standing positions.

A well-programmed examiner can intermingle his somatic, neurologic, and musculoskeletal examinations so as to minimize the changes in position. A simple sit-lie-stand sequence done only once should suffice. Bear in mind that the cardiovascular and abdominal examinations sometimes entail special positions to clarify murmurs or the presence of ascites. The entire examination should take only 10 to 15 minutes.

The foregoing orderly routine is for the patient who requires a complete traditional examination. If the diagnosis is already suspected on the basis of the history, any positional order may be followed, depending on what the examiner seeks.

For the patient who is very sick and cannot sit or stand, the examination must be done with the patient lying in bed at 30 to 45°. Some parts may have to be omitted. The back of the chest presents a difficulty which can be partially resolved by an attendant who turns the patient from side to side or helps him to sit by pulling on his arms (10).

Better Than a Physical. Tradition tells of many things which can be detected by the physical examination. Some of this is no longer true. Heart size and shape are best

determined by the chest x-ray, Auenbrugger's great art of percussion notwithstanding. Early pulmonary edema and beginning left ventricular failure are also best detected by the chest x-ray, since septal edema is noted before alveolar edema and rales occur. The tonometer, not the thumb, is the most reliable means of measuring intraocular pressure. And alveolar hypoventilation is best measured by arterial blood gases—not by the respiratory rate or cyanosis. Anemia is classically detected by a look at the skin, the conjunctiva, the tongue, the palms, and the fingernail beds. It may be overlooked in dark-skinned people, in whites with suntans, if conjunctivitis is present, or if normal muddy pigment discolors the conjunctiva and sclera as in some nonwhites. A blood count may surprise you. The reverse is true in shock, where the patient appears very pale on inspection yet is not anemic.

Those who argue that the eyes, ears, and hands are best for physical examination may have to retrench when it comes to some selected skills. Unless we can improve on the 19th-century techniques of French and German diagnosticians, we may have to rely more on the x-ray for diaphragmatic excursion, the isotope scan for liver and spleen size, and ultrasound for detecting small amounts of pericardial, pleural, and peritoneal fluid. Available facilities, seriousness of the situation, cost containment, and need for diagnostic certainty will help to determine how much technology to use in a particular case. And under certain circumstances, it may be more prudent to settle for less reliable modalities.

Unnecessary Parts. It is not necessary to do all aspects of the physical examination on each patient. If the patient has difficulty in hearing, then detailed hearing tests are in order; otherwise they are unnecessary. A coin test and whispered pectoriloquy are needed only if a pulmonary disease which gives either of these signs is suspected. Otherwise it is an exercise in futility. A detailed orthopaedic examination is indicated only if symptoms warrant it. In fact, there are still differences about what constitutes a complete physical examination and what a routine screening examination should include.

Paraclinical Studies

Under this heading are included the traditional serologic, immunologic, microbiologic, hematologic, and urine and blood chemical tests and studies. But also to be dealt with are the simple radiographic procedures, the electrocardiograms, pulmonary function tests, and other studies of body fluids and secretions.

Today's technological explosion has provided the physician with additional gourmet menus of diagnostic procedures which were until recently unknown and undreamed. These include expensive, exotic, and sometimes risky studies ranging through every specialty and every laboratory.

Over half the radiologic procedures done today were not done 10 years ago. Intrepid testers biopsy even the heart and brain—in addition to the liver, spleen, kidney, lung, pancreas, and small intestine. Catheters with dyes and drugs are insinuated into the cerebral, coronary, renal, adrenal, pulmonary, intestinal, and peripheral circulations. Radioactive isotopes define organs, detect defects within them, measure cardiac function and contractility, delineate ischemic myocardium, and assess blood supply to the heart and brain. Highly sensitive analytic techniques measure drug and hormone concentrations in ultraminute nanograms or picograms, a process that allows microminiaturized assays in the one billionth (10^{-9}) or one trillionth (10^{-12}) range. Thus the serum concentration of almost every known hormone is now assayable. Through only two natural orifices, the endoscopist can reach, image, or biopsy the entire gastrointestinal tract and its appendages. The new dimensions that have been added to diagnosis by the introduction of ultrasound, computed tomography (with or without dye enhancement), nuclear magnetic resonance, and positron emission tomography have not yet

been fully explored or delineated. The horizons for their applications seem boundless.

Just as a gourmet diet may be delicious but unhealthful, the formidable array of diagnostic studies available to the clinician may be a mixed blessing. While they are awe-inspiring, even mind-boggling, and often very helpful, sometimes they are not in the best interest of the patient, the public policy, or the pocketbook. Proper laboratory utilization has become a complex multi-faceted issue that justifies entire chapters. The numerous problems created by the large number of tests and procedures done in today's modern medical arena will be detailed in Chapters 6 and 7.

But in this section some fundamental information relating to tests and studies will be discussed. This is because the natural sequence of constructing a patient's data base is history-physical examination-laboratory. And it is by the processing of patient data obtained from these three sources that the problem list or differential diagnosis is formulated.

Resorting to Tests. At this time enough data have been obtained from the history and physical examination to provide a definite diagnosis, a tentative diagnosis, a list of hypotheses, or a ranked order of hypotheses, each with its own numerical probability. If you need additional data to make the diagnosis more certain, you may then turn to tests and studies. Bear in mind that a test is just another bit of information, another clue to help you evaluate a hypothesis, and is no more significant than an item in the history or physical examination. And, like any other clue, it may not be completely reliable.

But there can be no question that paraclinical studies often provide crucial information. An abnormal laboratory study, chest x-ray, or ECG may serve to confirm the problem or problems already implied by the rest of the data base. Conversely, it may negate a suspected problem or indicate that additional or unsuspected ones exist. A chest x-ray may show an infiltrate in a patient whose history and physical examination are unrelated to it. Unsuspected anemia, diabetes, or uremia may be uncovered in a patient who presents with symptoms of another condition that is not associated with these three laboratory abnormalities.

Routine Studies. Fifty years ago, every hospitalized patient received a complete blood count, urinalysis, Wassermann test, and chest x-ray on admission. This was done for screening purposes. The blood count no longer routinely includes the white blood cell differential because the latter is rarely of value if the white blood cell count is normal. The Wassermann test has been replaced by a more specific test—the Venereal Disease Research Laboratory test. This too is no longer routinely requested since unsuspected syphilis is so uncommon. Chest x-rays were performed to make sure patients with active tuberculous lesions were not admitted to open wards; today they are done primarily to exclude an asymptomatic neoplasm. The urinalysis was done because of reverence for tradition, its ease of performance, and for the valuable information it gave. This has not changed.

Several decades back, the blood sugar and nonprotein nitrogen were added to the routine list. It was deemed important to screen for diabetes mellitus and failure of renal function. Today these have been replaced by the serum glucose and blood urea nitrogen (or serum creatinine)—more specific determinants of the entities being tested. Note here and now that a normal glucose does not rule out diabetes mellitus, nor does an elevated glucose necessarily diagnose it. But a normal blood urea nitrogen *does* exclude renal failure while an elevated blood urea nitrogen indicates inadequate renal function; the reasons for the latter are many and are often unrelated to the integrity of the kidney.

In the past 10 to 20 years, remarkable advances in automation, computers, and laboratory management have permitted a large increase in tests at only a modest increase in cost. Now the potassium, sodium, chloride, and carbon dioxide are routinely done on admission. Yet electrolytes for screening purposes are rarely helpful except in patients where derangements might be expected; for example, the patient taking a diuretic, the patient with heart failure or renal failure, the patient with severe fluid loss, or the patient with a possible acid-base disorder.

Generally then, a 6-test chemistry profile includes the serum glucose, urea nitrogen, sodium, potassium, chloride, and carbon dioxide (or bicarbonate).

A battery of 12 additional tests is also seen on most charts since they are done for only an additional $17.50. So whether or not they are needed, the patient is tested for serum bilirubin, creatinine, protein, albumin, calcium, phosphorus, uric acid, lactic dehydrogenase, glutamic oxaloacetic transaminase, alkaline phosphatase, creatine kinase, and cholesterol. Some of these tests may have been sought anyway, but most are valueless and sometimes misleading. What constitutes a 12-test battery may vary somewhat from one hospital to another. The implications of reflexively ordering shotgun batteries of tests vs requesting hypothesis-driven tests will be discussed later. But we must not forget that complete studies may uncover problems not suggested by the rest of the data base—for example, eosinophilia, hypercholesterolemia, or hypercalcemia.

What Tests to Order. Aside from the fact that the "routine" tests may give you all the information you need, there are more select tests that may give yet more vital support to your provisional hypotheses. If liver disease is suspected, measurements of additional liver cell enzymes, coagulation tests, dye excretion studies, immunoelectrophoresis, and immunologic markers for hepatitis may be requested.

For patients suspected of having a disorder of blood coagulation, you might order a platelet count, prothrombin time, and partial thromboplastin time. But if you don't remember, don't wish to think, or prefer not to read, your laboratory may have an entire batch of coagulation studies available for you; just check the item marked "coagulation." You will have the results of 10 to 12 tests in a day or two, sometimes neatly labeled with a diagnosis.

The question is: Do we selectively cast a nylon line with a specific bait that catches only one kind of fish, or do we throw out a vast net that catches all? This question again raises the same important issues.

Consider a patient who has an *anemia* to be solved. Your favorite laboratory, on whom you have begun to rely more and more, can perform some 20 to 30 tests—all tests for all anemias. Just imagine! You needn't talk, examine, think, or read. The results may or may not give you the correct answer.

But, on the other hand, a few questions, a brief examination, and perhaps only two or three carefully selected tests may be all that are needed. Profuse menses in a 42-year-old woman, a hypochromic microcytic anemia, and a stool which is negative for occult blood tell you that the problem lies in the womb. High reticulocytes, high indirect bilirubin, normocytic anemia, Heinz bodies, and absence of sickle cells in a 24-year-old black man suggest that the problem lies in the genetic coding of glucose 6-phosphate dehydrogenase.

Cardiac patients being treated for congestive heart failure may need only electrolytes and a digoxin level. But for more complex cardiac problems numerous invasive and noninvasive studies are offered on yet another gourmet menu. And the decision to do which tests for what disease and in what order may be a difficult one and require consultation with the maître-d'hôtel. Gastrointestinal problems, suspected diseases requiring a series of radiographic procedures, and rare endocrine disorders may also require consultation from the authority who can tell you which tests to request and the order in which they should be done.

In general, the noninvasive studies with the least morbidity should be done before the invasive ones. The answer may come with less trauma. But there are occasions where you might go directly to the test with the most positive yield. If you suspect an impending massive myocardial infarct, you might go straight to coronary arteriography and bypass all else. Urgent surgical intervention may be indicated in other circumstances, and you would probably want to do the diagnostic procedure most apt to give you the go-signal no matter what its morbidity. A patient with massive upper gastrointestinal bleeding may need fiberoptic gastroduodenoscopy as soon as possible.

Then there is the situation where you find a lump in the neck or elsewhere. A direct approach with biopsy or resection might be the wisest tactic, since it is less taxing on the patient's nerves and bank account, and in the end you will probably do it anyway.

On Being Out of Order. While the sequence of data collection is usually *history-physical examination-laboratory data*, this is not always so. An ECG may be the first bit of data submitted since it is the reason for the patient's study. The same holds for a chest x-ray which may have discovered an asymptomatic abnormality. Then there is the patient who sees you for a lump in the neck. Naturally, you would examine the lump first and perhaps check a few other areas before embarking on the history. Or if the patient presents with severe chest pain, you might want a stat ECG even while recording the vital signs. So the order of gathering data is not fixed and may vary from patient to patient.

If an abnormality detected on physical examination or laboratory study has no relation to the history, do not hesitate to redo the history. After finding an enlarged prostate, further questions may reveal symptoms of mild lower urinary tract obstruction. A heart murmur may, in retrospect, reveal what sounds like rheumatic fever in childhood. Pyuria may recall a forgotten history of old gonococcal infection with a resultant stricture or prostatitis. A scar on the abdomen may remind your patient of a hysterectomy done a half-century ago.

Many times I have seen the radiologist alter his judgment or reading based on what the attending physician could add to the picture—so that he no longer needed to read in the dark. The ECG itself should be seen, not only the interpretation. It may have been read without the submission of adequate information, or the reader may be a third-year medical student who is just learning and whose tutor may have been too rushed to check it carefully. The thyroid scan should be reviewed because the alleged cold nodule seen by the radiologist may not be where it was felt by the clinician.

Check It Yourself. Ancillary studies should always be reviewed with the appropriate specialist. Reviewing my patients' x-rays with the radiologist each morning has proven most helpful to me, to the radiologist, and, foremost, to the patient. The physician learns how to read x-rays, has the results of yesterday's studies before making rounds, and does not have to wait for a written report (which may contain errors), and the radiologist has the advantage of knowing the clinical background—all of which is for the patient's ultimate benefit.

Should This Test Be Done? In our procedure-oriented medical community, physicians are turning more and more to diagnostic studies which are *complicated, discomforting, costly, or bear risk.* Included are arteriography of all types, venography, fiberoptic endoscopies with semiblind biopsies, radionuclide scans, and computed tomography. Before ordering a test of this sort, many factors must enter into the decision-making process: (*a*) What is the likelihood of diagnosis A over diagnosis B? (*b*) Will the test discriminate between A and B with 100% accuracy and reliability? (*c*) If not, what is the incidence of false positives and false negatives? (*d*) What are the risks of the test? (*e*) Will the results of the test alter treatment? (*f*) Is there a choice of treatment? (*g*) What are the risks and possible benefits of the treatment which may result from the test?

A common situation calling for such decision making is the case of the patient with chest pain in whom coronary arteriography is being considered. From the clinical picture, does this patient seem to have true coronary artery disease? Will coronary arteriography establish the diagnosis with reasonable certainty, and how often are you

misled? Are you considering the mortality and morbidity from the procedure as done in your hospital? If severe coronary disease is found, will your treatment be altered? Would the patient's general medical condition preclude surgery even if a surgically remediable lesion were found? Would the patient refuse surgery? What are the risks of surgery, the chances for improving the patient's condition, or the possibility of doing harm? Might medical therapy be the choice in this case no matter what the coronary anatomy? Are the patient's life style and other psychosocial conditions such that improvement of coronary circulation really does not matter? Numerous other questions could be asked. They vary from patient to patient. Decisions of this sort are not made lightly; but they should depend on whether the procedure will benefit the patient, not solely on whether a diagnosis will be made.

The decision-making process will be discussed in greater detail in Chapter 8, since it is too complex an issue to be covered before explaining probability theory and mathematical models of disease profiles.

To Come Later. Much to be learned about laboratory tests has not been discussed here, since an understanding of some of these matters requires a knowledge of probability, prevalence, sensitivity, specificity, predictive value, and the operating characteristics of combined testing. Later in this section (Chapters 6 and 7) we will discuss these issues, as well as other testing concepts important for the problem solver: the use, misuse, and overuse of tests; the concept of imperfect information; test reliability; sources for test errors; test interpretation; why tests are ordered; benefits and liabilities from unsolicited laboratory tests; the unexpected test result; and testing strategies for special clinical subproblems. From all this, you should learn how to orchestrate the proliferation of tests and procedures for the benefit rather than the detriment of the patient.

Data Processing

What It Is. Data processing in medicine is the method by which the data base is transformed into a problem list. It is the important step whereby information gathered about the patient is filtered and clues are selected and grouped into meaningful problems. Various clues are extracted from the data base by the brain as it calls upon its information base for help. We must repeatedly decide whether or not a positive or negative finding is related to the patient's complaints. Here the wheat is separated from the chaff, and you decide what is important. Most help is gotten from the history.

But throughout the collection of patient data, each bit of information is processed as it is acquired. Every item in the history, the physical examination, and the paraclinical studies is evaluated in terms of its *relevance* to the chief complaint, to the initial concept, or to the provisional hypotheses. Indeed, an item may indicate the presence of an additional problem. More important, a finding may tend to negate or eliminate the likelihood of an existing hypothesis, just as it may tend to diagnose or confirm its presence.

It has been emphasized that the collection, analysis, evaluation, processing, and synthesis of patient data take place simultaneously. Consequently, the discussion of data processing was included mostly in the preceding section on "Data Collection."

About Brain Waves. Little is known of the neurophysiologic codification of data input. *Evoked potentials* refer to measurable electrical impulses that are generated all over the nervous system by *visual, auditory*, and *somatosensory* stimuli. These electrical impulses quickly reach the brain stem and cortex where they register in the form of positive and negative waves. There are four principal waves—N_1, P_2, N_2, and P_3; they are detected and recorded all over the cortex by special equipment within a time frame of 60 to 300 milliseconds after the stimulus is applied. Individual waves can be identified with *perception, conceptualization, information processing, cognition, short-term memory*, and *decision making* referable to the stimulus.

Sensory input such as a sound, a word, a

sentence, or an image must pass through the stages of data registration just described before a decision is made to discard, remember, respond, ask a question, pass the salt shaker, turn the head, smell the breath, look at the eyes, etc.

Late occurring afterwaves are associated with additional information-processing transactions in the brain and are detected over associative and cognitive areas of the cortex.

Psychologic abnormalities, behavior disorders, and some organic diseases of the nervous system produce measurable abnormalities of evoked potentials. Such abnormalities may consist of alterations in the amplitude, shape, time domain, and interspacing of the various waves.

Tuning In. The brain must be specifically programmed to detect, receive, and acknowledge selected bits of information. In its infinite capacity, the brain can choose to ignore a sensory stimulus before it is received by tuning it out. You can be so intent on reading a book that you may not hear some one calling you. Even though a signal reaches your cortex, you may not perceive it if your attention is riveted elsewhere. Thus you can receive sound but not hear, look but not see, and touch but not feel. This is especially true in performing a physical examination.

Natural Intelligence. Information is transmitted from the examiner's sensory end organs (eyes, ears, fingers, nose) to cortical areas where it is received and acknowledged. Then it is transferred to subsidiary centers where it is evaluated, grouped, related to previously obtained data, accepted or denied, and used to confirm or negate impressions. Following this, the categorized and already qualified data are relegated to short-term memory, where they are registered, filed, and stored. There the data neurochemically and neuroanatomically communicate with other bits of recently acquired information and telecommunicate with long-term memory to conjure up new propositions and debate existing ones. But mostly the stored data stay in short-term memory where they await the arrival of additional bits of information with which they can be further correlated, matched, or unmatched. It may be that additional unsuspected problems exist or that the patient's constellation of clues represents two or more diseases.

This sequence of processes is a representation of natural intelligence—a higher cortical function which computer afficionados try to duplicate but with only limited success. Those who work on this project quite properly refer to it as *artificial intelligence.* But this author doubts that the most complex computer will ever match the highly sophisticated 100 billion-neuron human brain or that machines will ever capture the creativity, perceptiveness, imagination, and inspiration possessed by even an average physician.

Perceiving the Problem. The chief complaint, its allied symptoms, related physical signs, and confirmatory laboratory and x-ray information can usually be grouped into a diagnosis. If the underlying disease is in one organ, a knowledge of the symptoms and signs of diseases of the organ is helpful. In that case, the symptoms usually relate directly to malfunction or malstructure of that single organ. Clearly, not all the classical signs and symptoms need be present. There may be only a few. The patient with early heart failure may merely have dyspnea on exertion, orthopnea, enlarged heart, rales, and a confirmatory x-ray. On the other hand, a full-blown picture of florid congestive heart failure may be present. But a patient who has a complete textbook picture of a disease most often has been neglected or mistreated by himself, his family, or his physician. Classic cases are usually so because they are diagnosed late.

Data acquisition and data processing proceed simultaneously as experience and confidence are gained. If the patient's chief complaint is chest pain, the history and physical examination, while complete, are acquired in the light of this chief complaint. You look especially for symptoms and signs associated with these diseases which cause chest pain. Often a very few clues can be grouped with confidence into a single problem. Bilateral

pingueculae and an enlarged spleen in a Jewish child suggest Gaucher's disease; prove it with a bone marrow examination.

Does the Clue Relate? Deciding on relevance is not a simple determination. What seems relevant to one data retriever may not be considered so by another; the reverse also holds true. Sometimes a student will fail to see an obvious correlation; at other times, he may ingeniously relate two clues in a roundabout way even though they are truly unrelated. It is humorous to note how far a student will stretch to relate two clues which probably have nothing to do with each other, but which he can somehow pathophysiologically justify and explain. Even if incorrect, this is a good exercise in logic, and students should be encouraged to engage in such activity, for it cultivates correlative ability (see Chapter 13).

You must know how to select clues which relate. A patient has chest pain, dyspnea on exertion, and hemorrhoids. The first two symptoms probably relate, but the third is no doubt an independent problem. It is difficult to pathophysiologically connect hemorrhoids to the two other clues which are probably cardiac in origin. The next patient has angina pectoris, a recent myocardial infarction, and pain in the left big toe. The latter clue may or may not relate to the main problem. If the pain is chronic and antedated the cardiac episode it is unrelated. If it followed, it may be caused by thromboembolism and therefore may be related. But it could follow and still not be related—the patient may have gout, a bunion, or peripheral vascular disease, and further discerning evidence is needed.

Irrelevant material must be weeded out but not altogether disregarded, for it may relate to another problem. A chronic headache is probably not related to a chief complaint of tarry stools and syncope unless the excessive use of analgesics has caused gastric bleeding. It may, however, indicate that another problem exists (e.g. brain tumor) in addition to the one causing the presenting picture. Conversely, a recent backache may well be related to the presenting problem of nocturia, frequency of urination, and hematuria if you find a carcinoma of the prostate on rectal examination.

Often it is easy to note relevance, especially if the clues comes from the same system (e.g. cough and dyspnea). However, if this same patient also has a breast lump, the cough and dyspnea may be related by virtue of metastasis or may simply denote the presence of breast cancer in a patient who also has chronic obstructive lung disease. Your logic is frequently taxed in making decisions of this sort, and you may have to label a clue as *possibly* relevant. Consider a patient with weakness and pallor who has hemorrhoids—possibly related if bleeding; probably not related if not bleeding. The same patient has an inguinal hernia—not related. Suppose he also has chronic indigestion and a stool 4+ for occult blood—almost certainly related.

Fitting Clues Together. The clustering of clues into meaningful groups is also part of data processing. Symptoms and abnormal physical signs in the same system usually can be pooled. For example, nausea, vomiting, diarrhea, fever, and diffuse abdominal tenderness are related. So are weakness, weight loss, anorexia, abdominal pain, and black stools.

Cough, expectoration, dyspnea, and chest pain cluster quite nicely with signs of right lower lobe consolidation and fever; leg pain may or may not be related; leg pain with a tender calf probably *is* related. Additional information needs processing: the family pet is a healthy cat; the family pet is a sick cat; the family pet is a newly acquired parrot; the patient is an alcoholic; the patient's spouse had a similar illness last week; the patient is a male homosexual; and on and on. Each piece of information needs evaluation in light of what is already known.

Students often feel that only positive information is of value. But negative information may sometimes be even more helpful. The absence of a clue may be as important as its presence in helping you to decide. Patients with sarcoidosis usually have enlarged lymph nodes and an abnormal chest

radiograph. If these two features are absent, you lean away from diagnosing sarcoidosis. The absence of thyromegaly, no abnormal eye signs, and a normal pulse rate militate against a hypothesis of hyperthyroidism, even if the patient is nervous and has sweaty palms and a tremor.

Choosing the Subsets. Don't forget that the processing of data is in some measure dependent on the acquisition of data; data acquisition in turn is a reflection of the data collector's ability to selectively pursue only certain subsets of information. Therefore, we are dealing with an active rather than a passive process.

Given a 56-year-old man with chronic hoarseness for 3 weeks, you can immediately form your initial concept and hypotheses. These include chronic laryngitis, laryngeal cancer, or recurrent laryngeal nerve paralysis from lung cancer, aneurysm, etc. Your quest for additional data stems from these initial impressions, and data processing must of necessity follow the same course. The information you selectively seek includes this patient's occupation, hobbies, smoking history, pulmonary symptoms, chest examination, neck palpation, inspection for Horner's syndrome, chest radiograph, and vocal cord visualization. Each of these bits of information is acquired and processed in series and in parallel—consecutively and at the same time.

As the student evolves into a clinician, he soon learns which data set to pursue for each inquiry departure point and develops his own scheme of data acquisition that is invariant for each problem or subproblem.

Every Bit Helps. Note how many pieces of meaningful information the brain and the computer can process from a simple presentation. Suppose you see a *35-year-old woman whose only problem is recurrent symmetrical polyarthritis for several years.* Eight items are almost simultaneously evaluated:

1. The patient is female.
2. The patient is 35 years old.
3. The patient has arthritis.

4. The patient's arthritis affects many joints.
5. The patient's arthritis has been present for several years.
6. The patient's arthritis recurs and remits.
7. The patient's arthritis was not present when she was young.
8. The patient has no extraarticular manifestations of disease since it is stated to be her only problem.

Polyarthritis by itself can mean acute rheumatic fever, rheumatoid arthritis, systemic lupus erythematosus, gout, pseudogout, Lyme disease, sarcoidosis, and so forth. But given eight modifying factors stated in this patient's 14-word presentation, many inferences concerning exclusions, probabilities, and likelihoods can now be made. The fact that she is only 35 weighs heavily against pseudogout; the fact that she is 35 and a woman is against gout; being sick for several years at 35 tends to exclude acute rheumatic fever which begins at an earlier age; the absence of other manifestations points away from Lyme disease, sarcoidosis, rheumatoid variants, and lupus. More questions must follow, but the broad diagnostic field has already been considerably narrowed.

How Many Diagnoses? Always try to explain all clues by one diagnosis; but it is common to have two or more diseases in one patient, especially in hospitalized patients. All of Chapter 3 will be devoted to a discussion of clues, because the proper interpretation of clues is the essence of data processing.

Problem Lists

What They Are. The data base you have acquired is processed into a list of problems that tells you what is wrong with the patient. The first problem list is usually derived within 24 hours of seeing the patient and is placed at the beginning of the chart. It serves as a table of contents and quick reference source for all of the patient's afflictions. This list should represent the highest possible resolution of the patient's problems based on the data accumulated thus far.

Often a *diagnosis* may be clearly stated. At other times only a *syndrome* (such as hepatomegaly, ascites, and jaundice) may be listed since at this stage the physician may not yet be sure whether the patient has cirrhosis of the liver or metastatic carcinoma. Syndromes can also include pathophysiologic states or recognized entities, such as hepatorenal syndrome, nephrotic syndrome, Horner's syndrome, inappropriate antidiuretic hormone secretion, and respiratory acidosis. A *cluster* of clues which seem to belong together may be stated as a problem if you do not yet have enough evidence to make a diagnosis; e.g. nausea, vomiting, diarrhea, and fever or dyspnea on exertion, night cough, basal rales, and enlarged heart.

Also contained in the problem list are *isolated abnormalities* in the data base that do not seem to fit any of the other stated problems and were discovered in the course of routine data accumulation. These may come from the history, physical examination, or laboratory information and often designate uncategorized items, such as headaches, blurred vision, recurrent heartburn, rectal bleeding, internal hemorrhoids, a heart murmur, eosinophilia, or azotemia.

Psychosocial and *socioeconomic* problems constitute a last category to be included in the problem list; e.g. unemployment, poverty, recent divorce, alcohol abuse, and heavy smoking.

To summarize, a problem list can contain a:

1. diagnosis
2. syndrome
3. pathophysiologic state
4. cluster of clues
5. isolated abnormality
6. psychosocioeconomic issue.

Confusion sometimes arises when a diagnosis is labeled as a problem. Most people consider a problem as something to be solved and perhaps rightly so. Unfortunately, the word "problem" is used in two different contexts. The semantic distinction must be made between the patient's *complaints* which constitute his version of the problems and the *problem list* which outlines the physician's summation of what is troubling the patient. The latter list is composed of the diagnostic resolutions of the patient's complaints. As stated earlier, perhaps a problem list should more accurately be called a *diagnosis list* or *solution list*, bearing in mind that these solutions are simply diagnostic and do not refer to treatment.

Level of Resolution. Each diagnosis or problem on the problem list must be raised to the highest level of resolution with the information on hand. Examiners, especially students, will vary in their levels of confidence and amounts of basic knowledge. Thus the constellation of nausea, vomiting, diarrhea, and fever may be listed by some as "nausea, vomiting, diarrhea, fever;" by others as "acute gastrointestinal disorder;" and by those with more confidence as "viral or bacterial gastroenteritis." It is true that the third group may be settling for less than 100% certainty, but diagnostic infallibility may not be necessary in what is most likely a mild, self-limited illness. The more cautious examiner wants to see the results of a blood count and stool culture and wishes to observe the patient for 24 hours before attaching a definite diagnostic label. Each of the examiners is correct. But they vary in confidence and in the degree of diagnostic accuracy they require.

The presence of weakness, weight loss, anorexia, easy satiety, and an epigastric mass may permit one examiner to list the problem only by enumerating all the clues; the second examiner may label it as carcinoma "somewhere"; a third may boldly call it carcinoma of the stomach, especially if a Virchow node is palpated. The first and second examiners may prefer to await the results of gastrointestinal radiography, endoscopy, and biopsy before attaching a definitive diagnosis.

In this regard, students commonly make one of three errors. *First,* they may fail to assemble clues properly into one recognizable group and thus list each symptom and sign as a separate problem. *Second,* they may cluster clues properly, list them as an individual problem, but fail to raise the problem to as high a resolution as possible because of timidity. And *third*, they may make premature closure of a diagnosis and unjustified decisions before adequate information is available (11). Obviously there is a twilight zone where the level of resolution is not clear-cut and is debatable. (See Chapter 10 for more on this subject.)

How to Derive One. A 52-year-old alcoholic male patient with cirrhosis of the liver is admitted to the hospital with a massive upper gastrointestinal hemorrhage. After a 24-hour work workup concomitant with his emergency treatment, he is found to have the following problem situations:

1. chronic alcoholism
2. cirrhosis of the liver secondary to (1)
3. gastrointestinal hemorrhage
4. benign prostatic hypertrophy
5. hyperglycemia
6. infiltrate right upper lobe
7. unemployed
8. divorced.

Problems 1, 2, and 3 are quickly apparent. Note that problem 3 does not specify whether the bleeding is due to varices, ulcer, or gastritis, since at this stage it has not yet been clearly determined. Immediate gastroscopy was unsuccessfully attempted. Each problem must be formulated at a level you can defend (12). The prostatic condition is being recorded for the first time based on symptoms which have existed for 3 years plus the finding of a markedly enlarged prostate on rectal examination. It may or may not require attention in the near future and must be watched. Problem 5, the hyperglycemia, was found on routine blood studies. It may be related to the intravenous glucose the patient received while waiting for blood to be cross-matched; blood was drawn for chemical analysis at that time. But it was 300 mg/dl, higher than we would ordinarily expect from a slow intravenous drip. Listing it as a problem reminds us that it needs to be rechecked, especially after the patient is well. It may or may not indicate diabetes mellitus. Problem 6, an asymptomatic finding noted on chest x-ray, is probably a separate problem, but it too will require present and future investigation. Problems 7 and 8 probably relate to problem 1. In general the problem list will increase in complexity with the patient's age.

Initial and Final Lists. The *initial problem list* is based on the first 24 hours of information and may need considerable adjustment as the case develops. Each problem is assigned a number which remains permanent. The date or time of onset should be stated beside each problem. The order of number assignment may be determined by the sequence of pathophysiologic events as in the case just described. Another way, preferred by many, is the assignment of numbers based on the importance or seriousness of each problem. In that event, gastrointestinal hemorrhage (problem 3) would have been listed as problem 1.

The *final problem list* is completed when the patient is ready for discharge from the hospital, sometimes even sooner if satisfactory closure can be obtained for all problems possible. This may involve combining two or more originally listed problems into a single one, in which case they both assume one number and the other number is never used again. For example, hepatomegaly and ascites can become one problem: carcinoma of the liver. Another problem may be resolved; a statement to that effect and the date of resolution should be indicated. For example, problem 5 (hyperglycemia) turned out to be caused by intravenous glucose, and the patient did not have diabetes mellitus; in this way the problem was erased. The number 5 cannot be used again. Most important, the final diagnosis may now be stated at a higher level of resolution since more definitive and more diagnostic data were obtained. A problem originally listed as hyperglycemia may now be called diabetes mellitus without changing its number. What was thought to be hepatosplenomegaly becomes Hodgkin's disease after a biopsy; again, the number doesn't change. And so forth.

Assessment and Plan. After the initial problem list is formed, each item in the list must be assessed and a plan offered. The assessment may be written separately from

the plan, or the assessment and plan may be written together, but separately for each problem.

Included in the *assessment* of each problem should be the items in the data base which led you to label the problem as such, the urgency or seriousness of each problem, the pathophysiology of each problem, and the possible pathophysiologic relation between problems. A differential diagnosis for a problem may be stated here—not in the problem list. By reading a student's assessment, you can easily measure his understanding of the entire case.

The *plan* is the proposed management for each problem. It includes the diagnostic studies and why you want them done; the proposed treatment for each problem, including medication, nursing care, surgery, diet, consultations, etc; and what you aim to accomplish along the line of patient education.

The Need for Weed. It is no longer necessary to justify or defend the use of the Weed system. This method of record keeping demands that the physician think clearly, have integrity, and understand and justify his diagnoses, studies, and treatment. He has committed himself on paper. It makes assessment and quality control easy and computerization of data simpler. If another physician or consultant needs quick access to the patient's record, he can locate the problems without wading through a thick chart. Another bonus is that the treating physician is less apt to forget or overlook a concomitant abnormality which needs attention once the patient recovers from his primary problem.

Progress notes must be written so as to demonstrate a clear understanding of what is happening to the patient. "Status quo" and "patient improving" are no longer acceptable. In referring to a specific problem in a progress note, the Weed system requires attention to current subjective data, objective data, assessment, and plan for further management (S-O-A-P). For example, here is a progress note written on day 3 about the alcoholic patient described on page 35:

"Problem 3. The patient feels much better, is hungry, and complains only of the nasogastric tube. Bleeding has stopped, as there is no blood in the aspirate and the last stool was brown. The hematocrit is 34% and stable. All vital signs are stable and normal: P 84, BP 124/80, T 37.2 C, R16. Physical examination remains the same. The patient is doing nicely and the acute gastritis has subsided. The gastric tube will be removed, intravenous fluids tapered, and a pureed low-protein diet started." The note might also have been written with its component S-O-A-P parts clearly labeled.

The Loyal Opposition. While most medical schools teach their students to use the problem-oriented medical record, for many reasons this method has not received the widespread adoption that was originally expected. In fact, even the medical school's teaching hospital may not use it with enthusiasm; there the Weed system may be scrupulously used, modified, bastardized, or even rejected in favor of older methods. In nonteaching hospitals and in offices, the system is used even less. The mode of record keeping varies from office to office, from hospital to hospital, from one department to another within the same hospital, and even from one house officer to another within the same department.

And so the student is often faced with the dilemma of entering a health care delivery facility where he must quickly learn to do it like it's done *there,* not like it was taught. This should be an easy adjustment, although it raises doubts and questions.

Those who do not feel the need for the Weed system can keep good records according to their own methods. The use of the differential diagnosis is still a workable, effective way to manage the patient and has maintained its viability in many hospitals. Diagnoses, possibilities, rule-outs, and isolated unrelated findings may be substituted for problems in a less formal manner. But let nothing vital be omitted, forgotten, or irretrievable, and let progress notes really describe the progress of the patient.

Examples of data bases and their associated problem lists, assessments, and plans will be displayed in Section Two.

SELF-EVALUATION EXERCISES

(Don't look now, but answers appear following the last question!)

1. Which of the following requests for information is *not* open-ended?
   (a) Yes?
   (b) Go on!
   (c) So?
   (d) How badly did it hurt?
   (e) Tell me about that.
2. Which of the following is the only "don't" in relating to a patient?
   (a) Speak quietly.
   (b) Sit on the bed for comfort and rapport.
   (c) Address the patient by last name—e.g. Mrs. Jones.
   (d) Smile and be sympathetic.
   (e) Maintain frequent eye contact.
   (f) Preserve the patient's modesty.
3. Which part of the data base gives the most useful information?
   (a) history
   (b) physical examination
   (c) laboratory tests
   (d) scanning procedures.
4. Hypotheses for the causes of a presenting cluster are generally formed:
   (a) only after the complete data base is obtained
   (b) after the 18-test chemistry profile and x-rays return
   (c) early during the taking of the history
   (d) after the results of a highly sensitive and specific test are obtained
   (e) on first looking at the patient.
5. Regarding the order followed by the experienced data collector, which of the following is/are correct?
   (a) Get complete identification data first.
   (b) The history of present illness must precede the patient profile.
   (c) No order is necessary; selected data are requested.
   (d) Never start the physical examination until the history is completed.
   (e) The chief complaint is always obtained first because it is easy to do.
6. In obtaining data from a patient, an exclude-or-confirm strategy is often followed. Which statement is *untrue*?
   (a) The absence of a clue that is always present in a disease excludes the disease.
   (b) The presence of a clue that is always present in a disease confirms the disease.
   (c) The absence of three important clues that

are often present in a disease tends to exclude the disease.

   (d) The presence of three important clues that are often present in a disease tends to confirm the disease.

7. In doing a physical examination, one of the following is *not* correct:

   (a) Pay attention to one thing at a time.

   (b) Always examine in the same precise order.

   (c) You may first examine areas you expect to give the most help.

   (d) General inspection is often productive.

   (e) Avoid frequent changes of patient position.

8. Diagnosis may be made at a glance in all but one of the following:

   (a) myxedema

   (b) pheochromocytoma

   (c) acromegaly

   (d) Parkinson's disease

   (e) Cushing's syndrome.

9. Knowing what is normal helps you evaluate data. Only one of the following is *incorrect*:

   (a) Most patients urinate three to four times by day and zero to one time at night.

   (b) Most patients have *occasional* indigestion or head pain or backache.

   (c) Almost everybody has a few tiny angiomas on the skin.

   (d) Unequal pupils are frequently normal.

   (e) Upward gaze nystagmus is commonly normal.

   (f) Twenty-two respirations per minute is abnormal.

   (g) Blood pressure of 130/50 may be abnormal.

10. Diagnosis can be suspected by smelling the breath in all of the following except one:

   (a) hepatic coma

   (b) uremic coma

   (c) diabetic ketoacidotic coma

   (d) acute alcoholism

   (e) pneumonia.

11. Palpation is often underrated and not mastered. Which of the following is/are untrue?

   (a) Vibrations are best felt with the palmar aspect of the metacarpophalangeal joints.

   (b) Temperature is best appreciated by the dorsal aspect of the hand.

   (c) Thrills, friction rubs, gallops, and fremitus may be felt.

   (d) Fingertip palpation is best for abdominal tenderness.

   (e) Cardiac hypertrophy may be appreciated by palpation.

12. Parts of the physical examination best done with the patient standing relate to the search for each of the following except one:

   (a) hernias

   (b) carotid sinus syncope

   (c) orthostatic hypotension

   (d) posterior column disease

   (e) varicose veins.

13. Each of the following is better than a physical examination except one:

   (a) history for migraine

   (b) ultrasound for heart murmurs

   (c) isotope scan for precise liver and spleen size

   (d) chest x-rays for diaphragm mobility

   (e) ultrasound for small amount of ascites.

14. Tests for a disease (choose the one correct answer):

   (a) are better than clues gotten from the history and physical examination

   (b) are very dependable

   (c) diagnose the disease if positive

   (d) exclude the disease if negative

   (e) are valuable if they confirm preformed impressions.

15. Which of the following statements referable to the formation of a problem list raises the problem to the highest possible level of resolution?

   (a) consolidation right lower lobe

   (b) cough, chills, fever, chest pain

   (c) cough, chills, fever, rales and dullness at right base

   (d) pneumococcic lobar pneumonia, right lower lobe

   (e) pneumonia.

16. Which one of the following does not belong in the problem list of a particular patient?

   (a) infective endocarditis

   (b) fever, anemia, heart murmur, hematuria

   (c) poor oral hygiene

   (d) possible cerebral embolus

   (e) drug addiction.

17. Which one of the following fails to demonstrate a possible pathophysiologic relationship between its two components?

   (a) breast lump and pleural effusion

   (b) hemiplegia and chronic cough

   (c) good leg pulses and leg pain

   (d) leg injury and hemoptysis

   (e) good appetite and weight loss.

18. In each of the following clusters, which clue does not belong?

   (a) nausea, vomiting, dyspnea, cramps, diarrhea

   (b) headache, fatigue, depression, leg pains, insomnia

   (c) weight gain, weakness, anorexia, weight loss, pallor

   (d) cough, wrist pains, expectoration, hemoptysis, splenomegaly

   (e) thyromegaly, bradycardia, weight loss, tremor, good appetite.

ANSWERS

1. **(d)**	2. **(b)**	3. **(a)**	4. **(c)**
5. **(c)**	6. **(b)**	7. **(b)**	8. **(b)**
9. **(e)**	10. **(e)**	11. **(d)**	12. **(b)**
13. **(b)**	14. **(e)**	15. **(d)**	16. **(d)**

17. **(c)** These may coexist but are not related; (a) and (b) can represent metastatic cancer; (e) may signal hyperthyroidism.

18. **(a)** dyspnea **(b)** leg pains **(c)** weight gain **(d)** splenomegaly **(e)** bradycardia.

Note: Some questions may generate justifiably different answers from those given.

References

1. Ber R, Alroy G: The teaching of history taking and diagnostic thinking. *Med Educ* 15:97–99, 1981.
2. Koestler A: *The Act of Creation.* London, Hutchinson, 1964.
3. Barrows HS, Tamblyn RM: *Problem-Based Learning. An Approach to Medical Education.* New York, Springer, 1980.
4. Mueller JC: Independent history taking. *Ann Intern Med* 95:652, 1981.
5. Weiner S, Nathanson M: Physical examination—frequently observed errors. *JAMA* 236:852–855, 1976.
6. Engel GL: Are medical schools neglecting clinical skills? *JAMA* 236:861–862, 1976.
7. Hodder R, Langfield J, Cruess D, et al: Teaching concepts of clinical measurement variation to students. Presented at the annual meeting, Association of America Medical Colleges, Washington DC, 1982.
8. Williams TJ, Ahmad D, Morgan WKC: A clinical and roentgenographic correlation of diaphragmatic movement. *Arch Intern Med* 141:878–880, 1981.
9. Cattau EL, Benjamin SB, Kruff TE, et al: The accuracy of the physical examination in the diagnosis of suspected ascites. *JAMA* 247:1164–1166, 1982.
10. Morgan WL, Engel GL: *The Clinical Approach to the Patient.* Philadelphia, Saunders, 1969.
11. Voytovich AE, Rippey RM: Knowledge, realism, and diagnostic reasoning in a physical diagnosis course. *J Med Educ* 57:461–466, 1982.
12. Walker HK, Hall WD, Hurst WJ (eds): *Clinical Methods*, ed 2. Boston, Butterworths, 1980.

Chapter 3

Clues: The Building Blocks

PAUL CUTLER, M.D.

A clue* can be defined as any bit of information that seems to guide or direct in the solution of a problem. Chapter 2 spoke repeatedly of clues being the building blocks of problems, conclusions, and diagnoses. From time to time, clues were specified in case vignettes. But what are the principal clues we seek in the data base? Obviously they can be points in the history, the physical examination, or initial paraclinical data (laboratory tests, ECG, and chest x-ray).

This chapter is devoted to a dissection of the various aspects of clues, since a clue is of little value unless you understand its specificity, sensitivity, and importance. You must know the significance of its presence or absence, what to do when it does not fit

---

* "Clue" is used throughout this book even though many authors prefer "cue." The former word seems more appropriate in dealing with mysteries, whereas the latter recalls the theatrical world; e.g. *Sherlock Holmes* sought a *clue*, while *John Barrymore* awaited his *cue....*

or negates an impression, and how to select the most important of many clues.

Positive Clues. These are generally the most useful. Positive clues in the history might be chest pain, cough, chills, indigestion, impotence, or indeed anything the patient complains of. Positive clues in the physical examination might be rales in the lungs, a heart murmur, an enlarged liver, a nodular prostate, or any other abnormality that is noted. The chest x-ray can disclose a relevant positive bit of evidence, and the laboratory may tell you the patient has anemia, hyperuricemia, leukocytosis, or elevated serum gastrin.

The payoff of a positive clue can be dramatized by the following illustration. There are thousands of known medical diseases and conditions, 27 of which are characterized by nosebleeds. A positive history of nosebleeds directs you to only 27 diseases while at the same time it eliminates thousands. The absence of nosebleeds tends to exclude only 27 possibilites. Thus the diagnostic power of a positive answer is over 100 times greater than a negative response in this situation. *Every clinician knows this instinctively as he initially seeks positive data* (1).

Of the 27 diseases with nosebleeds, large lymph nodes will be present in only four. If these two clues are positive the diagnostic field is considerably narrowed. Thousands of diseases in which these clues do not coexist are ruled out as you reduce the possibilities to a finger count.

If you suspect the presence of a particular disease, search for positive clues known to exist in that disease. Such clues are usually far more apt to be positive, especially in combination, if the disease is present than if it is not present. Of course this depends in part on the frequency with which the clue is positive in the disease (true positivity) and the frequency with which it is seen in states other than the disease (false positivity). The more positive clues there are, the more likely the disease. The more clues are negative or absent, the less likely the disease. If pneumonia is suspected, you inquire about cough, fever, chills, and expectoration and search for rales and pulmonary consolidation. All of these clues, if positive, aid in making the diagnosis. If all clues are present, the diagnosis is likely. If only some are present, the diagnosis is possible. If none is present, the diagnosis is unlikely.

A *necessary* clue usually has various degrees of necessity. An absolutely necessary clue is one which is present in all cases of the disease (100% sensitive), and if it is absent the disease can be excluded. This situation is rare. More commonly, a clue is present in 20%, 50%, or perhaps 90% of cases; since a clue is of necessity either present or absent, it will be absent in, respectively, 80%, 50%, or 10% of cases of the disease in question.

The Importance of Being Negative. Pertinent negative clues may sometimes be as important as positive ones. If you expect a clue to be positive in order to further substantiate your hypothesis, yet it is negative, this can be helpful in several ways.

You would be hard pressed to establish a diagnosis of hyperthyroidism in a patient who is losing weight, is nervous, sweats profusely, and has a tremor, yet demonstrates no tachycardia or thyromegaly. If a patient has what you think may be carcinoma of the stomach, it would be important to note that there are no palpable supraclavicular nodes, that the liver is not enlarged, and that no anemia is detected. The known insulin-dependent diabetic who is admitted in coma certainly does not have a ketoacidotic coma if he is neither dehydrated nor hyperpneic and the urine is free of glucose and acetone.

It is more likely that he has hypoglycemia. In another vein, if you suspect thrombophlebitis it is important to note that chest pain, hemoptysis, and dyspnea are not present. If you think a patient has severe diabetes because he has frequent urination and has lost weight, the absence of thirst would be a strong negative factor against your suspicion. If thirst is present, it is another positive clue added to a picture which may be caused by diabetes mellitus as well as by other diseases. So the absence of a clue may tend to rule out a diagnosis just as a positive clue may tend to confirm it.

Conversely, the absence of a feature may militate in favor of a diagnosis and its presence be against it. You suspect that cirrhosis of the liver is the cause of the patient's ascites. The absence of distended neck veins would favor your impression, while their presence would indicate that heart failure might be the principal problem.

The Pertinent Negative. This leads us to a discussion of pertinently negative features in a data base and further exemplifies the importance of being negative. The fact that something is absent may be a strong indication that a particular disease in question does *not* exist.

When a student or intern presents a case, or when you read a case report in a journal, a list of pertinent negatives usually follows the chief complaint and history of present illness. These allegedly important negatives may sometimes be stated in the systems review. Why are they included? Obviously they are inserted for a very good and logical reason. On the basis of the chief complaint and history of present illness, certain provisional hypotheses have already been formed; the negative findings are stated in order to rule out or negate some of the competing hypotheses. This action may be called "pruning the differential."

Take the case of a 64-year-old man who has had a cough, expectoration, and exertional dyspnea for 15 days. A long list of negatives follows; each has special significance. "There is no history of chills, fever, night sweats, weight loss, anorexia, chest pain, hemoptysis, leg pains, peripheral edema, recent travel, or exposure to industrial dusts or toxins; the patient does not smoke and never did, does not frequent caves for fun, and has no family pets."

This list provides a wealth of information. On the basis of the initial clinical picture, many diagnostic possibilities exist. Each negative statement tends to exclude one or more possibilities. The absence of chills, fever, and night sweats points away from pneumonia or tuberculosis. No anorexia, no weight loss, no chest pain, and no hemoptysis are further points against tuberculosis and are also evidence against lung cancer. The fact that the patient has never smoked also goes a long way toward excluding lung cancer. No chest pain, no hemoptysis, no leg pains or leg edema, as well as no recent travel (prolonged or otherwise) all tend to exclude the possibility of pulmonary emboli. No recent travel is also against the presence of pulmonary fungal diseases which are endemic to the far west, the southwest, and the Ohio-Mississippi basins (coccidioidomycosis and histoplasmosis). So is the statement that he does not frequent caves where the spores in bat droppings might spread similar diseases. Furthermore, he has not worked in a coal mine, cotton mill, sugar cane mill, absestos plant, etc, where toxic inhalants can cause lung problems. The absence of family pets excludes the presence of sick or healthy psittacine birds and cats which transmit lung infections.

When such a list of negatives is presented, the implications are as just stated. And when a student reads a list of pertinent negatives, he should be sure he understands the significance of each one and not simply read a list that was written by the house officer. Frequently when students are asked to explain the meaning of such a list they are unable to do so. A similar list of pertinent negatives can be extracted from the physical examination and laboratory data. These negative clues do not tell you what disease the patient has, but they help tell you what disease he does not have.

A Bit of Sherlock Holmes. Remember that the clue gotten from the family, social, or occupational history may be the vital one. The patient with a bleeding or hemolytic disorder may tell you of similar illness in a parent or sibling. The man with diffuse pulmonary disease who works as a pigeon breeder may have histoplasmosis. Also, there is the patient who has a chronic recurrent fever caused by infective endocarditis, a diagnosis not considered until the telltale needle tracks are noted over the veins of the forearms. A seemingly insignificant clue may solve the mystery and find the guilty agent.

The decisive clue may, of course, be found in the initial laboratory workup. Some tests, like the sedimentation rate, are nonspecific and merely tell you that something is wrong. Hyperuricemia joins acute joint disease to indicate gout. But do not be fooled by the young man with known gout and hyperuricemia who develops a gonococcal joint from a night on the town. A high blood glucose and glycosuria would complete the picture in a patient with thirst, polyuria, and polydipsia—since some of the latter three can occur in diabetes insipidus, hyperparathyroidism, and compulsive water drinking too. A radiographic infiltrate in the right apex groups well with anorexia, cough, and low-grade fever. And a finding of elevated ST segments in leads 2, 3, and AVF of the ECG completes the clues needed to diagnose acute myocardial infarction in a man with severe chest pain radiating to both arms.

Primary and Secondary Clues. It is important to recognize that clues may be primary or secondary in putting together your picture; otherwise it may be difficult to relate seemingly unrelated findings to a single problem. You may think there are multiple problems when there is really only one. Primary symptoms or signs are those related to the disease process in situ. Secondary ones are usually at a distant site or may even seem to be physiologically unrelated. For example, a patient with carcinoma of the lung has cough and hemoptysis as primary symptoms. Secondarily, he may have hemiplegia from a brain metastasis or backache from a vertebral metastasis. Other secondary clues might be clubbing of the fingers, distal periostitis (hypertrophic pulmonary osteo-arthropathy), thrombophlebitis of the lower extremities, and a variety of other bizarre manifestations which are even today not clearly explainable. It is unclear why visceral carcinomas of all types are associated with thromboembolic phenomena, such as ve-nous thromboembolism and marantic en-docarditis. But this association of clues must be borne in mind.

Relations between Clues. Consider the fact that clues may be independent, inter-dependent, or mutually exclusive. Carci-noma of the lung can cause hemoptysis or chest pain, depending upon whether the le-sion is eroding a blood vessel or a rib. The two consequences are independent. Exam-ples of true interdependence are difficult to find; each clue must be the cause of the other. For instance, a patient has both acute coronary insufficiency with chest pain and ventricular tachycardia. You are not sure which came first. But a vicious circle has been set in motion. Coronary insufficiency causes arrhythmia, and in turn arrhythmia causes or worsens coronary insufficiency by decreasing coronary blood flow. Good pe-ripheral pulses and intermittent claudication are considered mutually exclusive; so too are almost all instances of loss of appetite and gain in weight. Increased appetite and loss of weight might at first glance seem to be mutually exclusive but they are seen together in hyperthyroidism where calories are rap-idly utilized, in severe diabetes where calo-ries are lost in the urine, and in malabsorp-tion where calories are lost in the stool.

Pinpointing the Diseased Organ. It is im-portant to distinguish between specific and nonspecific clues. Specific ones are those pointing directly to an organ or disease. A symptom may be specific or nonspecific, just as may be a physical sign. For instance, diar-rhea usually indicates an intestinal disease, whereas anorexia is not specific. Jaundice usually indicates disease in the liver or bili-ary tree. Fever, on the other hand, is a nonspecific though very important clue

which can be part of the picture in many diseases involving a variety of organ systems. So your clue can point directly at a trouble-some organ or may simply give you a general idea that illness is present.

The mere presence of headache tells you nothing about which organ is diseased; but papilledema, with rare exceptions, locates the lesion in the brain. Chest pain can be caused by a handful of problems, but chest pain on exertion is a different story. Fatigue is nonspecific and can arise from psychoso-matic as well as organic causes. But if an epigastric mass and anemia are found, the problem becomes localized to the upper ab-domen, and cancer of the stomach looms high on your list.

When the Clue Does Not Fit. What about the case where one clue does not fit the picture or may even seem to negate your provisional hypothesis? What if a suppos-edly necessary clue is absent? How are these situations reconciled?

First of all, you may be on the wrong track. However, you might still be on the right track in any of the above instances.

The usual simple problem-solving equa-tion is: $a + b + c = x$, wherein a, b, and c are clues and x is a problem. But suppose instead: $a + b + c = x + c$. This means that clue c is not part of problem x; c may be extraneous and unimportant or even indi-cate that another problem (y) exists—i.e. $a + b + c = x + y$. For instance, we have a patient with presumed hyperthyroidism who has, among other things, a large thyroid (a) and evidence of hypermetabolism (b). He has a good appetite but has not lost weight as expected. The absence of weight loss does not fit the picture. Perhaps his appetite makes him eat so much that he has main-tained or even gained weight. On the other hand, he may have congestive heart failure too and is retaining fluid. While weight loss is a prominent feature of hyperthyroidism, statistical studies show that it does not occur in all cases.

Even more perplexing, a single clue may be present which seems to contradict your diagnostic impression. This does not necessarily mean you are wrong. We have all seen patients with congestive heart failure who can sleep flat, duodenal ulcers that do not improve with alkali or a histamine H_2 receptor antagonist, and endocarditis without murmurs. There may or may not be a good reason for these paradoxical situations. Diseases do not conform to textbook descriptions, patients react uniquely, and the combination of disease manifestations and patient responses is often unpredictable. This is what adds spice to medicine and fun to making a diagnosis.

Do not forget that the clue which is contrary or does not fit may have been incorrectly obtained. Be sure the history was accurate, the physical examination properly done, or the laboratory result verified. A history of "no weight loss" may not be correct when checked with a relative. The pelvic mass may have disappeared with a bowel movement, and an abnormal blood count may become normal when rechecked.

The Key Clue. Suppose you see a patient whose data base gives you a large number of clues. They do not seem to relate, many are nonspecific, you cannot form a definite cluster, and you do not know where to begin. In this case, seek out the key clue and track it down.

Take the patient who presents with a variety of nonspecific constitutional symptoms like weakness, easy fatigability, malaise, and anorexia. He also has an enlarged abdomen and you determine that it is caused by ascites. This then becomes the key clue and you must start with ascites at the beginning of your algorithmic problem-solving process. Then there is the patient who has a variety of symptoms referable to several organ systems but you cannot make sense out of the clues presented. One thing is prominent: 16% eosinophilia exists. So you start with a list of conditions associated with severe eosinophilia and proceed from there.

The principal or key clue may be a symptom, a physical finding, or a paraclinical finding. If it is a big spleen, your line of reasoning and plan of attack are clearly mapped out. Asymptomatic bilateral hilar adenopathy would warrant a slightly different approach.

Common key clues which are the starting point for the pursuit of more information include symptoms like dyspnea, wheeze, cough, hemoptysis, swollen legs, swollen abdomen, chronic diarrhea, blood in the stools or urine, fever, cessation of menses, difficulty with urination, joint swelling, rash, itch, jaundice, abdominal pain, and so forth. Each one makes you think of a specific list of causes and a specific approach to solving the problem. Prominent physical findings which can serve as key clues include anemia, pulmonary congestion, enlarged heart, murmur, large liver, large spleen, large lymph nodes, ascites, jaundice, mass in the abdomen, nodular prostate, inflamed joints, and so on. Salient laboratory findings include polycythemia, anemia, leukocyte abnormality, low platelet count, and elevated alkaline phosphatase. Each of these can serve as a departure point.

You may compound several clues to form a pathophysiologic entity such as pulmonary hypertension, anuria, disseminated intravascular coagulation, or metabolic acidosis. This then becomes a key clue from which to begin your branching logic.

The Intersection of Clues. One more important issue. Suppose you have *two key clues which do not seem to relate* and each has a separate list of causes. For instance, a 48-year-old woman has fatigue and chronic diarrhea plus peculiar weak, sweaty, nervous spells. Fatigue and diarrhea bring to mind six or seven different diseases. The weak, sweaty, nervous spells could be caused by hypoglycemia, menopause, pheochromocytoma, simple anxiety, or hyperserotoninemia. Are we dealing with two separate problems, or do both diagnostic lists have a common denominator resulting in one diagnosis? Careful thought and further data disclose that the patient has Addison's disease, which can cause weakness, diarrhea, and hypoglycemic episodes. One disease has caused both key clues. However, she could have had two separate diseases. Track down each key clue and determine if they intersect at a common diagnosis.

A Clue in Three Dimensions. It is critical to know three things about a clue: *sensitivity, specificity,* and *relative importance. All three count.*

The *sensitivity* of a clue for a disease is a percentage expression of how often the clue is positive in the presence of that disease (true positive rate). It also tells you how often the clue is not present, because if it is not present, it is falsely negative; and the false negative rate equals 100 minus the sensitivity. The more sensitive a clue is, the more its absence will exclude a disease, since false negatives are rare under these circumstances.

The *specificity* of a clue for a disease is a percentage expression of how often the clue is negative in the absence of that disease (true negative rate). Likewise, it also tells you how often the clue is *present* in the absence of that disease (or in the presence of health or other diseases), because if it is present it is falsely positive; and the false positive rate equals 100 minus the specificity. The more specific a clue is, the more its presence will diagnose a disease, since false positives would be rare. In all cases, *decimals can be used instead of percentages* and 100 becomes 1.

The *relative importance* of a clue is an indication of how significant this clue is in the light of the whole clinical picture. Often it relates to the pathophysiology.

Take the clue of *weight loss.* If it occurs in 96% of patients with hyperthyroidism, it is a highly sensitive clue for that diagnosis, and only 4% of patients with this disease have false negatives (do not lose weight). However, the specificity of weight loss is not high since it occurs frequently in many other diseases.

Another illustration is the presence of *spider angiomas.* They are very common and have high sensitivity in patients with severe alcoholic cirrhosis of the liver, but they are also seen in rheumatoid arthritis and preg-

nancy. Therefore these angiomas also have high sensitivity but low specificity.

On the other hand, a clue may be uncommon in a disease but specific when present. Tophi in the ear would constitute such an example. They are not common in the gout population, but when seen they have great diagnostic significance because they do not occur in the absence of gout.

Another possibility is that a clue may be both highly specific (even pathognomonic) and highly sensitive. The *Kayser-Fleischer ring* is found in the cornea of essentially all cases of Wilson's disease and not in other diseases. But to demonstrate the futility of dogma in medicine, Kayser-Fleischer rings were reported in four cases of non-Wilsonian cirrhosis (2), thereby negating the absolute specificity of this physical finding.

The third critical factor in a clue is its relative importance. This refers to its role in the pathophysiology of the disease under consideration and the weight you attach to its presence or absence. For example, in hyperthyroidism fine silky hair may not be important, but an enlarged thyroid and evidence of hypermetabolism are. In mitral stenosis, the malar flush and palpitations do not even remotely approach the significance of the auscultatory findings. If hepatitis is suspected, jaundice has more relative importance than anorexia or nausea since it points in the direction of the pathophysiology.

A clue which has an amalgam of high sensitivity, high specificity, and high relative importance is the one we seek in our observance of Sutton's law, for it leads us directly to the diagnosis—"where the money is."

Suppose we have a patient with suspected cancer of the stomach. The clues are indigestion, early satiety, and weight loss. All three are nonspecific in that they occur in other medical problems. Often too the patient does not have all these symptoms early in the course of the disease. You would therefore not regard these as very important clues. However, the presence of a Virchow node in the left supraclavicular area would have very heavy weight. Its presence would point directly toward cancer and would certainly tip the diagnostic scale. An additional important clue would be an epigastric mass. The clincher might be a node biopsy, fiberoptic gastric endoscopy, or an upper gastrointestinal series. However, in choosing these tests, we must know how specific and sensitive they are. Why subject a patient to an expensive unpleasant procedure if both the specificity and sensitivity are low? A biopsy should be most specific and sensitive. But remember it is easy to miss the lesion with the use of fiberoptic biopsy, and barium studies are even more fallible.

You suspect a 40-year-old pregnant patient of having cirrhosis of the liver. A history of alcoholism may be helpful, but only 25% of alcoholics get cirrhosis, and cirrhosis sometimes has other causes. Spider angiomas, liver palms, and a distended abdomen are common to both cirrhosis and pregnancy. It may be difficult to feel her liver, but a huge liver might influence your thinking even though it is nonspecific. Probably the clue with the most reliability in this instance would be a positive liver biopsy—provided it were urgent to make the diagnosis promptly. During pregnancy might not be the wisest time to pursue the issue.

Obviously, the more specific and the more common a clue is in a particular disease, the more significant its presence becomes. And, conversely, the less specific and the less common a clue is, the less attention it merits in trying to pinpoint a disease associated with this clue. Turn the situation around: if we suspect a disease in which clue a is present in 98% of all cases and clue a is not present in this patient, the suspected disease is not likely. Carry it a bit further: suppose we suspect a disease in which clue a is found in 98% of cases and clue b is found in 92% of cases. If neither a nor b exists in this patient, the disease can be virtually ruled out. Here too the converse is correct. If both a and b do exist, then the diagnosis is almost certain—unless both these clues have low specificity.

False Clues. We must mention the instance in which a clue is found which could be related to the clinical picture but is not. Since a substantial number of elderly patients have gallstones, the finding of stones on x-ray does not necessarily explain the patient's indigestion or abdominal pain. It may be coincidental to an occult carcinoma or other disease. No wonder so many gallbladders are removed yet symptoms persist. A large heart seen on x-ray may not explain the patient's dyspnea if he is not in congestive failure, but he may have chronic obstructive lung disease which does explain it. Hypertrophic osteoarthritis of the spine seen on x-ray is a common finding in asymptomatic people. We cannot assume it is the cause of every kind of pain or discomfort starting in the back and radiating to the sides, the front, or the legs. A retroverted uterus is often unjustifiably blamed for many more symptoms than it should be, and "low blood pressure" is another common scapegoat.

Clues That Come and Go. The manifestations of a disease may be considerably altered by previous treatment. For instance, the patient with severe congestive heart failure may have no edema because of diuretics given to him. On the other hand, he may have symptoms of hypokalemia superimposed by the same diuretics. The patient with undiagnosed pernicious anemia may have received an injection of vitamin B_{12} in the recent past as part of indiscriminate therapy. His clinical picture, especially the laboratory aspect, will change after just one injection.

The stage of the disease is important. In early chemical diabetes the appetite is normal. If polyuria and thirst are present, the appetite should be excessive. But when ketoacidosis supervenes, anorexia is the rule.

The Sequence of Events. The relationship, timing, and sequence of events weighs our logic. If two symptoms develop close together in time they are probably related. But the sequence is important. Consider the patient who becomes dyspneic on exertion and several weeks later has ankle edema. Congestive heart failure is likely though chronic obstructive lung disease is possible. On the other hand, if edema precedes the dyspnea you might think of cirrhosis or the nephrotic syndrome where edema might occur first and pleural effusion later.

Leg pain followed by sharp chest pain suggests venous thromboembolism, while chest pain followed by leg pain suggests arterial thromboembolism—myocardial infarct with an embolus to the leg. The astute clinician, however, knows that the pain of pulmonary embolus may precede evidence of venous thrombosis or that the latter may not be present at all.

If a patient vomits blood, it is important to know if vomiting preceded or occurred simultaneously with the bleeding. For if it preceded the bleeding, we may have an esophagogastric mucosal tear (Mallory-Weiss syndrome). If not, the vomited blood was probably from some other source. While one event followed by another often constitutes cause and effect relationship, beware the non sequitur.

Three More Tips. Symptoms occurring in the same system are apt to be related. If they occur in different systems this may indicate the presence of two different diseases, a single multisystem disease, or diffuse spread of a single disease such as infection or cancer.

Bear in mind that the clinical picture of a single disease may be altered when another disease becomes superimposed. The diabetic patient who develops renal failure increases his glucose tolerance and seems to cure his diabetes. Angina improves as claudication develops since the patient cannot walk far enough to get chest pain. And the dyspnea and orthopnea of left ventricular failure improve when right ventricular failure supervenes.

And last we have the unusual situation where all clues point to a diagnosis which is statistically most likely and logically correct, yet the patient is found to have a diagnosis other than the expected one. Or the reverse happens; most clues point away from a particular diagnosis which turns out to be the correct one. Unfortunately, this does occur from time to time and serves to humble even the most cocky physician. But it does reemphasize that medicine and diagnosis are not precise sciences wherein mathematical problems can be solved by machines.

Quantitation of Clues. Precision and exact quantitation of clues are needed though almost impossible to attain. It would be desirable to have a system of grading symptoms. Claudication might be graded by the distance that can be walked before leg pain occurs; but the speed of walking, the length of steps, and different pain thresholds create immeasurable variables. Angina is also difficult to quantify. Is it measured in occurrences of pain per day or number of nitroglycerin tablets taken per day? What about the numerous variables, such as weather, emotional state, relation to meals, and duration and severity of the chest pain? How can we grade abdominal pain, headache, insomnia, frequent urination, or anorexia, without a multitude of questions bearing both qualitative and quantitative responses?

Do Not Be Misled. Physical signs may be equally unreliable. They differ from observer to observer and from day to day. An examiner may already be biased by the history and by his preformed impressions or hypotheses. He expects an S_3, so he hears it. Radiologic findings and interpretations are not always black or white. They vary with differences in technique of taking the film, from one reader to another, and sometimes even in the same reader confronted at different times.

As for the laboratory, imprecision abounds even with automation. This issue will be detailed in Chapter 6. Every physician has seen an unexpectedly abnormal result suddenly become normal on recheck. Quantitative tests can be high, low, or normal depending on the Gaussian curve, since 95% of all normal results lie within 2 SD of the mean. The other 5% are half above and half below the 95% area and should probably be called low normal, high normal, or borderline. Mainland (3), an American biostatistician, believes that many scientists are simply "addicted to the Gaussian standard deviation," and he advocates other procedures. In doing repeated measurements of a specific variant on normal individuals, distribution curves may be obtained which are quite different from a typical Gaussian curve. They may be excessively broad, bimodal, truncated, or skewed to the left or right. And, finally, Feinstein (4) has raised the heretical concept that the Gaussian curve may not be absolute dogma and talks about the need to "exorcise the ghost of Gauss."

SELF-EVALUATION EXERCISES

(Answers appear at the end of the exercises.)

1. Which *one* of the following has the greatest diagnostic weight in a single patient:
   (a) splenomegaly
   (b) no splenomegaly
   (c) enlarged lymph nodes
   (d) no enlarged lymph nodes
   (e) neither spleen nor nodes enlarged
   (f) both spleen and nodes enlarged
   (g) fatigue and weakness.
2. Two clues for a disease are 90% and 80% sensitive, respectively. Neither is highly specific. Which of the following has the greatest diagnostic significance?
   (a) both clues present
   (b) both clues absent
   (c) one clue present
   (d) one clue absent.
3. Contrive such a clinical situation (see question 2).
4. Select the *pertinent negative* clues: A 52-year-old man with a chronic cough and expectoration (a) does not drink alcohol; (b) does not smoke; (c) does not drink coffee; (d) denies venereal disease; (e) has no shortness of breath; (f) has no hemoptysis; (g) has anorexia; (h) has weakness; (i) has weight loss; (j) has no contact history for tuberculosis; and (k) has no family.
5. A 42-year-old, extremely obese, 350-lb man has severe dyspnea on exertion, somnolence, and fatigue. The physical examination is normal except for obesity, a widely split S_2 with a very loud pulmonic component, and a presternal lift. What is the key pathophysiologic entity that will serve as a takeoff point for your diagnostic search? (Questions 6 and 7 refer to the same patient.)
6. He has no cough or pulmonary abnormalities on examination. What kind of clues are these?
7. The pO_2 is low and the pCO_2 is high. What does he have?

8. Select the *key clue* in a patient with weakness, weight loss, anorexia, and black stools. She stopped menstruating at 52 and now has dyspareunia and occasional burning on urination. She has had mild diabetes and hypertension for 10 years.
9. Select the *key clue*: A 60-year-old man has anorexia, weakness, weight loss, jaundice, and dark urine. The liver is enlarged by percussion, but this enlargement cannot be confirmed by palpation. He smokes, takes medication for arthritis, eats raw seafood, and had an abdominal operation 1 year ago.
10. Select the *key clue*: For 3 weeks, a 28-year-old woman has had bloody diarrhea, weakness, easy fatigability, headaches, and feverish feelings. The abdomen is slightly distended and somewhat diffusely tender.
11. Form a pathophysiologic entity from which you may pursue a diagnostic quest. A 32-year-old woman delivers a child, has a severe postpartum hemorrhage, requires three blood transfusions, and over the next few days develops oliguria, nausea, weakness, and confusion.
12. Select the *key clue* in a patient with mild nausea, anorexia, abdominal cramps, headaches, and irritability. Examination is normal and laboratory results show normal electrolytes, blood glucose 148 mg/dl, serum uric acid 7.6 mg/dl, and 12,000 white blood cells/mm^3 of which 64% are polymorphonuclear leukocytes, 12% are lymphocytes, and 18% are eosinophils.
13. Which of the following is *not* a "scapegoat" clue (*false clue*)? (a) retroverted uterus; (b) hypertrophic osteoarthritis of the spine; (c) "borderline anemia"; (d) blood pressure 90/60; (e) blood glucose at lower limit of normal; (f) serum calcium 10% above upper limit of normal; or (g) "calcium deficiency."
14. What is the sequence of pathophysiologic events? (a) peritonitis, (b) albuminuria, (c) long-standing diabetes mellitus, (d) ascites, and (e) hypoalbuminemia.
15. What is the probable sequence of events in the following scrambled scenario? (a) hemoptysis, (b) pneumothorax, (c) percutaneous lung biopsy, (d) chest x-ray, and (e) 60 pack-year cigarette history.

ANSWERS

1. **(f)**
2. **(b)**—tends to exclude the disease
3. Many examples may be found. For instance, let the clues be dyspnea on exer-

tion and rales, and the diagnostic consideration be left ventricular failure.
4. **(b), (e), (f), and (j)**
5. Pulmonary hypertension
6. Pertinent negative. They tend to exclude chronic pulmonary disease as a cause of his pulmonary hypertension.
7. Anoxia and hypercapnia—the Pickwickian syndrome
8. Black stools
9. Jaundice
10. Bloody diarrhea
11. Acute renal failure
12. Eosinophilia
13. **(f)**
14. **(c)-(b)-(e)-(d)-(a)**
15. **(e)-(a)-(d)-(c)-(b)**

References

1. Blois MS: Clinical judgment and computers. *N Engl J Med* 303:192–197, 1980.
2. Fleming CR, Dickson ER, Wahner HW, et al: Pigmented corneal rings in non-Wilsonian liver disease. *Ann Intern Med* 86:285–288, 1977.
3. Mainland D: Remarks on clinical norms. *Clin Chem* 17:267–274, 1971.
4. Feinstein AR: Clinical biostatistics; XII. On exorcising the ghost of Gauss and the curse of Kelvin. *Clin Pharmacol Ther* 12:1003–1016, 1971.

Chapter 4

From Odds to Ends

PAUL CUTLER, M.D.

KEY WORDS

1. differential diagnosis
2. presenting symptom
3. mini-workup
4. midi-workup
5. maxi-workup
6. medical shortcuts
7. intuitive decision
8. diagnostic certainty
9. syllogisms
10. deductive logic
11. inductive logic
12. word quantification

We have talked of the selection of clues from the data base and how these clues are used as building blocks in the problem-solving process (Chapters 2 and 3). But before explaining the mathematical models for making diagnoses and making decisions (Chapters 5, 8, and 9), we need to clarify a number of miscellaneous important subjects. These include the application of bedside logic, depth of patient study, use of shortcuts, quantification of terms, decision-making process, science of diagnosis, tactics and strategies of reasoning, and reasons why clinical pictures differ for the same disease.

Application of Logic

How the Mind Works. It is difficult to teach somebody to think. You cannot give precise instructions on how to use the inter-neuronal processes involved in memory, thought, reasoning, and logic. Yet there are certain basic principles and maxims which can help you arrive at reasonable or logical conclusions. The following equation is an expression of how the physician's mind may work:

Data base + information base + logic

= problem list

The *data base* represents all the information about the patient. The *information base* is the knowledge of disease processes that you have or that is available to you. *Logic* was completely defined at the beginning of Chapter 1; it represents the application of correct principles of reasoning, predication, cause and effect, and various other techniques described and iterated throughout this book. The *problem list* outlines the diagnostic conclusions resulting from the factors on the left side of the equation; this subject was detailed in Chapter 2.

The problem solver employs logic when he considers the patient's age, gender, race, habitat, and the natural history of diseases. These factors alter probabilities in the quest for the most likely diagnosis.

On the Basis of Age. For instance, a patient of 21 with certain symptoms is much less likely to have cancer than a patient of 65. Some diseases are more common in the young, others in the old. Urinary tract symptoms in the 21-year-old male patient are commonly caused by venereal infection, while similar symptoms in a 71-year-old man suggest prostatic enlargement. Abnormal vaginal bleeding at age 21 is probably functional; at 61 it is probably neoplastic. Hypochromic microcytic anemia in an elderly person leads you to think seriously of a gastrointestinal malignancy, but in the 28-year-old multigravid patient with a history of two abortions and menometrorrhagia, excessive vaginal bleeding is the likely cause.

The Case for Sex, Race, and Place. The patient's gender is an important factor in the physician's diagnostic logic. Certain diseases are more common in one sex—for instance, systemic lupus erythematosus in the female and coronary disease in the male. Although statistics like these always influence our reasoning, a disease should not be ruled out solely on this basis.

Race too is important. Sarcoidosis is far more common in the young black woman than in a white woman of similar age. If you see a 28-year-old black woman with hilar adenopathy, sarcoidosis would be your first thought; in other races you might give more serious consideration to lymphoma. The predilection of certain anemias for ethnic or geographic origins is well known—pernicious anemia in the Scandinavian, sickle cell anemia in the black, thalassemia in the person of Mediterranean origin, and fish tapeworm in the Finn. Furthermore, carcinoma of the liver is more common in the Chinese, carcinoma of the stomach has a strikingly high incidence in Iceland and Japan, and diabetes is almost universal in some American Indian tribes.

Where you are might weight your logic. In the southwest United States, certain clues of pulmonary disease suggest coccidioidomycosis. The same clues signify histoplasmosis if the patient lives in the Ohio or Mississippi valleys. Hematuria in the United States warrants a detailed study for tumor and stone, whereas in Egypt schistosomiasis of the urinary bladder would be your first choice. A mass in the liver is an echinococcus cyst in Afghanistan, while in the United States you would think primarily of cancer.

Help from the Natural History. The clinical course of an illness is helpful in making a diagnosis, for many diseases have courses which fit specific patterns. For example, multiple sclerosis has exacerbations of varying symptoms, with long remissions at first and shorter ones later on, the illness eventually becoming continuous. A stroke has an acute picture from which it derives its apoplectic name; it may gradually improve. But a brain tumor begins gradually and gets progressively worse. Cancer too gets progressively worse, as do its accompanying symptoms. Duodenal ulcer has its ups and downs, is often symptom free, and may recur for many years. Asthma displays intermittent attacks of variable severity with symptom-free intervals; the disease may eventually become almost continuous. The same holds true for untreated gout or rheumatoid arthritis. The pattern, progression, and intermittency of the disease process must be documented in the history of present illness and are helpful in the formulation of a diagnosis.

You can now match the patient's history of present illness to the known clinical courses of suspected diagnoses.

A gastric problem which has been present intermittently for many years is not likely to be gastric cancer, but if symptoms have existed for only 6 months and are unremitting and progressive, cancer becomes a more serious consideration. A 46-year-old man with recurrent chest pain for 20 years is not apt to have coronary disease as the cause of his pain, but be wary of the chest pains he has had for only 1 or 2 weeks, especially if the character of the pain is suggestive. Cough and fever for 1 month may well be tuberculosis; for 2 days, pneumonia is more likely. The abrupt onset of relentless progressive wheeze and dyspnea does not sound like bronchial asthma. Other considerations are more likely.

Three Maxims. "*Common diseases occur commonly*" may seem elementary and redundant, but the phrase contains much wisdom. If you base your diagnostic reasoning on what is common, you will be right most of the time. Do not diagnose a rare disease when a common one fits the picture just as well. Three birds sitting in a row on a branch are more apt to be sparrows than canaries—unless you are in a pet shop. And if you hear the galloping of hooves, think of horses, not zebras—unless you are in East Africa.

"*Uncommon manifestations of common diseases are more common than common manifestations of uncommon diseases.*" For instance, a 56-year-old man presenting with the manifestations of superior vena cava obstruction is more apt to have lung cancer than Concato's disease or primary thrombosis of the vein. Though it is uncommon for cancer and common for the latter two possibilities to present in this way, lung cancer is by far the leading diagnostic contender since it is so much more prevalent than the other choices.

And an atypical presentation of coronary disease in a 56-year-old man with chest pain is more common than a typical presentation of mesothelioma of the pericardium.

I remember a resident in medicine who diagnosed systemic lupus erythematosus in almost half the women he saw; it was in the early 1950s and the disease was newly known. Since this disease presents in so many different ways, he could have been right all the time; instead he was wrong all the time—except once, which he never let me forget!

And do not forget: "*No disease is rare to the patient who has it.*" In our zeal to stay common, let us not overlook the rare possibilities. Think common—but remember rare.

This is especially true for the tertiary care specialist for whom common simpler problems have already been weeded out, and rare diseases have a higher prevalence. The same can be said for certain diagnostic conferences where only unusual cases are presented to confound the discusser and amuse the listeners.

Statistics Can Confuse. Our discussion has centered on the concept of probability based on the statistical frequency of diseases. We have rough guides as to how common certain diseases are, but they are not totally reliable. Disease incidences vary from continent to continent, country to country, state to state, and even from one physician's office to another. Mortality figures are not accurate, since they depend on the physician's being sure and complete when he fills out the death certificate. Any harassed practitioner knows how difficult that may be. If only the universe of disease were like a deck of cards! We know for certain that there are 26 red cards and 4 kings, 2 of which are red. But disease statistics are not so exact.

In Reverse Gear. Last, the principle of reverse logic merits some additional words. Medicine is generally taught in a manner and texts usually conform to a format whereby disease manifestations are emphasized. We learn separately about eight different diseases that cause hypertension. When confronted by a patient with high blood pressure, we must comb our knowledge base for all the causes—not an easy task. A patient hospitalized with acidotic coma could have one of four conditions: uremia, diabetic ketoacidosis, lactic acidosis, or respiratory failure. Before attacking the problem, you must know these possibilities; however, human retrieval mechanisms are neither perfect nor complete. Many students find it difficult to use this approach. While they may know diseases, they do not know much about patient presentations. Books and teaching might be more effective if they were patient-oriented rather than disease-oriented. And it is more important to know the various *causes of an effect* than to know the various *effects of a cause*.

In 1917, Richard Cabot did a remarkably good job in writing *Differential Diagnosis* (1) from a patient-oriented approach. He studied disease from the standpoint of presenting symptoms, wrote more than 300 case studies wherein each symptom introduced a detailed discussion, and stressed that we avoid treating symptoms. Furthermore, he had many things to say which are even today avant garde. "To state the symptoms of typhoid perforation" (then quite common) "is not difficult. To give a set of rules whereby the conditions which simulate typhoid perforation may be excluded is exceedingly difficult. Physicians are naturally reticent in such matters, slow to commit their thoughts to paper and very suspicious of any attempt to tabulate this method of reasoning." He was telling us that reverse logic is arduous but necessary. And as for good record keeping, he was also describing some impediments which the Weed system is designed to overcome.

The Presenting Symptom. If you were to look up the cause of *dyspnea* in Cabot's book or in any modern textbook of differential diagnosis, you would find a list of between 20 and 100 causes. This does not mean that a patient who presents himself to a physician with shortness of breath as his chief complaint can have that many possible causes. There are far fewer diseases whose *presenting symptom* is dyspnea.

For example, a patient with lobar pneumonia will have cough, fever, chills, expectoration, chest pain, and possibly even shortness of breath. But his chief complaint or presenting symptoms will in all probability be cough and fever. He may be dyspneic too, but that is not the complaint. Whenever I discuss a patient who presents with dyspnea on exertion, invariably some students will mention pneumonia as a possible cause. These students have read Cabot or French; they know the causes of dyspnea and answer accordingly, but they are not being logical. In this regard, a textbook containing lists of possible causes for symptoms may be misleading.

The male patient with secondary hypogonadism presents with loss of libido and impotence, not with loss of body hair, even though that may be present too. It is helpful to know how patients with certain diseases present themselves to a physician for care.

Depth of Study

A patient comes to you with a problem. Your job is to find out what is wrong and do something about it. Often this may require only one or two questions and a brief glance. At other times, you need an exhaustive history; a complete physical examination; extensive laboratory, x-ray, and other special studies; consultations; and at least 2 weeks before arriving at a solution. Between these two extremes, various gradations and complexities of workups are needed.

The Mini-Workup. For instance, the patient with an obvious head cold needs the most meager problem solving and treatment. He has had a stuffed, runny nose, watery eyes, and a slight sore throat for 2 days. Quick examination confirms the nasopharyngitis, and symptomatic therapy is given. Most patients fall into this category.

In working with ambulatory patients in the office and outpatient clinic, speed is generally required. Shortcuts should increase efficiency, though quality must not decrease. The physician must solve the problem of the patient with an acute short case in a few minutes (gastroenteritis, nasopharyngitis, infected finger). Monthly revisits by patients with known chronic disease should take no more than 10 or 15 minutes. Inquire about old and new symptoms, examine the few pertinent areas, and check the one or two crucial laboratory tests—allowing a minute or two for a chat about the patient's progress and treatment. Angina, hypertension, diabetes, asthma, and arthritis—indeed, most diseases seen in any medical clinic or office—can be so managed.

Shortcuts are not necessarily bad (2). Contrasted with hospital patients, ambulatory patients can usually be treated at an acceptable standard in the context of the realities and pressures of practice. You must learn to focus on the economy of time and money in patient encounters, bearing in mind that shortcuts have legitimate tradeoffs.

The Maxi-Workup. Then there is the patient with verified fever for 4 weeks who has been treated with antibiotics by two previous physicians. He is no better, so he comes to see you. A complete data base is obtained, and numerous laboratory studies reveal nothing. Consultants are of limited help. After a variety of noninvasive procedures, a liver biopsy reveals miliary tuberculosis. The process took 10 days, but treatment is now simple.

The Midi-Workup. Between these extremes is the 48-year-old man with chest pain suggestive of coronary thrombosis. A moderately detailed history is obtained. Examination shows cardiocirculatory evidence consistent with the history, and the diagnosis is confirmed by ECG and subsequent enzyme changes. Hypertension and new diabetes are also coincidentally uncovered. Appropriate therapy is promptly begun, possibly even before the diagnosis is verified.

Of 100 consecutive outpatients seen, many will be revisits; perhaps 1 needs a lengthy workup; 5 require an intermediary-length workup, and the remaining 94 need only a mini-workup. Of those seen in the outpatient department, clinic, or office, only a small percentage must have a complete physical examination. Most fall into the category of the "short case," or simple problem, and can be properly managed with a few questions and a brief examination.

For hospitalized patients, the percentage of maxi-workups increases greatly. There most medical problems warrant a complete study. Probably obstetric, gynecologic, surgical, and other inpatients need a complete workup too; but by custom, habit, or for practicality, many receive or perhaps only need a mini- or midi-workup. The price one may pay for treating only the principal illness is that, 3 months after the cholecystectomy, the patient may be found to have carcinoma of the breast—now too advanced for cure. Or, 6 months after treatment for acute myocardial infarction, he may be found to have inoperable carcinoma of the prostate.

This is not to say that every hospitalized patient needs an immediate complete physical examination. A pelvic examination in a patient having an acute myocardial infarction, or a rectal examination in a patient with a dissecting aneurysm is unnecessary at a time when we should be aiming for as much patient comfort as possible. Although we have learned that rectal examinations do not cause arrhythmias in patients with acute myocardial infarction, why introduce discomfort when enough already exists? A notation can be made in the chart that these parts of the examination have not yet been done and that they should be done prior to discharge.

The Complete Workup. Those who definitely need complete workups include: (a) new patients who are coming under your general care either de novo or from another physician, and for whom you should establish a baseline; (b) new patients who have a variety or complexity of illnesses, or those who have illnesses which are difficult to diagnose easily; (c) patients whose mosaic does not add up to a definite somatic problem and whose symptoms may possibly be functional or psychosomatic; (d) patients desiring or needing annual complete examinations, including the healthy patient who wishes to remain well or seeks reassurance that he is well, and the ill patient who should probably receive a complete reevaluation at least once a year (you want to know if his situation is stable, if complications have occurred, or if new problems have developed); and (e) the patient with a chronic disease whom you have not seen for the previous 6 to 12 months and who needs a new baseline for your continuing care.

There is another category of patients who need detailed workups. Assume you see a "short case" with a head cold or gastroenteritis. Most get well promptly, but your suspicions should be aroused and your concern increase if they do not recover quickly. Perhaps there is a more serious underlying disease. This category would include: (a) the patient with apparent acute gastroenteritis whose symptoms do not subside within the usual few days, (b) the patient with an alleged head cold which persists for well over a week, (c) the patient with the "grippe" or "viral disease" who remains febrile beyond 1 week, (d) the patient with "acute bronchitis" whose cough lingers, (e) the patient with "sore throat" which lasts for more than a few days, (f) the patient with "tension headache" which persists, and (g) the patient with superficial idiopathic thrombophlebitis. Additional examples might easily be included here.

Other factors must be considered. If you see a patient who has had a backache for a few days, a mini-workup and a prescription will suffice. However, if the backache is persistent or the patient has already seen two other doctors, a third presciption would be inadvisable. A child with a respiratory infection can be treated simply. But if infections recur frequently, his immunity may be impaired; a thorough study is clearly indicated, and a search must be made for more serious causes.

Shortcuts

Here are some tips and maneuvers that are often used to solve problems rapidly. While most are acquired with time and experience, many can be utilized early in a student's or young physician's maturation. First, the data base need not be collected in separate orderly blocks. We do not always complete each part, then go on to the next. It is often done all at once.

Zeroing In. Shortcuts may be taken as described in Chapters 1 and 2. Proceed from a few clues—filtering, processing, and sorting the incoming data in a dynamic, constant fashion. Two clues in the chief complaint and history of present illness may lead the physician to quickly examine a specific portion of the body and form an impression. For instance, when the patient complains of fatigue and lumps in the neck, an immediate feel for other nodes and the spleen will narrow the field to a very few possibilities. If this quick step yields nothing, return to the history and continue in the routine order.

Then there is the patient who sees the physician because he has been told he has a heart murmur. Who could keep his stethoscope off this chest before asking even a single question? One listen may solve the problem.

The 65-year-old woman with bone pains, anemia, and uremia probably has multiple myeloma. To be certain, she needs a urine study, protein electrophoresis, and bone marrow examination. Little is needed to diagnose cirrhosis in the heavy drinker who complains of a swollen abdomen and has distended abdominal veins and spider angiomas. A febrile 36-year-old woman with arthritis, a rash across the face, and a pericardial friction rub needs only an antinuclear antibody test for confirmation of sys-temic lupus erythematosus. The patient with dyspnea, markedly distended neck veins, low pulse pressure, and a large quiet heart probably has a pericardial effusion. Prove it!

Hypotheses and provisional diagnoses are continually tested all through the data-gathering process, beginning with the chief complaint. But problem-solving strategies actually begin immediately on seeing the patient, on shaking his hand, and on the first exchange of words. The handshake may disclose the fine tremor and warm, sweating hands of hyperthyroidism, the cold, clammy hands of severe anxiety, or the deformities of arthritis.

Diagnosis by a *coup d'oeil*, or *augenblick*, is popular among attending physicians—though treacherous. One glance can spot myxedema, Parkinson's disease, acromegaly, and numerous other disorders if the physician is thinking of them. At the door to the patient's room one can smell uremia even before seeing the patient, and older clinicians could smell typhoid fever on merely entering the room. But the former odor can be caused by incontinence, and older clinicians were often proven wrong as more precise diagnostic techniques were devised.

Nevertheless, even though we can often solve the main problem in a few minutes, this does not negate the importance of completing the data base in order to confirm the quick impression and rule out other diseases and concomitant problems. But this too has its shortcuts. Questions can be asked at the same time that you examine each system. Ask about all the usual gastrointestinal symptoms as you examine the abdomen, and so forth—elaborating only when you get a positive answer.

How Inspection Helps. Simple inspection of the patient at the beginning of the physical examination is a most neglected yet most useful skill. Here diagnosis can often be made with a glance. However, this inspection is usually sketchy, poorly done, and is where many oversights or errors occur (refer to "Physical Examination," Chapter 2).

You must set aside a full 2 minutes to look at the undressed patient: front, back, top, and bottom—programming your mind to look for a certain number of items in a definite order. If not, you may easily overlook the single clue that will give you the diagnosis.

Most textbooks of physical diagnosis devote only a paragraph or so to inspection; yet a proper inspection includes at least 18 items:

1. gait
2. how sick the patient looks
3. state of nutrition
4. state of hydration
5. apparent age
6. sensorium, state of consciousness
7. position, posture, tremors, movements
8. body type (ecto-, endo-, mesomorph)
9. hair distribution
10. endocrine appearance of face and body (thyroid, pituitary, adrenal)
11. genetic disease appearance
12. odor of breath and general odors
13. skin (pigmentation, rashes, cyanosis, pallor, plethora, jaundice, nodules, xanthomas, petechiae, ecchymoses, angiomas)
14. sweating pattern
15. edema
16. venous distention
17. breathing problems
18. deformities

Some Classic Examples. Take a chief complaint such as "dyspnea on exertion for several weeks." Three things cross your mind: heart disease, lung disease, and anemia. The last can be ruled out at a glance, since anemia severe enough to give dyspnea on exertion should be readily apparent. If there are no other cardiac symptoms, the heart is normal in size and exhibits no murmurs or gallops, and there are no fine basilar rales, heart disease is unlikely. The third possibility is quickly confirmed by the presence of chronic cough with expectoration, heavy smoking, faint expiratory wheezes, and a low immobile diaphragm. So you have quickly pinpointed chronic obstructive lung disease and will confirm it by x-ray, ECG,

and pulmonary function tests. Though the solution to the chief complaint was fairly easy, check the patient for additional problems.

Another example of quick problem solving is a 60-year-old man with pains in both legs for several months. You think of arterial insufficiency, venous insufficiency, and arthritis. The latter is ruled out by examining the joints. Venous insufficiency is unlikely since the legs are not swollen, there are no varicose veins, and the pain does not come on after the patient has been standing for a long time. However, the pain comes on walking, is relieved by stopping, and pulses are not felt in the lower extremities. It should take no longer than 1 minute to decide that this patient has atherosclerosis of the lower extremities. Since atherosclerosis is often a generalized disease, a complete examination is especially indicated here.

Coming to Terms

One of the most common shortcomings and causes for misunderstanding among physicians and especially among students is the failure to use simple quantitative terms properly. Few of us understand exactly what others mean when they say, "most of the time," "almost always," or "rarely." Students taking examinations are constantly asking what the examiner means in terms of percentages when such words are used in questions—since their answers depend on this interpretation. Dialogue between physician and patient can be a similar source of misunderstanding. Unfortunately, there is no uniformity of meaning of such terms for all people. What may signify 60% to one person may be 95% to another.

Communication would be markedly enhanced if likelihoods and probabilities were expressed in percentages rather than in words—just as in the weather report. The statement that a patient *probably* has a disease would be more meaningful if "probably" were assigned a 75% value by general agreement. Better yet, you could say that the patient has a 75% probability of having this disease. Similarly, there is no doubt in the patient's mind when he is told there is a 10% chance of postoperative complications. But the statement that "complications are uncommon" makes him wonder (3).

Causes for Confusion. Always have your patient quantify his symptoms if possible. If you ask a patient how frequently his headaches occur, he may say "all the time." He probably means "often," so you ask "are you having one now?" And he may answer "no" and further indicate that "all the time" really means "some of the time." And "frequent" to him means three or four times per day. "Now and then" to one patient may mean once a month, but to another it means two or three times daily. It behooves the history taker to nail down exactly what the patient means.

In an examination the student will ask you what you mean if your question reads "It is common for diabetics to have itching of the vulva: true or false?" First he may want to know the severity of disease and degree of control your diabetic patient has. Second he wants your definition of the word "common," since while this symptom does occur in the uncontrolled female diabetic, itching of the vulva is not common in the overall set of diabetic patients. So the answer depends in part on whether common means 5% or 45% of the cases.

Crichton (4) refers to the use of double negatives like "not uncommon," "not infrequently," and "not unusual" as outstanding examples of academic cowardice. These terms are equally confusing to physician, patient, and student.

On Being Precise. Quantitative ambiguities should be avoided whenever possible. Movements of the diaphragm and size of the liver, even though of questionable reliability, should be recorded in centimeters rather than fingerbreadths or rib interspaces. Centimeters never vary, but the width of fingers does. An apex beat should be located in terms of centimeters tangentially from the midsternal line rather than at an often ill-defined place, such as the midclavicular or anterior axillary line. Above all, the size of masses, tumors, or organs should be measured in centimeters rather than compared to fruit, nuts, and sporting goods.

A Study in Quantitation. We habitually use poorly quantifiable terms in everyday language. This is a source of confusion and faulty communication between doctor and patient, doctor and doctor, or teacher and student.

To demonstrate the individual variation in quantitatively defining words and terms, 45 commonly used words were submitted to 20 medical school faculty members for interpretation (5). Instructors from almost all departments took part in this pilot study. Included were easily quantifiable words like "never" and "always"—more difficult ones like "frequently," "often," "many," "few," "probably," and "commonly"—and most difficult ones (double negatives) like "not uncommonly," "not infrequently," and "not unusually."

The participants were asked to equate each term with a number from 0 to 100. Twenty valid observations were made on each word or phrase. The resulting data were tabulated and analyzed by computer. A sample of results including the mean, the range, and the standard deviation is shown in Table 4.1. Even though the sample is small, many tentative conclusions can easily be drawn from the data. First, it is obvious that there is nonuniformity of opinion for most terms—with wide differences between maximum and minimum evaluations (range) and almost intolerably large standard deviations. Next, it must be noted that the various terms fall into three broad categories. The first group ("always" and "never")—which should be 100% and 0% by dictionary definition—turn out to be pretty much so; the range and SD are small. But the fact that there is any range at all indicates how reluctant physicians are to be absolute; they have been indoctrinated to "never say never and never say always."

The second large category (3 to 17) demonstrates reasonable means but fairly wide ranges, yet SDs which are for the most part not very great. And third, all the double

Table 4.1
Terms Equated Numerically

Word	Mean (%)	Range (%)	SD (%)
1. never	0.1	10.0	2.0
2. always	99.1	15.0	3.4
3. rarely	6.5	19.0	5.4
4. uncommonly	10.4	18.0	5.8
5. frequently	64.5	70.0	19.2
6. usually	79.5	45.0	11.1
7. in most cases	78.6	45.0	14.1
8. probably	64.1	80.0	19.0
9. commonly	71.0	60.0	12.7
10. most likely	75.2	75.0	17.7
11. possibly	33.0	75.0	21.7
12. certainly	88.1	75.0	19.3
13. suggestive of	46.5	65.0	21.2
14. unequivocal	97.3	15.0	4.8
15. many	68.2	35.0	10.3
16. some	25.8	45.0	13.5
17. few	14.2	25.0	7.9
18. not uncommonly	44.2	80.0	28.3
19. not infrequently	50.2	85.0	23.6
20. not unusually	54.3	80.0	24.4

negatives (18 to 20) show very wide ranges and large SDs. Here the usual variability of interpretation was no doubt compounded by mistakes in recognition of the actual meaning of a double negative phrase.

If medical educators are imprecise in this regard, can we expect more from patients or students? There are no simple solutions to the misunderstandings and problems created by using quasiquantitative words. Numbers are exact and need no definition. Not so for words! Indeed, we are all guilty of the same inexactitudes ... for how else can we speak or write?

The Decision-Making Process

In Tres Partes. When it comes to making decisions, all mankind is divided into three parts. There are those who are bewildered when faced with decisions, have not the courage to make them, procrastinate, and pass the buck. Others make decisions quickly and with seeming certainty, but their decisions are not based on anything substantial. These people may not be correct but they are always certain. The third group, in

which all physicians should be, makes decisions either quickly or slowly, but these decisions are always based on data, careful thought, knowledge, experience, and judgment.

Decisions are made at each and every step in patient management: what branch of questions should you follow; are you on the right or wrong track; what parts of the examination are abnormal; which studies are helpful; what additional studies should be done; what are the problems; what needs prompt attention; is suicide imminent; is hospitalization indicated; what treatment should be given; and on and on for each patient.

An average physician may make decisions hundreds of times per day. He does it almost subconsciously. The teacher-academician is rarely faced with so many decisions per unit of time. But students must learn to make decisions as quickly as possible. They should not procrastinate by ordering more and more studies.

A Free Meal. Here is a story of rapid multiple decision making. Ten years ago, I attended a meeting in Seattle of teachers of Introduction to Clinical Medicine from medical centers all over the country. Many famous and prestigious educators were there but hardly any had ever practiced medicine or been on the front lines where decisions must often be made instantaneously.

One evening after the meetings some 30 of the registrants went to dinner at a well-known seafood restaurant. Suddenly, during dinner, a young lady sitting at a nearby table began to make violent jerking movements and became unconscious, with her mouth full of food and her head repeatedly banging against a glass partition. Everybody watched motionless. America's leading physician educators appeared unable to handle a relatively simple ambulatory emergency.

One of them, formerly a practicing physician, leaped into the arena making a series of rapid decisions. Clearly, the young lady was having a grand mal seizure. So he moved her chair away from the glass partition, then inserted a folded heavy cloth napkin into the side of her mouth between her upper and lower teeth so she could not bite her tongue or break her teeth. With a sweep of his index finger he emptied her mouth of food. Then he summoned two strong waiters to carry her, still in her chair, to the manager's private office where her convulsions stopped and she was laid down on a sofa to recover.

A quick history from her escort revealed past good health with no previous episodes. A branched examination showed no evidence of meningeal irritation, and a partial neurologic examination was normal. No examining instruments were on hand for further testing. Since this was her first seizure, another decision was made: hospitalization was indicated to rule out serious problems. And the last decision was whether the patient should go to the hospital by taxi or ambulance. She was now conscious and well, though bewildered and frightened, so a taxi was chosen. She was told what had happened and why hospitalization was necessary.

The others diners in the restaurant were much relieved to see this simple matter handled so efficiently, and personally expressed their gratitude to the lone physician. A fresh dinner was served to him free of charge by order of the manager and it seemed that, at least for this subset of the Seattle population, much had been done to improve doctor-public relations.

More on Decisions. In the past decade, mathematical precision has been added to the decision-making process with varying degrees of success. Statistics, data banks, decision matrices, and utility values are woven into diagrams which seem to add precision to intuitive decisions. It is deemed so important for the student and clinician to understand this new field that it will be discussed more fully in all of Chapter 8.

The Science of Diagnosis

A diagnosis can rarely be made with 100% certainty. The physician usually works with probability, likelihood, and weight of evidence. He can be certain only if a biopsy is 100% unequivocal or a test is unquestionably diagnostic.

How Certain to Be. The degree of diagnostic certainty that must be obtained in any particular case is arguable. Even in a court of law, proof beyond a reasonable doubt does not require 100% certainty. When do we decide that enough investigation has already taken place so that we can proceed with management? The threshold for arriving at diagnostic conclusions is an important part of clinical judgment.

To be considered are the seriousness of the disease; the age and otherwise general condition of the patients; the risks of further study; the already existing disease probability; and the costs to the patient in terms of inconvenience, money, and delayed treatment.

A search for evidence of a second diagnosis might be less diligent in an 85-year-old man with congestive heart failure than in a healthy 45-year-old wage earner. When contemplating a coronary artery bypass graft, 80% certainty is not enough. But if a patient wants to have coronary heart disease ruled out because of a contemplated vigorous adventure, a 10% likelihood does not yet give sufficient exclusion.

These interrelated factors are rarely subject to precise mathematical expression and articulation, though *decision theory* tries to deal with this issue (6).

A Wrong Label. Before making a diagnosis, you may sometimes have to *undiagnose* a patient. Such patients have been given labels on the basis of inadequate or inaccurate data and are then treated for those labels—sometimes for life.

Included are some who take digitalis for alleged heart failure but who may be dyspneic only from hyperventilation. The obese person is often given thyroid preparations for supposed hypothyroidism when thyroid function tests are borderline. Others who are nervous, shaky, and sweaty from simple anxiety may be treated for hyperthyroidism for years. Perhaps the most common false label is the "mild anemia" attached to psychoneurotic individuals whose blood counts are near the lower limits of normal and who complain of chronic fatigue. Vitamin B_{12} injections are often given in these instances. The tragedy of this latter situation is that, if mild anemia truly exists, the anemia may arise from a serious disorder that is unresponsive to vitamin injections.

In general, when wrong labels are applied, patients are treated for illnesses that are more serious than the ones they actually have. But the reverse can occur and a very serious yet treatable disease may be overlooked. Such situations must be managed with skill and diplomacy. Patients are often reluctant to relinquish their designer labels!

So what do you do? If you suspect that this situation may exist because the patient is not getting better or for some other reason, take the label off. Begin the diagnostic process over again. You may even tactfully have to discontinue the former treatment, cautiously observing the patient while you rediagnose him—it may be *you* who is wrong.

There is no more important field in medicine than diagnosis. Without it, we are charlatans or witch doctors treating in the dark with potions and prayers. Yet there is no field more difficult to teach. Strange that this art and science has not attracted innumerable theorists to make it more teachable! Thousands are studying membrane transfer, yet few strive to make a science of diagnosis.

When a physician sees a patient, how does he decide what is wrong? Ask him how, and he cannot really explain. He may use terms such as "hunch," "intuition," "judgment," "experience," "deduction," and so forth. He can explain the individual case but cannot give general rules and principles.

Only in the past 10 to 15 years have serious attempts been made to systematize the thought processes which the clinician uses every day but cannot define. The advent of the digital computer has been a great stimulus for these attempts. Mathematical theorems, new adaptations of traditional forms of algebra, some new concepts—all aided and abetted by the educator, the psychologist, the statistician, and the mathe-

matician—are being used in an effort to clarify and then teach the technology of the diagnostic process.

Tactics and Strategies

Before proceeding to problem-solving techniques, some of the tactics and strategies of basic logic and reasoning should be clarified.

The Greek Connection. Logic was a favorite topic for discussion among Greek philosophers, and axioms, postulates, theorems, and syllogisms were methods of argument and reasoning used by Euclid and Aristotle (7). A syllogism is the deductive scheme of a formal argument consisting of two premises (one major, one minor) from which a conclusion is drawn. The premises are axioms or postulates which are obviously true or have been proven true from a previous argument. There are many forms of syllogisms, and conclusions drawn from the basic premises may be valid or not, depending on the proper application of logic. Syllogisms are the essence of deductive logic and can also be aptly expressed by set theory, Venn diagrams, and Boolean algebra (Chapter 5).

A positive syllogism contains only positive statements. For example: "If a patient has coronary thrombosis he is seriously ill. This patient has coronary thrombosis. Therefore he is seriously ill." The conclusion is clearly correct. Had the minor premise and conclusion been: "This patient is seriously ill. Therefore he has a coronary thrombosis," the conclusion would have been invalid since it cannot be derived from the minor premise as stated. Not all patients who are seriously ill have coronary thrombosis.

Negative syllogisms may be sound strategies too. Usually a positive and negative premise lead to a negative conclusion. "To diagnose acute myocardial infarction, cardiac enzymes should become elevated and the ECG should show indicative changes in the first 3 days of illness. In this patient, the enzymes have not risen and the ECG has not changed during the first 3 days. Therefore a myocardial infarction has not occurred." The conclusion is valid; it would be simple to construct many invalid conclusions.

Deduction and Induction. Syllogisms are classic examples of *deductive reasoning*; a conclusion is drawn from established facts, and general statements are applied to an individual case. Conclusions are no more valid than the premises on which they are based; if two premises are correct, the conclusion should be correct if properly deduced. But the difficulty in stating 100% foolproof premises in medicine makes deductive logic not so useful or accurate as it might otherwise be. The accuracy of a premise is often debatable, and conclusions are often incorrectly drawn. Beware of inaccurate syllogisms which create Procrustean beds.

Inductive reasoning, on the other hand, is a tactic which is based on inference rather than fact. While it may not be completely accurate, it is often successfully used. The method is as follows: Study a set of individual cases, derive a general principle from this study, and then apply it to another case. For example, "A study of young patients with bleeding duodenal ulcers shows that almost all get well without surgery; a 42-year-old man is admitted to the hospital with a bleeding duodenal ulcer; he will get well without surgery." Although the premises and conclusion may not be absolutely true, the conclusion is correctly inferred. The fact that so many got well without surgery would lead you to conclude that this one will too.

Cause and Effect. Another tactic of logic and reason is the proper application of cause and effect in studying the interrelationship of events (7). Assume that there is no feedback between cause and effect, so that the effect does not repress or stimulate the cause. Numerous relationships can occur. But in order for two events to have a cause and effect association, one should follow the other in time sequence and they should have a clear-cut pathophysiologic relationship. Having a stroke after sipping a cola drink does not imply cause and effect, so beware the post hoc propter hoc philosophy.

Cause and effect may relate in many ways, but the most common and simple correlation is one wherein a cause brings about an effect $(C \rightarrow E)$. Some of the more complex interactions are depicted in Figures 4.1 to 4.11. In Figure 4.1 two causes have two effects that may or may not be separate. For example, decreased carbohydrate tolerance

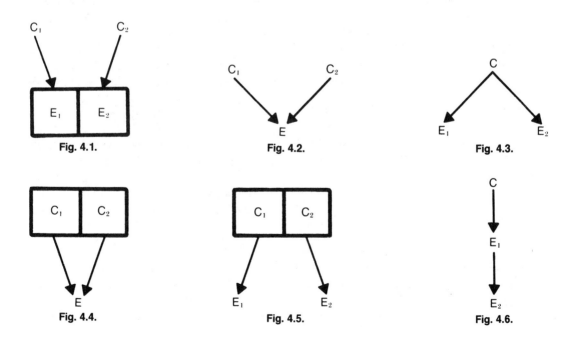

Fig. 4.1.　　　　Fig. 4.2.　　　　Fig. 4.3.

Fig. 4.4.　　　　Fig. 4.5.　　　　Fig. 4.6.

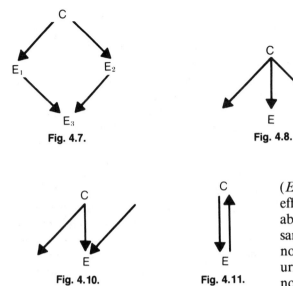

Fig. 4.7.   Fig. 4.8.   Fig. 4.9.

Fig. 4.10.   Fig. 4.11.

(C_1) and increased carbohydrate consumption (C_2) can cause hyperglycemia (E_1) and frequent urination (E_2). E_1 and E_2 are probably related, though E_2 could be unrelated and result from prostatic hypertrophy. In Figure 4.2 two unrelated causes have a single effect. Former acute rheumatic fever (C_1) and a current tooth extraction (C_2) can cause infective endocarditis (E). In Figure 4.3, a single cause can have two apparently unrelated effects. Diabetes mellitus (C) can cause vulvo-vaginitis (E_1) and retinopathy (E_2). In Figure 4.4, two related causes join to give one effect. A basic psychopathologic defect (C_1) plus use of heroin (C_2) results in infective endocarditis (E); or atheroma (C_1) plus fibrin clot (C_2) causes infarction (E). In Figure 4.5 two related causes give diverse effects. Alcoholism (C_1) plus malnutrition (C_2) can result in cirrhosis (E_1) or beriberi (E_2). While C_2 could cause E_2, it is unlikely that C_2 would exist in most American cultures without C_1. In Figure 4.6, one event causes a second which causes a third. The first could not directly cause the third. For example: diabetes (C) causes atherosclerosis (E_1) which in turn causes myocardial infarction (E_2). In Figure 4.7, one cause can result in an effect by either one of two pathways. For example: diabetes (C) causes blindness (E_3) via either cataracts (E_1) or retinopathy

(E_2). In Figure 4.8, one cause exists for the effect in question, but the cause can bring about other effects instead (8). C is a necessary determinant for E. Acute gout (E) cannot ordinarily exist without a high serum uric acid (C), though a high uric acid may not result in acute gout. Instead it may cause a renal calculus, a tophus, or nothing. In Figure 4.9, C is one sufficient determinant of disease E, but other causes too can bring E about. Diabetes mellitus (C) is the usual cause of hyperglycemia (E), though hyperthyroidism, acromegaly, and pheochromocytoma may also cause it. In Figure 4.10, C is only a contributory determinant of E and leads to an increased probability of E, though C does not always cause E, and E may be caused by something else. For example, diabetes mellitus (E) often results from obesity (C), though diabetes may occur without obesity, and obesity does not necessarily lead to diabetes. A common situation is shown in Figure 4.11. Two events occur together, and we do not know which is cause and which is effect. Circulating autoantibodies against human myoglobin have been found in polymyositis (9), but we do not know which came first. Does the patient's acute coronary insufficiency cause left ventricular failure, or is it the reverse? Problems such as this are very commonly encountered, and skill is needed to distinguish the chicken from the egg.

Why Clinical Pictures Differ

Before going on, it might be helpful to define *disease*. Literally, disease means "not at ease" or "a disorder of ease." Dictionary definitions are inconsistent but usually revolve around "a deviation from health or from normal organ or body function." Disease and the manifestations of disease result from two great forces: first, an environmental change, invasion from without, or an internal body derangement causes the disease; second, the body reacts to this derangement in such a way as to try to maintain homeostasis or normal milieu interieur. This homeostatic effort may be normal or exaggerated and varies from person to person. The initial derangement may be a bacterium, a cancer cell, a genetic abnormality, etc. The body's response is with fever, antibodies, renin-aldosterone, etc. These two forces combine to give the clinical picture.

Action and Reaction. It is no surprise that the signs and symptoms of a disease vary from person to person, that patients with the same disease can present differently, and that the usual clues for a disease may be present or absent. The disease *inoculum* may vary with the quantity and virulence of the bacterium, the aggressiveness of the cancer cell, or the genetic penetrance. The host may respond with his own pattern of behavior. He may be frightened, anxious, calm, stoic, dramatic, and have a different level of perceptiveness. He may procrastinate, deny, or report promptly at the first abnormal feeling. He may react organically with low or high fever; his renin-angiotensin-aldosterone mechanism may be sluggish or hyperactive.

Patients seen in office practice differ in their clinical manifestations from those seen in the hospital. The office patient is seen earlier, is usually in a less serious stage, and has fewer disease manifestations. Only later, when he is sicker, has more clues, or perhaps has had a delay in diagnosis, does he reach the hospital.

Symptom threshold is another factor. Some cirrhotics see the doctor when their abdomens enlarge. Others attribute this to beer and see you later for sexual problems related to testicular atrophy. It requires massive vomiting of blood or impending hepatic failure to get some cirrhotic patients into the medical care system. Obviously the clues and clinical picture will vary at each stage

and depend upon the cause and time of presentation. This accounts in part for the many faces of cirrhosis of the liver.

The patient's intelligence and intellect may be a factor. Would you expect both Einstein and a clod to present in the same manner even if they had the same disease?

You can easily see, then, why two patients with the same disease can give vastly different clinical pictures when first seen by a physician.

Unanswered Questions. The foregoing reasoning notwithstanding, we are still perplexed in many instances as to why pictures differ from patient to patient. Why are some diabetics who have had the disease for 20 years free of retinopathy, while others are blind after only 10 years? Why do some develop neuropathy almost at or even before the onset, while others never do? The same can be said of the patient with cirrhosis just described. Portal hypertension, hyperestrogenism, hyperaldosteronism, ascites, bleeding tendencies, anemia, and hepatic coma are some of the different groups of manifestations which may occur all together or in any combination. Only one or two may dominate the picture, and the others may be absent. The presence or absence of clues can be extremely chancy.

The fact that the many symptoms, physical signs, and laboratory tests for a particular disease have different sensitivities tells you that not every clue need be present in the patient who has the disease. Therefore the clinical picture of a disease will differ from patient to patient.

Osler (10) expressed this well: "Variability is the law of life, and as no two faces are the same, so no two bodies are alike, and no two individuals react alike, and behave alike under abnormal conditions which we know as disease. This is the fundamental difficulty in the education of the physician."

Conclusions

Science or Art. In spite of attempts to make a precise science of the skill of problem solving (Chapter 9), we are frequently left with indefinable though universally used techniques. The sharp clinician develops rapid and efficient diagnostic and management routines but is often unable to conceptualize them. A glance, a simple mathematical addition, a smell, intuition, experience, a hunch—and out comes a correct impression. The making of a masterful decision, often on the basis of scant or incomplete data, is not an art, not a science, but a disciplined amalgam of both.

The sequence of gathering a complete data base, then diagnosis, then action, is the one which is traditionally taught. However, this route is less traveled than the one by which a provisional diagnosis is based on the first few bits of information, and evidence for and against this diagnosis is then sought via a branching technique. The latter pursues a single line and gathers supportive data until confidence in a diagnosis has been attained—then action can proceed (11).

This narrower approach streams patients earlier into separate diagnostic categories or onto a branch of the diagnostic tree. The use of shortcuts may seem unsound to the student, but the sooner he masters the way it is done "in real life," the better for him. It is definitely worth trying to teach. After following one branch to its tip, we determine what other diseases may be present by exploring the rest of the tree.

Time Will Tell. It seems appropriate to close this chapter with a reminder that physicians are not omniscient, that humbleness is a virtue, and that there is inevitably a certain percentage of patient problems we are unable to solve without prescriptions for *essence of patience, tincture of time, and long-acting capsules of observation.* If you do not know what is wrong, consultants may be helpful. And if pressed for treatment you can always resort to a therapeutic trial and treat "as if"—bearing in mind that this is to be regarded only as a desperate measure.

The Bible speaks of man living three score years and ten. Public health measures and preventive medicine deserve the bulk of credit for man's present life span matching this expectation. If one considers the life expectancy of a 60-year-old today, not much has changed since Biblical times. Occasionally we do save a life with antibiotics or surgery. We may even prolong life a year or two with good care. But 70 still stands, give or take 10 years depending upon whether the genetic background does or does not include diabetes, hypertension, or atherosclerosis (12).

References

1. Cabot R: *Differential Diagnosis.* Philadelphia, Saunders, 1917.
2. Mechanic D, Parson W: Shortcuts are not necessarily bad (editorial). *JAMA* 50:638–639, 1975.
3. Robertson WO: Quantifying the meaning of words. *JAMA* 249:2631–2632, 1983.
4. Crichton M: Medical obfuscation: structure and function. *N Engl J Med* 293:1257–1259, 1975.
5. Cutler P: Quantification of words. Unpublished data, 1978.
6. Williams BT: *Computer Aids to Clinical Diagnosis.* Boca Raton, FL, CRC Press, 1982.
7. Murphy EA: *The Logic of Medicine,* ed 2. Baltimore, Johns Hopkins University Press, 1980.
8. Wulff HR: *Rational Diagnosis and Treatment,* ed 2. London, Blackwell Scientific Publications, 1981.
9. Nishikai M, Homma M: Circulating autoantibody against human myoglobin in polymyositis. *JAMA* 237:1842–1844, 1977.
10. Osler W: *Aequanimitas with Other Addresses,* ed 2. Philadelphia, Blakiston, 1930, p 331.
11. Cox KR: How do you decide what it is and what do you do about it? *Med J Aust* 2:62–64, 1975.
12. Kampmeier RH: Death and aging. *South Med J* 67:3–4, 1974.

Chapter 5

Digits, Decimals, and Doctors

PAUL CUTLER, M.D.

KEY WORDS

1. set theory
2. Venn diagram
3. Boolean algebra
4. Bayes' theorems
5. prevalence
6. incidence
7. probability
8. sensitivity
9. specificity
10. TP-FN-TN-FP
11. predictive value
12. 2×2 tables
13. stick diagram
14. likelihood ratios
15. operating characteristics
16. cohort
17. gold standard test
18. imperfect information
19. ROC curves
20. separator point
21. test efficiency
22. likelihood revision
23. product of probabilities
24. independent clues
25. interdependent clues
26. diagnostic likelihood
27. combination testing

Who Needs Math Anyway?

Most students of medicine are repelled by discussions of complicated mathematical concepts. Physicians are too. Such antipathy is both understandable and justifiable because medicine deals with people, not numbers.

While premedical students must undergo rigorous training in mathematical subjects, medical students soon learn that they neither need nor use much mathematics in clinical medicine. Aside from a few limited areas, such as pulmonary function and cardiac hemodynamics, it is considered irrelevant.

Unless your future course takes you into biostatistics, epidemiology, laboratory research, or clinical trial design, you need not know about linear regression, control limit theorem, confidence intervals, P value, and binomial, chi-square, and Poisson distributions, and so forth. The argument that such knowledge will enable you to judge the quality of medical literature is not sound, since even experts often disagree. Let's face the fact that most of us do not have the ability to scientifically evaluate the validity of articles that have already been preselected and judged publishable by editorial consultants.

However, the proposition that doctors don't need "math" is not entirely valid.

Modern medical economics, the rising importance of demographics, mathematical models of the diagnostic process, cost-benefit analysis, informed consent, scientific decision making, and the increasing use of computers in medicine—all mandate that the physician of the '80s and '90s know more about percentages, numbers, statistics, and mathematical methods.

How, then, does one make palatable the minimal amount of mathematics that *is necessary* for the 99% of students who will spend their lives treating patients? Over the past 10 years it has become increasingly evident that physicians must be familiar with some basic equations, theorems, and simple mathematical concepts in order to be able to: calculate the probability that a disease is present; be sure that a diagnosis exists; interpret the results of tests; determine how clues alter diagnostic likelihoods; render proper treatment; and much, much more. In large measure, reason, logic, intuition, and decisions are based on nonintellectualized internal mathematical operations.

What follows are the arithmetic essentials that a nonmathematical clinician-teacher thinks medical students need to know in order to be better physicians.

The Prototype Problem. You see a 65-year-old man who is being treated for chronic congestive heart failure with mild salt restriction, decreased activity, and .25 mg of digoxin and 40 mg of furosemide daily. He had been doing quite well for the past 6 months on this regimen, but for the preceding few weeks he complained of nausea and occasional palpitations. These symptoms had occurred from time to time in the past and were usually associated with clinically evident mild cardiac decompensation. Now, however, he has no dyspnea or orthopnea, there are no basal rales, jugular venous distention, enlarged liver, or ankle edema. He has lost weight. Cardiac abnormalities associated with his heart disease are present as before, but the first heart sound seems more faint than usual. The electrocardiogram shows no change from the one taken 6 months ago except for occasional ventricular premature depolarizations and a PR interval of .23 second which was .18 second when last recorded.

The questions: Are his complaints caused by his heart disease, by digitalis intoxication, or by something else? Does he need more or less digitalis? Does he need more or less diuretic? Does he need a search for another disease? Is the first degree heart block caused by his heart disease or the digitalis?

Serum electrolytes and creatinine are normal. He has no other symptoms. You predict that he has digitalis intoxication with an estimated probability of 50%. Now you wish to obtain a serum digoxin assay in order to revise the probability upward (1).

Assume that the cutoff point for this test which designates toxicity is 2.0 ng/ml in your laboratory. Moreover, you understand that in using any cutoff point you inevitably create false positive and false negative results. If the test result is normal (e.g. 1.5 ng/ml), how far down has the probability estimate of 50% fallen? If the test result is abnormal (2.5 ng/ml), how much more certain are you that the patient has digitalis intoxication? The decision on further management hinges on this issue. We shall return to this clinical problem after learning more about the calculations needed to deal with it.

A Pause for Orientation. The subjects of sensitivity, specificity, probability, predictive value, probability revision—and how these mathematical concepts may be expressed by words, symbolized by algebraic notation, and diagrammed by tables, formulas, and equations—are what this chapter is all about. You can easily see how these concepts relate to the common problem just presented and how comprehension of these concepts establishes a firm basis for the numerous clinical decisions made daily. Some of these subjects have already been introduced and others will be subsequently expounded. For example, the concepts of specificity and sensitivity were mentioned in the discussion of the clinical measurement in Chapter 2 and in the discussion of clues in Chapter 3; word quantification and the degree of diagnostic certainty were introduced in Chapter 4; and ideas related to disease probability will be further detailed in Chapter 8.

Questions That Arise Daily. Hundreds of times each day physicians ask themselves questions that need quantitative answers. For example, how certain am I that patient 1 has cancer? Does this test prove that patient 2 has coronary artery disease? Should I recommend surgery on that percentage of probability? Does the positive purified protein derivative skin test in patient 3 warrant chemotherapy? And does the negative test in her daughter guarantee that tuberculosis is not present? Given one positive clue, how sure am I that patient 5 has acquired immune deficiency syndrome? And if a second test is negative, how much reassurance can patient 6 be given that the disease is not present? The next patient has a sore throat; what are the chances it is streptococcal, and should I therefore give penicillin? Will further tests help, and how much? Here's an 18-year-old girl with a positive serologic test for syphilis; her mother has lupus; what is the likelihood of a false positive test, and should she receive antibiotic treatment? This 65-year-old nervous woman has abdominal cramps and gas; can she have cancer this time, and how can I be sure she doesn't? And on and on each day.

The physician proceeds to answer one question after another without precision. Not knowing the numbers game, he must usually make decisions that are based on imprecise premises. But an understanding of the application of *old* mathematical concepts to *new* medical information can give added dimension to diagnostic precision.

Boole à Bayes

Of Sets, Venn, Boole, and Bayes. The so-called "new" forms of mathematics—(*a*) set theory, (*b*) symbolic logic (Venn diagrams); (*c*) Boolean algebra, and (*d*) Bayes' theorems—are not really new at all. But they can be applied to various aspects of problem solving in ways which help us think clearly, deduce logically, weigh probabilities accurately, and draw conclusions correctly.

These mathematical concepts have made substantial contributions to reasoning in clinical medicine. They make a formal structure by which precise reasoning can be applied to diagnosis, prognosis, and treatment; and they offer an ideal way to distinguish or relate multiple properties that can be present or absent, alone or in combination (2). In medical diagnosis, these concepts guide our judgment of single clues, overlap of clues, absence of a clue, importance of a clue, and how many clues make a diagnosis definite.

They have become excellent tools for the analysis of clinical presentations and the synthesis of a problem list. In short, these mathematical concepts make for a more exact way of dealing intelligently with problem solving.

A *set* is a number of items, people, diseases, etc that have at least one characteristic in common—for instance, all humans, all birds, all birds with long beaks, all patients with heart disease, all patients with heart disease who have chest pain, or all patients with chest pain. Overlap is immediately noted in reference to the latter three sets, since patients with heart disease may or may not have pain, and patients with chest pain may or may not have heart disease. The set of patients with heart disease can be subdivided into subsets of those with chest pain and those without pain. On the other hand, if the set under consideration were all patients with chest pain, the subsets could be those with and those without heart disease.

In 1880, Sir John Venn introduced a graphic method for depicting overlapping sets of related but discrete and independent variables. He used overlapping geometric forms (circles, ellipses, polyhedrons, etc) to construct what are now called *Venn diagrams.*

Boolean algebra, proposed by George Boole during the late 1800s, is an algebraic means of relating sets to subsets and expressing Venn diagrams. It employs many algebraic symbols which are peculiarly Boolean.

Bayes' theorems are old too. But they are especially applicable to modern medical logic. They are the mathematician's concept of the total statistical diagnostic experience and deal with probabilities and likelihoods of diseases and their related symptoms.

Symbols, Circles, and Lines. A discussion of *sets and set theory* must inevitably include *Boolean algebra* and *Venn diagrams*; the three modes will therefore be described side by side.

Certain symbols must be introduced: if U represents the universe of all patients with cirrhosis of the liver, then $\bar{U}$ is the Boolean notation for all patients who do not have cirrhosis. In addition, ∪ means "and," and ∩ represents the intersection of or common area between two sets. $U \cup \bar{U}$ represents all patients, since it includes those who do and those who do not have cirrhosis.

In the universe of cirrhotics we have sets A, B, and C, representing those who have ascites (A), those who bleed (B), and those who develop coma (C). We will deal only with these three sets, though there are obviously more. Evident truths would be $A \cup \bar{A} = U$, $B \cup \bar{B} = U$, and $C \cup \bar{C} = U$. For example, the universe of cirrhotics is made up entirely of those who do and those who do not have ascites. Sets can overlap, so we may have cirrhotics who both have ascites and bleed ($A \cap B$), those who have all properties ($A \cap B \cap C$), and those who have none ($\bar{A} \cap \bar{B} \cap \bar{C}$).

Now regard only set B—those who bleed. Here we have three main subsets: those who bleed from (a) varices, (b) gastritis, and (c) ulcer. Subset b can be further subdivided into those who develop gastritis from (x) alcohol, (y) aspirin, and (z) other causes. Patient Bbx is a cirrhotic who is bleeding from alcohol-induced gastritis. Subsets a and c could also be subdivided.

Thus we have derived sets, subsets, and subsubsets (objects) from within a specific universe. Various combinations and overlaps can occur. For example, we can have a patient with ascites who develops alcoholic gastritis but does not bleed. Or there is the patient in hepatic coma who is bleeding from varices and has an ulcer too.

Set relationships become more complex when three or more sets are used, but the logic still holds true. Sets can be entered into relationship either by verbal expression, by diagram, or by algebraic expression. We can apply set theory to well-known clinical situations of cirrhotics who bleed from varices, cirrhotics who bleed but do not have varices, cirrhotics who have varices and bleed but the bleeding is not from the varices, and cirrhotics with varices and ulcer who bleed from alcoholic gastritis. Then there are cirrhotics who bleed and develop coma from the bleeding. Moreover, some cirrhotics with

ascites develop encephalopathy and coma from diuretic-induced hypokalemia. It is easy to think of dozens of possible permutations, combinations, and overlaps of sets and subsets as we regard the patient with cirrhosis, or indeed the patient with any disease.

Now consider *two overlapping sets—A and B*. This immediately creates four subsets: (*1*) both A and B, (*2*) A without B, (*3*) B without A, and (*4*) neither A nor B. In Figure 5.1 these relationships are depicted by Venn diagram and Boolean notation.

But sets A and B can have other relationships which can be diagrammed, expressed by Boolean notation, or verbalized by syllogism (Fig. 5.2). Overlap has just been discussed; it is the most common set relationship with which we deal in medicine. Complete containment or subordination may also occur; one set is contained within the other. This is not so common as overlap but is frequently seen. Here all of B is in A, but not all of A is B. $B \subset A$ is Boolean notation for "all of B is included in A," and $A \supset B$ means that A contains all of B; they say the same thing.

The third relationship—completely coinciding sets—is rare. The two sets must always be seen together, and neither can occur without the other.

Venn Diagrams. These are graphic representations of sets and subsets which permit us to diagram the relationship of overlapping

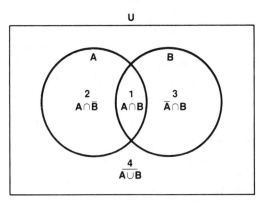

Fig. 5.1. Subsets created by two overlapping sets as expressed by a Venn diagram and Boolean notation.

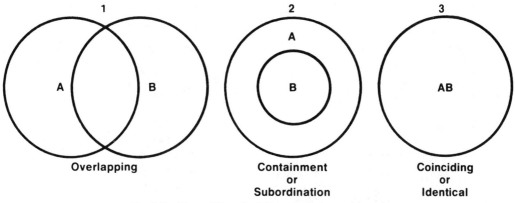

Fig. 5.2. Three different relationships between two sets.

variables. We have already seen how two sets can relate. The situation becomes more complex when there are three overlapping sets which create seven different subsets (Fig. 5.3). If all three variables, A, B, and C are needed to make a diagnosis, then only those in subset 7 would fulfill the criteria. Subsets 4, 5, and 6, in which only two of the sets overlap, might only make the diagnosis likely. The presence of only one set in a subset (1, 2, 3) might merely suggest a possibility.

For example, the three overlapping sets usually needed to diagnose Graves' disease are thyromegaly, eye signs, and tachycardia. All three should be present. A triad used to aid in the diagnosis of acute rheumatic fever might be chorea, carditis, and arthritis; one, two, or three of these might be present in a particular patient. Not all three are needed, provided other clues are present too. Thus, overlap may or may not be necessary. Three overlapping variables could easily be plotted in patients with acute myocardial infarction. These variables might be left ventricular failure, shock, and arrhythmias. In like manner, three criteria for the diagnosis, prognosis, and subsequent course of infarction could be diagrammed.

Four variables (A, B, C, D) which are sets, clues, etc, can be depicted by overlapping ellipses (Fig. 5.4). Note that 15 easily discernible subsets have been created. Each can be expressed in Boolean notation.

Four sets utilized in the diagnosis of cir-

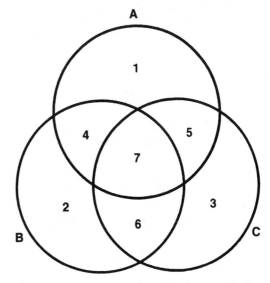

Fig. 5.3. Seven subsets created by three overlapping sets.

rhosis of the liver could be: (A) historical evidence, (B) physical signs, (C) abnormal liver function tests, (D) suggestive liver scan. Not all need be present to establish the diagnosis; in fact, several may be absent.

Consider the same diagram (Fig. 5.4), and try to think of other useful applications of four different clues which are necessary to make a diagnosis with certainty. Only those patients in subset 15 would fill these criteria. On the other hand, if only three of the clues were necessary, subsets 11, 12, 13, and 14, as well as 15, would fill the bill. The presence of only two clues in the population being

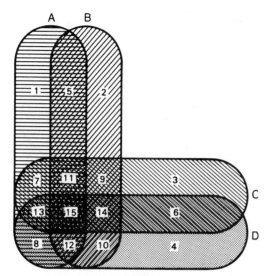

Fig. 5.4. Fifteen subsets created by four overlapping sets.

considered might merely arouse your suspicion of the disease's presence (subsets 5, 6, 7, 8, 9, 10). One clue might be negligible.

Thus, Venn diagrams may be useful in a variety of medical situations. They are good for classifying clinical manifestations of disease, especially where overlap is critical and where not all features of a disease are present in each patient. With these diagrams we can deal with clinical clusters, different types of clinical presentations, criteria for diagnosis, and clinical types of an illness. It can easily be seen how they might also be useful in the taxonomy of etiology, prognosis, clinical features, therapy, results of therapy, laboratory test reliability, and laboratory test results.

Note that *Venn diagrams are not quantitative*, though the insertion of numbers in each subset may help in this regard. For instance, the mode of presentation of 678 consecutive cases of carcinoma of the lung (2) can be diagrammed (Fig. 5.5). Cough, expectoration, and hemoptysis are some of the pulmonic features of lung cancer. Of the total number of patients, 29 presented solely because of metastatic problems such as gradual hemiplegia or backache. Systemic manifestations are common (348 patients), though they are infrequently the sole cause for seeing the doctor (14 patients); these

include weight loss, anorexia, hypertrophic pulmonary osteoarthropathy, and endocrine derangements. It is interesting to note that 40 patients were asymptomatic, and their diseases had probably been detected on routine chest x-rays.

Boolean Algebra. This is a system of algebra which can deal mathematically with sets, subsets, and Venn diagrams. Ordinary algebraic operations like addition, subtraction, multiplication, and division cannot be used. We have already learned to manage

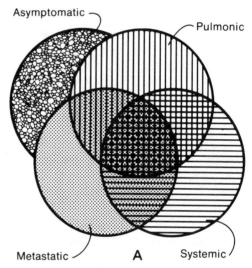

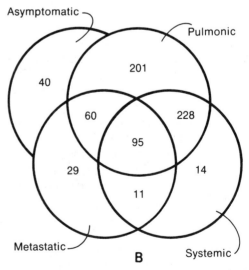

Fig. 5.5. (*A*) Varied modes of presentation in carcinoma of the lung. (*B*) Quantitation of overlapping presentations in carcinoma of the lung.

many Boolean symbols and operations such as U, A, B, C, $\cup$, $\cap$, $^-$, $\subset$, $\supset$, $=$, and $(\ )$. The parentheses and equal sign have the same meanings as in ordinary algebra.

Boolean notation serves the same purposes as sets and Venn diagrams but expresses them symbolically. It demonstrates the coexistence of combinations of clues in a patient and the presence or absence of clues. It is especially useful for processing patient data into a digital computer whose circuits are already organized according to the operational principles of Boolean algebra (2).

For example, contemplate the two overlapping sets of patients who bleed from the gastrointestinal tract (B) and patients who have proven duodenal ulcer (D) (Fig. 5.6). $D \cup B$ is the sum of all people who bleed and/or have duodenal ulcer. Four subsets are formed. $D \cap B$ is subset 1 and represents all patients who have both bleeding and ulcer. $D \cap \bar{B}$ is subset 2 and represents all patients with ulcer who do not bleed. $\bar{D} \cap B$ is subset 3 and includes all people who have gastrointestinal bleeding but do not have duodenal ulcer. Obviously only some patients with an ulcer bleed, and only some patients with bleeding have an ulcer. Subset 4 is the union of all people who neither bleed nor have ulcers and can be symbolized by $\bar{D} \cup \bar{B}$ or $\overline{D \cup B}$.

Now let us give *quantitative meaning* to some of the above notations. Suppose we have 1000 patients, of whom 98 have proven duodenal ulcer (D) and 108 have gastrointestinal bleeding (B):

$$U = 1000 \qquad D = 98 \qquad B = 108$$

Assume further that the overlap of those who have both D and B is 30. With a little thought, you can easily see the truth and logic of the following algebraic statements (n = number):

Set 1 $(D \cap B)$ is 30 *or* $n(D \cap B) = 30$
Set 2 $(D \cap \bar{B})$ is 68 *or* $n(D \cap \bar{B}) = 68$
Set 3 $(\bar{D} \cap B)$ is 78 *or* $n(\bar{D} \cap B) = 78$
Set 4 $(\bar{D} \cup \bar{B})$ is 824 *or* $n(\bar{D} \cup \bar{B}) = 824$
$U = (\bar{D} \cup \bar{B}) \cup (\bar{D} \cap B) \cup (D \cap \bar{B}) \cup$
$\qquad (D \cap B) = 1000$
$U = 824 + 78 + 68 + 30 = 1000.$

The same principles hold true for three or more discrete variables, though the algebra becomes more complicated. For example, we could consider all patients with ulcer and divide them into sets of those who bleed, perforate, obstruct, penetrate, do none of these, or combinations of these. These sets can then be qualitatively and even quantitatively expressed.

Bayes' Theorems. In 1763, Sir Thomas Bayes, a British minister and mathematician, devised a set of theorems which are mathematical expressions of statistical probabilities. His theorems relate disease prevalence and disease probability with the sensitivity, specificity, and predictive values of a test or clue. They are of great help and have done much to quantify medical judgment, but they also have serious limitations; both factors must be appreciated.

These precise old arithmetic methods have been resurrected in the past decade and applied to new methods of medical problem solving. Physicians deal with Bayes' theorems when they consider (a) the incidence of a disease in a population, (b) the incidence of a specific clue in a disease, and (c) the incidence of this clue in people who do not have the disease. Thus, the physician aims to relate individual clues or combinations of clues in order to make a specific diagnosis in a precise mathematical probabilistic fashion (3).

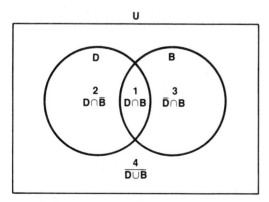

Fig. 5.6. Overlapping sets of patients who bleed (B) and patients who have duodenal ulcer (D).

Making Sense of Numbers

Prevalence and Probability. Simple Bayesian terminology must be understood before proceeding. D represents the presence of a disease, whereas $\overline{D}$ signifies the absence of a disease. C represents the presence of a clue (or the positivity of a test), whereas $\overline{C}$ signifies the absence of a clue (or the negativity of a test). P(D) symbolizes the probability that a disease is present in a given population. For example, if one person in 1000 has a disease, the P(D) or *prevalence* of the disease is .001. Diabetes mellitus has a 5% or .05 prevalence; essential hypertension has a 20%, or .20 prevalence in adults. The *prevalence* differs from the *incidence* in that the former represents the number of cases per unit of population that exists at any one time; the latter tells the number of cases that occurs per unit of population over a given period of time. They are not the same. At any one time, there may be 10 cases of influenza per 1000 people (prevalence), but the annual incidence of influenza may be 100 cases per 1000 people. On the other hand, in dealing with chronic diseases, such as diabetes mellitus, the prevalence may be .05 but the annual incidence of new cases only .005.

Not only does P(D) represent the prevalence of disease, but it has also come to signify the *probability* that a disease exists in an individual patient or in a cohort of identical patients. When we say thet the P(D) in a patient is .20, we also mean that in a cohort of 100 identical patients, 20 will have the disease and 80 will not. Given a lean patient with hypertension and dyspnea on exertion, the probability that he has left ventricular failure can be estimated at .40; the same P(D) would hold true for 100 similar patients. By the same token, there is a .60 probability estimate that he does not have heart failure—P($\overline{D}$)—since the probability that he does or does not must total 1.

Sensitivity and Specificity. Consider the following four statements about a disease and a related clue:

1. P(C/D) = .85
2. P($\overline{C}$/D) = .15
3. P($\overline{C}$/$\overline{D}$) = .95
4. P(C/$\overline{D}$) = .05

The first statement says that 85% of people with a certain disease will exhibit a stated clue. Stated differently, the clue has a *true positive (TP) rate* of .85, and the *sensitivity* of the clue (positivity in disease) is .85.

The second statement says that given the same disease the clue under discussion will be absent in 15% of cases; the *false negative (FN) rate* is therefore .15, and this is equal to 1 minus the sensitivity. Since a clue is either present or absent, the *"rule of ones"* can be readily understood.

The third statement says that 95% of people who do not have the disease under discussion do not have the clue. Those who do not have the disease in question may be healthy or have a different disease. Therefore, in 95% of those without the disease, the clue is *truly negative (TN)*; and the *specificity* of the clue, which is the TN rate, is .95.

The fourth statement falls quite naturally into place. If 95% of people who do not have the disease do not have the clue, it follows that 5% of those without the disease *do* have the clue. In these people, the clue is falsely positive (FP), and you may conclude that even in the absence of that disease, 5% of people do exhibit the clue. Note that the *false positive rate* also follows the "rule of ones"; even in the absence of the disease, the clue may or may not be present, and the *FP rate equals 1 minus the specificity.*

It follows that the TP rate plus the FN rate equals 1, and the TN rate plus the FP rate also equals 1. In the consideration just cited, if the disease is *tuberculosis* and the clue is *cough*, 85% of people with tuberculosis cough and 15% do not; 95% of people without tuberculosis do not cough, and 5% do.

Predictive Value. But in medicine we are less interested in how many people with tuberculosis will cough than in how many people with cough have tuberculosis. Put more dramatically, it is more helpful to know how likely is a person with hemoptysis to have lung cancer than to know how likely is a person with lung cancer to have hemoptysis. And how likely is a lesion not to be malignant if there is no associated hemoptysis. The doctor at the bedside wants to be able to prove a suspected diagnosis. Clearly we are now dealing with *the probability of a diagnosis given a clue* and the probability of the absence of a diagnosis given the absence of a clue—$P(D/C)$ and $P(\overline{D}/\overline{C})$. These are also called the *positive predictive value* (PV+) and the *negative predictive value* (PV−) of a clue. It follows that two other situations must exist—$P(\overline{D}/C)$ and $P(D/\overline{C})$. The first symbol represents the probability that a disease is absent even if the clue is present or positive; the second symbol represents the probability that the disease is present even if the clue is absent or negative. These are not so clinically significant as the others; the "rule of ones" applies here too, because, given a positive clue, a disease may or may not be present. Therefore $P(D/C)$ plus $P(\overline{D}/C)$ equals 1, and $P(D/\overline{C})$ plus $P(\overline{D}/\overline{C})$ equals 1 also.

If 10% of patients with hemoptysis have cancer of the lung, 90% of those with hemoptysis do not have cancer. The positive predictive value of hemoptysis for lung cancer is therefore .10 ($P(D/C) = .10$). The probability that cancer does not exist is .90 ($P(\overline{D}/C) = .90$). The calculation of predictive values is made from the prevalence or clinical probability and the sensitivity-specificity of the clue being considered; this mathematical operation will be explained shortly.

Tables and Sticks. The relationships between clues and diagnoses can be expressed by language, two-by-two (2×2) tables, Bayes' theorems, or stick diagrams. Language was the method just used. While Bayes' theorems and stick diagrams are frequently seen in medical literature, 2×2 tables are probably the easiest to understand, learn, and apply. All will be demonstrated in the following discussions.

To start, the reader must understand that

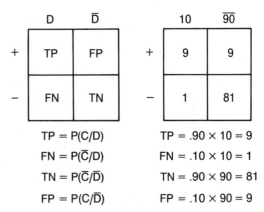

$$TP = P(C/D)$$
$$FN = P(\overline{C}/D)$$
$$TN = P(\overline{C}/\overline{D})$$
$$FP = P(C/\overline{D})$$

$$TP = .90 \times 10 = 9$$
$$FN = .10 \times 10 = 1$$
$$TN = .90 \times 90 = 81$$
$$FP = .10 \times 90 = 9$$

Fig. 5.7. 2×2 tables relating a clue to a disease.

"*test*" and "*clue*" are used interchangeably for this and subsequent related discussions. The same mathematical models may be applied to any feature in the history or physical examination, to laboratory tests, and to diagnostic procedures.

Figure 5.7 shows the results obtained in each cell of a 2×2 table where a clue is either positive or negative in the presence or absence of a disease. Inspect the left half and note the derivation of TP, FN, TN, and FP (true positive, false negative, true negative, and false positive). Then study the right side of the diagram where numbers are substituted for symbols. This represents a hypothetical case where the disease probability is .10 and the clue's sensitivity and specificity for that disease are both .90. A patient with a 10% likelihood of having a disease is represented schematically by 100 identical cases of whom 10 will have the disease and 90 will not. Calculations of the exact TP, FN, TN, and FP values are made on this basis. Of the 10 patients with the disease, 90% will evidence a positive clue; thus there will be 9 TPs and 1 FN. Of the 90 patients who do not have the disease, the clue will be absent or negative in 90%, and there will therefore be 81 TNs and 9 FPs.

Note also that there are 18 positive results in 100 patients; 9 of the 18 are truly positive. This means that the predictive value of a positive clue (PV+) is 50%, and that a positive clue in this case raises the likelihood of disease from 10% to 50%. In addition, note that there are 82 negative results, of which 81 are truly negative. This means that the predictive value of a negative clue (PV−) is approximately 99%, and a negative clue in this case reduces the likelihood of disease from 10% to 1% (or increases the *unlikelihood* from 90% to 99%).

As was just demonstrated, the predictive value (PV) of a test will vary with the initially estimated disease probability—P(D). Had the disease probability been 50%, the PV+ would have been 90% and the PV− also 90% (Fig. 5.8). Note that the PV+ equals the ratio of TPs to the total number of positive tests (TPs plus FPs); the PV− equals the ratio of TNs to the total number of negative tests (TNs plus FNs). It can be seen that the higher the P(D), the higher will be the resulting PV+, and the lower will be the resulting PV−.

These interdependent variables—P(D), PV+, and PV−—can be accurately graphed, assuming that the sensitivity and specificity remain constant for the test being applied (Fig. 5.9).

When a test is performed on a patient with an estimated pretest P(D), *the resultant PV becomes the posttest P(D)*. The difference between the pretest P(D) and the posttest P(D) is equal to the incremental gain (or loss) in the probability that the disease is present.

Study the figure and note how the P(D) is altered by a positive or negative test. If the

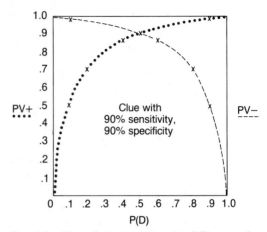

initial P(D) is low, a positive test increases the disease likelihood; a negative test diminishes the likelihood and confirms the low probability. If the initial P(D) is high, a positive test merely confirms the disease's presence and increases its likelihood only a little. The test may sometimes not even be worth doing. But if it is *unexpectedly* negative, the disease likelihood is greatly diminished.

These well-known clinical truisms are borne out by further careful inspection of Figure 5.9. The greatest incremental gain in disease probability—the difference between the pretest P(D) and the posttest P(D)—results from a *positive* test when the initial P(D) is in the .10 to .50 range. The greatest decremental fall in disease probability—the difference between the pretest P(D) and the posttest P(D)—results from a *negative* test when the initial P(D) is in the .50 to .90 range.

For example, if the pretest P(D) is .10, a positive test raises the disease probability (PV+ or posttest P(D)) to .50 and a negative test reduces the disease probability to .01 (PV− is .99). If the pretest P(D) is .50, a positive test results in a new P(D) of .90; a negative test reduces the P(D) to .10 (PV− is .90). And if the pretest P(D) is .90, a positive test raises the disease probability to .99, not a great change; a negative test reduces the P(D) to .50, a substantial reduc-

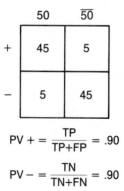

$$PV + = \frac{TP}{TP+FP} = .90$$

$$PV - = \frac{TN}{TN+FN} = .90$$

Fig. 5.8. Calculation of predictive values.

tion. By regarding the slopes of each curve, you can see that the greatest impact of a positive test occurs when the P(D) is between .10 and .50. The greatest jolt of a negative test results when the initial P(D) is between .50 and .90.

The Operating Characteristics. Although this concept has been previously mentioned and will be expanded later in this chapter and in Chapter 6, it will be reintroduced here. The operating characteristics of a clue, test, or diagnostic procedure are its two most important features—*sensitivity* and *specificity.* They have a profound influence on the overall usefulness and predictive value of the clue, test, or procedure.

The higher the sensitivity and specificity, the better the procedure, and the more effect it will have on the diagnostic probability. *Test efficiency* is measured by the sum of the sensitivity and specificity divided by 2. If the sensitivity is .90 and the specificity is .90, then the test efficiency is 1.8/2.0 or 90%. This is a "decent" test, clue, or procedure. If the sensitivity and specificity total 1.0, the efficiency is 1.0/2.0 or 50%; this is a worthless test, and it will have no effect on the initial probability.

Do a series of simple studies yourself and see that this statement is true. Assume the initial P(D) is .10; apply varied sensitivities and specificities that total 1 (.40 and .60; .50 and .50; .30 and .70; .60 and .40); then calculate the PV+ based on these figures. The calculations all determine that the PV+ or P(D) resulting from the application of the test is the same as the original P(D). The PV− of a negative test is the same as the initial P(D̄). No benefit is derived from a test of this type.

But if a test raises the probability of disease from .10 to .60 or from .30 to .90, it is a good test. Likewise, if it reduces the probability from .30 to .01 or from .60 to .01 by virtue of being negative, it is also very helpful. The matter boils down to the degree of positivity and negativity you seek before making a further decision.

How to Derive the S and S. We have spoken repeatedly of *sensitivity* and *specific-*

ity, and their application to the P(D) in a 2×2 diagram. Now let's explain where these values are obtained, whether they can vary, and how they help the diagnostic process.

The sensitivity of a clue for a disease is its *true positivity* (true positive rate or TP). The specificity of a clue for a disease is its *true negativity* (true negative rate or TN). These operating characteristics of the clue or test are obtained as follows. Select a population known with absolute certainty to *have* a disease, and a population known with absolute certainty to *not have* that disease. This degree of certainty can be attained only by a biopsy, surgery, or arteriography, though doubt exists as to the absoluteness of even these tests. Assume then that we have performed coronary arteriography upon 1000 men with chest pain of various types. Assume further that arteriography is able to separate those with and those without "significant" coronary disease according to predetermined criteria of cross-sectional narrowing. Such a perfect test is commonly called a "gold standard test". As a result of these tests, it is determined that 600 men do and 400 men do not have significant coronary disease.

Now apply a *new test* to this cohort so that you may evaluate its performance and determine its sensitivity and specificity. The test is inexpensive, noninvasive, seems fairly reliable, and you wish to establish its operating characteristics for future clinical use. Criteria for positivity and negativity are decided, and the test is performed on both groups. Results are seen in Figure 5.10. Of those with proven coronary disease, 540 had a positive test (TP) and 60 had a negative test (FN). Therefore the sensitivity of the test is 540 divided by 600, or .90. In men without coronary disease there were 320 negative results (TN) and 80 positive results (FP). Therefore the specificity of the test is 320 divided by 400, or .80.

Knowing the operating characteristics of the test, you can now apply it to any individual who needs further study and for whom you can form a fairly reliable clinical estimate of disease probability.

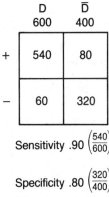

Sensitivity .90 $\left(\frac{540}{600}\right)$

Specificity .80 $\left(\frac{320}{400}\right)$

Fig. 5.10. Determining the operating characteristics of a new test.

Applying the S and S. A 36-year-old man consults you for vague chest pain which has been intermittently present for 3 days. He smokes heavily, his father died of a heart condition at age 42, and the patient is most apprehensive. The pain does not sound like coronary pain, but you're not sure. Aside from the blood pressure of 160/94, his examination is normal. So is the ECG. You assign him a clinical P(D) of only .10 and perform the special new test. Executing the test on a cohort of 100 patients with the same picture would produce the 2×2 table seen in Figure 5.11. The PV+ is .33, less than you might think, because the original P(D) was low. A positive test would increase the likelihood only a little, but a negative test would rule out the disease with 99% certainty. The test is negative.

The same man consults you 10 years later. His pain is different and more closely resembles angina though it is still not typical. Everything else is the same. A serum cholesterol is 350 mg/dl. You revise the P(D) to .40 and do another test. A positive test increases the P(D) to .75, and a negative test reduces it to .08 (Fig. 5.12). Depending on the results in either instance, you might give reassurance with caution, treat medically, or do arteriography in contemplation of surgery, considering all the other factors that go into the decision. Remember that a test has little value if its PV+ is little more than the existing P(D), and, as stated earlier, note

that the PV+ increases and the PV− decreases by an amount that depends on the originally estimated P(D).

Can the S and S Change? Bear in mind that the operating characteristics of a test never vary once established—or almost never vary. But there are instances where sensitivity and specificity may be varied by altering the criteria of abnormality. If 3 mm rather than 2 mm of ST segment depression is the requisite for a positive exercise tolerance test, the sensitivity is decreased and the specificity is increased. (The implications of this maneuver will be explained later in this chapter.) Other factors, such as whether dig-

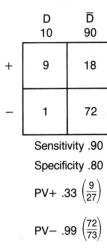

Sensitivity .90

Specificity .80

PV+ .33 $\left(\frac{9}{27}\right)$

PV− .99 $\left(\frac{72}{73}\right)$

Fig. 5.11. Changing the probabilities by a test with known operating characteristics.

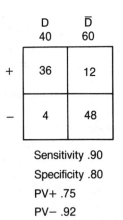

Sensitivity .90

Specificity .80

PV+ .75

PV− .92

Fig. 5.12. Alteration of probabilities when the P(D) is more likely.

italis is being taken and the population sub-set under consideration, may also alter the sensitivity and specificity of this test.

The operating characteristics of a purified protein derivative skin test will vary with the criteria for positivity. So will the operating characteristics of a hypertensive pyelogram that seeks renal vascular ischemia; it de-pends on whether you require one, two, or three abnormalities to declare positivity. The operating characteristics of serum transam-inases to detect viral hepatitis are altered if the patient is alcoholic too. The stage or severity of a disease being tested, the pres-ence of coexisting diseases, the gender of the patient, and other patient-specific features may also cause changes.

Pas de Deux

The varied and complex interrelationships between a clue and a disease can be com-pared to the intricate related movements of two ballet dancers.

Diagrams give a more readily understand-able concept of the relationships of sensitiv-ity, specificity, clue, and disease (Fig. 5.13). These four graphic representations portray the various relationships (*a, b, c, d*) that exist between a *disease* and a *clue* for that disease. Read the following statements carefully, study the diagrams, and understand the cor-relations, for they are important at the bed-side.

In (*a*) you see a clue which is *100% sen-sitive* for a disease. The clue is always but not only found in the disease. Sometimes it occurs in people who do not have the dis-ease, in which case it is falsely positive (FP = C/D̄). Note that while there are FPs, TPs, and TNs, there can be no FNs. There-fore, if the clue is absent or negative, it must be a TN, and the disease can be *absolutely ruled out*.

(*b*) shows a clue which is *100% specific* for a disease. It is always negative or absent in the absence of the disease, and it is only but not always found in the presence of that disease. While some persons with the disease may not exhibit the clue, it is never present

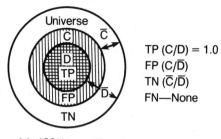

(a) 100% sensitive clue;
     no false negatives

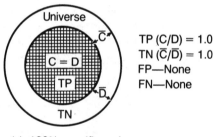

(b) 100% specific clue;
     no false positives

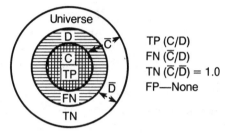

(c) 100% specific and
     100% sensitive clue;
     no false results

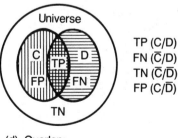

(d) Overlap;
     four subsets exist

Fig. 5.13. Relations between a disease and a clue.

or positive in persons who do not have the disease. No FPs exist; if the clue is positive, it must be a TP, and the disease is therefore *diagnosed with absolute certainty.*

Clues that are 100% sensitive or 100% specific are not common. Even more uncommon is the clue that is *both 100% sensitive and 100% specific.* This is a utopian clue, a "gold standard" clue, an ideal clue! Such a clue might be exemplified by a properly obtained, carefully examined biopsy, but even this on rare occasion may be misleading. Figure 5.13(*c*) represents such a clue. The clue is *always and only* present or positive in the disease, and there can be no FPs or FNs. *If positive, the disease exists; if negative, it does not.*

The fourth representation (*d*) is the usual situation seen in medicine. The clue is *often* but *not always* positive in the presence of disease, and is *sometimes* but *not often* positive in the absence of disease. Clearly there is an overlap, and therefore there are TPs, FNs, TNs, and FPs. As the ellipses approximate each other and overlap more and more, the clue becomes more sensitive and more specific and approaches but never reaches the ideal situation. The more sensi-

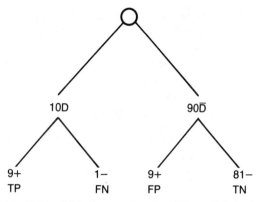

Fig. 5.15. Stick diagram denoting .90 sensitivity and .90 specificity of a clue for a disease. Let P(D) = .10.

tive the clue, the less the FNs; the more specific the clue, the less the FPs. Such clues give relative but not absolute support in making a diagnosis.

Instead of using Venn diagrams, the same four situations can be simply represented by 2×2 tables. Assume the disease probability is .10, and 10 people have the disease and 90 do not. (*a*), (*b*), (*c*), and (*d*) in Figure 5.14 tell the same story, denote the relationships between a clue and a disease, and demonstrate that the same conclusions can be drawn therefrom.

The matter of *stick diagrams* is easy to explain at this point. They can portray the same relationships and are preferred by some authors and teachers. Only one representative diagram is shown (Fig. 5.15). It demonstrates the same circumstances seen in Figure 5.14(*d*).

It is important that patients as well as doctors understand the *concept of imperfect information,* and that they do not have the false perception that a test which is positive or negative concludes the story.

Where to Draw the Line. Until now we have dealt only with dichotomous tests and clues which are either positive or negative, or present or absent. But other tests show a linear distribution of values, and a cutoff point between normality and abnormality must be established. The ideal test of this type clearly separates health from disease and is illustrated by Figure 5.16 where there

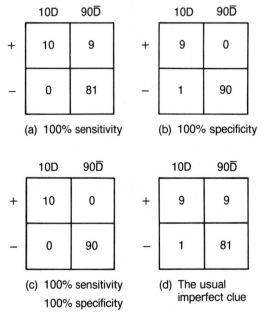

Fig. 5.14. Relations between a disease and a clue as expressed by 2×2 tables.

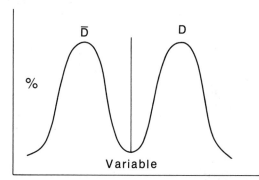

Fig. 5.16. Distribution of values for the ideal test. No overlap is present and there are no false results.

is no overlap of values; consequently there are neither false positive nor false negative results.

Unfortunately, such tests are rare or nonexistent. The usual situation is depicted in Figure 5.17 where there is an overlap of values between healthy people and those with a disease. In fact, this diagram aptly describes the situation that is seen with serum uric acid levels in normals and in patients with gout. The overlap of values between 5 and 8 mg/dl determines that some normals have what is regarded as elevated serum uric acid (FP), while some patients with gout have normal serum uric acid (FN). The cutoff point determines the incidence of false negativity and false positivity. If the separator is set at 6.5 mg/dl (c) the FN and FP rates are about equal.

However, by moving the cutoff point to the left (from c to b to a), all patients with gout will have a positive or abnormal test result. In so doing, the sensitivity of the test has been markedly increased; but this was done at the expense of decreasing the specificity since many normal people will now have "abnormal" serum uric acids.

Similarly, if the cutoff point is moved to the right (from c to d to e), normal people will almost always have normal test results. The specificity of the test has been markedly increased, but the sensitivity is diminished since many more patients with gout will have normal serum uric acids according to the new separator. There are obvious trade-

offs when moving in either direction. This generalization holds for all tests.

At this point we must clarify the confusion resulting from the use of antonymous terms under varying circumstances. For example, a clue in the history or physical examination is either *present* or *absent*. A test or procedure is either *positive* or *negative* if the result is dichotomous, or it is *abnormal* or *normal* if the test result is measured by continuous variables.

Thus "cough is present but hemoptysis is absent." A test for occult blood in the stool is either positive or negative. But a chest x-ray, electrocardiogram, serum glucose, serum bilirubin, or computed tomographic liver scan is either abnormal or normal. In the interpretation of some procedures, *positive* and *abnormal*—or *negative* and *normal*—may be used interchangeably.

As ill luck would have it, some tests and procedures needing expert interpretation may yield equivocal results. They are neither positive nor negative for sure. This all-too-common occurrence causes doubt and concern for the diagnostician and compels decisions that require further actions.

ROC Curves. Because changes in the separator point alter the sensitivity and specificity of a test, these alterations can be plotted on a graph whose coordinates are the true positive rate (sensitivity) and the false positive rate (1 minus the specificity). A plot of these two related variables is called an ROC

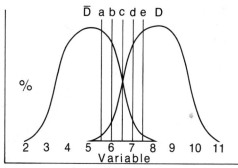

Fig. 5.17. Distribution of values for the usual test. Overlap is present. False positive and false negative results exist. Operating characteristics vary with the location of the cutoff point.

Table 5.1.
Sensitivity and Specificity of Serum Uric Acid Levels for Gout; Variation with Separator Point

Separator (mg/dl)	Sensitivity (TPs)	Specificity (TNs)	1-Specificity (FPs)
5.5	.95	.70	.30
6.0	.93	.80	.20
6.5	.88	.90	.10
7.0	.80	.95	.05
7.5	.70	.97	.03

curve (receiver-operating characteristic); this is an indicator of test performance (4).

Take the case of serum uric acid levels and gout. Assume that the specificity and sensitivity for this test referable to gout vary with the separator variable according to the data in Table 5.1. The operating characteristics of this test will vary depending on the selected separator point. When the value of 5.5 mg/dl is used, the test is highly sensitive but not very specific. The reverse is true when a level of 7.5 mg/dl is chosen. Note the operating characteristics at intervening serum uric acid levels. When the related variables (sensitivity and 1 − specificity) are plotted on a graph, the resulting curve is the ROC curve (Fig. 5.18). By convention, you plot the sensitivity (TP rate) against 1 minus the specificity (FP rate). Quite naturally, the higher the true positive rates and the lower the false positive rates the better the test. By the same token, the better the test, the higher and the more to the left the curve will be. The best test ("gold standard") will occupy the upper left corner of the graph; it will be 100% sensitive and 100% specific at essentially all separators (TP rate = 1.0; FP rate = 0).

A "good test" will proscribe a parabola whose apex approaches the upper left corner. A "fair test" will trace a parabola which is lower and approximates the 45° diagonal which is a "poor test." It is poor because the TP rate and FP rate are always equal; thus the sum of the sensitivity and specificity equals 1, the predictive value at any separator point is equal to the original P(D), and the test has added nothing. A test can there-

fore be ranked by its distance from the diagonal.

An ROC curve could just as easily be plotted by using values for the sensitivity and specificity. The curve would simply have occupied the upper right corner. Note too that according to the data in Table 5.1, the separator of 6.5 mg/dl yields the test with the *greatest efficiency* since the sum of the sensitivity and specificity is 1.78, the highest of any of the conditional separators; the test efficiency at 6.5 mg/dl is 1.78/2.00 (89%).

The decision on which separator point to use, as with any test, is made on the basis of the clinical situation, the maximal efficiency, a careful analysis of what you seek most, and what will be the outcomes and consequences of missing a disease or diagnosing one that does not exist. Knowing that your choice of a separator point will cause trade-offs between TPs and FPs, determine which is most important. If you fail to diagnose gout when it actually exists, no great harm will result. Gout would remain untreated because of a false negative test result. Other clues in the history, physical examination, and joint fluid aspiration will put

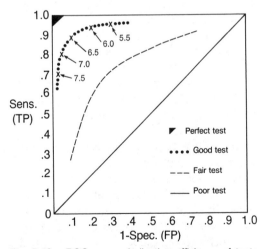

Fig. 5.18. ROC curves indicating efficiency of tests and operating characteristics at various cutoff points. The "good test" represents the data referable to the serum uric acid and gout. (Modified from Weinstein, MC, Fineberg, HV: *Clinical Decision Analysis*. Philadelphia, Saunders, 1980, 118.)

you back on the right track if the patient does not improve.

On the other hand, if, because of a false positive test result, you diagnose gout when it does *not* exist, much harm may result. The patient is treated with potentially toxic drugs, and you may fail to treat a serious disease (such as acute suppurative arthritis) that may be present.

Therefore avoid false positives as much as possible by moving the separator point to the right. Establish a higher cutoff point of 7 or 7.5 mg of uric acid/dl. The test is now less sensitive but more specific.

Such decisions and analyses must be made in determining the separator point for every test that measures continuous variables. In measuring the digoxin blood level, what is the cutoff point for digitalis toxicity? A false positive result would only cause digitalis to be withheld for a few days—not a life-threatening action. A false negative result would cause you to continue digitalis in the presence of toxicity—not a desirable strategy and possibly very harmful.

In this case, try to avoid false negative results by moving the separator point to the left. This creates a lower cutoff point for determining toxicity and makes the test more sensitive though less specific.

Consider the situation where you are trying to decide whether or not a patient has serious coronary heart disease by using a standard treadmill exercise test. The sensitivity and specificity of this test may depend on whether you regard 1.0, 1.5, 2.0, 2.5, or 3.0 mm of ST segment depression as the separator point. If 1.0 mm is used, the sensitivity will be very high and the specificity low. While almost all patients with coronary heart disease will have a positive test, so will many people without coronary disease. This can result in overdiagnosis and needless treatment, thus causing serious psychosocial problems, overutilization of the coronary catheterization laboratory, and increased patient and public expense. On the other hand, if 3.0 mm of depression is used as the cutoff point, the sensitivity is decreased and the specificity is increased. The result is that

many cases of coronary disease will be missed, and only the more serious forms (e.g. main left coronary disease) will be discovered. This too has its pros and cons. Patients with FNs (of whom there will be many) will not receive proper treatment, but those with TPs will get prompt angiography and perhaps urgently needed surgery. There will be few if any FPs. Therefore you use the separator point which is deemed most appropriate for the clinical situation and subsequent plans.

To summarize, in deciding on a separator point, consider the consequences of false negative and false positive results. The trade-offs revolve around two questions. Is it serious if the disease is missed and left untreated? Is it serious if the disease is overdiagnosed? In the final analysis, it depends on whether you wish to minimize the FP results or the FN results.

The Ways of Bayes

Explaining a Theorem. We are now in position to easily understand what Bayes was telling us over 200 years ago. One of the simplest equations for the use of Bayesian statistical inference in medical diagnosis follows (2):

$$P(D/C) = \frac{P(C/D) \cdot P(D)}{P(C)} \qquad 1.$$

This says that the probability of a disease, given the existence of a certain clue, is equal to the probability of this clue existing in the disease, multiplied by the prevalence of the disease, and divided by the total statistical incidence of this clue. Analyze each part of the equation. $P(D/C)$ is the positive predictive value of a clue, or "how likely is the suspected diagnosis, given a positive clue?" The numerator of the fraction on the right represents the sensitivity of the clue for the disease multiplied by the prevalence of disease; this is equal to the incidence of true positive clues. The denominator of the fraction represents the incidence of all positive clues (true positive and false positive). Another way of stating the same equation would be:

$$PV+ = \frac{TPs}{TPs + FPs} \qquad 2.$$

Now substitute Bayesian terminology for TPs and FPs in the denominator of equation 1. The following restated equation results:

$$P(D/C)$$

$$= \frac{P(C/D)\cdot P(D)}{P(C/D)\cdot P(D) + P(C/\overline{D})\cdot(1-P(D))} \qquad 3.$$

The incidence of false positives is gotten by multiplying the false positive rate (1 − specificity) by the probability of the disease being absent: $P(\overline{D}) = 1-P(D)$ according to the "rule of ones." Obviously a disease is either present or absent.

Knowing the P(D) and the sensitivity and specificity of the clue, the positive predictive value of the clue can now be calculated using Bayes' theorems. Assume a P(D) of .10, a sensitivity of .90, and a specificity of .80; substitute the proper values in the last equation:

$$P(D/C) = PV+$$

$$= \frac{(.90 \times .1)}{(.90 \times .1) + (.20 \times .90)} = \frac{.09}{.27} = .33$$

The probability of this patient having the disease in question has been raised from one chance in ten to one chance in three by virtue of the positive clue. The 2×2 table would have been simpler, but all three methods should be understood.

Negative or absent clues can be treated in the same way, because the predictive value of a negative clue is equal to the incidence of true negatives divided by all the negative results. By calculation and by inference, the following equation (which can easily be translated into Bayesian terms) is also true:

$$PV- = \frac{TNs}{TNs + FNs} \qquad 4.$$

Applying a Theorem. The application of Bayes' theorems to solving problems involving the use of one clue or test can be illus-

trated by many practical examples. For instance, assume the probability that 10% of people in a nursing home have congestive heart failure (CHF). Let a third heart sound (S_3) be the diagnostic clue, and it may be reasonable to state that it can be heard in 90% of those with CHF and is not heard in 95% of those without CHF. The clue is 90% sensitive and 95% specific. There will be 10% FNs and 5% FPs. Figure 5.19 considers such a cohort.

If you listen to the heart of any resident, the presence of an S_3 indicates the diagnosis of CHF with 66⅔% certainty—9 true positives out of 13.5 total positives. If an S_3 is not present, then you can be 99% certain that CHF is also not present. The negative predictive value is determined by the ratio of TNs to all the negatives (TNs plus FNs): 85.5 to 86.5.

Bear in mind that if your patient has dyspnea on exertion, orthopnea, and basal rales, you are beginning with a higher probability, e.g. .50; in this case the presence of an S_3 will have a much greater positive predictive value and will raise the likelihood of CHF to .95. Applying Bayes' theorem (equation 3) in the latter example:

$$PV+ = P(D/C)$$

$$= \frac{(.90 \times .5)}{(.90 \times .5) + (.05 \times .5)} = .95.$$

Simple Clinical Uses. Now consider clues which are 100% specific. You often hear someone say "this test is specific for that

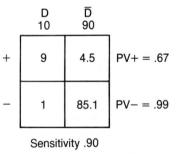

Sensitivity .90

Specificity .95

Fig. 5.19. Relationship of S_3 and congestive heart failure.

disease." The underlying logic is that the test or clue is found *only* in that disease, and if the clue is present, the disease must exist. A tophus in the ear is specific for gout. With one exception (see Chapter 3, reference 2), a Kayser-Fleischer ring is specific for Wilson's disease. Free air under the diaphragm is specific for a ruptured or perforated viscus. Few clues are completely specific. But if a clue is specific, there can be no FPs; the presence of the clue or positivity of the test has a predictive value of 1.0, and the disease is present with 100% certainty.

Neither are 100% sensitive clues common. The clue must be present in every instance of the disease, and if the clue is absent, the disease cannot exist. Albuminuria in the nephrotic syndrome, azotemia in renal failure, and tachycardia in hyperthyroidism are examples of clues which are always present when the stated diseases exist. Note how nonspecific these clues are; each can occur in many other diseases. This allows for many false positives but no false negatives. You can only venture a guess about the PV+ of each of these clues; however, the PV− is 1.0.

Let's venture for a moment into the realm of more than one clue. Suppose there are two clues for a disease, each of which has high but not 100% sensitivity. If both clues are present, the disease *may* be likely, depending on the degree of specificity of the clues. If both clues are absent, the disease is most unlikely to be present, though it is not ruled out. Suppose clue A is 90% sensitive and clue B is 80% sensitive, yet neither is present. The disease is therefore unlikely because by simple arithmetic—.90 + (.80 × .10)—98% of people with that disease have at least one of those clues present. This means that only 2% of patients with that disease would present without either symptom—a rare occurrence. The properties of combined testing will be explored in greater depth later, since physicians deal with multiple entries and must know how to combine clues into a single expression of diagnostic likelihood.

But a striking example of how a disease may exist in the *absence* of two sensitive clues can be found in a recent case study (5). Even in the absence of skin pigmentation and diabetes, the patient under discussion turned out to have hypogonadism secondary to hemochromatosis. These two absent clues are ordinarily so prominent in hemochromatosis that the disease is often called "bronzed diabetes." The clinician discussing the case stated that the patient was neither bronzed nor had diabetes, and therefore the diagnosis was unlikely. He was right, but he was wrong. According to data banks, excessive skin pigment occurs in 90% of cases and diabetes in 65%. Either one of the clues should be present in 96.5% of cases—hence the correct *clinical* conclusion. But clinical pathological conferences are frequently selected for their unusual qualities, rare manifestations, and rare diseases. Such was the case here.

More Practical Benefits. Numerous practical applications of the various principles just discussed exist in the current literature. More and more, clinical investigators—and clinicians too—are using Bayesian modifications to reach precise conclusions.

One paper discusses the use of HLA-B27 testing to increase the diagnostic probability of ankylosing spondylitis in white men (6). The test is of very little value in screening because the P(D) is so low, but in a white male who has backaches, generalized aches and pains, and a high erythrocyte sedimentation rate, the P(D) is much higher and the test is more helpful. In white men, the test is 92% sensitive if disease is present; but normal white men have a 7% false positive incidence, and the specificity is therefore 93%. Assume the P(D) in the patient just described is .50 and apply the test (Fig. 5.20). If positive, the revised probability of ankylosing spondylitis is now greater than 90%. The sensitivity of the HLA-B27 test is much lower in black men with ankylosing spondylitis, resulting in different operating characteristics and less usefulness of the test.

Contemplate the use of the fluorescent antinuclear antibody test (7). Its sensitivity in systemic lupus erythematosus is 98%; its

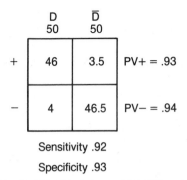

Sensitivity .92

Specificity .93

Fig. 5.20. Relationship between HLA-B27 and anky-losing spondylitis in white men.

specificity is 90%. When applied to any individual in whom the P(D) is extremely low, it is of little value because of the high number of FPs that might occur. The test has its maximal value when five clinical criteria are already present, and the P(D) is moderately high. The marginal benefit of a test is the difference between the pretest and posttest P(D)s. When the P(D) is very low or very high, the marginal benefit (incremental gain) is small; when the P(D) is intermediate, the marginal benefit (incremental gain) is greatest. This is readily demonstrable by graphing techniques (Fig. 5.13). But what these examples demonstrate is that tests are ordered with a *diagnosis already in mind.*

Regard the intersection between Bayes' theorem and the Wassermann test for syphilis (8). FPs first came to be recognized in the 1940s, when it was discovered that other diseases could give positive tests too, and more specific tests therefore came into use. Before then, anyone with a positive test and a negative history for sexual contact was regarded as a liar and treated for syphilis. The PV+ of a positive test varies with the prevalence of disease in the population being screened. In North Dakota, where the TP rate and the FP rate are the same (.03% or 30 cases per 100,000), a positive test has a PV+ of .50. In areas where the P(D) is higher, the PV+ is also higher; the FP rate remains the same, while the TP rate goes up. In the Selective Service, the TP rate was 4,530 per 100,000; the PV+ was therefore .99. In San Francisco, the TP rate is 263 per

100,000; the PV+ is .90. The same reasoning applies to a negative result. This entire paragraph centers around the question: "Given a positive Wassermann test, what are the chances that the patient has syphilis?"

In an attempt to eliminate "hedging" on some biopsy reports, it has been suggested that pathologists utilize the clinical probability to revise and quantify their final reports (9). The use of terms like "consistent with" or "cannot exclude" is difficult to deal with on a clinical basis. It is felt that the use of probabilistic reasoning combining the clinician's and pathologist's efforts will substantially improve interpretation and reporting. This holds for radiographic and imaging techniques too. But pathognomonic findings and normal findings do not need such maneuvers.

Perhaps the finest work on the subject of mathematical models for test interpretation was recently published; it should be slowly and carefully digested by all those interested in the subject (10). This should include all medical students who are beginning to deal with patients. The many examples these authors offer are impressive. An exceptionally good one deals with mammography (Fig. 5.21). Assume that the prevalence of breast cancer in women over 50 is .003 or 3 cases per 1000 women and that the mammogram is 66⅔% sensitive and 99% specific. Accordingly, the cells of the 2×2 diagram are appropriately filled. Should a patient ask you for the significance of a positive mammogram done on a routine survey, you can calm her somewhat by telling her that the

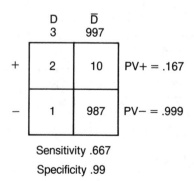

Sensitivity .667

Specificity .99

Fig. 5.21. Mammography and breast cancer.

chance of having cancer is only 16⅔%. If the test is negative, she can be 99.9% sure she doesn't have the disease. On the other hand, if her mother and sister had breast cancer, she is in a different subset, and her P(D) is more likely to be .012 than .003. In this case, a positive mammogram would have a PV+ of about .50. Note how these calculations translate into the practicalities of doctor-patient interaction.

The Prototype Problem Revisited. Now let's get back to the problem presented at the beginning of this chapter and apply the mathematical logic that has just been learned. The clinical estimate of digitalis toxicity is .50. It has already been determined in your laboratory that with a cutoff point of 2.0 ng/ml the digoxin assay is 90% sensitive and 80% specific for toxicity. The 2×2 table (Fig. 5.22) tells us that the PV+ is .82, and the PV− is .89. The assay reports 2.5 ng/ml; this is abnormal. Therefore the probability of digitalis toxicity has risen to 82%; digoxin is stopped and the patient should improve in several days, at which time he will start on a smaller dose. Had the digoxin assay shown normal values (e.g. 1.5 ng/ml), the probability of digitalis toxicity would have fallen to 11% (i.e. $P(\bar{D})$ = .89). In this instance, progressive heart disease or another underlying disease, such as cancer, would have to be considered.

The operating characteristics of this test are as just stated. But they could be altered by changing the cutoff point, by abnormal fluctuations of serum potassium or calcium,

Table 5.2.
The Revision of Disease Likelihoods by a Positive Clue

Disease	P(D)	P(C/D)	P(D/C)
D_1	0.20 (200 pts*)	0.10 (20 pts)	0.80
D_2	0.01 (10 pts)	0.50 (5 pts)	0.20

* patients.

by the testing procedure, or even by the nature of the underlying heart disease.

From all that has just been said, an important conclusion to be drawn is that most information we receive about patients is imperfect. And this *concept of imperfect information* applies to historical data, physical diagnosis, and almost all the tests we do. This includes the venerable blood count, blood gases, and blood chemical studies, and ranges all the way up to cytology and complex imaging techniques.

Revision of Likelihoods. So far we have seen how a positive or negative clue or test can revise the likelihood of a disease being present or absent. But what if the resolution must be made between *two disease probabilities* (D_1 and D_2) by the clue or test (C). Here too we apply simple Bayesian logic. Clue C is present *only* in two diseases, D_1 and D_2, and is not found in nondisease ($\bar{D}$). D_1 is common and occurs in 20% of a given set of 1000 people. D_2 is uncommon and occurs in only 1% of that set (Table 5.2). Therefore 200 people have D_1 and 10 people have D_2. Clue C is uncommon in D_1 (10% incidence) and common in D_2 (50% incidence). Thus 20 people with D_1 have C, and 5 people with D_2 have C. A total of 25 people will have C, so if C is found to be present in a particular patient, there is an 80% chance the patient has D_1 and only a 20% chance that he has D_2.

Assuming that C is a major diagnostic determinant, note how the incidence of C alters the probabilities of D_1 and D_2. In the presence of C, D_1 could be more likely, as likely, or less likely than D_2, depending on the P(D) and P(C/D) for each disease.

Table 5.2 shows how an uncommon manifestation of a common disease can be more

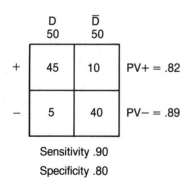

	D 50	$\bar{D}$ 50	
+	45	10	PV+ = .82
−	5	40	PV− = .89

Sensitivity .90

Specificity .80

Fig. 5.22. Solving the prototype problem of digitalis toxicity.

common than a common manifestation of an uncommon disease.

A revision of probabilities may also be accomplished by a normal or negative test. Regard another form of the practical application of Bayes' theorems. Suppose a clinician decides that a patient with a given cluster has a 75% likelihood of having disease D_1 and a 25% likelihood of having disease D_2. A further diagnostic procedure (x-ray, scan, laboratory test) is done, and the result is negative. The fact that it is negative may give much useful information (11). A negative test does not simply make a disease less likely; it may make another possibility more likely and must be weighed on a balance of clinical judgment.

The pathologist or radiologist (the test expert) tells us that this test is negative in 20% of patients with D_1 and in 60% of patients with D_2. In a cohort of 100 patients with this given cluster there will be 30 negative results: 15 in D_1 and 15 in D_2. Therefore, given a negative result, the revised likelihoods of D_1 and D_2 are 50%–50% (Table 5.3).

Knowing the likelihoods of diseases in a clinical situation and knowing the incidence of positivity and negativity for subsequent diagnostic procedures in each of these diseases, this type of mathematical logic can alter likelihoods when a procedure has a positive result or a negative result. The same mathematical logic applies when dealing with a multiplicity of disease likelihoods or a multiplicity of diagnostic procedures, although the computations may be more extensive.

For example, on the basis of clinical evidence you decide a patient has a 50%–25%–

25% chance of having pulmonary tuberculosis, cancer, or sarcoidosis, in that order. The results of a purified protein derivative skin test, fiberoptic bronchoscopy, and laminograms alter the computed likelihoods to 5%–5%–90%. A good physician performs these calculations many times daily, though he uses quick mental maneuvers instead of precise figures and formulas.

Given correct statistical data, formulas and equations can be written for all combinations and probabilities. For instance, in the presence of three clues and the absence of a fourth, how likely is a diagnosis? Physicians approximate such statistics and probabilities many times daily as they solve their patients' problems, without writing equations for Bayes' theorems—indeed, without being aware of their existence.

Confronted by a 65-year-old man with crampy abdominal pains and bright red blood in the stool for 2 weeks, the physician finds a constricting lesion in the descending colon by barium enema. He might have predicted it even before seeing the x-ray. Carcinoma of the colon is a frequent serious diagnostic consideration in 65-year-olds. The two symptoms stated are common in left-sided colon carcinomas and together are uncommon in other diseases. The odds are therefore high that the patient has carcinomas of the descending colon, even before the corroborative x-ray is taken. Absence of tenderness is against diverticulitis, which might be a close contender.

Why "Cushing's" Is Rare. A further example of Bayesian bedside logic! I have searched for Cushing's disease in all my obese female patients and have found only one case in 35 years. The following statistics tell me why. Consider the universe of all women between 30 and 60 years of age. Assume that the figures shown in Table 5.4 are approximately correct and that the criteria for establishing the presence of the clues have been met. A patient in this age group who had these four clues should be more likely to have Cushing's disease than not. But note that these clues are relatively common in non-Cushing's disease too. Also re-

Table 5.3.
The Revision of Disease Likelihoods by a Negative Clue

Disease	Initial Likelihood	Negative Test per Cohort of 100 Pts*	Revised Likelihood
D_1	75%	20% = 15 pts	50%
D_2	25%	60% = 15 pts	50%

* patients.

Table 5.4.
Incidence of Clues in a Population Subset with and without Cushing's Disease

Clue	Cushing's Disease	Non-Cushing's Disease
Hypertension	.40	.20
Obesity	.90	.30
Diabetes	.88	.08
Hirsutism	.50	.10

member that in the universe of 30- to 60-year-old women Cushing's disease has an approximate incidence of 1 per 100,000 (0.00001).

If the four clues stated in Table 5.4 were independent of each other, by the law of the *product of probabilities* (see p. 90), all four clues would be seen together in .16 or 16% of the cases of Cushing's disease (.40 × .90 × .88 × .50). But there must be some mutual interdependence since a high cortisol level is the pathophysiologic mechanism underlying much of what is seen. However, even with *maximal* interdependence, the combined incidence of all four clues in Cushing's disease cannot exceed the clue with the lowest sensitivity (.40). Therefore, when all four clues are seen together, the tetrad has a combined sensitivity ranging between .16 and .40.

On the other hand, in the absence of Cushing's disease there is no or possibly only slight interdependence. All four clues can be seen together with a *coincidental* concurrence rate of .00048 (.20 × .30 × .08 × .10)—5 women per 10,000, or perhaps a few more in order to account for some interdependence.

Since the prevalence of Cushing's disease is .00001, for each 100 cases of Cushing's disease, there will be slightly fewer than 10,000,000 women who do not have the disease. Of those with the disease, between 16 and 40 will have all four clues; compare this with the 5,000 women who have the four clues in the absence of Cushing's disease (5 per 10,000). It becomes readily evident that, given these four clues, the likelihood of Cushing's disease is at most one in a hundred and probably far less.

This is why so many women with these four clues turn out to be obese, hirsute women with diabetes and hypertension, not Cushing's disease. The solution to the problem—"given a set of clues, how likely is the diagnosis?"—is often managed "intuitively" in this manner.

Why "Cancer" Is Common. Visualize a population subset of 50- to 60-year-old men for whom coal mining is the job, cigarette smoking is the pleasure, and cough is almost the rule. Try to relate these men statistically to cancer of the lung. In Table 5.5, approximations of P(D), P($\overline{D}$), and the sensitivities for each clue are stated. The prevalence of cancer is .05; 95% do not have cancer. Note that the four stated clues occur to a much lesser degree in those without cancer, but they *do* occur. At a quick glance it can be seen that a 60-year-old smoking miner who has all four clues given in the table has a much greater possibility of having cancer of the lung than did the previously discussed lady of having Cushing's disease. The P(D) is much higher, and the incidences of the four clues in $\overline{D}$ are much lower. Such conclusions can be easily deduced using logic and common sense, but they can also be expressed by complex derivations of Bayes' theorems and the application of rules governing independent and interdependent variables.

The *mini-max* probabilities of all four clues occurring in lung cancer are .013 (.85 × .20 × .75 × .10) if the clues have virtually no interdependence to .10 (the clue with the least sensitivity) if the clues have maximal interdependence. In the event that there is maximal interdependence, we must assume

Table 5.5.
Incidence of Clues in a Population Subset with and without Carcinoma of the Lung

Clue	Cancer P(D) = .05	No Cancer P($\overline{D}$) = .95
Cough	.85	.35
Hemoptysis	.20	.01
Weight loss	.75	.05
Clubbing	.10	.01

Table 5.6.
Likelihood Ratios Determined by Prevalence, TPs, FPs, and Degree of Interdependence

4 Clues +	Cancer 5 Patients	No Cancer 95 Patients	Likelihood Ratio D:$\bar{\text{D}}$
Independent	TPs (5×.013) .065	FPs (95×.175 × 10⁻⁵) .00017	400:1
Maximally interdependent	TPs (5×.1) .5	FPs (95×.01) .95	1:2

that clubbing always occurs together with the other three clues, certainly not an absolutely valid assumption. If the person does not have lung cancer yet has these four clues, either another disease exists or there may be a combination of problems which may or may not have a common substrate. The possibility that all four clues can occur in the absence of lung cancer is .00000175 (.35 × .01 × .05 × .01) or .000175%. The figure may be as high as .01 if there is maximal interdependence of clues. As stated, the P(D) is .05, and the incidence of TPs and FPs for the existence of all four clues can be calculated. When this is done, the likelihood ratio of cancer:no cancer for people with all four clues is 400:1 if the clues are totally independent and 1:2 if the clues are maximally interdependent for both D and $\bar{\text{D}}$ (Table 5.6). Somewhere between these two extremes is the correct likelihood. In any event, cancer of the lung probably exists if the four clues are present.

The Nays of Bayes

Its Limited Utilities. Bayesian logic has great value in solving medical problems. But it has its limitations too because statistics and incidences of clues and diseases often differ. While in a deck of cards you know the exact probability of picking a red card, a heart, a court card, or a red seven, it is *not so for medicine.* Here ideal precision is rarely possible, since medicine itself—diseases, incidences, and clues—is not precise.

The preceding section on Boolean algebra dealt with the relation between ulcer and gastrointestinal bleeding. If the exact incidence of ulcer, bleeding with ulcer, and bleeding without ulcer were known, the statistical likelihood in a specific case might be calculable. But such figures are seldom available; they vary from physician to physician, hospital to hospital, one geographical location to another, and one decade to another.

Diagnostic procedures vary in their negativity or positivity depending on the quality of equipment, the technique of performance, the skill of the operator, and the population sample being tested. This holds true for a simple serum uric acid as well as for complex endoscopic or imaging procedures.

While statistics about the incidence and clues for Cushing's disease and hyperthyroidism are uniform in different series, many other diseases vary in this regard. Sarcoidosis is one example. Its incidence is not known since so many cases remain asymptomatic or undiagnosed. Quantitative data regarding clues vary with who sees the patient first— the dermatologist, pulmonologist, ophthalmologist, rheumatologist, hematologist, or generalist. Figures from a sarcoidosis clinic should be most reliable, but these too can be skewed because undiagnosed and "simple to treat" cases might be managed elsewhere.

Look at the incidence of various clues in paratyphoid fever. First of all, the occurrence of the disease is quite variable. Five different series of cases (12) compare the incidence of specific clues: diarrhea ranges from 14 to 68%, cramps from 29 to 97%, enlarged spleen from 2 to 74%, and rose spots from 2 to 50%.

Another reason for lack of precision in the application of probability theory is the inability to define a disease clearly. Criteriology for diagnosis is in its infancy. Except for acute rheumatic fever, rheumatoid arthritis, and disseminated lupus erythematosus, there are no fixed criteria for diagnosis. Diseases are described but not clearly defined so as to eliminate all other possibilities. This holds for common problems like ulcer, hypertension, diabetes, and angina, as well as for less common ones like Crohn's disease. No wonder the incidence of regional enteritis varies so from one center to another!

Bedside Hazards. The hazards of bedside Bayes (13) are nicely demonstrated by reviews of many diagnostic procedures performed in various medical centers; significant variability was found in the sensitivity and specificity of supposedly reliable tests. Four or five published studies for seven commonly used tests were compared. Included were the exercise stress ECG, lung perfusion scan, gallbladder ultrasound, lymphangiography for Hodgkin's disease, and xeromammography for breast cancer. "Gold standard" tests were performed first. Then the test being evaluated was applied. The results showed significant differences in operating characteristics between various studies in almost all instances, and the tests were therefore considered not satisfactory. A few tests such as postexercise thallium scanning for coronary disease and rapid sequence intravenous pyelogram for renal artery stenosis were felt to be satisfactory because no significant differences were found in various studies ($P > .05$).

Therefore those who rely on Bayesian methods for making decisions may be depending on test data which are not reliable and possibly not even obtainable. Furthermore, when many separate bits of information must be applied, the mathematics and formulas become complicated and unwieldy at the bedside. This is especially true when the interdependence of separate items is not known—usually the case.

Adding by Multiplication

Combination Testing. The concept of the effects of multiple pieces of information on the diagnostic process has already been introduced. Not all historical, physical, and laboratory clues need to be present in any single instance. So in testing for the presence of a disease, we commonly do more than one test or procedure, hoping to become more and more certain with each positive or abnormal result. This approach may be *a help or a hindrance*, and the outcomes must be carefully measured.

For example, you suspect gallstones in a 55-year-old woman with recurrent right upper quadrant pains and consider doing a cholecystogram, ultrasound, or computed scan. Then there's the patient with suspected cirrhosis of the liver; do liver function tests, a nuclear scan, or a biopsy. For the 50-year-old man with suspected angina pectoris, you wonder about a simple ECG, ECG with stress, ECG with stress and thallium scanning, or coronary arteriography. In each instance, is one procedure enough? Which is best? Are two tests better than one? Are three better than two? What if one test is positive and the next is negative? Two positive and one negative? Suppose the first is negative; should a second be done at all? How likely is the disease to begin with, and what degree of diagnostic certainty must we achieve? All these questions arise frequently as you enter the *domain of multiple testing.* This subject will be expanded in the next chapter, but since many of the answers revolve around mathematical computations, it is being discussed here first.

Interdependence of Clues. Assume there are two important clues (A and B) existing in a disease (D). Each clue is found in 50% of cases of D. This does not mean that the two clues must necessarily be found in the same patient or in all patients with the disease. Various relationships may exist (Fig. 5.23).

The first situation (*a*) indicates that the two clues are *never seen together.* This is mentioned as only one of many theoretical possibilities, though it is in effect an impossible happening and is not seen in clinical medicine. It is not logical that two important clues for a disease be mutually exclusive.

The second situation (*b*) wherein two

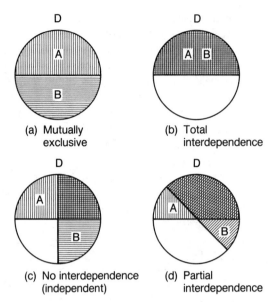

(a) Mutually
exclusive

(b) Total
interdependence

(c) No interdependence
(independent)

(d) Partial
interdependence

Fig. 5.23. Degrees of interdependence of clues A and B in disease D.

clues are *always seen together*, one never without the other, is quite possible, though not seen with great frequency. It represents total interdependence.

The third situation (c) and the fourth situation (d) are the ones most commonly seen. Our discussion will dwell primarily on these. If the two clues are mutually independent (c) there is no interdependence, and the *presence or absence of one clue has nothing to do with the other.* This situation occurs frequently. If 50% of patients with D have clue A, then 50% of those with A will also have clue B. Therefore only 25% of patients with D will have both A and B. The probability of both clues existing together is equal to the product of the individual probabilities (.50 × .50 = .25).

To exemplify and clarify this important point further, if clue A is present in 90% of cases and clue B is present in 80% of cases and there is no interdependence, then *both A and B will be present in 72% of cases.* Only 80% of the 90% with A will also have B (.90 × .80 = .72). But recall that 80% of the 10% who do not have A will also have B. Therefore *either A or B will be present in 98% of cases.* The sensitivity of the coexist-

ence of both clues has diminished while the specificity has increased. If it is established that both clues A and B must be present for D to exist, then the absence of either one will negate the diagnosis and indicate a state of nondisease (98% specific).

The last situation (d) is most common. The pathophysiologic abnormality underlying a disease often creates a degree of *interdependence among clues.* For example, high cortisol levels cause most of the manifestations of Cushing's disease, and it is easily understandable that clues would occur with some interdependence. The *circle* in Figure 5.23 (d) has been drawn so that the degree of interdependence may be varied by rotating the *semicircle* of B around the center of the *circle.* Thus the degree of interdependence can vary from none (c) to all (b). Obviously, the precise location of *semicircles* in (d) lies somewhere between (c) and (b), and the limits can be calculated (see Table 5.7).

Note that values for (d) always lie somewhere between those in (b) and those in (c). The degree of interdependence which varies from *none to all* is the determining factor. When dealing with three or more clues, the same relationships apply but the calculations become more complex.

Comparing Likelihoods. Suppose four clues are associated with a disease according to the frequencies cited in Table 5.8. These clues are also seen as FPs in the stated amount. Note that the concurrence of all clues (Σ) ranges from .04 to .4 depending on

Table 5.7.
Varying Degrees of Interdependence for Two Clues (A and B) in a Disease (D)*

	(b)	(c)	(d)
A	.5	.5	.5
B	.5	.5	.5
Only A	0	.25	0–.25
Only B	0	.25	0–.25
Both A and B	.5	.25	.25–.5
Either A or B	.5	.75	.5–.75
Neither A nor B	.5	.25	.25–.5

* Decimal tabulations are derived from situations (b), (c), and (d) in Figure 5.23.

Table 5.8.
Diagnostic Likelihoods in the Presence and Absence of Four Clues

+	D	$\bar{D}$
C_1	.5	.05
C_2	.4	.04
C_3	.5	.05
C_4	.4	.04
Σ	.04–.4	.000004

$D:\bar{D} = 100,000:1$ or $10,000:1$
If $P(D) = .10$, $D:\bar{D} = >1,000:1$
If $P(D) = .01$, $D:\bar{D} = >100:1$
If $P(D) = .001$, $D:\bar{D} = >10:1$

the degree of interdependence. The concurrence of all clues (Σ) in the absence of disease is .000004 or $.4 \times 10^{-5}$ since no interdependence may be assumed. If all four clues are present, the likelihood ratio of $D:\bar{D}$ is between 10^4 and $10^5:1$. If the disease prevalence is .10, $D:\bar{D} = >10^3:1$ and so forth as noted in the table. Given a $P(D)$ of only .001, the disease is 10 to 100 times as likely to be present as not. Even if one clue is absent, the likelihood is reduced by a factor of only 10 and its absence is therefore not that significant. If two clues are absent, the disease exists with only moderate certainty. In the example being cited, the high specificity of each clue seems to be a greater diagnostic determinant than the moderately high sensitivity. Recall that the FP rate is equal to 1 minus the specificity.

Estimating the Likelihood. As has been previously discussed, $P(D)$ means the *prevalence* of a disease or the probability that it is present in a particular patient based on the clinical evidence on hand. The $P(D)$ changes as each new bit of evidence is added.

It is surprising to note that physicians, given only the barest of clues, show only little or modest differences in their original estimates of disease likelihood. Consider a 34-year-old woman with polyarthritis, a 26-year-old woman with periodic dyspnea at rest, a 56-year-old man with severe substernal pain, or a 3-year-old child with a large tumor in the left abdomen. Most would agree that the respective likelihoods are in the vicinity of rheumatoid arthritis .80, hy-

perventilation .90, coronary heart disease .50, and Wilms' tumor .50.

Then as additional data are gathered the likelihood increases or decreases, especially in comparison with a competing diagnosis. If you see a youngish woman with recurrent polyarthritis, the differential diagnosis rests almost entirely between rheumatoid arthritis and systemic lupus erythematosus. Knowing that the former disease is 20 times more common than the latter, you can begin with these relative likelihoods (Table 5.9). Each additional clue alters the relative likelihoods so that you end with a reversed ratio. The values stated are approximations. More exact figures can be determined if the operating characteristics of each clue are known for each of the two diseases. Each $P(D)$ is revised by a clue whose resultant PV turns out to be the next $P(D)$ for subsequent testing ($P_1 \rightarrow P_2 \rightarrow P_3 \rightarrow P_4$, etc).

A second example concerns a 68-year-old obese woman who complains of dyspnea on exertion. You estimate that the $P(D)$ for left ventricular failure is .30; but other conditions may exist. Note in Table 5.10 how the probabilities fluctuate up and down with each additional clue. Eventually, left ventricular failure becomes almost certain.

Two Separate Tests. Consider another circumstance. You see a 60-year-old man in whom the clinical likelihood of unstable advancing angina pectoris is .50. In considering surgical intervention, you wish to be more sure of the diagnosis. Test A is simple, non-invasive, and inexpensive, but only 80% sensitive and 80% specific. Test B is 95%

Table 5.9.
Alteration of Likelihoods by Adding Clues*

	RA		SLE
1. Initial P(D)	.95	P_1	.05
2. Pleurisy	.70	P_2	.30
3. Rash	.50	P_3	.50
4. Albuminuria	.30	P_4	.70
5. RF test +	.50	P_5	.50
6. ANA test +	.05	P_6	.95

* RA, rheumatoid arthritis; SLE, systemic lupus erythematosus; ANA, antinuclear antibody; RF, rheumatoid factor; P, probability.

Table 5.10.
Fluctuation of Likelihoods in an Obese Woman with Dyspnea on Exertion

		LVF*		Other
1.	Initial likelihood	.30	P_1	.70
2.	Chronic hypertension	.50	P_2	.50
3.	Chronic cough—2 packs/day	.30	P_3	.70
4.	Orthopnea	.50	P_4	.50
5.	Basal rales, no wheeze	.60	P_5	.40
6.	S_3 at apex	.80	P_6	.20
7.	Large heart, Kerley-B lines	.95	P_7	.05

* LVF, left ventricular failure.

sensitive and 95% specific, but it is invasive, expensive, and dicey. *The tests are conditionally independent.* You decide to do test *A* first; it is positive. The revised or posttest probability (based on the PV+) is .80 (Fig. 5.24). Had the test been negative, the disease probability would have fallen to .20. As a clinician, you wish to be as certain as possible before recommending surgery, so you perform test *B*. This is also positive and the revised probability is now .985 (Fig. 5.25). A surgeon is consulted.

Two tests are better than one if both are positive or both are negative. If one is positive and one is negative, the results are confusing and the P(D) reverts to somewhat more or less than where you started. In the suspected case of severe angina pectoris, had test *B* been performed first, the resultant P(D) would have been .95. Buf if test *B* were followed by test *A*, and both were positive, you would have obtained the same final likelihood of .985. The order of testing has no impact on the final diagnostic probability. The PV of both tests combined is not derived by adding the two separate PVs. It is obtained by doing *two separate operations.* Apply one test and use the resulting PV as the P(D) for the next test.

There are very few reliable figures available for the operating characteristics of combination testing, but this issue will be addressed in Chapter 6.

Aiming for Certainty. Suppose a disease exhibits three independent clues, each of

which is present in 75% of patients with the disease. While each clue is common in the disease, only 42% of patients will have all three clues (.75 × .75 × .75). A diagnostic study that is positive in only half the cases further reduces the concurrence of clues to 21%. As each additional independent procedure is done, the likelihood of all being positive or present in the same patient approaches zero. Even though partial interdependence of some clues may tend to slow the downward spiral, these statistics are the basic reason *why classic cases are rarely seen.*

As the number of clues either needed or present increases, the sensitivity of the *combination* decreases, the FP rate for the combination *decreases,* and the specificity and PV+ *increase.* Fewer cases of the disease will have more and more clues, but if the clues

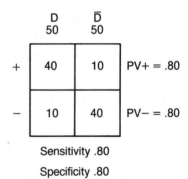

Fig. 5.24. Revision of likelihood by test *A*.

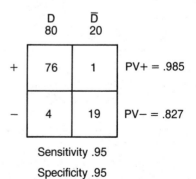

Fig. 5.25. Revision of likelihood by test *B* performed after test *A*.

are present, a weight of evidence is building for a more perfect tableau of the disease. Persons without the disease are far less likely to have a combination of falsely positive clues and exhibit a false face. These are some items from the bag of tricks of the diagnostic trade. The clinician uses these concepts and mechanisms without thinking about them; students should be able to do likewise.

Some Final Reflections

From Words to Numbers. During this entire chapter, I have tried to relate medical logic, words, and symbols to numbers, decimals, and percentages. In translating everyday medical language into precise numerical meaning, you must *avoid getting trapped in your own words.* When you say that "gross ventilation-perfusion mismatches are never seen in patients without pulmonary emboli," you are saying that there are no FPs and the specificity of this abnormality is 100%. The statement that "perfusion scans are always abnormal in patients with a pulmonary embolus" means the test is 100% sensitive. Additionally, if "one never sees a negative antinuclear antibody test in the presence of lupus," it means there are no FNs and the test is 100% sensitive. "One often sees a positive test even if the suspected disease is not present" means there are many FPs and the test is not very specific. "If the test is positive, the disease is much more likely to be present" speaks of the PV+ of a test. "A normal treadmill test is against the pain being coronary artery in origin" says that the PV− in this instance is high. And on and on.

Numerical meaning has also been given to current diagnostic decision-making terms such as sensitivity, specificity, separator, trade-offs, ROC curves, predictive value, test efficiency, gold standard test, prevalence, incidence, probability, likelihood, 2×2 tables, and stick diagrams.

Mathematical Models for Intuition. The previous discussions and examples of medical logic have demonstrated many important clinical concepts and hopefully have taken some of the mystery out of what is euphemistically called "medical intuition." We usually regard intuition as an instinctive mystical direct perception of a truth obtained without recourse to inference or reasoning. But intuitive judgments, on the whole, are probably not at all intuitive. They may very well be precise conclusions reached by complex calculations performed in a flash by billions of connected cortical cells—much like the previously described simple mathematical models that mimic basic intuitive processes. Models will be further described in subsequent chapters.

Some of the concepts of intuitive logic which have already been given mathematical meaning are the:

1. Estimation of probability
2. Degree of probability required
3. Product of the probabilities
4. Degrees of interdependence
5. Likelihood ratios of D:$\bar{D}$
6. Revision of likelihoods
7. Notion of imperfect information
8. Construction of a weight of evidence
9. Rarity of textbook cases
10. Principles of combination testing.

SELF-EVALUATION EXERCISES

(Answers appear following the last question.)

1. On clinical evidence, you suspect that a patient you are treating for congestive heart failure may have digitalis toxicity, though you think it isn't likely; P(D) = .20. A digoxin level is 2.5 ng/ml. According to your laboratory, the separator point is 2.0 ng/ml, and the test is 80% sensitive and 80% specific under these circumstances.
   (a) What is the revised likelihood that digitalis toxicity exists?
   (b) What decision would you make about continuing digoxin?
   (c) What is the revised likelihood if the result were 1.5 ng/ml?
   (d) Would you continue the same digoxin dose?
2. If 20% of peptic ulcers eventually bleed and 40% of gastrointestinal bleeds are caused by peptic ulcer:
   (a) What is the likelihood that a peptic ulcer will never bleed?
   (b) What is the likelihood that a bleed is not caused by a peptic ulcer?

(c) If a bleed occurs, how likely is it to be caused by a peptic ulcer?

3. How many subsets are created by three overlapping sets: a, b, and c?

4. In a certain hospital there are 360 patients, 40 of whom have clinically proven cirrhosis of the liver. An expert in abdominal palpation determines that 32 of the 360 patients have palpable spleens, of whom 16 have cirrhosis. In this hospital:
   (a) What is the sensitivity and
   (b) the specificity of palpable splenomegaly for cirrhosis?
   (c) What is the predictive value for cirrhosis in a patient with palpable splenomegaly?
   (d) What is the probability that a different problem exists in those with palpable spleens?
   (e) Is the presence of a palpable spleen a good clue for cirrhosis?
   (f) What is the probability that a patient whose spleen is not palpable does not have cirrhosis?
   (g) What percentage of patients with cirrhosis have palpable spleens? What percentage do not have palpable spleens?

5. A certain test for the presence of cancer exhibits 80% true positives and 2% false positives.
   (a) Given 25 patients with known cancer, how many will have negative tests?
   (b) Given 50 patients in good health who are known not to have cancer, how many will have negative tests?
   (c) If this test is used for screening purposes on 5000 people of whom 1% can be expected to have cancer, how many positive tests will be found?
   (d) Of these positives, how many will have cancer?
   (e) How many will not have cancer?
   (f) What is the PV+ of this test in the stated population?

6. Only sarcoidosis and tuberculosis are under consideration in a patient. The P(D) of each is .50. A test is performed which is positive in 80% of tuberculosis patients and negative in 80% of sarcoidosis patients. It is positive.
   (a) What is the revised probability of tuberculosis?
   (b) Of sarcoidosis?

7. A combination of neurologic symptoms and signs suggests that a patient has either a brain tumor or a demyelinating disease. The relative likelihoods are 3:1. A diagnostic procedure that is negative in all cases of demyelinating disease and negative in one-third of brain tumors is done. The test is negative.
   (a) What are the new relative likelihoods?

(b) What are the relative likelihoods if the test is positive?

8. After a health survey of a town with 5000 adult inhabitants, 1000 are found to have hypertension, 250 have diabetes mellitus, and 3850 are free of both diseases.
   (a) What is the prevalence of hypertension?
   (b) What is the prevalence of diabetes?
   (c) If these two diseases were completely independent, how many adults would have both diseases?
   (d) How many adults *actually* have both diseases?
   (e) Are the two diseases interdependent?

9. A 60-year-old man with an 80 pack-year cigarette history develops a severe cough, expectoration with streaks of blood, weight loss, weakness, and anorexia over an 8-week period of time. There is a faint expiratory wheeze heard only in the left upper lung field. He has a left-sided Horner's syndrome.
   (a) What is the probability that he has lung cancer: .20, .40, .60, .80, or .95?
   (b) Approximate a new probability for lung cancer in the absence of wheeze and Horner's syndrome, and in the presence of a normal chest x-ray except for increased basal markings.

10. A 52-year-old man has had recurrent indigestion for 10 years. He has 2-hour postprandial heartburn and epigastric pain relieved by alkali. The present episode has lasted 4 weeks and is worse than the usual attack in that the pain wakes him at night. There has been no weakness, weight loss, or anorexia. The probability of stomach cancer is:
   (a) .80
   (b) .60
   (c) .40
   (d) .20
   (e) less than .10.

11. Assume the P(D) in problem 10 is .05. An endoscopic procedure with biopsy is performed. This test is 90% sensitive and 98% specific for cancer of the stomach; it is negative. Cancer is ruled out with a certainty of:
   (a) 85%
   (b) 95%
   (c) 99%
   (d) 99.5%
   (e) 100%.

12. Suppose that 10 mm of erythema and induration is required for absolute positivity of a purified protein derivative skin test in your hospital. The chief of infectious diseases decides that henceforth 12 mm is needed for positivity. In so doing, he has:
   (a) decreased the sensitivity
   (b) decreased the TN rate

(c) increased the specificity
(d) increased the FP rate
(e) done none of the above.

13. A kidney disease has two *independent* clues; clue A is present in 90% of patients with this disease, and clue B is present in 80%. Which one statement is *incorrect*?
   (a) Both A and B will be present in 72% of cases.
   (b) Both A and B will be absent in 2% of cases.
   (c) If both A and B are present, the disease is diagnosed with 72% certainty.
   (d) Either A or B will be present in 98% of cases.
   (e) If both A and B are absent, the disease is virtually ruled out.

14. Refer to Figure 5.21. But now consider another woman with a positive mammogram who excitedly telephones you. In view of the fact that both her mother and sister died of breast cancer, you estimate that she is five times as likely to have cancer than any other woman.
   (a) What is her pretest P(D)?
   (b) What is her posttest probability?
   (c) What do you advise?
   (d) Why does the mammogram have a greater positive predictive value in this case?
   (e) Had her test been negative, how much reassurance could you give?

15. Four clues exhibit the following sensitivities for a disease: .8, .6, .1, and .5.
   (a) If the clues are completely independent, how many of 100 patients with the disease will have all four clues?
   (b) What is the maximum number of patients who could exhibit all four clues if the clues are interdependent?
   (c) The four clues are also found in normal people with a sensitivity of .08, .06, .01, and .05, respectively. What is the likelihood of a healthy patient's having these four independent clues?
   (d) Given a P(D) of .01, approximate the likelihood ratio of D:$\bar{\text{D}}$; again assume that all clues are present and independent.

16. Tachycardia is always present in patients with hyperthyroidism. Which of the following statements is/are therefore true?
   (a) The clue is 100% specific.
   (b) The clue is 100% sensitive.
   (c) The presence of the clue diagnoses the disease.
   (d) The absence of the clue excludes the disease.

17. There is a 50–50 chance that a patient has a serious disease which is curable by surgery. But the surgeon requests at least a 95% likelihood of disease before he will operate. Three tests are available to you. Test A has 80% sensitivity and specificity; test B has 90% sensitivity and specificity; test C has 98% sensitivity and specificity.
   (a) What is the PV+ of each test done separately?
   (b) Which test or tests will be satisfactory if positive?
   (c) However, test C cannot be done because it is precluded by an abnormal prothrombin time and severe vascular disease. If you do test A followed by test B and both are positive, will the resultant revised probability be satisfactory for surgery? What is it?

18. Translate the statement that follows into a symbolic expression: "If disseminated intravascular coagulation is present, split fibrin products cannot be normal."
   (a) There are no TPs.
   (b) There are no FPs.
   (c) There are no TNs.
   (d) There are no FNs.

19. A combination of clues is 100 times more common in disease A than disease B. But disease B is ten times more common than disease A. Given a patient with this combination of clues, what is the relative likelihood of A:B?
   (a) 100:1
   (b) 1:100
   (c) 10:1
   (d) 1:10
   (e) 1:1.

20. A disease may be excluded from consideration because:
   (a) it is rare
   (b) a 100% specific test is negative
   (c) a 100% sensitive test is negative
   (d) a test for a competing disease is positive
   (e) a test for it is negative.

21. The presence of a disease may be absolutely confirmed if:
   (a) it is very common
   (b) a 100% specific test is positive
   (c) a 100% sensitive test is positive
   (d) the clinical template resembles the disease
   (e) a test for it is positive.

22. In an adult male population of 8000, .25% have gout, of whom 95% have hyperuricemia (over 7.0 mg/dl). Account for the fact that only approximately 5% of males with hyperuricemia have gout.
   (a) Hint! What is the false positive rate that permits such a ratio to exist: 1%, 2%, 5%, 10%, or 20%?

(b) If an individual has a serum uric acid level of 10 mg/dl, is he more, equally, or less apt to have gout than the male whose serum uric acid is 8.0 mg/dl?

ANSWERS

1. (a) .50. Make a 2×2 table. There are 16 TPs and 16 FPs.
   (b) Stop digoxin for several days.
   (c) .06. From the same 2×2 table, the PV− is equal to the TNs divided by TNs + FNs (64 ÷ 68 = .94); P(D) = .06.
   (d) yes.
2. (a) .80   (b) .60   (c) .40.
3. Eight: a, b, c, ab, ac, bc, abc, abc.
4. Draw another 2×2; let P(D) = cirrhosis and the test be palpable splenomegaly.
   (a) sensitivity .40 (16 per 40 patients)
   (b) specificity .95 (304 TNs plus 16FPs; 304 ÷ 320)
   (c) PV = .50 (16 TPs and 16 FPs)
   (d) .50 (those with splenomegaly have cirrhosis or something else)
   (e) No—it is no better than a tossup.
   (f) .93 (calculate the PV− from the 304 TNs plus 24 FNs; 304 ÷ 328)
   (g) 40% (the sensitivity); 60% (those with cirrhosis without palpable spleens).
5. (a) 5 (20% of 25)
   (b) 49 (98% of 50)
   (c) 139 (80% of 50 plus 2% of 4950)
   (d) 40
   (e) 99
   (f) PV+ is .29 (40 ÷ 139).
6. (a) .80. Revised probability = .50 × .80 for tuberculosis and .50 × .20 for sarcoidosis = 4:1 = .80.
   (b) .20 since P(Tb) + P(Sa) = 1.00 by original consideration.
7. (a) 1:1 or 50-50. Original P (tumor) is .75; P (other) is .25. The revised likelihoods are (.75 × ⅓) : (.25 × 1.0) = 1:1.
   (b) 1:0. The patient *must* have a tumor because a positive test cannot occur in the other disease. Under the circumstances, since by original contention no other disease is possible, the test is 100% specific for brain tumor.
8. (a) .20 (1000 ÷ 5000)
   (b) .05 (250 ÷ 5000)
   (c) 50 (.05 × .20 × 5000)—the product of the probabilities
   (d) 100. Construct a Venn diagram with two overlapping circles. Those with diabetes alone plus those with hypertension alone plus those with both diseases equal 1150. Let x = those with both diseases. Then (250-x) + (x) + (1000-x) = 1150. Solve, and x = 100.
   (e) yes.
9. (a) .95

(b) .40 or less.
10. (e) is correct (less than .10).
11. (d) 99.5% certainty that cancer does not exist. The 2×2 diagram demonstrates that the PV− is 93.1 ÷ 93.6 (.5 FN + 93.1 TN).
12. (a) and (c) are correct. By creating more stringent criteria, the test becomes less sensitive but more specific. The TN rate goes up, and the FP rate goes down.
13. (c) is the incorrect statement. Construct a stick diagram starting with 100 cases of D. Apply clue A; 90 will be positive and 10 will be negative. Then apply clue B to all patients. The 90 A-positives will yield 72 B-positives and 18 B-negatives. The 10 A-negatives will yield 8 B-positives and 2 B-negatives. It can be seen that (a), (b), (d), and (e) are all correct statements. Only (c) is incorrect. The fact that both A and B are present merely states that 72% of patients with D have both A and B present and has nothing to do with the calculation of disease probability.
14. (a) .015 (5 × .003)
   (b) .50. Draw another 2×2 table; 15 have disease and 985 do not. Then apply the same operating characteristics; there will be 10 TPs and 9.85 FPs, resulting in a PV+ of .50.
   (c) Examination and biopsy
   (d) The initial P(D) was higher, the TPs are more, and the FPs are slightly less; but the latter has only slight impact on the equation.
   (e) 99.5% (975 ÷ 980). This is slightly less assurance than you could give another person who had not had a mammogram and whose P(D̄) is .997.
15. (a) 2.4 (.8 × .6 × .1 × .5 × 100 patients)
   (b) 10—the least sensitive clue
   (c) 2.4 × 10⁻⁶ (.08 × .06 × .01 × .05 × 1 patient) or 2.4 chances in a million
   (d) 100:1 (.024 ÷ .0000024 ÷ 100). This is calculated on the basis of a single patient whose P(D) is .01 and who is then found to have the four clues present.
16. (b) and (d) are correct.
17. (a) .80, .90, .98. Construct 2×2 tables for each test. Note that, because the P(D) is .50 and the sensitivity-specificity are the same for a test, the PV is equal to the sensitivity (or specificity).
   (b) Test C will suffice.
   (c) Yes. It is .973. First calculate the revised probability if test A is positive; it is .80. Now use .80 as the new P(D) and perform test B. There will be 72 TPs and 2 FPs, resulting in a PV+ (or new P(D)) of .973 (72 ÷ 74). Test B followed by test A would yield the same result.

18. **(d) is correct.** The clue is 100% sensitive for the disease; the implication is that given a patient with disseminated intravascular coagulation, the test for split fibrin products must always be abnormal.
19. **(c) is correct** (10:1). Disease *A* is ten times as likely as disease *B*. This may seem paradoxical at first glance.
20. **(c) is correct.** Other answers are only partially or possibly correct.
21. **(b) is correct.** Other answers are only partially or possibly correct.
22. (a) 5% is correct. This allows for 19 TPs and 399 FPs, roughly a 1:20 ratio.
    (b) Gout is more likely. This is intuitively correct. The subject of the *degree of abnormality* of a test that measures continuous linear variables will be explained in Chapter 6.

References

1. Ingelfinger JA, Mosteller F, Thibodeau LA, et al: *Biostatistics in Clinical Medicine.* New York, Macmillan, 1983.
2. Feinstein AR: *Clinical Judgment.* Baltimore, Williams & Wilkins, 1967.
3. Lusted LB: *Introduction to Medical Decision-Making.* Springfield, IL, Charles C Thomas, 1968.
4. Weinstein MC, Fineberg HV: *Clinical Decision Analysis.* Philadelphia, Saunders, 1980.
5. Case Records of The Massachusetts General Hospital; Weekly clinicopathologic exercises. *N Engl J Med* 308:1521–1528, 1983.
6. Khan MA, Khan MK: Diagnostic value of HLA-B27 testing in ankylosing spondylitis and Reiter's syndrome. *Ann Intern Med* 96:70–76, 1982.
7. Richardson B, Epstein WV: Utility of the fluorescent antinuclear antibody test in a single patient. *Ann Intern Med* 95:333–338, 1981.
8. Waring GW Jr: False-positive tests for syphilis revisited. *JAMA* 243:2321–2322, 1980.
9. Schwartz WB, Wolfe HJ, Pauker SG: Pathology and probabilities. *N Engl J Med* 305:917–923, 1981.
10. Griner PF, Mayewski RJ, Mushlin AI, et al: Selection and interpretation of diagnostic procedures. *Ann Intern Med* 94:553–600, 1981.
11. Gorry GA, Pauker SG, Schwartz WB: The diagnostic importance of the normal finding. *N Engl J Med* 298:486–489, 1978.
12. Meals RA: Paratyphoid fever. *Arch Intern Med* 136:1422–1428, 1976.
13. Harris JM Jr: The hazards of bedside Bayes. *JAMA* 246:2602–2605, 1981.

Chapter 6

How to Use Tests

PAUL CUTLER, M.D.

KEY WORDS

1. screening
2. targeted screening
3. sequential strategy
4. tandem strategy
5. profiles, batteries, panels
6. referent values
7. dichotomous results
8. unsolicited data
9. unexpected test results
10. testing strategies
11. diagnostic protocols
12. combination testing
13. parallel testing
14. series testing

Modern concepts of using diagnostic tests and procedures were introduced in the section on paraclinical studies in Chapter 2, and the mathematical notions of tests' operating characteristics and predictive values were detailed in Chapter 5. In the present chapter, we deal mainly with the very practical aspects of testing—the whats, wheres, whens, hows, whys, and why nots—as well as the interpretation of test results.

There is an urgent need to overhaul some patterns for ordering diagnostic tests. Medical students must learn new, more effective, and more efficient trends before they fall into the same bad habits that are often passed on from one generation of house officers to the next.

A staggering array of information has become available with the mere puncture of a vein; with the ability to dissect every body fluid into picograms; with the skill to biopsy virtually any tissue; with the use of new imaging techniques that reflect the anatomy, physiology, and biochemistry of most organs; and with the wizardry to employ altered genes, electrons, positrons, magnets, and computers to track almost everything. The marriage of immunology and genetics at the biochemical altar has given birth to magic bullets, disease tracers, chemical factories, and yet more tests—all of which are as awesome as *Star Wars.*

Couple this diagnostic explosion with a new religion that deifies the measurement and looks upon simpler clinical methods with impiety. The result is an exponential increase in the ordering and performance of diagnostic tests and procedures with only little knowledge of and little consideration for their necessity, cost, risk, benefit, and reliability. *It's easier, simpler, and more glamorous to order tests than to talk, examine, or think.*

We don't even know if patients have benefited or if medical care has improved as a result of this new technology. Numerous anecdotes, both humorous and otherwise, portray the opposite result. The fact that too many tests are ordered is undeniable. The fact that many tests are unnecessary, not helpful, and often misleading is well established. The fact that the shocking rise of health care cost is in large part related to tests and procedures is a statistical reality.

Our challenge is to do whatever is possible to improve this situation without affecting quality care—to orchestrate the proliferation of procedures for the patient's benefit rather than his detriment. To do this, *you must know* how your laboratory and procedure departments operate, why tests are ordered, how to order tests, how to interpret single and multiple test results, and how to decrease testing and avoid diagnostic overkill.

That is what this chapter is all about.

Why We Use Tests

In the Beginning. Twenty-four hundred years ago, Hippocrates not only gave us his immortal oath, but he also smelled and inspected the urine of sick people. This may have been the primordial laboratory test. Today the properly performed simple urinalysis produces more reliable information than any other single test. Just give the patient a clean container and have him urinate into it; then you smell it, look at it, float a urinometer, insert a dipstick, and examine a drop of sediment under the microscope. It's simple; it's easy; it's cheap; it's noninvasive; it's quick; and it's very informative. You can even do it yourself. If all tests had the same attributes, there would be no need for this chapter.

Today the situation is vastly more complex for the many reasons already stated. Considerations of expense, wasted time, imperfect information, cost-benefit analysis, risk, and the need for help in deciding between alternative treatments—all have made very important issues of the selection of tests and the interpretation of their results.

Reasons for Testing. The fundamental reason for doing tests in conjunction with or following the history and physical examination is to help find out what is wrong with the patient. But in truth there are many other reasons. Some say that tests are done simply for purposes of *discovery, confirmation,* or *exclusion.* To be more complete, we can list the following reasons for testing: (*a*) diagnosis, (*b*) prognosis, (*c*) screening, (*d*) monitoring, (*e*) baseline data, and (*f*) decisions.

Diagnosis is most important; a test or procedure helps to detect, confirm, document, or exclude a disease. The aim is to increase certainty and decrease uncertainty. *Prognosis* can be determined, for example, by noting the degree of test abnormality or the extent of metastases. *Screening* is more complex. Here we search for illness in healthy patients or look for diseases other than the principal one. *Targeted screening* is the ordering of a single test on a single person or an entire population, aiming to discover or rule out a single disease. Venereal Disease Research Laboratory tests for syphilis, or purified protein derivative skin tests for tuberculin sensitivity are specific examples. On the other hand, multiphasic screening, or the ordering of entire profiles or batteries of tests to be done by automated techniques, is an example of screening for many diseases. At one time, we search for liver, kidney, bone, muscle, adrenal, and prostatic diseases, as well as electrolyte, lipid, and diabetic disorders.

The use of tests for *monitoring* has many purposes. You may wish to measure progression or regression of disease, response to treatment, or drug levels of medication being used. Tests obtained for *baseline data* tell you what is *not* wrong with the patient and establish patterns of normality; these permit you to detect additional problems that may crop up later during the course of the primary disease or as a result of its treatment. A *decision* on treatment may depend on the result of a test; whether or not to use anticoagulants can hinge on a ventilation-perfusion scan; whether to continue or withhold digoxin may depend on a blood digoxin level. Not included in the list, but also important, is the fact that tests are ordered for patient and doctor reassurance and for defensive medicolegal reasons. And, outside the hospital, it is unfortunate that tests are sometimes ordered merely to generate income.

On Being in Order. The sequence in which tests are ordered depends on many factors. If the situation is critical, the test with the highest yield is done, even though there may be some risk. But if there is time, perhaps lower yield, less risky procedures can be done first. If a massive myocardial infarction is impending, angiography might be the initial test. But if the situation is less fragile, an ECG and cardiac enzymes come first, perhaps a treadmill test next, and a thallium scan thereafter.

Ordinarily the order of testing is (*a*) from cheap to costly; (*b*) from less to more risky; and (*c*) from simple to more complex. Within the constraints of time, risk, and cost, try to do the test or procedure with the most efficiency as soon as possible; that is, use the procedure with the highest sensitivity, specificity, and predictive values.

Ideally, all the preceding objectives should be observed in deciding which tests to request first and the sequence in which they should be ordered. But this is not always practical. One or more objectives may be sacrificed for speed, convenience, accuracy, parsimony, a waiting list for procedures, time needed to await the results, and the condition of the patient. Sometimes it may be best to get the costly test first; it may solve the problem quickly and save money by cutting hospital days. Or if you must wait 3 days for a certain x-ray study, you might do other tests in the meantime.

Traditionally, however, routine studies are ordered first. These include a urinalysis, blood count, one or two profiles of 6 or 12 blood chemistry tests, a chest x-ray, and an ECG. Or the treating physician may order the routine tests as well as many special ones at the same time. At admission, the doctor often orders everything he thinks will be necessary and reevaluates the patient when all the information is in. The nursing staff and the various laboratories and diagnostic units involved then work out the sequence. Or it may simply evolve by chance. These methods are not always in the best interests of the patient, the costs, and the making of a diagnosis.

Assume the patient has a solitary thyroid nodule. The special studies might include a thyroid function profile, a radioisotope scan, an ultrasound study, and needle aspiration biopsy. The blood tests can be done immediately, the echo in 2 days, and the scan in 3 days, but the surgeon is immediately available. You can see how the "correct" order of testing might require a summit conference and could differ from place to place, from person to person, and from time to time. Problems of this sort arise daily. Often there is a well-conceived intelligent strategy for doing tests in a specified order, since if one is positive or negative, subsequent tests may or may not have to be done. Thus you may use a *sequential* strategy as just described, or a *tandem* strategy that permits many tests and procedures to be done before evaluating their total impact upon completion.

Know Your Lab

The discussions in this chapter do not relate only to what is commonly called "the lab." Included in the laboratory are the subdivisions of hematology, immunopathology, microbiology, histopathology, chemistry, etc. In addition, reference to "tests" includes all those procedures done by radiologists, cardiologists, gastroenterologists, and pulmonary disease specialists. So what is said for a simple blood chemical test applies to computed tomographic (CT) scans, ultrasound studies, arteriography, programmed cardiac electrical stimulation, endoscopic procedures, and pulmonary function tests as well.

Familiarity Breeds Respect. One of the first things the beginning clinical person must do is visit the laboratory. Learn the tests that are available, how they are requested, what preparation is needed, the costs, the turnaround time, and the operating characteristics. The same should be done in the radiology and cardiology departments. Become familiar with all diagnostic procedures, their indications and contraindications, their operating characteristics, their risks and complications, and who does them. Tactfully find out about the reliability of the results and the reliability of the performer. You are now well on the way toward understanding what help you can expect from paraclinical sources.

Learn the Menus. Just as you would in a fine restaurant, carefully inspect the various offerings in each department. Become acquainted with the hematology, chemistry, endocrinology, cytology, microbiology, and immunopathology menus. Which tests are done in each subdivision? Learn what the 6-test and 12-test chemistry profiles include in your hospital. Usually it's the serum sodium, potassium, chloride, bicarbonate, glucose, and urea nitrogen for the former; and it's the serum protein, albumin, calcium, phosphorus, cholesterol, uric acid, creatinine, total bilirubin, alkaline phosphatase, creatine phosphokinase, lactic dehydrogenase, and glutamic-oxaloacetic transaminase for the latter. You may be offered 18, 20, or 24 tests by the sequential multiple analyzer.

There is much to be gleaned as you inspect the request forms for each division. On the hematology form, the tests are listed, normal values are stated, and special procedures and entire profiles are grouped. Should you have a patient with a coagulopathy, one check mark generates a battery of 4, 6, 10, or even 15 tests. The presence of "fibrinogen degradation products" cues you to the fact that you've forgotten what this test is and why it's done. So naturally you look it up in your reference textbook and relearn all about disseminated intravascular coagulation.

A look at the endocrinology menu gives similar information. Here the tests are grouped for each endocrine gland. All four thyroid tests can be requested if you suspect a thyroid problem. Under the adrenals, there are 11 tests; if a problem is suspected here, order them all; better yet, order à la carte—only what you want. It might surprise you to learn that in your hospital the vitamin B_{12} level and drug assays are done in endocrinology. Memorize the drug levels that are available, and know which ones are not.

Profiles, batteries, and panels of tests are available with a simple check mark. You may order one or more, depending on the area you wish to investigate. A *coronary risk profile* includes the serum cholesterol, high- and low-density lipoproteins, and the cholesterol:high-density lipoprotein ratio. If the

problem suggests arthritis of some sort, an arthritis profile will produce the rheumatoid factor titer, C-reactive protein, erythrocyte sedimentation rate, uric acid, and antinuclear antibody. The *Torch profile* includes the toxoplasma antibodies, rubella titer, cytomegalovirus antibodies, and herpes virus I and II antibodies. Other available grouped studies include comprehensive viral agglutination titers, heavy metal screens, hypnotic profiles, and prenatal profiles.

Microbiology is startling. The large number of specimen sources is notable. Review the list of identifiable bacteria and the special culture techniques needed in some instances. This form is filled with surprises. Costs may be astonishing.

Other things must be learned. Which tests are available on an emergency basis? Which are not available on weekends? Which are done only once weekly, and on which day? Which tests must be sent to a distant laboratory because your hospital doesn't do them? Which drugs does a toxic drug screen screen? How long does it take for a result to reach the chart? A blood count? A blood culture? Indeed any test! You will be surprised by the huge amount of information on the urinalysis request form.

Ask your laboratory for the small pamphlet or instruction booklet that lists all tests alphabetically, tells you how much blood is needed for each test, what color-cap tube is used, and the cost of each test. Know what each test you order costs, and *calculate the expenses* every time you write some orders. Do you really want to measure the angiotensin converting enzyme for $26.50 or the α-fetoprotein for $40.75? What about a daily serum bilirubin at $15.50 a day? Is it that helpful? Think three times before ordering a vitamin B_1 level for $49.00; and even if absolutely necessary, how reliable are the results? By the time you read this book the prices may be much higher.

If you are not already impressed, peruse the CT scan, ultrasound, x-ray consultation, and cardiac study request forms. There you see not only what studies are offered, but you also get a good review of the possible uses for each procedure. The various nuclear scans are listed, but you don't know their operating characteristics, nor are the charges usually printed. Inquire, and you'll understand why not. The multiple uses of ultrasound are impressive; the sensitivity and specificity for each use are not included, for rarely are they known. Costs are not stated either. Would you order these tests less often if you knew that the cost for doing the procedure and the cost for reading the results are separate—each being in three figures? Sometimes even four! The same can be said for computed tomographic scans, digital subtraction angiography, endoscopies, and the multitude of specialized cardiologic studies.

The foregoing is not meant to be antiintellectual, but is rather a plea for prudence, deliberation, and consideration before ordering tests and diagnostic procedures. If the need and benefit far exceed the cost and risk, the test should be done. If the data derived are of questionable value, some risk, and high cost, *don't order the test*. The sparse but adequate diet of a county jail may be more healthful than the gourmet feasts served in a fine continental restaurant.

The number of tests ordered seems to be roughly proportional to the number of tests available. And the ultimate decisions that have such profound effect on the cost of health care depend on the physician or house officer who checks off the items on the menu.

Reporting Techniques. Know the method by which tests are reported back to you, the nursing office, or the chart. When certain specifically predesignated dangerous abnormalities are detected in the laboratory, somebody in authority is immediately notified by telephone. The level at which a blood glucose, digoxin assay, or electrocardiographic abnormality becomes a notifiable emergency is preset in each hospital.

Aside from this, the laboratory communicates by hard copy, television, or computer. Most routine tests are usually back on the chart by late in the day or the next morning. Those tests which take more time

should be well known to you. Results of chemical tests are usually reported by simple tables, graphic displays, or computer-assisted radial plots (1). Normal values are stated, abnormalities clearly flagged, and their degrees of abnormality easily observed. Sometimes several abnormalities can be grouped together to suggest a disorder. For example, an elevated serum bilirubin, normal liver enzymes, and elevated alkaline phosphatase suggest obstructive jaundice. The concept of interpretive reporting may bring the pathologist into the diagnostic process. Given a group of abnormalities, the physician who oversees the test results may render an opinion.

What Are the Risks? Before requesting a diagnostic procedure, the ordering physician must consider the risks as well as the costs and benefits. Other than the trauma of venipuncture, the possible damage to veins which may be needed later, and the contribution to iatrogenic anemia, there are no risks attached to doing blood tests. In this regard, do we really need "lytes" daily, 12-test chemistry profiles daily, or cardiac enzymes every 4 hours?

Certainly there are no risks involved in obtaining a urinalysis or culturing body fluids, unless the urine is obtained by catheter, the sputum by transtracheal needle, and the spinal fluid by lumbar puncture.

Scans and ultrasound are generally harmless. However, if a computed scan is dye-enhanced, renal damage may result, especially if there is diabetes mellitus or preexisting renal disease.

As for the more invasive procedures involving introduction of tubes and needles into tissues, arteries, and veins for pictures or biopsies, there are definite though poorly quantified risks. In fact, a recent study showed that accurate information on risks of procedures is not available (2). Thus, decisions on doing such diagnostic studies are rendered more difficult. Twenty-five procedures were studied in 434 published reports. Many reports were not well designed and were incomplete, and the quality of the data obtained was not acceptable. Complications and risks were listed for lumbar puncture, Swan-Ganz catheter placement, marrow aspiration, thyroid aspiration biopsy, transbronchial biopsy, kidney biopsy, stress ECG, etc. Not only were the complications staggering, but wide variations from place to place were noted in all instances.

This bears out a common-sense appreciation of the fact that complications will vary from one institution to another and even from one operator to another, depending on case selection, skill, and frequency of performance.

What Normal Is

There are at least seven different definitions of "normal." They vary from "average" to "mean" to "usual." A test result that is either positive or negative is usually normal when negative. But a test which measures a biologic distribution of variables is normal when the result falls within a predetermined range of values. These are called the "referent values" or "cutoff points." They represent the range of normal values as determined by performing large numbers of measurements in healthy young people. The mean value is then determined, and the upper and lower limits of normal are set by calculating two standard deviations above and below the mean. By mathematical edict, only 95% of normal people will have normal values; 2.5% will be below normal and 2.5% will be above normal. This latter 5% will be falsely positive or falsely abnormal.

If the referent values for blood urea nitrogen are 10 to 20 mg/dl, a value of 200 mg/dl is definitely abnormal. So is 40 mg/dl. But what about 25 mg/dl? Could this be a false positive? And how far above the referent interval must the result be to indicate the presence of disease? This becomes a very important issue, especially in the consideration of other tests like the transaminases or alkaline phosphatase. How much above normal must the test result be before an intensive chain of studies is set into motion to determine the cause for the alleged abnormality?

On the other hand, what difference does it make? It depends on the penalty inflicted for ignoring a true positive vs the penalty for exhaustively working up a false positive. By the same token, there are penalties for not being aware of, or ignoring the possibility of, a false negative. Trade-offs occur in either direction; this issue was discussed in Chapter 5. But the clinician who is seeking a "decision level" want to know at which point above or below the referent values a test result becomes definitely abnormal and indicates the presence of disease. If so, what disease (3)?

You must understand the effect of increasing the "degree of abnormality" of a test with nondichotomous results. How abnormal must a test result be before you become concerned? Common sense tells you to ignore a slightly abnormal result if the implied diagnosis is clinically highly unlikely but to regard it seriously if the implied diagnosis is clinically likely. Of course, you must raise an eyebrow if the result is markedly abnormal even if unexpected.

At each increment of abnormality, the test has different operating characteristics, resulting in different true positive and false positive rates. Thus the likelihood ratio (TP rate:FP rate) is generally proportional to the degree of abnormality of the test result. The more abnormal the test result, the more likely it is to be truly positive and the less likely it is to be falsely positive.

The cutoff point between "worry—don't worry" will vary with the seriousness of the disease under consideration, the P(D) before the test is done, the otherwise general health and age of the patient, the aggressiveness of the physician, and the decision level with which he can feel comfortable.

The Perfect Test. In order for a test to be perfect, it must be: (*a*) accurate, (*b*) precise, (*c*) discriminating, (*d*) pain free, (*e*) risk free, (*f*) inexpensive, and (*g*) useful. The accuracy of a test refers to its ability to give *correct* results and hit the bull's-eye on retesting. Precision refers to reproducibility of results on replicate measurements, even though the results are not necessarily accurate. Ideally, a test should be both accurate and precise, though the two don't necessarily go hand in hand. For a test to be discriminating, it must be able to distinguish between health and disease. There should be a minimum number of false negative and false positive results. The other attributes of a perfect test need no further explanation. Obviously, there is no such thing as a perfect test!

You must appreciate the inherent limitations of the test, vis-à-vis its specificity and sensitivity, and the incidence of false positives and false negatives. A test has 100% *sensitivity* if all patients with the disease being tested have abnormal results and there are no false negatives. A test has 100% *specificity* if there are no false positives; this means that the test result is never abnormal in those who do not have the disease (see Chapter 5).

Actually, tests which measure continuous variables, such as serum uric acid, white blood cells, and PR intervals, do not clearly distinguish between health and disease.

It was once thought that all patients with active tuberculosis had positive skin tests. But this is not so because false negative results exist in overwhelming fulminant tuberculosis, in some patients on steroids, and in those who are otherwise anergic. Since large numbers of people without active tuberculosis have positive skin tests, the purified protein derivative test is neither specific nor sensitive for active tuberculosis. However, it is much more sensitive than it is specific.

On the other hand, a positive sputum test for acid-fast bacilli is found in only some cases of active tuberculosis. Such bacilli are even found in a few patients who do not have active tuberculosis since the bacillus may not be *Mycobacterium tuberculosis*. So all these variations must be carefully considered when interpreting a test. Venn diagrams and Boolean algebra clearly depict these interrelationships.

Remember that when new tests are first discovered many are thought to be specific for certain diseases. This was true for rheumatoid factor, lupus erythematosus cell preparations, the Widal test, serum glu-tamic-oxaloacetic transaminase and serum glutamic pyruvic transaminase, serum leucine aminopeptidase, α-fetoprotein, and carcinoembryonic antigen. These tests were originally thought to be specific for rheumatoid arthritis, lupus erythematosus, typhoid fever, acute myocardial infarction (or liver cell necrosis), carcinoma of the pancreas, etc. However, subsequent studies showed them to be nonspecific and positive in other diseases which were either closely related or not related at all. Also, some tests are negative in diseases where positivity would once have been considered sine qua non. So beware of allegedly pathognomonic tests when they are first released.

Knowing What Is Normal. To interpret a laboratory test result properly you must know the referent values. This is frequently difficult since they vary with age, gender, race, populations, time of day, method of performing the test, and other interrelated factors.

For example, the upper normal limit of serum uric acid in men varies from 5.5 to 8.0 mg/dl depending on some of the factors mentioned. Sometimes the physician is unaware that test results are being measured in new unfamiliar units. Currently, much effort is being directed toward expressing all units in molar terms or SI (*systeme internationale*) units. Such a uniform system would eliminate much confusion, but its adoption is still in the debating stage. The physician must also know the test method and units being used before he can interpret the results of a sedimentation rate, alkaline phosphatase test, or even a serum glucose determination. Values for normal serum creatinine are constantly being revised and vary with age and size of the patient. Because of mass determinations of serum bilirubin, the upper normal level has been so revised that Gilbert's disease may not even exist. A glucose tolerance test does not give valid results unless the patient has been properly prepared. The validity of other tests, such as aldosterone, renin, urine and serum electrolytes, and urine vanillylmandelic acid, may be altered by the position of the patient, his preceding diet, or the taking of certain medications.

Never diagnose a serious disease on the basis of an unpredicted or unexpected laboratory test result. Always repeat the test. One elevated fasting blood glucose does not establish a diagnosis of diabetes, nor does the presence of glycosuria necessarily indicate diabetes if the urine was collected in a poorly rinsed cough syrup bottle.

When Normal Is Not So. The range of variability for normal laboratory values in a particular patient or in an entire population may be a source of misinterpretation. You can have difficulty telling whether a result is normal or abnormal because of the wide range of normality rather than because of overlap.

If the normal blood urea nitrogen is 10 to 20 mg/dl, a patient who usually has 10 mg/dl and then rises to 20 mg/dl is twice his normal. Yet he is still "within normal limits" even though his kidney function may already be compromised. Similarly, a rise in bilirubin from 0.4 to 1.0 mg/dl would indicate a profound disturbance in bilirubin metabolism. Yet both values are within normal limits. The range of variability is wide in both instances.

Contrast this with the fasting blood glucose, where a rise from 70 to 122 mg/dl must be viewed with great suspicion even though the increment of rise is smaller. If 70 mg/dl were to more than double, as in the aforementioned case of serum bilirubin, the patient would clearly have diabetes. Calcium limits are even narrower (8.9 to 9.3 mg/dl). Here a slight rise is very significant.

Consider too the male patient whose hematocrit was 52% (top normal) and is now 42% (bottom normal) because he lost 2 to 3 pints of blood internally. You might not know it. The hematocrit of 42% could be considered low and abnormal only if you knew his usual hematocrit, since normal is 47% (±5%). In each case described it would help to know the patient's usual value before the change of clinical status occurred or the borderline value was obtained.

Watch for Errors. Since many human beings and machines are involved in doing tests and procedures, it is only natural to expect a certain percentage of errors. Never forget that the more tests are ordered, the more "red herrings" and errors may be introduced into the data base, and the more physicians may be misled.

Mistakes are made at all levels—before the laboratory, in the laboratory, and after the laboratory.

Prelab errors include improper preparation of the patient (e.g. diet, fasting state), the *taking of drugs* which interfere with accurate test performance, mislabeling of tubes, and obtaining poor specimens. Notable in this latter regard is the collection of unsterile urine and what is allegedly sputum for cultures.

Intralab errors are said to occur at a frequency of 3.65 per 100 tests. These include misplacing of specimens, errors in recording and filing, illegible reports, and poor referent values and referent intervals. And even if the referent values are well selected, by their very construction there will be an additional 5% false positives. If six unrelated tests are done, you can expect at least one test result to be falsely positive in 26.5% of normal healthy individuals (1 minus $.95^6$ = 1 minus .735 = .265). If 12 independent tests are done, at least one test result will be abnormal in 46% of normals (1 minus $.95^{12}$ = 1 minus .54 = .46). Whether these abnormal results represent false positives and what to do about them will be discussed later in this chapter.

Once the results leave the laboratory, they may be placed on the wrong chart. If a test result does not jibe with the clinical picture, always compare the name on the report with the name on the chart. The final error may be made by the physician himself who does not interpret results correctly because he either does not know or does not look. *There is no excuse for ordering a test and then ignoring or overlooking the result—commonly done.*

Correct Test Usage

A test for a disease cannot be properly used and its result compounded into the diagnostic process unless all its aspects are clearly understood. First you must know when the test is indicated and what it measures. In addition to a test's referent values (normal limits), you should also know the possible sources of error, the conditions required for proper specimen collection, and any concurrent medications that can interfere with the test's accuracy. If available, you should also know the operating characteristics of the test or procedure, so that you can approximate the incidence of false negatives and false positives; then assess the overall test reliability or efficiency. For a procedure, know its modus operandi, indications, contraindications, risks, cost, and possible benefits. You should also be able to make a reliable estimate of the suspected disease's prevalence or the clinical probability of the presence of the disease before the test is done. Given this information, you can then calculate the predictive value or posttest probability of a positive or negative (abnormal or normal) result, always bearing in mind that every test gives imperfect (not 100% accurate) information. A test, at best, is just a test (see Chapters 2 and 5).

Divergent Strategies. A theme which pervades this chapter—indeed this book—is the argument over the *use of test batteries vs the use of selectively chosen studies.* Those who favor entire batteries, profiles, and relatively indiscriminate testing are not without justification. For multiple tests often cost little more than a single one, and additional occult problems may be uncovered.

On the other hand, shotgun testing *is* more expensive, *the need for individualized thought is lessened*, there is a tendency to order more than is necessary, and unexpected false positive results often lead to long, unending, fruitless quests for diseases which do not exist.

It might be imprudent to take sides in this ongoing dispute—but the two strategies (battery testing and selective testing) will be detailed and their pros and cons discussed so that readers may steer courses for themselves. Practicality would seem to favor the former plan, while intellection urges the latter approach.

Once upon a Time. A certain internist was

a patient in one of America's finest university hospitals. He was hospitalized for 5 weeks during which he was studied for a malignant ventricular arrhythmia associated with coronary heart disease. Six intraarterial cardiac catheterizations were done, and 12-test profiles were ordered almost daily. Additional blood tests were also done. During the fifth week, he developed orthostatic syncope and was found to have a moderately severe anemia. The house staff asked no questions, did no examination, and proceeded to order an "anemia workup." This battery of more than ten tests included a serum B_{12}, serum folate, Schilling test, and others. Still no questions were asked, no examination done, nor were the stools or red blood cells checked. Was it possible to develop pernicious anemia or folic acid deficiency in 5 weeks? Obviously not! The hapless patient had developed a *nosocomial anemia* caused by subacute blood loss resulting from multiple procedures and tests.

The same patient in the same hospital was subsequently given an "infectious disease workup" because of several elevated leukocyte counts. Again there were no questions or examination! But of course a urine culture, several blood cultures, a chest x-ray, and repeated blood counts were done. The fact that the leukocytoses were *on the wrong chart* was the incidental ultimate irony.

La Fontaine derived truths from fables. The lessons learned from true stories like the foregoing are even more meaningful, and they distill into principles that are taught and preached. Ask questions and examine the patient! Then do carefully selected tests. Avoid the reflexive ordering of shotgun batteries.

Which Tests to Order. The actual ordering of tests is usually simple. First the "routine tests" are requested. These often include a blood count, urinalysis, a 6-, 12-, or 18-test blood chemistry profile, chest x-ray, and ECG. But as will be discussed later, hospital quality assurance and cost-containment personnel and third-party insurers are raising serious questions about the need for so many routine tests in all cases.

Additional tests are problem-oriented. If jaundice is the principal problem, you can begin with a direct and indirect bilirubin, alkaline phosphatase, and hepatic cell enzymes (whichever transferase you prefer). But on the basis of clinical evidence there is already an established likelihood of obstruction or hepatic cell disease. The test results will decrease or increase an existing probability. Thus when clinical judgment is used in ordering laboratory tests, the patient suspected of having a disease is placed in a new population with a higher P(D), and the test therefore has a greater positive predictive value.

Should anemia be the problem, the clinical setting and study of the red blood cells help you decide whether to look for chronic blood loss from the gastrointestinal tract, a macrocytic anemia, altered marrow production, and so forth. At this point you can order all tests for anemia in robot fashion or intelligently select those that are appropriate for the most likely diagnosis. For example, for weight loss, anorexia, indigestion, and microcytic anemia, order stool studies for occult blood, serum iron and iron-binding capacity, and gastrointestinal tract visualization. If the history, examination, and red blood cells suggest macrocytosis, folate and vitamin B_{12} levels are indicated. In other circumstances, bone marrow aspiration, reticulocyte count, glucose 6-phosphate dehydrogenase levels, transferrin, etc might be indicated. And this reasoning goes on and on for each clinical likelihood. *If the initial batch of tests does not confirm the prime clinical impression, tests may be ordered for the second likelihood.*

The other strategy, subject to some criticism though perhaps having timesaving benefits, is to order tests for all leading likelihoods at once and wait for all results to return. But it would seem wasteful and distasteful to aspirate the bone marrow for what is almost certainly an anemia caused by chronic blood loss. Similarly, it would be premature, inappropriate, and fruitless to order a biopsy, CT scan, or endoscopic retrograde cholangiopancreatography if the clinical picture and initial few tests indicate that hepatitis almost certainly exists.

The Value of Special Tests. With the passage of time, certain tests become obsolete, some are proven valueless, and others assume greater value. You should be aware of such changes as they appear in the medical literature.

For example, a Gram's stain of the stool is 43.5% sensitive and 99.4% specific for *Campylobacter* enteritis (4). This microbe has become an important cause of infectious diarrhea and needs unique antibiotic therapy. The very high specificity makes a positive stained smear essentially diagnostic. A negative smear is reasonably dependable at P(D)s between 5 and 20%; the predictive value of a negative test remains high because of the low ratio of FNs to TNs. Treatment can be intelligently directed by this simple test requiring basic staining techniques.

For years, clinicians have pondered the best way to detect acute myocardial necrosis. The standard procedure has been to obtain the SGOT-CPK-LDH triad on 3 consecutive days. More recently, studies have demonstrated that the parallel and series testing of the CPK, its MB isomer, and LDH isoenzymes every 12 hours for 48 hours is preferable. The CPK rises and its MB fraction goes above its normal 5% portion; this rise is slightly preceded by an LDH "flip" whereby the LDH 1 fraction becomes greater than the LDH 2 fraction. Together, these two changes are essentially 100% sensitive and 100% specific for myocardial infarction—perhaps *the perfect test*. Remember however that new investigations may make even such excellent protocols obsolete.

Let us remember that abbreviations for body chemicals are often changed. This may lead to confusion. The SGOT is the serum glutamic-oxaloacetic transaminase; many now call it the AST or aspartate aminotransferase. Most cardiologists now prefer creatine kinase (CK) to creatine phosphokinase (CPK). The lactate dehydrogenase (LDH) remains unchanged—so far. Keep these changes in mind when reading case studies.

Other clinical studies make us revise previous axioms. When seeking its cause, we often categorize an anemia by the red blood cell size and hemoglobin concentration. It is surprising to learn that, in this regard, the hematologist's review of a peripheral blood smear is not so dependable as the measured red blood cell indices (5). However, the finding of sickle cells, target cells, Howell-Jolly bodies, spherocytes, teardrops, etc may indeed be helpful.

It is also helpful to know that the predictive value for the presence of the Epstein-Barr virus is 100% if the heterophile antibody titer is elevated, and that virtually all patients with infectious mononucleosis have abnormal white blood cell differential counts. By knowing these facts, and knowing that adenopathy is 100% sensitive in this disease, testing can be minimized.

The carcinoembryonic antigen has a sensitivity of .72 and a specificity of .80 for colorectal cancer. As a screening test it would be worthless because of the high number of false positives. But in a patient whose $P(D)$ is already elevated by the clinical picture—e.g. $P(D) = .50$—a positive test raises the probability to .78; a negative test reduces the likelihood to .26. It has value, though limited.

An acid-fast stain for tubercle bacilli has always been regarded as having questionable reliability. But studies which used a positive culture as a gold standard have revealed that a carefully and properly performed smear is highly specific (approaching .999) and moderately sensitive (.39) (6).

Well-done studies of this type help us decide whether to use a test. And having used it, we know how to interpret the results. Data of this sort are needed for all tests and procedures. Most tests used today have never received critical evaluation at the medical decision level, and their predictive values remain unclear.

A Very Special Test. Take the very important issue of whether serious coronary artery disease exists or not as measured by the treadmill test. Few matters are more serious than the decision on whether a patient's chest pain means nothing or may lead to surgery or death. For a "positive" test

often leads inevitably to surgery, while a "negative" test results in medical treatment or nothing. Sensitivity and specificity must be carefully predetermined and the consequences of false negatives and false positives weighed (7).

Before performing this test, the test protocol must be carefully designed. This includes the method of performance and the establishment of the criteria for positivity. The latter can be determined by a discriminant function analysis score that takes into account not only the slope and degree of ST segment depression (or elevation) at the peak of exercise, but also the heart rate, the heart rate-pressure product, the presence of and duration of symptoms, ECG abnormalities, arrhythmias, and so forth. Usually only ST segment abnormalities at a heart rate of 85% of the predicted maximum are the principal criteria for abnormality.

The sensitivity hovers between .55 and .75 for severe coronary disease, and false negatives can occur with single vessel disease, with less stringent criteria for positivity, because of indefinable abnormalities in coronary anatomy, and for unknown reasons. The specificity is high but not high enough to exclude numerous false positives that can result from hyperventilation, mitral valve prolapse, and abnormal left ventricular depolarization and repolarization (e.g. left ventricular hypertrophy, digitalis, or Wolff-Parkinson-White syndrome).

In order to quantify the predictive value of a positive or negative test result, an estimate of disease probability—$P(D)$—must be made. This clinical estimate depends on the presence and type of chest pain, gender, age, family history, blood glucose and cholesterol, and associated symptoms.

These are the multiple considerations required to make this or *any test* worthwhile. Included are test performance, criteria for abnormality, efficient operating characteristics, and a reasonable approximation of disease probability prior to doing the test.

Misuse of Tests

It may be difficult to distinguish between use, overuse, and misuse of tests and procedures. There may be sincere and genuine differences of opinion between physicians as to whether a test is indicated or whether a procedure should be done.

Patients' charts already bulge with laboratory data. The annual growth in the test rate is 15%. Extrapolated statistics predict that *$50 billion* will be spent on hospital laboratory tests and procedures in 1985. This does not include tests done in doctors' offices. Laboratories contribute a large fraction to the rising costs of medical care. Small alterations in test-ordering attitudes could reverse this frightening trend.

Reasons for Overuse. There are many (1). First is the greater availability and variety of tests resulting from technologic advances. Next, more and more, diseases are diagnosed and their treatment is being monitored by lab tests. The ability to monitor drug levels and to do toxicologic studies has also increased laboratory use. For medicolegal reasons, too, tests are often unnecessarily done. Someone in the emergency room who has had an automobile accident may have an x-ray study performed wherever there is an ache or pain in order to rule out fractures. This is one example of the widespread practice of defensive medicine brought on in part by a litigious society.

Older physicians may be reluctant to give up outmoded tests, and there are still protein-bound iodine tests and liver flocculation tests being done.

Younger physicians tend to rely more on laboratory tests and procedures. Residents and interns may order large numbers of tests out of curiosity, in the interest of one-upmanship, according to established behavior, or because of the need to "be complete." Too often, the "chief" is more apt to criticize the house officer for a possibly helpful test that *wasn't* ordered than for an unnecessary test that *was* ordered. Omission is a greater sin than commission, so every conceivably related study is requested. These same house officers are then replaced by new ones who tend to *follow the leader.* Tests are especially overdone in teaching hospitals.

Some examples of questionable and probably unnecessary ordering patterns are: (*a*)

electrolytes daily; (*b*) 18-test chemistry profile daily; (*c*) arterial blood gases every 4 hours; (*d*) chest x-ray daily; (*e*) sputum cultures daily × 3; (*f*) SGOT, CPK, LDH daily × 3; (*g*) CT scan, ultrasound study, and isotope scan of liver; (*h*) CT scan for vague abdominal pain or headaches; etc. Some institutions tend to encourage package ordering. This may change!

Consider the 6-test chemistry profile which is done almost routinely for screening purposes. It includes the serum sodium, potassium, chloride and bicarbonate. Electrolytes are rarely abnormal in healthy patients not taking medication (8). Here the ratio of false to true positives may be as high as 20:1, and the tests therefore may be misleading. In diseased patients taking medication the ratio would be drastically altered. Electrolytes should be ordered only if the clinical background suggests a reason for a possible abnormality.

Admission studies may have been done once before, or they may be ordered twice the first day (once by the student, once by the intern) and then done twice the next day. Often the tests are done by the referring physician or in the attending physician's office—then repeated the next day in the hospital.

The lack of physician education in the proper use of tests, their operating characteristics, and their predictive values may be another root cause of misuse. Also, students are inadequately educated in most medical schools; courses in laboratory medicine have for the most part been eliminated from the curriculum.

The fact that most patients do not directly pay their own bills gives the physician an implied freedom to order tests. Another unfortunate situation is that diagnostic procedures are done by different departments in different specialties, each of which may be biased in favor of its own procedure. The patient may have three procedures done when one would suffice. Or the test done first may not have been the wisest choice, but it was done because its performer was more convincing. Not to be ignored is the realization that most procedures generate much income, and that, in a few instances, dishonesty rather than bias may be the governing factor.

A final cause for the overuse of tests is the frequent need to follow up a false positive result. The more procedures and tests that are done, the more false positives occur, and the more the need to track them down with yet more tests. Unfortunately, false positive results may even lead to harmful interventions, such as biopsies and exploratory surgery.

Unexpected Test Results. An inevitable outcome of multiple tests and *unsolicited data* is an unexpectedly positive test result. This presents the physician with problems and decisions. Is it a false or true positive? Does another problem exist? What additional studies need be done?

First, we must realize that a slightly abnormal test result may merely represent the 2.5% on either end of the reference interval. A hemoglobin of 11.5 g/dl, a lactate dehydrogenase 10% above upper normal, or indeed any test result which is just outside the "normal range" may trigger a long search for nonexistent disease. We have all seen many needless probes of this sort.

Next, the degree of abnormality must be considered. Nobody gets excited about a white blood cell count of 4,500 or 11,000, but what if it's 1,500 or 28,000? An alkaline phosphatase slightly above normal might merely raise an eyebrow, but if it's three times normal, you worry and then search. A blood glucose of 58 mg/dl or 116 mg/dl would be disregarded, but 40 mg/dl or 160 mg/dl would not (3). Both the true and false varieties of "chem profile disease" are common.

Given an unexpected abnormal test result, it may be ignored or acted upon. The basic approach for the action option would be: (*a*) repeat the test; (*b*) if normal, forget about it; (*c*) if still abnormal, consider the role of any drug the patient may be taking; (*d*) if still unexplained, consider a differential diagnosis for the abnormality; (*e*) if a workup is deemed appropriate after carefully weighing all aspects of the situation, track it down.

There are literally dozens of drugs that can cause each chemical aberration. And there are dozens of diseases that can do so also. You can easily develop or research a protocol to track down any abnormality. At times, the job will be easier if a group of abnormalities is uncovered which points to one organ or one disease. A distinctly increased alkaline phosphatase requires an isoenzyme study, some type of liver scan, and a bone survey; in this setting, a γ-glutamyltransferase may help separate liver from bone disease. Hypercalcemia demands a detailed study for hyperparathyroidism or malignancy.

The investigation of every case of unexpected hypercalcemia opens Pandora's box. The public cost is over \$100 million/year. A detailed voyage of discovery is indicated, resulting in either surgery or inoperable cancer. Recent studies show that the removal of asymptomatic, unexpectedly discovered parathyroid adenomas may not be indicated in the long run. The question of surgery— now, later, or never—has not yet been resolved.

Then there's the patient who has an ultrasound study for gallstones and in whom an abnormal area is noted in the liver. Or the patient with abdominal or back pain whose CT scan produces yet another quandary about adrenal lumps and bumps. These apparent abnormalities may be congenital liver cysts or benign functionless adrenal tumors completely unrelated to the prime problem. But they *trigger prolonged odysseys* that often end in shipwrecks rather than in safe harbors.

Whether the worship of unsolicited laboratory data can result in more trouble than benefit is a matter to be decided on the basis of all the evidence in each individual case.

Alteration of Testing Formats

Nobody denies that tests and procedures help in the management of patients. On the other hand, nobody denies that tests are overused, misused, and that they may create as well as solve problems. Furthermore, nobody denies the need to restructure the pattern for ordering tests. Can this necessary change best be accomplished by education, supervision, example, coaxing, incentive, or edict?

Those who write the orders in the chart are in large measure responsible for the control of hospital costs. The attending physician must set a good example by ordering only necessary and useful diagnostic and therapeutic measures. He must practice as he preaches and teaches.

Admission Studies. Routine studies are done on every hospital admission. These are established by hospital policy, physician habit, and house officer perseveration. They may change from year to year, from hospital to hospital, from medical to surgical patient, and according to the patient's age. Regulatory agencies, including third-party insurers and hospital quality assurance programs, mandate changes from time to time.

For example, the elimination of the complete blood count and its replacement by the white blood cell count and hematocrit have cut costs without altering quality. Routine ECGs are not recommended for patients under 35. The need for chest x-rays and chemistry profiles must be documented on the chart. More and more tests will require notations explaining their need. Attempts are being made to eliminate "standing orders" and preprinted uniform order sheets emanating from the attending physician's office. Duplication of tests just done on an outpatient basis should be avoided. Reimbursement for some tests is denied if they are not indicated. These are all steps in the right direction.

Special Patterns. The most important test-ordering pattern to be established is that there be *no* pattern. As far as is humanly possible, the ordering of batteries should be abolished, and only those tests that are specifically indicated should be selected. It might be preferable to provide a blank order sheet rather than long printed lists. The former requires thought; the latter needs only mindless check marks.

A *separate catalog of tests* which lists everything in the paraclinical supermarket should always be available. But the catalog must be only a reference and not the sheet upon which tests are ordered. Everyone knows that those who shop in supermarkets buy more than they need since they are tempted by the vast array of goodies. Only the most budget-conscious shopper will precisely purchase only what is absolutely needed. The same is true of the person who orders tests.

Nevertheless the order writer must be aware of or know where to retrieve selected subsets of available studies if a particular diagnosis is suspected or if there is a need to eliminate a possible diagnosis. This information either has already been taught, is becoming available in textbooks, or can be learned from material furnished by each diagnostic subunit. Note that standard textbooks usually merely list the tests that may be abnormal in a given disease without suggesting strategies.

If the problem is either jaundice, melena, hypochromic anemia, suspected hyperthyroidism, sore throat, chest pain, dyspnea on exertion, or backache, etc, there are a limited number of *high-yield studies* to be done in each instance—after or during the extraction of data from the history and examination. The initial tests and any needed additional studies are usually well known. If not, you can read about them, discuss them with your peers, or consult appropriate experts. Section Three of this book includes the diagnostic approach to many such common problems.

Today's best way to order tests for a suspected myocardial infarction has been established. It may be different tomorrow. If so, your hospital should communicate this advice to you.

The patient suspected of having adrenal insufficiency needs only three or four well-selected tests, not a dozen to cover all aspects of adrenal dysfunction. If panhypopituitarism is under serious consideration, only a handful of studies is needed to make sure; you need not do all tests for all endocrine abnormalities. Most thyroid problems need only two tests, not the complete four-test thyroid panel that is frequently requested. While there are currently ten serologic markers for viral hepatitis, they must be ordered in meaningful small groups depending on the clinical situation. Because of rapid advances in this field, the clinician may not know which tests to order first and which may possibly be needed later. Advice on current usage must be available. It seems that a problem-oriented request form might be preferable to either a blank form or one listing all available tests (9). Sample protocols are discussed later in this chapter.

Bear in mind that if tests and studies are ordered in sequential batches rather than all at once, laboratory expenses may be reduced, but costs for hospital days may increase. Again we must deal with the issue of trade-offs.

Students, not yet committed to concrete-cast routines, must learn all about tests and procedures. Medical schools should teach concepts of sensitivity, specificity, predictive value, and cost-risk-benefit factors. And clinical pathology courses should be restored to their rightful place in the second-year curriculum.

Is Change Easy? Having identified the problems and some of the solutions, you might think it would be a simple matter to apply the cure. But it isn't. Numerous studies have proven both the success and failure of remedial measures.

One group demonstrated that 80% of complete thyroid panels ordered were judged unnecessary (10). Education was not instrumental in changing the pattern of ordering these tests, but an alteration in the test request form was very effective. A change was made to a problem-oriented format wherein the tests to be ordered for each special thyroid problem were indicated. This caused a 50% reduction in the number of thyroid function tests ordered. The same investigators were unable to alter established patterns for ordering cardiac enzymes by using educational tools alone.

Others maintain that educational intervention, incentives, careful supervision, and daily feedback can bring about a 50% decrease in the number of tests ordered (11).

Some pessimism is expressed by different investigators who were only somewhat successful in their attempts to change test-ordering patterns. They question whether the fox can "learn to guard the chicken coop" (12).

It appears that change is possible though difficult to achieve and maintain. The setting up of specific diagnostic protocols seems to be helpful.

The Effect of DRGs. The present implementation of the diagnosis related groups (DRGs) system throughout American hospitals may be most effective in reducing the overall amount of diagnostic testing. This system pays a hospital a stipulated sum for the care of a patient according to the patient's diagnosis. The optimal use of laboratory tests, drugs, and beds will be in the hospital's best interests. In whatever ways possible the hospital will see to it that costs do not exceed payments—hopefully without compromising quality care.

Strategies for Testing

Whenever a patient tells you his chief complaint, you should immediately formulate and follow a protocol for getting more data. Usually this format is self-designed, and each physician generates his own special protocol for each clinical problem he sees. For common problems, the physician develops his own sequence. Less common problems may require some ingenuity or acquisition of additional knowledge from printed material or consultants.

Once the history and examination are completed and initial hypotheses are formed, further tests, studies, and procedures are often necessary. Generally the physician has a preconceived problem-driven sequence for obtaining added information. This sequence is based on many of the principles discussed in previous sections. Which tests shall he order first? Which later? All at once? Is one procedure enough? Are two better? Should all available tests and procedures be ordered? What if some are positive and some are negative? All these questions need careful consideration when tests are ordered.

In Series or Parallel. The first decision to make is whether to order several studies at once or await the results of one before ordering the next. Each strategy has its pro's and con's. If you decide to order tests sequentially you may find that as a result of the first test the second may not be necessary. This would occur if the first study resulted in a positive or negative predictive value deemed sufficient for your purposes. The revised disease probability would have excluded or confirmed a diagnosis with enough certainty. However, if additional security or confidence is sought, a second study could be ordered. The predictive value resulting from the first study becomes the new P(D) for calculating the performance and results of the second study.

The enigma of parallel testing (or, for that matter, series testing as well) arises when one test is positive and the other is negative. Often patients are seen who have a positive ultrasound study and a negative CT scan or vice versa. This causes confusion, and retests or additional tests must be done to add clarity. Always present is the disconcerting effect of "an equivocal test result." But, on the other hand, if tests are either all positive or all negative, great confidence is established.

Combination Testing. If two tests or procedures (*A* and *B*) are to be done on a patient, the clinician must observe certain guidelines. He may require that both tests be positive, or he may require only that either of the two be positive to establish reasonable diagnostic certainty. Most clinicians prefer the security of two tests over one, or three over two.

But as you deal with the combined operating characteristics of two tests, you must be aware of alterations in sensitivity and specificity created by combination testing. If the clinical guidelines by which you abide require that both tests be positive before diagnostic confidence is established, sensi-

tivity diminishes as specificity increases (Tables 6.1 and 6.2.). If only *A* or *B* need be positive, the combined sensitivity increases, while the specificity decreases (13). It is important to note that the precise mathematical relationships denoted in the two tables are true *only if* the two procedures are *mutually independent.*

First note Table 6.1. Tests *A* and *B* are both performed on 100 patients known to have a disease and on 100 people known not to have the disease. Test *A* is 90% sensitive and 80% specific. Test *B* is 70% sensitive and 90% specific. Note the number of diseased patients who will test positive for one, both, either, or neither of the tests. Now note the figures in those without the disease. It is readily seen that, in diseased patients, 63% will be positive for both *A* and *B*, 97% will be positive for either *A* and *B*, and 3% will be negative for both tests. By doing two tests, you have decreased the sensitivity of the combination. But if both tests are posi-

Table 6.1.
Combination Testing in Diseased and Nondiseased Populations (Numbers Represent Percentages)

	D		D̄	
A	90+	10−	20+	80−
B	63+ 27−	7+ 3−	2+ 18−	8+ 72−
A+ *B*+	63		2	
A+ *B*−	27		18	
A− *B*+	7		8	
A− *B*−	3		72	
	100		100	

Table 6.2.
Effect of Combination Testing on Sensitivity and Specificity (Numbers Represent Percentages)*

Test	Sensitivity	Specificity
A	90	80
B	70	90
A or *B*+	97	*A* and *B*− 72
A and *B*+	63	*A* or *B*− 98

* (Modified from Griner PF, Mayewski RJ, Mushlin AI, et al: Selection and interpretation of diagnostic tests and procedures. *Ann Intern Med* 94: 553–592, 1981.)

tive the disease is more apt to be present, since you have increased the specificity at the same time. Only 2% of nondiseased persons will be falsely positive for both tests. Also heed the fact that 3% of patients with the disease will be falsely negative for both tests. All final figures would be the same whether A or B was done first. Study these results and note both the clarification and confusion that can result from multiple testing.

From Table 6.1, the figures in Table 6.2 can now be understood. They represent the combined operating characteristics of two tests, each of whose sensitivity and specificity are known. Note that if only one positive test is required, the sensitivity is high—97%—but the specificity is reduced—72%. If both tests must be positive, the sensitivity is diminished—63%—but the specificity is markedly increased—98%. Put simply, two independent tests are less apt to both be positive in a patient with disease, but if they *are* positive, the disease is much more likely to be present.

If only one test need be positive to diagnose the disease, the sensitivity is high, since 70% of the 10% of patients who test negative for A will be positive for B (90% + 7% = 97%). But in this circumstance, the specificity will be markedly reduced (72%) because of the greater number of false positive results (2% + 18% + 8% = 28%).

Observe that the rule for the product of probabilities has been invoked (90% × 70% = 63%; 80% × 90% = 72%). Also be aware that when only one test need be positive to determine the sensitivity rate, the corresponding specificity rate is ordained by the requirement that *both* tests be negative. Contrariwise, if both need be positive to determine combined sensitivity, then the specificity rate depends on *either one* of the tests being negative. Carefully think about these two statements; they are true, though difficult to comprehend at first. For if both tests need be positive to diagnose a disease, then the negativity of either will establish the absence of disease. And if either test's being positive diagnoses a disease, then both tests

must be negative to establish that the disease does not exist. Think about that.

Economy or Accuracy. At this point a decision must be made. If the previously discussed disease is suspected, both tests may be done. This will increase accuracy at the expense of economy. On the other hand, you can apply only one test, and then do a second test on either those who test positive for A or only on those who test negative for A. If B is applied only to those who were positive for A, you are seeking the security of both tests being positive. If B is applied only to those who were negative for A, you are seeking those who are positive for only one of the two tests, and some accuracy is being sacrificed.

Take 100 patients, each of whom has a 50–50 chance of having a disease for which there are two tests—A and B. Assume that tests A and B have the operating characteristics stated in Table 6.2. All patients are given test A. The resulting incidence of positive results (true and false) and negative results (true and false) is stated in Table 6.3 (line 1). Then all 100 patients are given test B. The results are noted on line 2. An analysis of those who are positive for A, negative for A, positive for B, negative for B, positive for both A and B, negative for both A and B, and positive for either A or B is presented on lines 3 to 9, respectively. At the extreme right of each line, the predictive value of each situation has been calculated. Note that two positive tests and two negative tests almost eliminate false positives and false negatives, and thus give very high predictive values. Also note that the positivity of only one test does not give nearly so much assurance as the positivity of two tests. And as was previously portrayed in Chapter 5, the higher the initial P(D), the higher the resulting positive predictive value and the lower the resulting negative predictive value. All in all, 200 tests were done for a cohort of 100 patients.

Be aware of the fact that the various numbers and predictive values displayed in the foregoing discussion apply either to a single patient whose P(D) is .50 or to a cohort of

Table 6.3.
Results of Parallel Testing Using Tests *A* and *B* in a Subset with a 50% Probability of Having a Disease*

	50D		50D̄			
1. *A*	45+	5-	10+	40-		
2. *B*	31.5+ 13.5-	3.5+ 1.5-	1+ 9-	4+ 36-		
3. *A+*	45 TP		10 FP		PV+	.82
4. *A-*	5 FN		40 TN		PV-	.89
5. *B+*	35 TP		5 FP		PV+	.88
6. *B-*	15 FN		45 TN		PV-	.75
7. *A+ B+*	31.5 TP		1 FP		PV++	.97
8. *A- B-*	1.5 FN		36 TN		PV--	.96
9. *A or B+*	48.5 TP		14 FP		PV+	.78

* TP, true positive; TN, true negative; FP, false positive; FN, false negative, PV, predictive value (positive or negative for one or two tests). Test A is 90% sensitive and 80% specific; test B is 70% sensitive and 90% specific.

100 similar patients, 50 of whom have the disease in question and 50 of whom do not.

The foregoing illustration is an example of *parallel testing* wherein every suspect got two tests. A more economical method that promotes less tests follows. If two positive tests are required by the clinician, then apply test *B* only if test *A* is positive. If only one positive test is deemed adequate for reasonable diagnostic certainty, then apply test *B* only if test *A* is negative. This is *series testing.*

Now put series testing into operation on the same 100 patients, in each of whom P(D) is .50. Table 6.4 demonstrates the results obtained *when you seek positivity of both tests A and B.* Note that the same results are obtained, and the predictive value of two positive tests is the same. Those who tested negative for *A* were not tested for *B*. Diagnostic accuracy was not compromised, but the number of tests done on a cohort of 100 patients was reduced from 200 using the parallel method to 155 with the series method.

If the clinician requires that *only one of the tests need be positive* for adequate diagnostic certainty, test *B* is done only on those patients who test *negative* for *A*. Under these circumstances, the figures in Table 6.5 apply. Note that 48.5 patients with the disease will be positive for either *A* or *B*, but 14

Table 6.4.
Series Testing in a Cohort of 100 Patients Whose P(D) = .50; Two Positive Tests Are Required for Diagnosis; Only Those Who Are Positive for *A* Are Tested for *B*

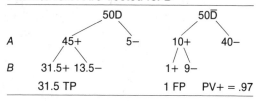

Table 6.5.
Series Testing in a Cohort of 100 Patients Whose P(D) = .50; Only One of Two Tests Must be Positive to Establish a Diagnosis; Only Those Who Are Negative for *A* Are Tested for *B*

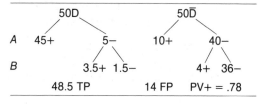

people without disease will also be positive for one of the tests. *Sensitivity* has been increased, but *specificity* and *predictive value* have been decreased—heavy prices to pay for the advantage of decreasing the number of tests to 145. An interesting sidelight is that the bottom lines are the same regardless of which test is used first in the diagnostic plan. But if test *A* (the one with the higher sensitivity) is done first, fewer tests need be done—145 rather than 160. It should be noted that alterations in the P(D) have a small but distinct influence on the total number of tests that need to be done for any cohort.

While the foregoing discussions involved only two tests, the same logic applies when more are used, but the calculations become more complex. The astute clinician usually utilizes several tests, trend analysis, and judgment to permit him to exceed the predictive value of a single test (14).

Which of Two to Do. If you should wish to do only one of a choice of many available tests, you may be faced with the question of doing the test with the greatest sensitivity or the test with the greatest specificity. Choose the one with the highest sensitivity if you cannot afford false negative results. Choose the test with the highest specificity if you cannot afford false positive results. As discussed in detail in Chapter 5, the matter distills to a trade-off between the harm of missing a disease in a patient who has it, and the harm of diagnosing a disease in a patient who doesn't have it. To be considered are the seriousness and treatability of the disease, the chances of detecting the disease by additional tests, the psychologic and economic harm of a false diagnosis, the moral issues revolving around treating somebody for a disease he doesn't have, and so forth.

All in All. Some simple truths to be deduced from the preceding discussions are:

1. Two tests are better than one if both are positive or negative.
2. Parallel testing is costly but informative.
3. Series testing is less costly and gives comparable information if both tests must be positive for diagnostic certainty.
4. Series testing has higher sensitivity but lower diagnostic value if only one of two tests must be positive.

Specific Clinical Problems. Physicians have always had their favorite strategies for

the diagnostic management of most problems. But as new procedures and tests become available, strategies have changed, are changing, and will continue to change. This will be especially true when the applications and properties of newer procedures become defined. Several examples of specific diagnostic protocols will be presented here, but many more examples can be found in the case studies of Section Three. Emphasis will be placed on the sequential ordering of tests and procedures on the assumption that as much help as possible has already been harvested from the history and physical examination.

Consider a patient with blunt abdominal trauma in whom intraabdominal bleeding is being considered. The choice lies between CT and peritoneal lavage. CT visualization is highly sensitive, can detect as little as 100 to 200 ml of blood in the peritoneal cavity, and can also note retroperitoneal trauma to the pancreas or duodenum. But it is costly and may not be immediately available. Needle lavage is simple, cheap, done in the emergency room, and essentially risk free. The presence of bile, amylase, or leukocytes may signal complications not yet suspected. But lavage may be overly sensitive and not quantitative; it is best for liver and spleen injury but is not good for retroperitoneal trauma. *The clinician must now make a choice.*

If a multiphasic test is unexpectedly abnormal, you can devise or research a protocol for follow-up. Opinions may differ. An elevated transaminase in a patient with no history or physical findings to suggest liver or heart necrosis requires retesting and a careful drug history. A slight elevation may warrant no action, just observation and recheck. A modest or severe elevation sets a train of tests into motion. This may include a radioisotope liver-spleen scan, ultrasound, CT, and possibly even a biopsy.

Should the alkaline phosphatase be surprisingly high, isoenzymes should help determine the organ source of the elevation— bone or liver. From there, you can either do bone radiographs (conventional or isotopic), search for a primary malignancy anywhere, or study the liver with added function tests, a CT scan or ultrasound, and biopsy if indicated. It is difficult to decide when to get off the *diagnostic treadmill* once you are on it. Multiple considerations enter the equation, and diagnosis cannot go on indefinitely. How important is it to track this isolated laboratory abnormality in the face of compounded risks and costs?

If acute pancreatitis is suspected, parallel and serial measurements of serum amylase, serum lipase, and urine amylase are still very helpful. The amylase:creatinine clearance ratio may not be as good as was first thought. Chemical tests available in most 18-test profiles are good indicators; electrolytes, glucose, urea nitrogen, calcium, and bilirubin are included. Coagulation profiles are indicated on alternate days. Beyond the laboratory, ultrasound and CT aid in the diagnosis. Not all these tests are necessary in each case, but the diagnosis can be substantiated, treatment can be directed, and the severity of disease can be gauged by some of the results.

Liver disease provides an inexhaustible stimulus for diagnostic tests and procedures. But here the *concept of substrategies* should be introduced. Since there are separate batteries to measure hepatic viral infection, liver cell injury, cholestasis, metabolic derangement, and liver anatomy, you must select the tests that fit the clinical problem. For hepatitis, only three or four antigen or antibody selections are enough. Liver cell injury is detected by the released enzymes (GGT, GOT, GPT, LDH). Cholestasis is measured by the alkaline phosphatase, 5'-nucleotidase, and bile acids. To detect metabolic derangements resulting from liver disease, assay the total proteins, albumin, prothrombin, choline esterase, etc. The transition from acute to chronic liver disease is monitored by protein electrophoresis, immunoglobulins, and coagulation factors. Anatomic delineation and histologic abnormalities can be detected by numerous more complex techniques that include scintigraphy, sonography, angiography, laparoscopy, biopsy, transhepatic cholangiography, and endoscopic retrograde cholangiography. Clearly, *not all tests are done for every liver problem*. The chosen substrategy depends on what information you need for the particular situation.

Printed Aids. Most strategies are well known and rapidly integrated into the physician's knowledge base. But there are excellent resources wherein organ panels and diagnostic strategies may be found (1). There you can research the protocols for acute renal failure, acute myocardial infarction, carcinoma of the prostate, hemolytic anemia, pulmonary embolism, and on and on. Then decide on your own course of action, remembering that the exact niche for each new procedure has not yet been carved and there is always room for disagreement.

References

1. Speicher CE, Smith JW Jr: *Choosing Effective Laboratory Tests.* Philadelphia, Saunders, 1983.
2. Flegel K, Oseasohn R: Adverse effects of testing. *Arch Intern Med* 142:883–887, 1982.
3. Statland BE: *Clinical Decision Levels for Lab Tests.* Oradell, NJ, Medical Economics, 1984.
4. Ho DH, Ault MJ, Ault MA, et al: *Campylobacter* enteritis; early diagnosis with a Gram's stain. *Arch Intern Med* 142:1858–1862, 1982.
5. Jen P, Woo B, Rosenthal PE, et al: The value of the peripheral blood smear in anemic patients. *Arch Intern Med* 143:1120–1125, 1983.
6. Murray PR, Elmore C, Krogstad DJ: The acid-fast stain: a specific and predictive test for mycobacterial disease. *Ann Intern Med* 92:512–513, 1980.
7. Goldschlager J: Use of a treadmill test in the diagnosis of coronary artery disease in patients with chest pain. *Ann Intern Med* 97:383–388, 1982.
8. Griner PF, Glaser RJ: Misuse of laboratory tests and diagnostic procedures. *N Engl J Med* 308:1336–1339, 1982.
9. Wong ET, Lincoln TL: Ready! Fire! ... Aim! An inquiry into laboratory test ordering. *JAMA* 250:2510–2513, 1983.
10. Wong ET, McCarron MM, Shaw ST Jr: Ordering of laboratory tests in a teaching hospital: can it be improved? *JAMA* 249:3076–3080, 1983.
11. Schroeder SA, Martin AR: Will changing how physicians order tests reduce medical costs? *Ann Intern Med* 94:534–536, 1981.
12. Eisenberg JM, Williams SV: Cost containment and changing physicians' practice behavior. *JAMA* 246:2195–2201, 1981.
13. Griner PF, Mayewski RJ, Mushlin AI, et al: Selection and interpretation of diagnostic tests and procedures. *Ann Intern Med* 94:553–592, 1981.
14. Galen RS, Gambino SR: *Beyond Normality: The Predictive Value and Efficiency of Medical Diagnosis.* New York, Wiley, 1975.

Chapter 7

The Impact of New Technology

PAUL CUTLER, M.D.

KEY WORDS

1. endoscopy
2. tumor markers
3. imaging techniques
4. diagnostic protocol
5. hardware
6. software
7. ultrasound
8. real time
9. computed tomography
10. nuclear imaging
11. digital subtraction angiography
12. magnetic resonance
13. positron emission tomography

In the foregoing discussions on diagnostic protocols in Chapter 6, much was said of new high-technology techniques. These consist mainly of ingenious imaging devices. Serious consideration must be given to the impact of these new techniques on the diagnostic process. In some instances, previous testing sequences have been made obsolete.

For example, computed tomography (CT) and ultrasound studies of the kidney have almost relegated retrograde pyelography to the past. Ultrasound has virtually replaced the cholecystogram. The first step in the management of upper gastrointestinal bleeding is fiberoptic endoscopy, not contrast radiography. In many cases, dye-enhanced CT brain scans have replaced cerebral arteriography.

Studies which have become prominent in the past decade include: (*a*) *fiberoptic endoscopy* with extension into the distal bronchi, the pancreatic and biliary trees, and the entire colon; (*b*) *biopsies* of lung, brain, heart, and pancreas—formerly considered very risky, but now less so under radiographic guidance; (*c*) *tumor markers* (immune-mediated or otherwise); (*d*) *radioisotopic studies* of infinite varieties, including measurements of blood flow and cardiac function, organ imaging, abscess location, proof of pulmonary emboli, etc; (*e*) *CT* of the head, chest, spine, abdomen, and pelvis; (*f*) *ultrasound* for cardiac anatomy, function, and disease, neck tumors, liver and gallbladder disease, pelvic tumors, tubal pregnancies, etc; (*g*) *magnetic resonance imaging* whose uses are still to be delineated; (*h*) *positron emission tomography* which also awaits evaluation; (*i*) *evoked brain potentials* to measure specific neurologic and behavioral deficits; (*j*) hosts of new radiographic techniques, such as *digital subtraction angiography*.

The full comprehension of each technique warrants the reading of a textbook. However, for medical students, a lecture or review article explaining the procedure and its mechanism, uses and indications, operating characteristics, and costs and risks should suffice. Physicians need greater depth of comprehension, but a short primer is enough. Specialists and procedure performers, on the other hand, must know all there is to know.

Complex Considerations

Some generalizations must be understood about recently adopted procedures. As new techniques appear on the horizon, old ones may fade into obsoletion. But new procedures must first be evaluated for reliability, and their operating characteristics must be established. Cost-benefit-risk factors must be appreciated. The precise and proper position of each procedure in the array of diagnostic weapons will change from time to time. New applications for each procedure will appear in the literature, and each new application must pass stringent inspections. And as always for any new test, the pendulum will swing back and forth several times before the test's proper niche is found.

It is important to remember that in this decade of diagnostic revolutions, the situation concerning the various aspects of new technologic procedures is in a hyperdynamic state of flux. *Yesterday's discovery can become today's dictum and tomorrow's relic.* What is considered correct diagnostic traffic flow may be detoured, rerouted, bypassed, short-cutted, or even firmly established as a major highway. Keep in mind that not all new techniques are better than old ones. Some start out with great expectations only to be proven inadequate by further experience.

In selecting your diagnostic protocol in each case, always consider the skill of the procedure performer, the concept of imperfect information, and the availability of technology at your work site. It is one thing to read of nuclear magnetic resonance in a leading medical journal, another to realize that it is not available in your community hospital. How intellectually stimulating to know that coronary artery graft patency can now be determined with noninvasive techniques in selected centers—but sobering to know that the hospitals in your area have neither the hardware nor software (personnel) to duplicate this process. Even if your

hospital can afford a million-dollar scanner, what benefit if your radiologist hasn't the skill to interpret the color-coded or shaded gray digital or analog signals he sees?

There can be no question that many formerly used diagnostic plans have been radically altered by new imaging techniques. In most cases the trend has been in the direction of using an expensive procedure that reaches the bottom line of a diagnostic problem while bypassing less efficient, time-consuming techniques. Generally, this *reduces costs* by decreasing the number of days needed. But recall that false positive results may require repeat studies and additional studies that increase hospital costs.

To this moment, debates still exist over a wide range of medical and surgical problems. Consider a patient with cholestatic jaundice whose ultrasound study shows dilated intrahepatic ducts. The subsequent procedure of choice in most medical centers is a percutaneous transhepatic cholangiogram; in others the endoscopic retrograde cholangiogram is preferred. Some will do both.

For other hepatic problems, the CT scan is preferred by some, ultrasound by others, isotopic scans by still a few; all three are used where indecision exists. Each technical expert will tell you why his procedure is the one of choice. Unless you know better, the decision is a difficult one. Eventually huge properly compiled data banks for each diagnostic study may be of help.

In hospitals where CT, ultrasound, and nuclear medicine sections have separate staffs, budgets, and scheduling arrangements, those who perform these procedures may become advocates and may compete for patients (1).

Given the same diagnostic problem, it can be seen why and how different doctors and different hospitals may pursue varied procedural sequences.

With some notable exceptions, CT and ultrasound give similar information and one study tends to reinforce the other. In many instances the superiority of one technique over the other is still to be firmly established.

Newer procedures under development must find their place in the system of strategies for specific clinical problems. Much research remains to be done in order to define the most appropriate strategies and to understand the merits of alternative routes. Yet more work is needed to decide if one test, two tests, or multiple tests are best in any special circumstances.

The nation-wide adoption of Diagnosis Related Group Systems (DRGS) will be a strong force in designing economical strategies that diminish procedures, shorten hospitalizations, and cut costs. Possibly they may compromise quality care. While combinations of CT, nuclear imaging, angiography, and ultrasound should do much to elevate predictive values and diagnostic likelihoods in cases where certainty is required, such combinations may not be in the best interest of hospital budgets. As noted in Chapter 6, they are often not in the patient's best interests, either.

Ultrasound

Images obtained from the reflection of high-frequency sound waves have proven their tremendous usefulness over the past decade—even though their usage got off to a slow start and was primarily in cardiology. Now echos are successfully used in *diagnostic problems from head to pelvis*. The technique is inexpensive, noninvasive, harmless, without radiation exposure, simple to perform, and can be done at the bedside. It is available in all hospitals and even in some private offices. However, the interpretation and reading of the black, white, and gray images do require considerable skill and experience, and obesity and intestinal gas render the test less valuable. Furthermore, an accurate rendition is in great measure dependent upon the technical skill of the operator who performs the test.

The M-mode method is used primarily in heart disease. A single stationary ultrasound beam documents the activity of a linear needle-like projection of underlying tissue. Sound is reflected from each interface of tissues having different acoustical impedances, and the time between sending and receiving the signal is converted into distance between the reflecting surface and the transducer. A rolling drum synchronized with a simultaneous ECG records continuous motion along the probe line in real time. Therefore this mode's chief value lies in its precise delineation of motion and thickness of underlying cardiac tissues during the cardiac cycle.

Two-dimensional ultrasound (2D) uses a sound beam that rapidly sweeps across the chest, abdomen, or pelvis and generates a cross-sectional image in the plane traversed. Dynamic imaging at 30 or more frames/second can observe motion and 2D detailed anatomy in *real time*.

Combinations of both modes often best serve the patient. It is likely that computer-generated constructs will soon pile body slices to form more perfect three-dimensional images; this will yield quality information.

The uses for such techniques are legion. Ultrasound is the procedure par excellence for demonstrating gallbladder stones, dilatation of hepatic bile ducts in obstructive jaundice, ascites, and subphrenic abscesses. It is especially good in cardiac diagnosis where motion is a factor and anatomic and functional abnormalities can be detected. For example, some clinicians consider this diagnostic modality to be 100% sensitive for subphrenic abscess, 95% sensitive for demonstrating the dilated intrahepatic ducts of obstructive cholestatic jaundice, and 95% sensitive for gallbladder stones. In these instances, it is highly specific too.

In cardiovascular diagnosis, 2D and M-mode techniques are very helpful in confirming ventricular wall contraction abnormalities, valve defects, congenital ailments, pericardial effusions, aneurysms, mural thrombi, myxomas, mitral prolapse, vegetations, etc.

Always an enigma, cancers, inflammations, and pseudocysts of the pancreas are rendered more diagnosable. Retroperitoneal nodes and masses can be detected, and lymphoma staging may be done too. The liver, spleen, and kidneys can be measured for size; and stones, tumors, metastases, cysts, and congenital abnormalities may be detectable in these organs.

Differentiation can be made between cyst and tumor of the thyroid, kidney, or ovary. Pelvic masses can be outlined and sometimes diagnosed. In obstetrics, where x-rays or isotopes are taboo, the expected date of delivery, placenta previa, and fetal gender and abnormalities can be noted. However, questions have recently arisen about the absolute safety of ultrasound in pregnancy.

These are only some of the myriad ways in which ultrasound waves may help the clinician.

Computed Tomography

Since its introduction in 1972, CT has revolutionized the science of diagnosis perhaps more than any other procedure. It has proven to be most versatile and is widely accepted and used. X-ray signals from a body-encircling source are collected and computer-synthesized into a cross-sectional image of a body slice. Different tissues and different pathologic processes in the same tissue will display varying shades of gray. These variations may be enhanced by the intravenous injection of iodinated radiographic contrast material which not only increases density differentials between types of tissue, but also dynamically visualizes vascular structures. In this way the sensitivity and specificity of the procedure are increased; the dye not only helps in the detection of lesions, but aids in their differentiation and analysis.

CT is superior to conventional radiography in that the gray scale is more widely spread; thus the radiographic densities of various types of juxtaposed soft tissue, air, and fat can be more clearly discerned, defined, and interpreted. The ability to visualize total accurate 2D transverse cross-sections rather than traditional flat pseudo-3D films is a decided plus.

The minuses follow. The procedure is costly, must be done in the radiography department, and requires a skilled interpreter and $1 million worth of hardware. X-ray exposure is equal to that of a barium enema, so it should not be used in pregnancy. With dye enhancement, consideration must be given to the discomfort of an intravenous injection, possible nausea and vomiting, and depression of renal function in diabetics and those with already damaged kidneys. Also, CT has only limited value in uncooperative patients who move, in cardiologic problems where heart motion is rapid, and in the rare very obese patient whose girth is too large.

New-generation CT scanners are faster and have larger numbers of detectors. Thus scan time is markedly shortened and images are rapidly constructed. Eventually, as motion is stopped by "camera speed" or by ECG gating, CT will be as useful in cardiac problems as it is elsewhere.

This modality has *outstanding* merit in the following diagnostic situations: brain disorders where distinctions must be made between trauma, types of strokes, hemorrhages, and tumors; adrenal tumors suspected by the clinical picture (but beware the incidence of benign nonfunctioning adrenal adenomas); possible herniated intervertebral discs or spinal stenosis where intrathecal dye studies are often no longer needed; mediastinal masses where aneurysms, nodes, larger vessels, and tiny thymomas can be differentiated; lung lesions whose malignant or benign nature may often be determined; abdominal suppuration when suspected; retroperitoneal tumors, nodes, or metastases; and the detection, staging, and resectability of malignant disease.

What a formidable accomplishment! Not only does CT do these positive things, but by so doing it often decreases or eliminates the need for more invasive tests, such as laparotomy, angiography, lymphangiography, biopsy, myelography, or endoscopic retrograde cholangiopancreatography (2). The patient who is unconscious following head trauma can be spared invasive and risky cerebral arteriography; the scan can detect and discern intracerebral, subdural, epidural, and subarachnoid hemorrhage, as well as edema or contusion. Even though the procedure is expensive, it may result in shortened hospital stays and reduced costs, elimination of surgery or additional procedures, and improved patient care.

Other highly beneficial uses for CT scans include the detection of serious trauma to the liver, spleen, or kidney; the confirmation of dissecting aneurysms; the diagnosis and characterization of unusual or difficult to detect fractures of the vertebrae or pelvis; the distinction between cyst and tumor when a mass lesion is noted on renal pyelography; the identification of cancer and acute inflammation of the pancreas; and the fathoming of other abdominal masses.

But a word of caution must be added. CT scans must not be used to supply repetitive and redundant information. When scans are used strictly for screening vague problems, such as nonspecific abdominal pain, fever, or weight loss, very little significant information is obtained. But if the study is *goal-directed* with a more specific problem in mind, the positive yield is much higher (3). Not all fevers, coughs, headaches, indigestion, or backpains need CT scans! If medicine were practiced in that way, costs would be astronomical and the diagnostic yield extremely low.

Nuclear Imaging

This is a procedure whereby chemicals tagged with radioactive isotopes are given intravenously. Radioactivity is then measured over the special site to which the chemical is selectively attracted. Such scintigraphic techniques have been successfully used for two decades. The number of chemicals and dyes has multiplied, and all sorts of practical applications are now in use.

For example, the size and shape of the liver and spleen can be precisely delineated; tumors, cysts, and deformities detected; and even histopathologic abnormalities suggested. The ventilation-perfusion scan is highly sensitive for pulmonary emboli. Cere-

bral blood flow can be measured with serial scans. Multiple gated acquisition (MuGA) scans measure ventricular ejection fractions as a determinant of cardiac function. Ischemic areas can be detected in the heart, lung, brain, or kidney. Postexercise thallium heart scans are highly sensitive for coronary artery insufficiency and myocardial ischemia.

Other popular uses include total body bone scans for inflammation or metastases, ^{99m}Tc-labeled compounds (e.g. diisopropyl imidodiacetic acid (DISIDA)) to diagnose or rule out acute cholecystitis; radioiodinated fibrinogen to locate acute thrombosis; tagged erythrocytes to study their survival and sequestration, and to pinpoint the site of gastrointestinal bleeding; tagged leukocytes to locate occult abscesses; and on and on.

Such procedures are fairly simple to do but require skill and strict criteria for performance and interpretation, expose the patient to radiation, require an intravenous injection, and are moderately expensive.

Biopsies

These too are being done with increasing frequency. Brain, heart, liver, kidney, spleen, thyroid, and pancreas are all accessible to the probing biopsy needle. Aspiration biopsy and cytologic study of thyroid nodules may replace more formal biopsy procedures, eliminate nuclear scans, bypass ultrasound, and avoid many instances of surgery.

Transthoracic and transbronchial lung biopsies are done almost with impunity under simple fluoroscopic guidance. Cervical mediastinoscopy for carinal node biopsy helps to determine operability of lung cancers.

Perhaps the greatest encouragement for biopsy of formerly inaccessible or dangerous sites is given by CT and ultrasound. With the precision and accuracy of guided missiles, real time ultrasound or rapid sequence CT scanning can quickly direct a probing biopsy needle to a tiny 1-cm target or a drainage catheter to an occult abscess. This is an expensive, skill-requiring procedure, but it can bypass other less fruitful attempts at diagnosis and can save time and money in the long run.

Newer Radiologic Modalities

Insofar as new diagnostic techniques are concerned, the great majority involve the radiology department under whose aegis all types of imaging are done. The radiologist's role in the medical universe is undergoing evolution. In many cases he still deals with shadows and reads the films requested by the attending physician. But more and more the radiologist is serving as a consultant (4). After being given the suspected clinical problem, he can suggest the most suitable diagnostic procedure or procedures and the order in which they should be done. Usually he knows which procedure is best suited for each clinical situation. A conference between the clinician and the radiologist is often very productive. In hospitals where such consultations are mandatory before CT scans are done, the number of procedures decreases, and the number of true positive results increases.

On the cutting edge of expanding diagnostic facilities are: three-dimensional reconstruction, computer-assisted ultrasound, computed digital subtraction angiography, nuclear magnetic resonance, and positron emission tomography. Each will be briefly described.

Adjacent body slices obtained by ultrasound or CT scan can be built into *three-dimensional images*. This is already of use to maxillofacial surgeons considering major reconstructions, and it may be infinitely valuable in depth perception of organs from any direction.

Computer-assisted ultrasound purports to achieve the accuracy of other imaging procedures with the bonus of eliminating radiation exposure. At present it is an adjunct in the examination of the breast and may be of help in determining liver and other tissue abnormalities.

Digital Subtraction Angiography. This computerized system for visualizing arterial trees by the intravenous injection of a contrast material may eliminate the need for and risk of some intraarterial dye injections. Formerly, dyes reaching the arteries after intravenous injection were so dilute that they gave unsatisfactory images; the vessels could not be distinguished from the background soft tissue densities. But the computer stores the digitized preinjection image and subtracts it from the postinjection image, leaving only the dye in the arteries to be seen. This filmless system, which is stored and displayed by computer, dramatically increases the signal:noise ratio and *permits clear visualization of arteries*. It demonstrates flow and perfusion defects. So far its greatest use has been to visualize carotid artery stenosis. It is reported that pulmonary artery occlusions by tiny emboli are detected with 100% sensitivity and rare false positivity. Renal circulation, coronary artery pathways, cerebral artery circuits, and other visceral and peripheral vessels may become clearly delineated by this almost harmless, slightly invasive procedure. The values of such visualizations are boundless.

Magnetic Resonance Imaging. This radiologic technique offers images that reflect not only anatomy but also biochemistry. Energy is released by certain elements in body sites that have been subjected to giant circumcorporeal magnetic fields and then bombarded with short bursts of radiofrequency waves. These energy signals from stimulated atomic nuclei, such as hydrogen and phosphorus, can be computer-imaged. This gives *structural and biochemical information* about tissue, thus tending to fingerprint some disease processes by performing "body chemical analyses" in the liver, brain, spinal cord, and neoplastic tissue. Some of the known beneficial applications of this totally noninvasive diagnostic procedure are the detection of areas of cerebral edema, the delineation of the spinal cord, the discrimination of white from gray matter, the differentiation between liver disorders, and the early detection of neoplasms.

Positron Emission Tomography (PET Scan). This is another real time imaging device, used primarily in brain disorders. Tracer amounts of biochemically important substrates are labeled with very short half-life positron-emitting radionuclides. The in vivo distribution of these tracers is measured by special scanning devices. Thus you can measure cerebral blood flow, oxygen consumption, glucose metabolism, and protein synthesis, depending on the chemical substrate used. Regional brain physiology and biochemistry can be observed, and areas of metabolic derangement can be pinpointed. Implications for the diagnosis of stroke, schizophrenia, epilepsy, and multiple sclerosis become evident. For example, the abnormal biochemistry in the plaques of multiple sclerosis and the glucose metabolic defect in an epileptogenic focus can be detected when other diagnostic methods are nonproductive. It has been noted that schizophrenics do not metabolize glucose equally in all areas of the brain. Cardiac, pulmonary, and abdominal disorders are still on the research agenda.

This diagnostic and research tool is necessarily *limited to large institutions* for two reasons. First, the cost of the hardware alone is several million dollars. Second, since very short half-life radioisotopes are needed, they must be manufactured on site and cannot be transported elsewhere. It follows that only medical centers with cyclotrons or linear accelerators can do PET scans.

Other procedural diagnostic techniques described early in this chapter will be mentioned and detailed in Section Three where specific case studies are presented. What is considered to be the current state of the art of test selection will be presented in the individual case studies where diagnostic decisions are being made.

Are We Better Off?

Are the patient and clinician in a more advantageous position because of the newer diagnostic techniques? This question has three possible answers—yes, no, and maybe.

Confusion, complications, and costs escalate. The accuracy of resulting diagnostic and therapeutic decisions may be enhanced or diminished in any individual case. Always present is the grim specter of imperfect information, since false negative and false positive results exist for complex as well as simple tests. The skill of the procedure performer is a variable that must be considered.

Then too the clinician is often confounded by conflicting or indeterminate results which are "suggestive of" or "compatible with." In fact, uncertain tests or reports that neither exclude nor confirm a diagnosis only provoke the physician to order yet another test. And rapidly advancing technologies often leave him befuddled as to the appropriate test for a given problem; so he may order one, two, three, or all, hoping for a uniformity of results. When they are not in accord, he is understandably stumped.

For the Opposition. The following case study demonstrates the pitfalls, snares, and entanglements that can result from reliance on new procedures (5).

A 55-year-old man with 10 months of malaise, jaundice, dark urine, and light stools is presented. He has had no weight loss, and his liver is slightly enlarged.

In the 1960s and early 1970s, such a patient would have received a few liver function tests, possibly a liver biopsy, a gastrointestinal x-ray series, a barium enema to exclude a neoplasm, and then surgical exploration for obvious obstructive jaundice. Cancer, stone, or sclerosing cholangitis were the preoperative possibilities.

In the 1980s, *the same patient* had additional multiple diagnostic procedures before a decision to operate was made. The carcinoembryonic antigen was strongly positive. Ultrasound showed subtly dilated intrahepatic ducts and a thickened gallbladder wall. But the CT scan revealed no dilated intrahepatic ducts and no gallbladder wall thickening. Percutaneous transhepatic cholangiography (PTC) showed constrictions of the hepatic ducts at their confluence. A liver biopsy was "consistent with obstructive jaundice." Endoscopic retrograde cholangiopancreatography (ERCP) showed normal distal ducts but gave no information about trouble higher up. Repeat PTC confirmed strictures in the proximal hepatic ducts but also suggested a mass in the porta hepatis. The mass was confirmed by transfemoral selective arteriography.

Surgery was performed. Sclerosing cholangitis of the upper biliary ducts was found, and the mass was not there. The preoperative impressions, the decision to operate, and the operative findings were the same in the 1960s, 1970s, and 1980s.

But the CT scan and ultrasound were at odds. The carcinoembryonic antigen was falsely positive. ERCP was not helpful. The liver biopsy showed what was easily predictable. And the mass seen in PTC and arteriography was not present. In short, these additional complex procedures were confusing, added little helpful information, were redundant, were mostly not needed, and altered no decisions. They did, however, expose the patient to repeated dangers and to 47 rem of radiation (the equivalent of six barium enemas), and added $5745 to the hospital bill (cost of procedures plus extra hospital days).

On the Flip Side. On the other side of the coin, there's no denying that the intelligent, appropriate use of new "hi-tech" tests can greatly benefit the patient. Diagnoses are often made more easily, more quickly, more correctly, and more cheaply, and surgery may be simplified or exploration avoided. Not only will more diagnoses be made, but disease processes will be better categorized and understood.

Consider, for example, the patient with *obstructive jaundice* just discussed. Assume that the initial study, ultrasound, had clearly shown dilated intrahepatic ducts and stones in the gallbladder. Assume further that the second study, a PTC, had shown a stone obstructing the common bile duct. No further studies would have been needed, and the therapeutic decision path would have been clear. Had the second test been an ERCP, the same necessary information might have been garnered.

Consider also a patient in whom *you suspect a pulmonary embolus*. Before starting

expensive, lengthy, and risky anticoagulant treatment, you want to be more certain of the diagnosis because the patient also has chronic liver disease and mild hypertension. The chest x-ray and ECG are both normal. There are many tests and procedures to choose from: arterial blood gases, perfusion scan, ventilation-perfusion scan, pulmonary arteriography, and digital subtraction angiography. Some clinical groups routinely perform pulmonary arteriography in such situations. After all, it is essentially a gold standard procedure and invades only the right side of the heart. However, the most universally used test is the ventilation-perfusion radionuclide scan. It is barely invasive, relatively inexpensive, universally available, and has high sensitivity and specificity. Therefore put your eggs in that basket. But if therapeutic surgical intervention is contemplated and 100% certainty is needed, arteriography should be done (6).

As a corollary, should you need to know if *iliofemoral venous thrombosis* is the source of the embolism, you can do a venogram, a plethysmogram, Doppler studies, or a radioiodinated fibrinogen scan. The choice is not clear-cut and will vary from patient to patient.

For the detection of silent impalpable *carcinoma of the breast*, there is mammography, xeromammography, magnification, CT, xonics, ductography, ultrasound, computed ultrasound reconstruction, and so forth. While mammography is still the method of choice, the state of each art may change so that another technique may be preferable in the future (7).

A 60-year-old man with weight loss, anorexia, glucose intolerance, and no family history of diabetes mellitus is suspected of having *carcinoma of the pancreas*. Conventional radiography has been fruitless. You must now decide whether to order a CT scan, ultrasound, radionuclide scan, duodenal drainage cytology, ERCP, selective arteriography, serum markers, or a guided needle biopsy. Each test has its approximate operating characteristics, risk, cost, and availability. So you consult your friendly unbiased radiologist, who will help you decide. One or two tests should suffice. Perhaps the best sequence is either ultrasound or CT scan followed by ERCP. The sensitivity and specificity of either combination are in the 95% range. If one neoplastic area is delineated, a guided needle biopsy may raise the predictive value to 100%. No room for further doubt!

The next decision concerns a 64-year-old man with *transient ischemic attacks* and a right carotid artery bruit. Before suggesting surgery, you would like to perform the gold standard test for carotid stenosis—arteriography. But this procedure carries a 1% risk of causing a stroke. So you consider less invasive though not so accurate studies, such as oculoplethysmography, ophthalmodynamometry, ultrasound, and digital subtraction angiography. If one test is positive and the second is negative, you must now order a "tie-breaker." Even with its attendant risk, arteriography might still be the best choice if surgery is anticipated. So do it first since it will probably be all you need.

In some instances, we can unequivocally state the best procedure for a prospective diagnosis. The "best test" for gallbladder stones is ultrasound; for acute cholecystitis it is a radionuclide scan with a substance like DISIDA; for carotid stenosis it is arteriography; for pulmonary emboli, it's the ventilation-perfusion scan; for suspected intracranial bleeding do a CT scan. But for many other problems it's a tossup or a slight edge for one procedure here and now but for another procedure there and later.

This section begins and ends with the same question and the same answers. Are we better off as a result of new diagnostic procedures? Yes? No? Maybe? *Ça depends.*

References

1. Griner PF, Glaser RJ: Misuse of laboratory tests and diagnostic procedures. *N Engl J Med* 307:1336–1339, 1982.
2. Wittenberg J: Computed tomography of the body (two parts). *N Engl J Med* 309:1160–1165, 1224–1229, 1983.
3. Kapoor W, Hemner K, Herbert D, et al: Abdominal computed tomography: comparison of the usefulness of goal-directed vs. non-goal directed studies. *Arch Intern Med* 143:249–251, 1983.
4. Baker SR: The operation of a radiology consulting service in an acute care hospital. *JAMA* 248:2152–2154, 1982.
5. Case records of the Massachusetts General Hospital; weekly clinicopathologic exercises. *N Engl J Med* 306:349–358, 1982.
6. Hull RD, Hirsh J, Carter CJ, et al: Pulmonary angiography, ventilation lung scanning, and venography for clinically suspected pulmonary embolism with abnormal perfusion lung scan. *Ann Intern Med* 98:891–899, 1983.
7. Kopans DB, Meyer JE, Sadowsky N: Breast imaging. *N Engl J Med* 310:960–966, 1984.

Chapter 8

Making Medical Decisions

PAUL CUTLER, M.D.

KEY WORDS

1. decision theory
2. decision tree (matrix, scenario)
3. strategies (options)
4. decision nodes
5. probabilistic events
6. chance nodes
7. outcomes
8. utilities
9. foliating the tree
10. averaging out and folding back
11. optimal strategy
12. sensitivity analysis
13. threshold determinations
14. QALYs
15. DEALE
16. benefit-cost analysis
17. cost effectiveness analysis
18. risks-costs-benefits
19. estimating the P(D)
20. informed consent
21. public policy
22. Diagnosis Related Groups

On Zen, Zoos, Zealots, and Zeitgeist

Monkey Business. In the south of India, the monkeys are prolific and ubiquitous, frighten the children, steal the food, and in general are a nuisance. So the natives try to get rid of them by building monkey traps (1). These consist of hollowed-out coconut shells filled with rice and tied to the ground with a stake. The hole in the coconut is large enough to admit a monkey's hand but too small to permit the withdrawal of a monkey's hand filled with rice.

When the monkey cannot withdraw his hand he is trapped, and the angry villagers descend upon him with sinister motives. Seeing the villagers running toward him, the monkey is frightened and must speedily make a decision. He can let go of the rice, withdraw his hand, and run for the nearest tree; he can struggle to free his full hand or dislodge the coconut; or he can hold on and be caught. Actually he is trapped between hunger and fear of capture, but is confused by a value rigidity that rates rice above freedom. Not being able to calculate the likelihoods quickly, to distinguish clearly between alternative pathways, and to make a rational decision to do something, he is captured and disposition is made.

Seven-Eleven-Twenty-one. Let's move now to a more sophisticated zoologic arena—the gaming tables of your favorite casino. If you take your chances at the craps table, you can bet more intelligently if you understand that each die has 6 sides, and that the chances are 1 in 36 of rolling a combination of 2 or 12; 4 in 36 of rolling a combination totaling 5 or 9; and 6 in 36 (1 in 6) of rolling a lucky or unlucky 7.

Then try your hand at blackjack. If you count the number of low cards and court cards that come out of the dealer's shoe, you can predict with some degree of accuracy whether the next card will be high or low. This helps you gamble with more wisdom and less chance.

But what does all this have to do with the practice of medicine? Certainly medicine is not like a deck of cards where you know the exact number of diamonds, red cards, court cards that are hearts, and black kings. Nor can we in medicine quickly estimate the combinations and likelihoods as we do in the game of dice.

More and more, however, quantitation, precision, probabilities, likelihoods, numbers, and percentages are being attached to what we read, how we think, and how we decide. The mathematical modeling of patient care and a systematic approach to making medical decisions under conditions of uncertainty may become the vogue of the decade.

Decisions! Decisions! Whoever makes a decision makes a choice among competing options after considering the various *tradeoffs between benefits and risks.* Political decisions are often made on the balance of votes vs good of country. Economic decisions decrease interest rates at the cost of greater unemployment. Military leaders decide if the capture of a hill is worth 100 lives. But medical decisions should be made only for the individual patient's welfare after a consideration of the benefits and risks. If public policy mandates that costs to society be considered too, a revision of moral-ethical issues concerning the fundamentals of medical practice may become necessary.

Physicians make hundreds, even thousands, of decisions daily. These concern both themselves and their patients. For, as with anybody else, their personal decisions begin on awakening: choice of clothes, choice of breakfast, which route to travel to work, and quick almost thoughtless choices between various options that are part of everyday living. But when they enter the world of medicine, decisions are made almost by the minute or second. How to greet a patient? What to say first? Is this bit of information important? What questions do I ask next? What parts shall I examine? What's wrong? Am I sure? Are tests needed? What treatment is indicated? Shall we operate? And on and on for each patient.

The answer to each question requires multiple entries into the decision maker, and many items are quickly considered and tac-

itly weighed before a decision is made. Even simple decisions such as whether to give penicillin to a patient with a sore throat require the consolidation of many items. Look at the throat, take the temperature, feel for cervical nodes, estimate the streptococcus-virus likelihood, weigh the risks of renal, rheumatic, and peritonsillar complications caused by the streptococcus vs the cost of penicillin and possible penicillin allergy, and make your decision. You may decide to decide later after a throat culture report. And almost buried in all these peripheral issues is the need to make the patient well as soon as possible.

Decisions acquire a more precise mathematical aura when we consider the likelihood of a disease in the presence of a positive clue, three positive clues, or perhaps a negative test result. Given certain data, how likely is a diagnosis, and given a certain diagnosis, how likely are selected bits of data to be present? Can treatment be given on the basis of an estimated P(D), or must the disease probability first be increased by a test or procedure? Indeed, given the concept of imperfect information, what is the net benefit to be derived from this diagnostic step?

Generally even complex decisions are made by quick *subconscious* mental maneuvers and computations which are euphemistically called "intuition" or "logic." Actually these decisions are at least in some part based on experiential and acquired semiquantitative information stored in the brain's circuitry. Here too we may have another example of boiling ephemeral "intuition" down to computed brainwork. But, admittedly, many decisions are made on the basis of guess, hunch, mimicry, or protocol.

The big questions are: Can the use of precise numbers, percentages, equations, algebra, diagrams, and computers lend greater accuracy to our decisions, make us better doctors, and improve health care delivery? Can reliance on quantitative data bases help us make decisions on individual patients? And can we make wiser major health policy decisions that affect *all* people?

For example, given a 28-year-old woman

with arthritis, pleuritis, and a facial rash, does a negative antinuclear antibody test rule out systemic lupus erythematosus? Does a positive test diagnose it with certainty? Can we proceed with treatment under either circumstance?

Given a nonalcoholic patient with severe liver disease and a positive hepatitis B surface antigen, can we treat with steroids or must we biopsy first? What are the benefits, costs, and risks of biopsy and steroids? What if the biopsy gives imprecise information?

And given a patient with a 20% likelihood of having a pulmonary embolus, should we proceed with heparin, or should additional confirmatory evidence be sought? What is the risk of heparin? Of re-embolization? Of death? And would the presence of concomitant liver disease alter the decision? What if the likelihood of embolus were 5%, 50%, or 90%? Where is the line drawn?

What should public and professional policy be regarding immunization with hepatitis B vaccine for male homosexuals, intravenous drug users, blood transfusion recipients, and exposed professionals?

And suppose a purified protein derivative test turns positive in a 35-year-old nurse? Considering the risk of drug-related hepatitis, should isoniazid be given to prevent a disease that may never flourish?

What of the patient with a loud carotid bruit and an episode of syncope? Are the two related? How much stenosis exists? Should ultrasound or arteriography be done? What is the patient's annual risk of stroke? Of permanent neurologic damage? Of death? Should surgery be done? Now or later? Can medication help? Help!

What Decision Theory Is

Decision theory is the credo that some decisions can be made in an explicit and hopefully superior fashion by *the careful structuring of alternative pathways* and the *assigning of quantitative estimates* to disease probability, test information, risks, benefits, and outcomes.

This chapter is devoted to a discussion of decision theory, decision analysis, and the mathematical logic of making medical decisions. Since the subject is controversial, pros and cons will be presented. For sure, this matter is not the phlogiston of the '70s, '80s, and '90s. But its exact role is yet to be defined, and decision theory must still be regarded as a clinical adjunct, not a curative elixir for diagnostic and therapeutic problems.

Who Are the Infidels? Hundreds of eminent educators ardently believe that decision analysis has value in a variety of clinical situations. Many others have been converted to their faith. One cannot deny the significant contributions being made to medical science by this new breed of medical decision makers. For example, it should be pointed out that the American Cancer Society's current recommendations for screening cervical, breast, and colon cancer are derived from mathematical models based on decision analysis (2).

But in contrast to those who believe in the value of decision analysis, there are competent educators who feel that decision theory and its applications are not practical, that it is merely a toy based on shoddy information, and that it cannot be applied to the individual case which almost always has some feature that makes it unique.

However, since literary and educational circles are becoming replete with information derived from decision-assisting devices such as decision analysis, today's medical student must become familiar with this zeitgeist—this new spirit of our current times. Still, even though it has the promise of becoming more tool than toy, its proponents emphasize that decision theory is not a substitute for but a supplement to clinical judgment.

Medical decision making is a rapidly evolving sophisticated field in which the attempt is made to combine scientific, economic, ethical, and personal considerations into a framework that permits the physician to make a wise choice in an explicit manner. We try to formalize and structure the combined objectives of the doctor, the patient, and society. These may conflict. In this regard, I have never met a patient who gave a hoot about benefit:cost ratio (if he was well insured!) nor many health care administrators whose prime concern was patient welfare. If possible, the physician must artfully blend the interests and policies of all concerned. This may become more difficult as public and administrative policies come into conflict with the individual patient's welfare, and the physician is trapped between the horns of hospital regulations and the sacred doctor-patient relationship.

Mainly, *clinical decisions focus on whether to wait, to treat, or to test; to test and then treat; and how to treat.* Decision theory allows these problems to be represented in the form of decision trees. Since this book is concerned with diagnosis and not with therapy, subsequent discussions will deal principally with *diagnostic* decisions. But because decision analysis must often deal with *diagnosis and treatment* in the same scenario, both will be discussed in order to broaden the reader's overview of the subject.

With the advent of the Orwellian era, many new MEDSPEAK terms are in common usage. Some of these new words and phrases have been discussed in previous chapters, but others will be introduced here because they are vitally related to the anatomy and physiology of decision trees. Included are such terms as: P(D), sensitivity, specificity, predictive value, decision tree and scenario, utilities, decision nodes and chance nodes, averaging out and folding back, strategies, threshold determinations, sensitivity analyses, benefit:cost ratios, QALYs (quality-adjusted life years), and the DEALE (declining exponential approximation of life expectancy).

A decision tree is a flow chart format that depicts the options and outcomes of a clinical situation requiring a decision. It tells you what can happen if you opt to go in one direction rather than another. The tree deals mainly with such issues as the likelihood that a disease is present, the various strategies that may be applied and the efficacy of each, the possible need for a test or procedure that alters the P(D) and permits an optimal choice, and the fact that the test's ability to lend a hand depends on its operating characteristics.

The terminology used by decision analysts may sometimes be confusing. Clarification may be in order. The decision tree itself portrays the entire road map, which includes the structural matrix, the various choices that can be made starting with a clinical picture requiring a decision, and the events, subsequent decisions, and final outcomes of each. Take a moment *now* to look briefly at Figure 8.1.

Alternative option, action, and *strategy* are synonyms for the various choices available to the decision maker at the time of making a decision. These three terms are interchangeable.

And last, the *scenario* or *path* depicts the sequence of actions, events, and outcomes that follows only one particular option. Thus, a scenario represents only one portion of a decision tree.

To illustrate: If, in taking an automobile trip, you come to a fork in the road, you must decide whether to go right or left. These are the two options. If you go left, the path or scenario is 68 miles long; you will cross a bridge, travel a muddy road, pass two intersections, and encounter an additional fork in the road, but there will be no traffic. On the other hand, if you choose to go to the right, the path is 108 miles long, follows a paved road that is often congested, and goes through four traffic lights and three towns. You are in a hurry to reach your destination, there are 20,000 miles on your tires, and your automobile is not new. Knowing each path or scenario and the possible decisions, events, and consequences you may encounter, which option do you choose?

Structuring the Decision Tree. The formation of a decision tree that is based on a clinical picture depends on the inclusion of all alternative actions that the clinician is considering. Not only the options but the sequential events and all important clinical outcomes must be dealt with. What will happen if action 1 is pursued? What may

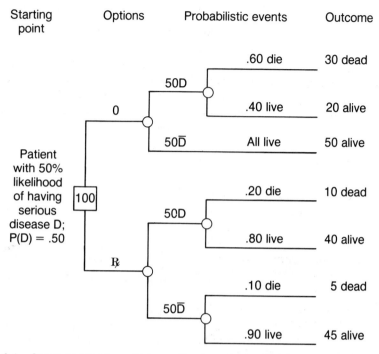

| Starting point | Options | Probabilistic events | Outcome |

Fig. 8.1. Simple decision tree with two paths; the outcome of each path is predictable.

result if action 2 is chosen? The tree must consider all important options, possibilities, outcomes, "what-ifs," and "on the other hands." Try to mimic the master of socio-political decision trees—Alexander Solzhen-itsyn—as he dissects every action path and its consequences on his way through the Gulag (3). Fortunately, not all medical decisions are so complex.

The *elementary* decision tree in Figure 8.1 is based on a patient who has a 50% like-lihood of having a serious disease whose mortality rate is 60%. Treatment reduces the mortality rate to 20%. Ordinarily there would be no question that this patient should be treated. But the risks and lethal side effects of the treatment are such that 10% of nondiseased as well as diseased pa-tients die if they are treated. The decision is now not so simple.

Figure 8.1 is a diagram of the two op-tions—to treat or not to treat. The outcome is measured in terms of life or death. A cohort of 100 individuals having the same clinical background as the propositus is un-

der consideration. The "don't treat" option is labeled "0"; the "treat" option is labeled "℞."

The *small square* at the extreme left is the starting point or **decision node.** Here the clinician is in control of the decision. The alternative options (treat or don't treat) that emanate from this decision node are clearly delineated, and the ensuing probabilistic events and outcomes are printed. *Small cir-cles* indicate **chance nodes**; these are pathway dividers that do not require decisions. Chance nodes are places where the patient's status is revealed, test information becomes established, or other events beyond the cli-nician's control take place.

Note that a P(D) of .50 (50% disease likelihood) implies that in a cohort of 100 similar patients, 50 would have the disease and 50 would not. Thus in treating a patient for a disease there is always a possibility that we are treating one who does not have the disease. And if we don't treat the patient, there is a possibility that we are withholding treatment from one who does have the disease. Due to the uncertainty of diagnostic probability based on clinical information, the imperfection of tests, and the deficiencies of treatment, judgments in medicine are for the most part probabilistic. Decision trees permit us to *make explicit* the probabilistic nature of medical information and the medical decisions made therefrom.

By inspecting the decision tree in Figure 8.1, you can see that giving treatment is the correct way to go in this case. This would doubtless have been your intuitive judgment anyway. Those with disease have their mortality rate reduced from 60% to 20%. Those without disease encounter a 10% mortality rate. In terms of a single patient with a 50-50 chance of having the disease, the mortality rate is cut in half by treatment.

It cannot escape your eye that while saving lives of people with disease, you may inadvertently cause death by treating somebody who does not have the disease. Since we rarely deal with 100% diagnostic or therapeutic certainty in medicine, such unfortunate outcomes must inevitably result from the management of health problems.

But it must be made clear that decision analysis does not *cause* ethical problems; it merely *mirrors* or *reveals* them by reflecting some of the facts of life. Giving treatment to patients without disease may be harmful. Consequently, the less likely the diagnosis the less likely you are to treat. The more likely the diagnosis the more likely you are to treat. In turn, these actions depend on mortality rates with and without treatment and the risk of the treatment itself.

And that is what decision analysis is all about.

Note that intuitive decisions are simple when dealing with clinical situations such as the one just described. Other situations may require a closer call. In that event, a more complex decision tree with fully foliated scenarios may be helpful before choosing an option.

In the case just set forth and exemplified in Figure 8.1, it is useful to know the exact probability of disease—P(D)—where either option would produce the same likelihood

of mortality. This enables you to select an action according to your clinically estimated P(D).

In calculating the P(D) where different options have equal outcomes, you are doing a *threshold analysis.* It can be simply done by setting up simultaneous algebraic equations. Let x equal the P(D) and y equal the P($\bar{\text{D}}$).

$$x + y = 1 \text{ or } y = 1 - x \qquad\qquad 1.$$

$$.6x = .2x + .1y = .2x + .1(1 - x) \quad 2.$$
$$.6x = .2x + .1 - .1x$$
$$.5x = .1 \text{ and } x = .20$$

Equation 1 states merely that the probability of disease plus the probability of nondisease equals 1. Equation 2 represents the situation whereby *the mortality* from no treatment equals the mortality from treatment; the numbers are obtained from Figure 8.1. The P(D) and P($\bar{\text{D}}$) are the x and y unknowns to be solved. By substituting simultaneous equations we learn that when the P(D) is .20, either pathway yields the same outcome. Therefore, if the clinical P(D) is less than .20, don't treat. If the clinical P(D) is greater than .20, do treat. We have just performed a threshold analysis and have determined that the "treatment threshold" is .20.

If you now substitute .20 for P(D) and .80 for P($\bar{\text{D}}$), calculations will determine that either pathway leads to 12 deaths/100 patients (Fig. 8.2). If you don't treat, all 12 deaths are in diseased patients. If you do

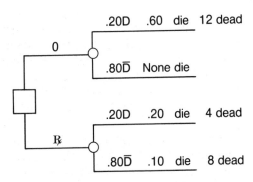

Fig. 8.2. Simple decision tree with two paths; P(D) is such that each path has the same outcome. O, don't treat; ℞, treat.

treat, 4 deaths occur in diseased patients, but 8 deaths occur in nondiseased patients.

Translating this information into terms of a *single patient* whose P(D) is .20, the mortality rate is 12% whether you do or do not treat. If you decide *not to treat*, there is a 12% chance the patient will die of a curable disease. But if you decide *to treat*, there is an 8% chance of causing the death of a patient who is not even sick. Which is the greater sin? Many moral and ethical issues are revealed here.

How a Test Can Help. There are tests and procedures that can help you decide whether to treat or whom to treat. If a disease is likely and the test result is positive, or if the disease is unlikely and the test result is negative, you can proceed with greater confidence because your clinical opinion is reinforced. But if the test result is *unexpectedly* positive or negative, your confidence is shaken. You now question your judgment as well as the test, so you repeat the test, consider another diagnosis, and/or do yet other tests.

But since very few (if any) procedures are 100% reliable, the possibility always exists that a positive test result represents a false positive or that a negative test result may be a false negative. You are faced with the ever present though diminished possibility that you may be treating a patient with no disease and not treating a patient who has the disease. The likelihood that such unfortunate events may occur decreases when you use tests with high operating characteristics. The better the test, the more favorable the outcome!

Suppose you decide to recommend a diagnostic test for the patient previously described. The clinically estimated P(D) is .20 and you don't know which way to go. Perhaps a test will raise or lower the P(D) and help you decide. The test is 90% sensitive and 90% specific. Using a 2×2 table, the TP, FP, FN, and TN rates can easily be calculated. From these figures, you can then determine the positive and negative predictive values. In turn, the PV+ provides the revised P(D) or true positive rate if the test is positive, and the PV− provides the revised P($\overline{D}$)

or true negative rate if the test is negative. All this information has been entered into the 2×2 table and decision tree of Figure 8.3.

By treating only those who test positive and not treating those who test negative, the mortality rate is markedly decreased. The P(D) of the positive testee is raised from .20 to .69 (18/26); the P($\overline{D}$) of the negative testee is raised from .80 to .97 (72/74). And the decision to treat only those with positive tests results in a mortality rate of 5.6%; 4.8% occur in patients with disease who test truly positive and falsely negative, and 0.8% occur in patients without disease who test falsely positive. If the test is negative and no treatment is given on that basis, the mortality rate is 1.2%, all deaths occurring only in diseased patients who test falsely negative.

Observe that in the "test and decide" option, the mortality rate has been decreased from 12% to 4.4% of those with positive tests and to 1.2% of those with negative tests. These are dramatic results. Clinical situations do not always lend themselves to such happy outcomes. Not only have you decreased the mortality rate but you have lessened the chance of wrongfully giving or withholding treatment. Most of those who die are sick.

In essence, you have simply made yourself more confident of the diagnosis before instituting treatment—a wise medical principle.

Now inspect Figure 8.3 more carefully. Study the 2×2 diagram at the extreme left and see how the predictive values are determined. Pay attention to the three optional paths, and in particular examine the "test and decide" path. Note the invariant requisite that the sum of all decimals in the divided trails following a chance node must equal 1.0. The outcomes in this case are *life or death*; they are arbitrarily assigned numerical values of 0 and 1, respectively. It is evident that bad outcomes—death—are being measured. Conversely, had respective values of 1 and 0 been assigned, you would be measuring good outcomes—life—rather than bad. This is an arbitrary determination, and the subject of outcomes as measured by

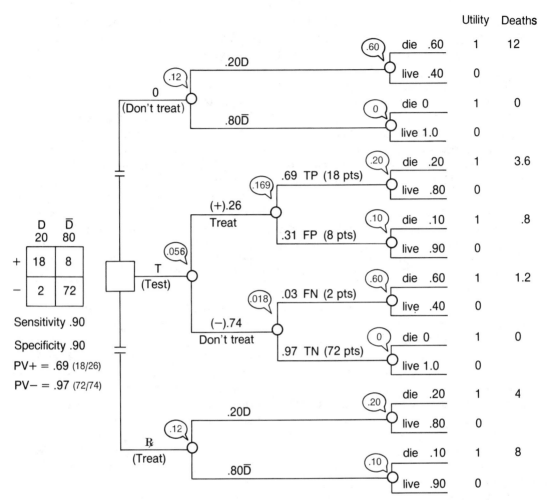

Fig. 8.3. Decision tree with three paths—treat, don't treat, test and decide. Note the 2×2 table used to calculate test results. Observe how a good test decreases the mortality.

utilities and utility scales will be discussed later. The numbers of deaths listed on the extreme right are those that would occur if a cohort of 100 patients were under consideration. If you regard only one patient, the numbers in the right column can be changed to percentages—the chances that one patient will die as a consequence of following either path.

Next trace each route from left to right. You should be able to understand what happens at every chance node, why the numbers are as stated, how the scenarios are constructed, and why the outcomes are as they are. The figures in the ovals inserted above each chance node are averaged-out values,

and their derivation will be explained shortly.

Foliating the Tree. After the entire decision tree and its component strategies and outcomes have been carefully mapped, numbers must be inserted into the appropriate places. As already partially noted, these numbers include estimates of P(D) and P(D̄), mortality rates, utility values, complication rates, operating characteristics of tests, and figures reflecting TP, FP, FN, and TN rates. In the jargon of decision analysis, this is "foliating the tree."

Averaging Out and Folding Back. First formulate the tree; determine the outcomes of optional strategies and scenarios, assign numerical values to them, and then calculate from *right to left* in order to obtain numerical values at each node.

Averaging out is the step whereby we collapse and summate the probabilities for all branches emanating from a chance node. This process is carried out all the way back to the beginning at each alternative option emanating from the principal decision node. By performing these calculations we derive an *expected mortality rate* for each available option.

Compute backwards in Figure 8.3 along the "no treatment" path to the first chance nodes where the averaged-out values are inserted in the form of oval *"thought balloons."* The values at these points are .60—(.60 × 1) + (.40 × 0)—and 0—(0 × 1) + (1 × 0). Then compute farther left to the next chance node where the averaged-out value is .12—(.20 × .60) + (.80 × 0).

The same can be done for each path. Special care must be given to the more complicated "test and decide" path, but the same principles apply. The computation of the values for the first set of chance nodes is simple. The final value of .056 for the "test and decide" option is derived as follows: .26 [(.69 × .20) + (.31 × .10)] + .74 [(.03 × .60) + (.97 × 0)] = .056. In this sweeping calculation we have included the averaged out values obtained at two "chance-decision nodes"—treat if positive and don't treat if negative.

We are now in a position to make an intelligent choice between optional tracks (4). In Figure 8.3, the calculated expected values for each option are .12, .056, and .12, respectively. Since we have chosen to measure bad outcomes and have arbitrarily assigned higher numerical values to death than to life, the path with the lowest numbers represents the path that will result in the least mortality. Therefore the .056 option is the one to choose—test and decide. It causes the least mortality.

To those stalwart and compulsive readers who have actually calculated the predicted outcome (expected mortality rate) for the "test and decide" option, it must be men-

tioned that slight mathematical discrepancies were introduced by rounding the predictive values at the second digit after the decimal point.

Folding back is the step whereby each strategy is pruned, except the one with the best expected value. Having decided which is the best option to pursue, cut off all others by drawing a double line perpendicular to and disruptive of each undesirable action. The decision has been made!

Remember that this basic demonstration (Fig. 8.3) becomes more complex as the scenarios become more intricate and develop many more branches and twigs. This depends on the clinical problem with which you deal. Outcomes are often expressed in more sophisticated ways than simply life or death. Computations may be time-consuming, and a calculator or computer may offer great assistance to the decision analyst.

Sensitivity Analysis. In general this type of analysis depicts how changing the assumptions in a decision tree may affect the desirability of options being considered. Such analyses probe the different structures, outcomes, risks, mortality rates, test predictive values, and disease prevalences incorporated into the tree. Each analysis permits a graphic display of the effect of changing a variable on the expected value of each strategy.

For example, what is the effect of varying the P(D) upon the expected values of three alternate strategies? Or what is the effect of varying a test's predictive value upon the decision to test or treat without testing? Graph the alterations in the risk of a diagnostic or therapeutic procedure with the averaged-out value of its related decision path.

A sensitivity analysis, then, is actually a "test of the stability of conclusions of an analysis over a range of structural assumptions, probability estimates, or value judgments" (4).

In particular, draw, construct, or print out a graph whose coordinates are: the clinical probability of colon cancer and the PV+ of a stool that is positive for occult blood; the 2-year survival probability of an untreated patient with advanced undiagnosed liver disease and the initial probability of chronic hepatitis; the surgical mortality rate for coronary artery bypass graft and the operation's cost effectiveness; and the mortality of an invasive diagnostic procedure and the averaged-out value of the "biopsy then decide" strategy. In each case the numerical values on the ordinate vary in a precise curved or linear manner with changing values on the abscissa.

Threshold Determinations. This is a technique whereby you determine at which P(D) two options result in equal expected outcomes (or averaged-out values). Such an analysis was made earlier in determining the P(D) at which the "treat" and "don't treat" paths had equal mortality rates (Fig. 8.2).

Very often the physician must decide whether to withhold treatment, give treatment, or perform a procedure or test first and then decide. The physician's estimate of disease probability is a prime factor in making such decisions. Intuitively, if the disease is very unlikely, he *will not* treat. If the disease is very likely, he *will* treat. Between these extreme probabilities there is a twilight zone, a specific P(D), where either path leads to the same outcome. This is the "treatment threshold" that was derived in Figure 8.2.

Frequently, a test that substantially increases or decreases the probability that a disease exists may help the physician decide on a course of action or inaction. The "test threshold" is the precise P(D) where the decision to "don't treat" and the decision to "test first and then decide" have equal outcomes. The *"test-treatment threshold"* is the precise P(D) where the decision to "test first and then decide" and the decision to "treat without testing" have equal outcomes.

These thresholds are derived in the same way that the *treatment threshold* was calculated. Allow x and y to equal P(D) and P($\overline{D}$), respectively. Then determine the P(D) where the expected outcomes (mortality rates in this case) for the "don't treat" and "test first and then decide" options are equal. This represents the *test threshold*. Using the same technique, determine the P(D) where the

expected outcomes for the "treat without testing" option and the "test first and then decide" option are equal. This represents the *test-treatment threshold.*

To summarize: In a clinical setting where you are faced with diagnostic uncertainty and the options to do nothing, treat directly, or perform a test and then decide, the thresholds of interest are:

1. *The treatment threshold*—the P(D) below which treatment should be withheld and above which treatment should be given;
2. *The test threshold*—the P(D) below which a test need not be done and treatment may be withheld, and above which a test should be done;
3. *The test-treatment threshold*—the P(D) below which a test should be done before deciding, and above which the test need not be done and treatment should be given (5).

Having obtained such thresholds, it may be possible to construct a simple bar graph which shows, for example, that if the P(D) is less than .25, don't treat; if it is between .25 and .75, do a test first and then decide; and if it is greater than .75, then treat. Among other things, these thresholds will vary with the accuracy and risks of the test. The greater the accuracy and the less the risk, the wider will the testing range be; the less the accuracy and the greater the risk, the narrower will the test's range of applicability be. Under certain circumstances, testing may never be preferable to other options. This is especially true if the test is very risky and/or has low predictive value, or if the disease is almost certainly absent or present.

If you carefully consider what has just been said, you will realize that a good clinician performs all these calculations intuitively as he proceeds to act. Executing these maneuvers with pencil and paper or by computer adds mathematical precision to the clinician's actions.

Practical decisions about patients with chest pain are often made in the preceding manner. If the P(D) of angina pectoris is only .01, no treatment is given. If the estimated P(D) is .25, you might wish to perform a stress ECG. And if the P(D) is .75, you might begin treatment without benefit of a test. Actually, the high P(D) is probably derived from the fact that, in effect, the patient performs a similar test every time he suffers anginal pain on exertion.

There are other valuable threshold determinations. By the mathematical expedient of varying only one factor in your analysis and keeping the other variables in the decision tree constant, you can determine at what precise value a single variable results in equal expected outcomes along two option paths.

For example, at a given P(D) you can calculate the threshold values for the surgical mortality rate, the mortality rate of a diagnostic procedure, the predictive value of a test, the benefit:cost ratio, the risk of hepatitis resulting from drug treatment, and so forth. In each case you determine the numerical value of the variable that would make the choice between competing options a tossup.

Here are some practical applications. If the surgical mortality is greater than the threshold value, treat medically. If the risk of drug-induced hepatitis is lower than the threshold value, proceed with the use of the drug. If the test's predictive value is greater than the threshold value, do the test; if it is less, choose another option. And on and on.

Sometimes the determination of thresholds is more complex and they must be performed in accordance with the number and quality of the remaining years of life and hospital or public policy.

Where the Numbers Come From

In previous sections, we have written about numbers, percentages, statistics, mortality rates, treatment success rates, test performance characteristics, and disease probabilities. Where do these numbers come from, how are they obtained, and how are they methodically inserted into a decision tree? The following discussion deals mainly

with the P(D), outcomes or *utilities*, and procedure performances.

Estimating the P(D). Much space was devoted to this subject in Chapter 5 on the mathematics of problem solving. The P(D) depends on your evaluation of the clinical picture based on the known data. The greater your experience and the better your judgment, the more accurate the P(D) will be. You may also be aided in assigning a correct number to this important symbol by reading published sources, by consulting your colleagues, and by deriving an overall opinion by polling a group of experts—the Delphi technique. There is disagreement on how accurate simple clinical evaluation is in this regard. In some instances, computer software programs are alleged to be as capable as the clinician in estimating diagnostic probabilities based on clinical information (Chapter 9).

On the other hand, you may be surprised by the narrow range of P(D) estimates given by clinical experts or even by medical students when presented with just a few essential bits of evidence.

For example, when told that the patient is a 60-year-old male smoker with a chronic cough, recent hemoptysis, and weight loss, estimates of the P(D) for lung cancer are all close to .50. Analogous classroom "experiments" with brief vignettes yield similar results. But what may not be so readily appreciated is that when you raise the P(D) from .80 to .96 by a procedure or test, you are increasing the disease likelihood from 4:1 to 24:1.

Outcomes and Utilities. The sample decision tree constructed earlier used strategies that terminated in either life or death. These are commonly considered outcomes in any clinical decision. But often there are different kinds of consequences that can result from contending strategies.

Outcomes that concern you will vary with the clinical situation. In deciding whether to biopsy the temporal artery in a suspected case of polymyalgia rheumatica, loss of vision must be one possible end point. Depending on the illness being considered, the outcomes may include: temporary to permanent neurologic sequelae; loss of speech; quality of remaining life; permanent disability vs ability to play golf; subsequent annual mortality rate; loss of a limb below or above the knee; worsening, stable, or completely relieved angina pectoris; and so forth.

Consider a patient on anticoagulants for a mitral valve prosthesis who develops a spontaneous subdural hematoma which is appropriately managed. The decision to stop or continue anticoagulants will be derived in part from a quantitative estimate of the comparative harms of recurrent intracranial hemorrhage vis-à-vis prosthetic thromboembolism.

Then contemplate a patient who you suspect has developed hepatitis B. In deciding on this patient's diagnostic and therapeutic management, the outcomes to consider are: patient gets well; patient becomes carrier; patient develops chronic hepatitis, cirrhosis, or liver cancer; or patient may die.

The utilities of a decision tree are simply the value of the outcomes expressed in numbers. We quantify the values of each possible outcome of a clinical decision according to a *utility scale.*

It is commonly recognized that the process of establishing a scheme for quantifying utilities (the utility scale) may well be the Achilles heel of decision analysis. There must be some way of assigning values to clinical outcomes that is in keeping with what's important for both the physician and the patient. But the universally accepted way to design utility scales has not yet been formalized. You can use a scale consisting of positive or negative numbers, a 1-to-100 ordinal scale, fractions, decimals, and so forth. But you must have some *reasonable* way of assigning numbers to outcomes. For example, negative values may represent bad outcomes, and positive numbers may represent good outcomes. If -1 represents a bad outcome, -2 may signify a very bad outcome, and -3 or -5 may denote a disaster.

Thus, after you have established the important outcomes in a decision analysis, utilities must be assigned. Parenthetically it

should be noted that the simple act of *constructing* the decision tree for a clinical problem may serve as an organizational device that helps the clinician think more clearly and may render a quantitative approach unnecessary.

Proceed now with the determination of utilities. A simple scale using positive numbers might assign 2 to life, 1 to life with residual disability, and 0 to death. Here you would be rating good events higher on the scale, and the averaged-out value of the optimal strategy would be represented by the highest number. These are arbitrary assignments, and you could as easily use 10, 5, and 1. Just so you understand the ranking of numbers and the significance of what you are doing! The ordinal scale may not be the best way to express utility values, but future studies will establish better ways to structure utility scales.

Now you can enter these utilities into the averaging-out process, deriving averaged-out values at each chance node in retracing the tree from right to left (from the branch tips to the main trunk). This procedure will be demonstrated in "A Case in Point" that follows on page 141.

Always to be kept in mind is "who determines the utilities?" Whether medical purists like it or not, utilities are both private and public. The outcomes to be valued depend on the doctor, the patient, the patient's family, the hospital administrator, and/or public policy. And the utilities may vary in each circumstance. While the physician may be primarily concerned with life and death and the administrator with benefit-cost analysis, the patient's main concern may be for the quality of life. Value trade-offs inevitably arise, and the patient may be more interested in how happy his remaining years will be than in whether he will die or live.

The subject of utilities cannot be concluded without at least mentioning the innovative ways in which some medical decision makers have begun to deal with the outcomes of *altered life expectancy* and *quality of life.*

The declining exponential approximation

of life expectancy (DEALE) is a convenient way of providing a patient with a specific estimate of his life expectancy. This is performed by a simple calculation that takes into account his life expectancy if he were healthy, life expectancy with the illness or illnesses he has, and life expectancy that might result from competing strategies (6). Fundamental to this tactic is the assumption that there is a simple reciprocal relationship between the annual mortality rate and the life expectancy.

Quality-adjusted life years (QALYs) is another way of assigning utilities to outcomes. For example, 1 pain-free year of life may be equal to 3 years with angina. Two years of active life may be equal to 6 years in a wheelchair. Clearly, the patient must play a large role in this determination because his values and yours may not be the same.

These are some of the factors that make a decision analysis complex.

Test Operating Characteristics. The derivation of the sensitivity and specificity of a test or procedure has already been discussed in Chapter 5. A gold standard test must always be available as a basis for determining who certainly has a disease and who certainly does not.

But the truth of the matter is that the operating characteristics of any particular test are never clearly established for all institutions, for all patient subsets, and for all times. A literature search for the attributes of any selected procedure used for a special purpose reveals different numbers emanating from different investigators. The data bank is very far from being complete in this regard.

Consider the use of ultrasound to detect intrahepatic biliary duct dilatation, or the use of a CT scan to detect pancreatic carcinoma. Figures for sensitivity and specificity are not yet clearly established. This is true for almost all tests and procedures.

Should you wish to know the performance characteristics of any procedure, you may have to search out some articles in the *Index Medicus.* The articles need careful scrutiny. Look at the authors, the institutional source,

and the experimental protocol; then decide for yourself if the results seem dependable. Or you may consult the procedure expert in your hospital. In any event, the numbers you use may not be absolutely correct, even though they are the best approximations available to you.

Take a test that is 95% sensitive-98% specific in one reported study and 97% sensitive-96% specific in another. This is not a significant difference. But if two studies reveal operating characteristics that are 98%-95% in one and 90-60% in the other, their respective impacts on the P(D) are widely divergent.

Risks, Costs, Benefits

Definitions. Previous discussions have included mention of risks, costs, and benefits, though they have been nowhere defined. Their explication varies depending on the sphere in which they are being applied. In the realm of medicine, these terms are defined as follows:

Risk always involves the patient and includes possible damages such as the side effects of drugs, morbidity of procedures, mortality from treatment, and the hazard of doing nothing.

Cost, in a medical sense, refers to the total expenditure of health resources in providing a service (4). The cost of a service (test, treatment, surgery, intensive care, etc) encompasses professional care, nonprofessional labor, the use of buildings, facilities, equipment, and other forms of overhead. *Charges* may be poor reflections of *costs* since for some services charges exceed costs in order to make up for other services where costs exceed charges. Because reimbursement of these costs is made by the patient or insurance companies, the government, and eventually the public, the matter of *whose dollars pay the costs* may be critical in making decisions. With just a little thought, you can predict the inevitable conflict between the interests of society and the interests of the individual.

Benefit signifies the good that accrues as

the result of an action. It may be measured in terms of improved health, survival, better quality of life, relief from pain, and the reestablished ability to work and earn a living.

Relating the Three. The ideal intention is to achieve the greatest benefit for the patient at the least risk and the lowest cost. These three objectives are rarely attainable together; some "give and take" is required, and trade-offs between options always enter the equation.

As in the conduct of any business, the first thoughts that often occur in the making of a decision are: "what can I gain, and what can I lose?"; "will my decision do the patient more good than harm?"; and "is it worth taking the calculated risk?"

Decision analysis purports to help quantify the answers to these questions. In this regard the following discussions will apply certain principles of economics to medicine.

Cost Effectiveness Analysis. This type of analysis aims to establish the cost (days, dollars, physician time, etc) that will accomplish an objective (find cancer of the colon, prevent hepatitis B, discover breast cancer, save lives, etc). Costs and health outcomes using different strategies are described in the analysis. Often such an analysis entails the determination of an optimal screening strategy after comparing the cost per case discovered by using different techniques. The more lives saved or the more disease discovered, the greater the total cost. But what is the *cost per life saved or per disease discovered* for each method? Knowing this, you can then decide on the optimal strategy within the constraints of available resources. Therefore the analysis serves as a means of determining the most efficient allocation of limited resources.

A good example is the use of various screening procedures for the detection of carcinoma of the colon in an elderly male population known to have a P(D) of .001 (1 case/1,000) (4). Various diagnostic strategies are used. These include digital examination (DE) only, occult blood in stool (OB) only, OB plus DE, OB plus DE plus barium

enema (BE) if OB is positive, etc. The cost of each strategy is calculated for each case of cancer discovered in a population of 100,000 persons in this subset. Entered into the calculations are the total costs, the total number of cancers found, and the average cost per cancer found. The figures show that the most cost-effective and the most cancer-discovering strategy is OB followed by BE if OB is positive. In this instance, 80 cancers were discovered at a cost of a little over $10,000/cancer found. To find an additional 17 cancers, extra strategies would be required; these would quadruple the total expenditure and increase the cost per cancer found to $34,000. Two and one-half million dollars were spent to find 17 additional cancers. The cost of finding each additional cancer was $150,000. Was it worth it? Does it depend on whether the cancer was found in me, in you, or in him? Who decides?

Benefit-Cost Analysis. This term is often confused with "cost effectiveness analysis." It is not the same. Executives and economists calculate benefit-cost analyses by reducing everything to dollars. Then they decide whether the benefit is sufficiently greater than the cost before embarking on a project. Medical analyses of a similar nature can also be done on a monetary basis, but many intangible factors must first be reduced to dollar values—a formidable task. For not only must real dollar costs be included, but quality of life, health benefits, restored vision, greater longevity, and renewed earning ability must be translated into dollars too. This type of analysis helps to establish the most efficient allocation of limited resources.

Such an analysis can be portrayed by the plight of a patient in whom a coronary artery bypass graft is contemplated. The cost is approximately $50,000, but rightfully the cost should also include the risk of surgical mortality and the risk of being made more sick. Benefits must be measured in increments of slight improvement, great improvement, disappearance of symptoms, and the associated alterations in quality of life, length of life, and ability to work. Then transpose these benefits into monetary values. So in the event of the best possible outcome, the patient may have 10 high-quality extra years of life and earn an additional half-million dollars. A year of high-quality life may be worth $50,000. So all in all, your cost has been $50,000 and your benefit $1 million— a 20:1 benefit:cost ratio. The ratio diminishes if surgery is less than successful.

As society becomes more concerned with the efficient allocation of health care resources, the kinds of analyses just discussed will have an increasingly important impact on policy decisions. Can we afford to give everybody the highest quality of health care? Screening procedures, immunization protocols, the quest for diagnostic certainty, unlimited use of high technology, organ transplants for everybody—all need careful scrutiny and evaluation in the light of *limited financial resources.* During this decade, society may very well decide to systematically ration certain categories of patient care.

A Case in Point

When confronted with a patient who has possibly just had a pulmonary embolus, the physician usually has a gut feeling about whether to give or withhold anticoagulants. He knows that such treatment is inconvenient, costly, lengthy, and may cause serious hemorrhages. On the other hand, he does not wish to risk the reembolization that carries a substantial mortality rate.

So if the likelihood of a pulmonary embolus is low, he withholds treatment. If the likelihood is high, he anticoagulates the patient. But there must inevitably be a twilight zone within whose boundaries of probability he cannot decide. This is where he orders a test or procedure to help him make an intelligent choice.

While some physicians request a diagnostic procedure (e.g. ventilation-perfusion scan, pulmonary arteriography, or iliofemoral venography) on either the slightest suspicion or even a high degree of diagnostic certainty, this may not be the wise thing to

do. In the case of a possible pulmonary embolus, *threshold analysis* can indicate the P(D) below which no treatment should be given and the P(D) above which treatment should always be given. Under these circumstances a test may not needed. But when the disease likelihood is well inside the outer limits of probability, a diagnostic study is usually performed.

Since most patients' cases have certain aspects that make the clinical picture unique, we will present such a patient, draw a decision tree, and choose an optimal management by precise mathematical methods rather than by "clinical judgment." In doing so, decision analysis will be demonstrated in vivo.

The Case. A 55-year-old woman is admitted to the hospital with cough, expectoration, fever, and pleuritic chest pain. Ten days ago, a hysterectomy was performed for uterine fibroids. She was ambulatory on the second day, had an uneventful hospital course, and was discharged on the fifth postoperative day.

At home, her husband had had a bad chest cold. For the past 2 days the patient has had a cough, expectoration, and low-grade fever. Shortly before admission she developed right chest pain that was worse on breathing and coughing.

Additional historical information reveals that she had an active duodenal ulcer 2 years ago though there are no symptoms to suggest activity now. She has on occasion been mildly hypertensive but has never taken medication. Each night for years she has drunk several bottles of beer, as does her husband; on weekends some additional highballs are consumed.

Examination on admission shows a moderately ill woman with shallow rapid breathing; respirations are 30/minute, pulse is 110/minute, temperature is 38.3 C, and blood pressure is 160/90 mm Hg. Fine inspiratory rales are heard at the right base, but no friction rub is noted. The calves are not tender, Homans' sign is negative bilaterally, the abdominal incision appears adequately healed, there are two small spider angiomata noted on the chest, and the examination is otherwise entirely normal.

The chest x-ray, blood count, urinalysis, and 18-test blood chemistry profile are all normal except for a slightly elevated serum glutamic-oxaloacetic transaminase. Prothrombin time and partial thromboplastin time are normal.

The Judgment. Consideration is given to an early pneumonic process resulting from a transmitted respiratory infection or a pulmonary infarction caused by iliofemoral or pelvic thrombophlebitis and embolization.

Recent pelvic surgery, respiratory tract symptoms, and pleuritic chest pain in the presence of a normal chest x-ray suggest a pulmonary embolus, but the preponderance of evidence favors a respiratory tract infection.

The admitting physician estimates the probability of pulmonary embolus to be .20 and considers the use of heparin even though he believes pulmonary infection to be more likely. Ordinarily, when the P(D) for pulmonary embolus is .20, this physician would not hesitate to give heparin together with treatment for the other diagnostic possibility whose "P($\overline{D}$)" is .80. But now he is cautious. He is concerned about the increased risk of bleeding from anticoagulants because of the ulcer history, mild hypertension, and possible liver disease.

In order to help him decide whether or not to use anticoagulants in this case, he constructs a decision tree. He inserts into the matrix a diagnostic procedure that will alter the P(D) enough for him to make a safe decision (Fig. 8.4).

Foliate and Prune. The tree is constructed to portray three possible paths: (a) don't treat; (b) test and decide (treat if positive and don't treat if negative); (c) treat with anticoagulants. The possible outcomes of each decision node and chance node are clearly set forth in terms of branches and twigs.

Consider the "don't treat" option; the possibility of reembolization exists. Now regard the "treat" option; reembolization may occur but at a lower rate. You have also introduced the risk of serious hemorrhage resulting from treatment.

Last, look at the "test and decide" option in the middle of the diagram. The test has the operating characteristics and predictive values as noted in the 2×2 diagram at the lower left. If the test is positive, the patient is treated, since the P(D) has been raised from .20 to .83; but you may also be treating a patient whose test is falsely positive and who doesn't have a pulmonary embolus. On the other hand, if the test is negative, the P(D) is lowered to .01; anticoagulants are not given, even though there is a very slight chance (1:100) that treatment is being withheld from a patient who does have an embolus.

Note that the tree has already been pruned of dead branches. In the absence of an embolus ($\overline{D}$), reembolization cannot occur; and if anticoagulants are not given, hemorrhage cannot occur. Carefully trace each branch, note each node, and understand the chance events that follow each dividing point.

The Test. Various procedures to determine the presence or absence of pulmonary embolism are well known. Their operating characteristics are not (7). Arteriography is as close to a gold standard test as possible. But for the patient under discussion, we have chosen a less invasive, less risky, and less expensive test—a ventilation-perfusion scintillation scan. Criteria for determining the test's positivity are predetermined. The test's operating characteristics were previously established by comparing its performance to that of the gold standard test—pulmonary arteriography. For the case under discussion, we assume that the test is 95% sensitive and 95% specific; these numbers are subject to some contention. Given a P(D) of .20, the TP, FN, FP, and TN rates, as well as the PV+ and PV−, are calculated as noted in the 2×2 diagram.

The Probabilities. Certain assumptions that are validated by only soft evidence must be made. The reembolization rate for an untreated pulmonary embolus is .40. The reembolization rate for a pulmonary embolus that is properly treated with anticoagulants is .15. Here we shall skirt the knotty problem of what constitutes proper anticoagulation.

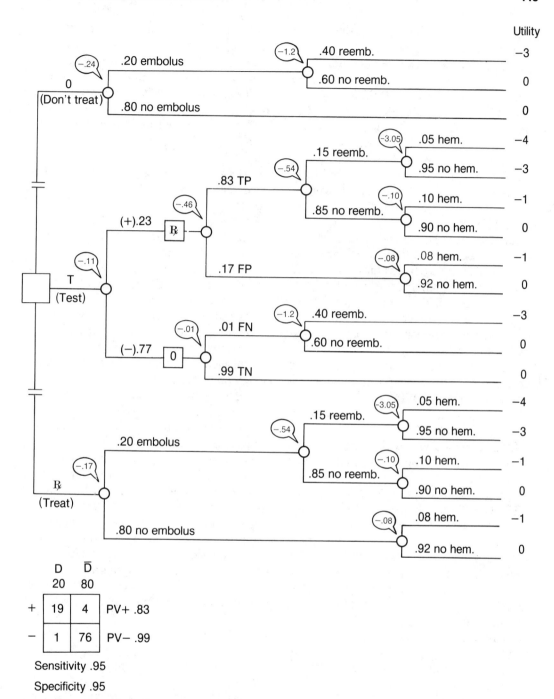

Utility

.20 embolus
−.24
0
(Don't treat)

−1.2 .40 reemb. −3
.60 no reemb. 0
.80 no embolus 0

.15 reemb.
−3.05 .05 hem. −4
−.54 .95 no hem. −3
.83 TP
−.46
(+).23
℞
.85 no reemb.
−.10 .10 hem. −1
.90 no hem. 0

.17 FP
−.08 .08 hem. −1
.92 no hem. 0

−.11
T
(Test)

.01 FN
−1.2 .40 reemb. −3
−.01 .60 no reemb. 0
(−).77 0
.99 TN 0

.15 reemb.
−3.05 .05 hem. −4
−.54 .95 no hem. −3
.20 embolus

−.17
℞
(Treat)
.85 no reemb.
−.10 .10 hem. −1
.90 no hem. 0

.80 no embolus
−.08 .08 hem. −1
.92 no hem. 0

	D	D̄	
	20	80	
+	19	4	PV+ .83
−	1	76	PV− .99

Sensitivity .95

Specificity .95

Fig. 8.4. Decision tree for case discussion in text; choice between three alternative pathways in management of suspected pulmonary embolus. Note associated 2×2 table for test characteristics. *Reemb.*, reembolization; *no reemb.*, no reembolization; *hem.*, hemorrhage; *no hem.*, no hemorrhage.

Generally accepted statistics state that 5% of patients on anticoagulation therapy have serious hemorrhagic complications in the brain, gastrointestinal tract, or kidneys. While this percentage seems a bit high to this author, we will accept a yet higher rate in this patient because of the mild relative contraindications she may have to anticoagulants. Bear in mind too that there is an inverse relationship between the incidence of emboli and the incidence of hemorrhage. A "well-anticoagulated" patient is less apt to embolize and more apt to bleed, and vice versa. Therefore we can assign hemorrhagic complication rates of .10 to those who do not reembolize, .05 to those who do reembolize, and .08 to those who never had an embolus to begin with. In the latter instance, reembolization cannot occur so we can accept an intermediate hemorrhagic complication rate.

The Utilities. Numerical values are assigned to the possible outcomes. Bad outcomes are given negative values, and a good outcome (no reembolization and no hemorrhage) is assigned a value of zero. Reembolization is considered to be much more serious than hemorrhage since approximately half of those with the former but only one-fifth of those with the latter die of these complications. Therefore reembolization is given a -3 utility, hemorrhage is given a -1 utility, and the coexistence of both is given a -4 utility.

These arbitrary values have been chosen for simplicity. The reader who wants a more detailed explanation of utilities and their selection should consult reference 4.

The Best Path. Now average out the utility values back to the initial chance node. The more negative the value at each option path, the worse the outcome, since by initial agreement negative values represent bad events. The values in each "thought balloon" have been rounded out at the second number after the decimal point. See if you agree with the arithmetic. It is a good learning experience.

It can be seen that the averaged-out utility value for the "don't treat" option is $-.24$, the "test and decide" option is $-.11$, and the "treat" option is $-.17$. Obviously, in this case the best results are obtained if we test first, then treat if positive and don't treat if negative. Now, fold back the two undesirable options by drawing double lines through each one.

If we follow the optimal path, fewer complications will occur, and most of those that do occur will be in patients who have had an embolus. Very little trouble will result in those who had no embolus from the start.

Thresholds. In this patient, or in any subset of patients, the precise P(D) that would yield equal expected utilities between paths 1 and 2, 2 and 3, and 1 and 3 can be calculated. Just let $x = P(D)$ and $y = P(\bar{D})$, set up simultaneous equations as done earlier in this chapter, and perform the simple algebra.

Back to the Patient. The ventilation-perfusion scan is performed, and according to the criteria that have been established the test is positive. The revised diagnostic likelihood is now .83. Treatment with continuous intravenous heparin is begun, and the therapeutic level of coagulability is carefully maintained. Had the test been negative, anticoagulants would not be given and the patient would be treated for probable early pneumonia. The revised diagnostic likelihood for pulmonary embolus would be .01; the probability that another disease exists therefore would be .99. Even with a positive test, some physicians would give antibiotics too in order to "cover all possibilities."

Also recall that many clinicians prefer pulmonary arteriography in such situations since its operating characteristics are close to gold standard performance. If the clinical situation is such that vena caval ligation is under consideration or embolectomy is deemed necessary, arteriography and/or venography is the way to go. For under these circumstances, 100% certainty is desirable.

Uses, Pros, and Cons

Over the past decade, decision analysis has assumed a position at the busy crossroads of clinical practice, medical research, biostatistics, and public health.

More and more, decisions are made on the basis of explicit reasoning, quantitative data, and mathematical models. Yet the properties of implicit inference and experience—combined with the almost chimerical and indefinable powers of intuition, judgment, and hunch—still play a very important role in decision making. Side by side, these two grand strategies continue their tug of war in a quest to dominate the arena of patient care. There is both room and need for all tactics. The good physician must learn to intertwine hard facts with soft intellect for the combined benefits of patient and public.

And while decision analysis is the "systematic articulation of common sense, the mind of the expert is a miraculous synthesizer and the quality of intuitively made decisions may at times be better, quicker, and more practical" (4).

Trees As Lovely As Poems. Literally scores of high-quality and clinically meaningful programs for the management of common medical problems have been generated by decision analytic methods. These include decision trees that deal with: (*a*) strategies in the diagnosis and management of coronary artery disease; (*b*) optimal timing of repeated medical tests; (*c*) management of temporal arteritis; (*d*) treatment of enterococcal endocarditis in the presence of penicillin allergy; (*e*) diagnosis and treatment of dyspepsia—a cost effectiveness analysis; (*f*) criteria for diagnosing chest pain; (*g*) treatment of sore throats in the emergency room; (*h*) need for kidney biopsy in a nephrotic patient; (*i*) management of the incidentally discovered adrenal adenoma; and on and on.

These subjects and others were included in just two issues of *Medical Decision Making*, a new medical journal. Reports that use similar analytic methods to reach conclusions are being published in all medical journals regardless of specialty. These include topics like: whether to operate on suspected appendicitis or wait 6 hours and then decide; what the proper timing is for abdominal aortic aneurysm resection; how to treat transient ischemic attacks; and whether to do cholecystectomy for asymptomatic gallstones.

You can see how the precise quantitation of such important clinical decisions may be

of tremendous help to the decision maker as he decides whether or not to cross the Rubicon.

Felling the Tree. Objections have been offered concerning the accuracy, dependability, and use of decision analysis. There are numerous criticisms, some of which appear valid. These will be set forth here, but rebuttals will be presented in the next section.

Many consider the discipline too time-consuming and therefore not applicable at the bedside, where urgency often exists.

Then there is skepticism that an intelligent decision can be made on small differences in predicted outcomes (e.g. 2%).

Further drawbacks revolve around difficulty in establishing accurate utility scales, lack of uniform information about tests' operating characteristics, and precise data on the outcomes of alternative choices. For example, is the incidence of reembolization 40, 50, or 60%? Does anticoagulant treatment really reduce the incidence to 15%? And don't these figures depend partly on the doctor, the laboratory, and the patient?

As for tests, the sensitivity and specificity of diagnostic procedures are known to vary with the performer, the subset of patients being tested, and the criteria for test positivity. The operating characteristics of these procedures are often based on a study of a small number of *selected cases* that represent only the tip of the iceberg. The figures obtained are not accurate for all patients who will undergo the procedure because the complexities of the assembly process eliminate most members of the subset being studied (8). It seems evident that the quality of test evaluation research must improve and that those who do the research must be more critical.

Other complexities enter the picture. Each clinical situation is unique, the matrix of the decision tree may have to include multiple diseases and tests, and you may have to deal with many bits of information that are mutually interdependent. Decision trees can become labyrinthine jungles.

Simple cases do not need decision trees.

Complex cases do, and it is precisely here that decision analysis seems to be or is actually impractical for the clinician. While clinicians are intrigued by the principles of decision analysis, they are turned off by time factors, unavailability of data, and lengthy intricate scenarios.

There exist arguments that decision analysis deifies the number and dehumanizes patient care, that it takes the art out of clinical judgment, that it creates ethical-moral-socioeconomic issues, and that it is insensitive to the dictum of primum nolo nocere.

In fact, isn't it really true that, contrary to our claims, we really do not treat all patients alike? The rich, the poor, the black, the white, the homosexual, the addict, the alcoholic, the criminal, the young, the old, and the famous ... ! Sociocultural factors and our own biases inevitably and subconsciously enter into the decisions we make.

It is also true that the decision tree may be chopped down in one fell swoop by the patient or the patient's family, who—in spite of careful analyses and predictions—make the decision for you by such unequivocal statements as: (*a*) Do what you will, but absolutely no surgery. (*b*) Do everything possible to keep my wife alive regardless of the risks and costs. (*c*) I'll risk anything to be able to play tennis again. (*d*) No more procedures, doctor—I've had enough. (*e*) I'd rather be dead than alive and blind. (*f*) Even if there's only a 1% chance of cure, take it. (*g*) Let no stone be unturned.

Clearly, we have ventured into the deep dark realm of patients' and families' values. And when patients' values are dominant, decision analysis may be futile.

Physicians as well may act illogically and emotionally. When they proceed with high-risk treatment for a disease with low probability, their defense is: "I refuse to let my patient die of a curable disease." This represents a bastardization of the old extinct cliché, "better to remove ten normal appendices than to leave one bad appendix in!"

Under other circumstances, needed treatment may be withheld because "errors of omission are better than errors of commission."

And so it appears that medical decisions often stem from interactions between individuals and may involve the unique attitudes of human beings—both doctors and patients. In these situations, statistics derived from manipulated populations and clinical studies may play only a limited role (9).

Propping the Tree. The prevailing sentiments today are in defense of decision analysis. Even though many of the polemics just described are clearly correct, sound arguments can be made against most of the chief complaints mentioned (10).

Estimates of probabilities are reasonably sound, and slightly different figures do not appreciably alter the numbers that determine decisions. The fact that there may be only a 2% difference in outcomes regardless of the option you choose only serves to emphasize the fact that decisions are sometimes close calls or tossups. Accurate numbers for test performances and clinical information will become reality as good research studies deposit their statistics into expanding data banks. When these data banks become available and accessible, and when microcomputers are as usable as stethoscopes, the analytic exercise of making decisions will require only minutes. Furthermore, decision analysis doesn't claim to make data more precise; it is only a tool for eliciting your best guesses based on *available* data.

Many of the objections to decision analysis are not objections to decision analysis itself. On careful examination, you can see that the analysis per se does not create problems; it merely brings them into focus. The problems already exist. For example, we are compelled to come to grips with the reality that good decisions may lead to bad outcomes and vice versa. Occasionally a patient is treated for a disease he doesn't have and death may ensue. Such ethical dilemmas are exposed, not caused, by decision analysis.

Furthermore, this system of making decisions seems to compel consideration for patients' values more than ever before. The physician must be aware of the patient's feelings in establishing utilities and discussing available options. This is certainly not a dehumanizing process; it merely blends additional science into the art of medicine.

One of the inevitable desirable results of decision analysis is the more appropriate use of "informed consent." Society no longer automatically bestows unquestioned wisdom on the bearer of the Aesculapian wand. Arbitrary decisions are neither expected nor accepted by some enlightened people. Explanations and information are requested from the plumber, electrician, roofer, teacher, and clergyman—as well as from the physician. Many patients want to know about their illnesses—the causes, treatment, prognosis, reasons for procedures, medication, and surgery, and a rough quantitation of the benefits, costs, and risks. They want to take part in the decision-making process—and rightly so! Other patients will rely on the physician's advice, because they may not be able to cope with all the numbers and values in a decision tree. "What do you suggest, doctor?"

A further consequence of decision analysis may be cost containment. The analyst often aims toward decreasing unnecessary tests, treatment, and surgery and increasing benefit:cost ratios. At times, however, the analysis may indicate the *need* for a test or treatment.

Last, the science of decision analysis demands that the clinician, the teacher, and the student think clearly and be accountable for their thoughts, their logic, and their decisions. The most junior student may expect logical explanations from the most senior

faculty. The teacher should demand the same from house staff and students. What's more, the patient should get the same from any of the above.

If soundly applied, decision analysis should be a means of promoting better medical care for satisfied patients by concerned, thinking doctors. And that's what the practice of medicine is all about.

Note: Exercises referable to clinical decisions and decision analysis follow Cases 22 and 39 in Section Three.

References

1. Persig RN: *Zen and the Art of Motorcycle Maintenance.* New York, Morrow, 1974.
2. Eddy DM, Schwartz M: Mathematical models in screening. In Schottenfeld D, Fraumeni JF (eds): *Cancer Epidemiology and Prevention.* Philadelphia, Saunders, 1982, pp 1075–1090.
3. Solzhenitsyn AI: *The Gulag Archipelago* (trans.). New York, Harper & Row, 1975.
4. Weinstein MC, Fineberg HV; *Clinical Decision Analysis.* Philadelphia, Saunders, 1980.
5. Pauker SG, Kassirer JP: The threshold approach to clinical decision making. *J Engl J Med* 302:1109–1116, 1980.
6. Beck JR, Kassirer JP, Pauker SG: A convenient approximation of life expectancy (the DEALE). Part 1. Validation of the method. Part 2. Use in medical decision making. *Am J Med* 73:883–897, 1982.
7. Hull RD, Hirsh J, Carter CJ, et al: Pulmonary angiography, ventilation lung scanning, and venography for clinically suspected pulmonary embolism with abnormal perfusion lung scan. *Ann Intern Med* 98:891–899, 1983.
8. Philbrick JT, Horwitz IR, Feinstein AR, et al: The limited spectrum of patients studied in exercise test research. *JAMA* 248:2467–2470, 1982.
9. Brett AS: Hidden ethical issues in clinical decision analysis. *N Engl J Med* 305:1150–1152, 1981.
10. Schwartz WB: Decision analysis; a look at the chief complaints. *N Engl J Med* 300:556–559, 1980.

Chapter 9

Problem-Solving Methods

PAUL CUTLER, M.D.

KEY WORDS

1. early hypothesis generation
2. clusters
3. pattern recognition
4. syndrome
5. key clue
6. pivotal clue
7. forming the differential
8. hunch
9. intuition
10. lanthanic
11. dendrograms
12. decision path
13. algorithm
14. flow chart
15. proof by exclusion
16. proof by suppression
17. pattern building
18. template matching
19. weight of evidence
20. computer assistance

The idea that experienced clinicians use complex indefinable tactics to unravel diagnostic problems is a myth. Medical intuition and clinical judgment can be fragmented into clearly described, recognizable, and duplicable heuristic strategies.

In this chapter we will conceptualize, describe, and simplify the many commonly used diagnostic techniques. Hopefully, much of the mystery surrounding the clinician's seemingly magical skills will be lifted so that students can begin to use them with facility. These problem-solving techniques are listed on page 150, and each one will be discussed at length. Most are used every day by the practicing physician though he may not recognize them by name. He may use some more than others by habit or preference. Often he varies his techniques from patient to patient and problem to problem, depending on which seems best or most practical for the particular case.

Before dissecting each problem-solving method, it may be profitable to explore some preliminary concepts.

First, we want to know what the criteria are for making a diagnosis in any particular case. Certainly not all the features of a disease that are listed in a textbook need be present. But how many are needed, and which ones? Must the diagnosis be clinical, chemical, or histologic? Indeed, we have already decided that in most cases the diagnosis must not necessarily be made with 100% certainty.

The sad truth is that, except for acute rheumatic fever, rheumatoid arthritis, and systemic lupus erythematosus, precise criteria for diagnosing diseases do not exist. And even the criteria for the three diseases mentioned undergo frequent revision. Diseases cannot be *diagnosed* with certainty because they cannot be *defined.* It is easy to list the many clinical features of a disease. We may be able to attach a number to each feature indicating the frequency with which it occurs; moreover, the number may be accurate. But that is *description*, not *definition.*

To define a disease, we must outline its borders, clearly identify and describe it, and exclude all other possibilities. We must establish a set of criteria which are fulfilled by *all* patients alleged to have a particular disease and by *no* patients without it. By analogy, a cube is a regular three-dimensional object having six equal square sides. Nothing else meets these criteria; therefore nothing else is a cube, and a cube is nothing else.

Textbooks describe diseases but do not define them. Clinicians do the same. However, computers that demand definitions should serve as a further stimulus toward the delineation of diseases—not an impossible task and certainly a worthy one. Such an accomplishment would go far in distinguishing between diagnostic look-alikes.

The fact that patients with the same disease can present differently has been amply covered in Chapter 4, but it warrants repetition at this point. Also worth rementioning is the fact that textbook cases are rare and probably exist only in textbooks. Books list all the manifestations of a disease; sometimes they even describe a fairly "typical case." But patients do not conform to books, and common features are often absent. In fact, with few exceptions, no two cases with the same disease are identical; each has at least one feature which is peculiar to that particular patient and absent in the others. Diseases differ as do people.

Establishing the degree of diagnostic certainty needed in any particular case may be difficult. This subject too was discussed in Chapter 4, but needs further clarification here. Recall that 100% certainty is seldom attainable, and therapeutic decisions must often be made even if you are less than sure. Diagnosis and treatment may proceed simultaneously. Chest pain needs treatment even before diagnosis. Diarrhea can be treated symptomatically before determining the underlying disease. So can urinary frequency and dysuria. These interventions are determined by the seriousness of the case, the time required for more and more studies, the urgency for needed action, and the level of certainty humanly possible in each instance.

Often only minimal problem solving is needed. Little is required for the patient with glycosuria or hypertension if diabetes mellitus or essential hypertension is easily established. But the situation becomes more complicated if genetic diabetes or essential hypertension is not the diagnosis and a specific cause must be sought. Nosebleeds, sore feet, and simple infectious processes of the skin, fingers, toes, and upper respiratory tract are not usually problems requiring diagnostic skills. Nose picking, foot strain or poor shoes, cuts, wounds, injuries, and transmitted nasopharyngeal secretions are the usual underlying causes. But such seemingly simple benign problems can sometimes turn into riddles. Nosebleeds may signify multiple myeloma; repeated infections can presage either diabetes mellitus or the altered immunity of lymphomas, agammaglobulinemia, or acquired immune deficiency syndrome. Beware of complacency in what seems like a simple matter.

One of the first things to decide in the course of harvesting patient data is whether the principal problem is limited to one organ or one system, involves several systems, or if indeed more than one disease exists. The decision about one organ or one system is usually easy since the symptoms and physical signs are apt to be thus confined. But the distinction between a multisystem disease and multiple diseases is not simple and requires added information and skill. Duodenal ulcer is a one-organ disease in most cases; occasionally it is associated with an endocrinopathy. Systemic lupus erythematosus and sarcoidosis are multiple system diseases. Diabetes mellitus, essential hypertension, and cerebral thrombosis are multiple diseases that may occur in the same person.

Before delving into the list of problem-solving methods that follows, the concept of disease prevalence and disease probability must be reexplored.

The prevalence of a particular disease is represented by the number of cases of the disease per population unit at any particular time. Thus the prevalence of diabetes mellitus is .05 or 5%, of hypertension in adults is .20 or 20%, and of breast cancer in women over 50 years of age is .003 or .3% (3 cases/1000 women).

The probability that a disease exists in a particular patient is a decimal or percentage estimate based on available data. For example, the clinical picture may suggest a .25 or 25% probability that the patient has coronary heart disease. This also means that in a cohort of 100 similar patients, 25 would have coronary heart disease and 75 would not.

Both the prevalence and probability of disease are expressed by the Bayesian symbol P(D).

Given a patient with a clinical P(D) of .25, you may wish to increase or decrease the likelihood of disease before embarking on a planned course of treatment. To alter the P(D) and thus establish greater negative or positive certainty, more clinical information must be obtained. A revised P(D) can be calculated after each procedure or clue, provided you know the prior probability and the sensitivity and specificity of the clinical information or paraclinical procedure used to alter the likelihood or probability. This subject was discussed in Chapter 5 and will be met again in the description of some problem-solving methods.

But probability revisions are simply done by adding clinical information. Suppose you see a 65-year-old man who has dyspnea on exertion and a long-standing hypertension. It is surprising how students and clinicians, even on the basis of scant information, can estimate the P(D) with reliability, consistency, and only small interobserver variation. Most would estimate the likelihood of left ventricular failure at 50 to 75%. Then add the fact that there are no pulmonary symptoms; the P(D) rises to 75 to 85%. Next you note grade 2 hypertensive fundi, blood pressure 210/120 mm Hg, basal rales, an enlarged heart, and a third heart sound. The P(D) rises to 95%; left ventricular failure is virtually certain. Similar situations presented to students produce strikingly little variation in P(D) estimates; their evaluations are essentially as good as those of clinicians

and groups of experts using the Delphi technique. This is a good teaching and learning exercise.

In gathering more data, we are able to raise the P(D) to an acceptable level by probability revision. We may also be obliged to reject the diagnosis because negative information has lowered the P(D) to a point where the diagnosis may be essentially eliminated. In this way, probability revision enables us to make consequent patient-management decisions.

Now that these preliminary concepts have been set forth, we can proceed with a discussion of problem-solving methods. Note that some of the tactics and strategies discussed in Chapters 4 and 5 are often used as supplements to any of the methods listed below. Also be aware of the fact that the problem-solving methods listed and described here will be exemplified and noted in the clinical cases solved in Section Three.

List of Problem-Solving Methods.

1. Traditional method
2. Early hypothesis generation
3. Clusters
4. Pattern recognition
5. Syndromes
6. Key clue
7. Pivotal clue
8. Formation of a differential
9. Suppression of information
10. Hunch and intuition
11. Lanthanic method
12. Anatomic method
13. Maneuvers with clues
14. Mathematical operations
15. Dendrograms
16. Decision path
17. Algorithms
18. Flow charts
19. Computers.

Traditional Method. Much has already been said of this method in Chapters 1 and 2. A complete orderly data base is constructed from the history, the physical examination, and the laboratory, which are treated as three discrete data sources. Clues are selected from each of them, then fitted together to form a diagnosis, just as you would complete a jigsaw puzzle. From the leftover clues, you elongate the problem list.

This method is tedious and time-consuming, though frequently necessary in obscure cases, in complicated or multisystem diseases, or when multiple diseases exist in one patient. It is especially helpful for the beginner who may feel uncomfortable about forming early hypotheses and may hesitate to depart from time-honored sequences. Even the seasoned clinician may find this method necessary at times.

Some facetiously call this the "method of exhaustion," since so much detailed and often useless information must be obtained. It is said to resemble the process of looking through all the M's in a telephone directory for a name you have forgotten except for the first letter. But it is useful when simpler timesaving methods cannot be readily applied, or when you don't remember the second and third letters of the name beginning with M.

Early Hypothesis Generation. This is the single most commonly used and most effective method of solving problems. It is often called the *hypothetico-deductive* method and has already been discussed in Chapters 1, 2, and 4 which relate to the collection and processing of data. The problem solver forms tentative impressions early in the data-gathering process; these impressions are rapidly rejected or accepted as specific data are acquired. Various maneuvers govern the rejection or acceptance of hypotheses. These include case building, pattern building, template matching, weight of evidence, proof by exclusion, mathematical operations, and so forth. Such maneuvers as they apply to the hypothetico-deductive process will be further described as separate problem-solving methods later in this chapter.

Educational experiments have challenged clinicians with simulated clinical cases and subsequently analyzed their verbalized problem-solving behaviors. The idea that clinicians methodically gather facts about patients and reserve judgment about the underlying problems until later is put to rest.

However, the idea that clinicians rapidly generate hypotheses that orient them and guide them in inquiry is well established (1).

The origination of hypotheses may be triggered by pairs or combinations of symptoms, by an initial concept based on age, gender, and chief complaint, by mention of a cause or complication of a disease, or by a string-together technique (2).

When a patient suddenly develops double vision and you note a third nerve palsy, you hypothesize diabetes mellitus, intracranial aneurysm, or brain tumor. A 56-year-old woman develops intense vulvovaginitis with itching, burning, and discharge; you postulate diabetes mellitus. The string-together technique for hypothesis generation can be exemplified as follows. A 36-year-old man has hematuria, pyuria, and fever; he says he passes clumps of tissue as well as blood; you think of necrotizing papillitis; he is not diabetic so you consider analgesic abuse; this suggests there may be a cause for analgesic abuse; there is—chronic worsening headaches; eventually you hypothesize and later prove the existence of a brain tumor. Note how you have gone from one hypothesis to another by chain reaction.

Sometimes less likely hypotheses are considered first because they are curable, whereas the more likely hypothesis, if incurable, will not activate so avid an interest in the problem solver.

While a novice may have ill-defined plans for managing each hypothesis, the seasoned clinician develops fixed deductive patterns. These patterns become integrated as templates into his cognitive structure and can be recalled on demand for any predicated hypothesis (3). If disease A is suspected, there are five precise bits of evidence to be sought. For disease B, there are eight. To distinguish A from B, three studies must be done—and so forth.

Clusters. The use of recognized clusters, patterns, and syndromes is a popular, practical, and economical method of diagnosis and is often employed by the more experienced physician. From two or three clues he can formulate a provisional diagnosis which subsequent data prove correct. But even beginners are quick to group the findings of diarrhea, abdominal cramps, and weight loss; or those of dyspnea, orthopnea, weakness, and swollen legs. Also, they soon learn that "moans, bones, and stones" equal hyperparathyroidism. The formation of clusters is most helpful in the generation of hypotheses (4).

There are many *classical triads and tetrads* which are easily mastered and committed to memory. Thyromegaly, tremor, tachycardia, and eye signs form a cluster which is unquestionably caused by hyperthyroidism. Cirrhosis, diabetes, and bronzing of the skin equal hemochromatosis. And on and on.

Cluster diagnosis is widely employed and works quite well when a given cluster is pathognomonic for a single disease. Sudden severe abdominal pain, rigidity, and subdiaphragmatic air equal perforated peptic ulcer in almost every case. On the other hand, pain, tenderness, and rigidity in the right lower quadrant usually mean acute suppurative appendicitis. But this triad could also signify acute pelvic inflammatory disease, perforated cecal carcinoma, severe regional ileitis, etc. So consider patterns and clusters with caution.

If you must formulate your own cluster in a particular patient, decide if all the symptoms and signs in the cluster apply to a single diagnosis or to several (5). Check to make sure you are not dealing with two or more simultaneous diseases. You can easily be misled at this stage of the diagnostic process. Also, the *cluster components should be clearly related*, if not by region or system, then by a pathophysiologic process or chronologic sequence. Concurrent tooth abscess and eosinophilia are obviously not related and do not form a cluster. But when dyspnea and cough occur with eosinophilia, look out—especially if you are in the tropics or subtropics. *Ascaris lumbricoides* migrating through the lungs is possible.

In general, the more clues that form a cluster suggesting one diagnosis, the more reliable your conclusion. A cluster of five clues, all of which fit together and point toward one disease, is apt to yield higher diagnostic accuracy than a cluster of only two clues. Dyspnea and edema can have many causes. But dyspnea, edema, orthopnea, distended neck veins, and an enlarged laboring heart can be explained by only one problem: congestive heart failure—which, in turn, can have many causes. Polyuria and polydipsia present many options, but polyuria, polydipsia, polyphagia, and weight loss almost invariably mean severe diabetes mellitus.

One large rubbery node in the neck leads you to suspect lymphoma. If the spleen is palpable it becomes more likely. The presence of anemia too makes it even more likely. And if the patient also has generalized pruritus and intermittent fever, you can be reasonably sure. This could be called "the weight of evidence." One clue is suggestive, but put five together and there is little doubt. In the 55-year-old male heavy smoker who has developed a cough, sputum, hemoptysis, and weight loss—and, in addition, has clubbing of the fingers, a left upper lobe expiratory wheeze, and a large hard left supraclavicular node—carcinoma of the lung appears certain.

Remember that the cluster technique, like others, is only a part of the game. Having formed your provisional hypotheses by this method, you must still prove them with additional data.

Pattern Recognition. This method allows you to make a diagnosis with a single glance. If you were to see Abraham Lincoln on the street, you would know him at once. You would not analyze his eyes, hair, nose, and mouth separately. In the same way, you can instantly identify your friends without consciously knowing the color of their eyes or hair. It is the overall pattern that counts. This is recognition by gestalt.

Many diagnoses are made this way. For example, an elderly man with an oily expressionless face and a coarse tremor shuffles into your office with small steps, bent over, his arms and legs slightly flexed. You recognize Parkinson's disease by one look.

There is no mistaking it, provided you have seen it before and have the picture in your mind. The recognition of myxedema, acromegaly, Cushing's disease, and Turner's syndrome occurs in the same way.

For example, a patient you have known for many years may have myxedema, yet you have never diagnosed it. But a new physician may spot it at first glance. With a quick look at the head and face (puffy eyelids, dull expression, slight pallor, coarse sparse hair, dry skin), he knows what is wrong without analyzing the individual features. While he recognizes it because he is seeing the patient for the first time, you missed it because the changes occurred over a period of years under your very nose.

Mitral stenosis can be diagnosed similarly by a single "listen." You do not have to analyze each of the six or seven separate auscultatory findings and put them together. Just place the bell of your stethoscope over the apex and listen to the song of mitral stenosis. It's diagnostic. You should know it and recognize it as readily as the Star-Spangled Banner. The gestalt of a melody is distinct from its separate notes.

The gestalt technique can be used to play the game of "sidewalk diagnosis." Look at the people who pass and pick out those with obvious thyroid disease, acromegaly, Paget's disease, and Marie-Strumpell arthritis. In modern civilized cultures this game is not very fruitful because people usually see physicians early and may have the course of their diseases changed. But in undeveloped lands, where diseases abound in advanced untreated states, it is a different story. Moreover, the disease spectrum shifts. There you can spot leprosy, lymphoma, far-gone obstructive lung disease, draining scrofulous glands, textbook heart failure, nephrotic syndromes—just by a glance.

Syndromes. A syndrome is a concurrence of manifestations seen frequently enough to be more than a chance relationship (6). This group of clues may be simply part of a disease, may be seen in several different diseases, or may actually be a disease which has not yet been labeled as such. If you spot a syndrome, you may be well on your way to making a diagnosis.

The presence of sinusitis, bronchiectasis, and situs inversus is called Kartagener's syndrome; its cause and pathophysiology are unclear. The nephrotic syndrome consists of the coexistence of edema, hypoalbuminemia, and marked albuminuria. It can be caused by a dozen diseases affecting the kidneys in such a manner as to bring about this triad. Horner's syndrome is a combination of ptosis, myosis, enophthalmos, and anhidrosis occurring on one side of the face; it is not a disease in itself, but it can be caused by a variety of diseases affecting the superior cervical sympathetic nerves anywhere from their origin in the spinal cord to their upward course in the neck. Thus it may be a consequence of cerebral thrombosis, spinal cord diseases, cancer of the lung, or cancer of the thyroid, among other possibilities.

Cavernous sinus syndrome is composed of edema of the lids, proptosis of the eye, and paralysis of the third, fourth, and sixth cranial nerves. It is caused by cavernous sinus thrombosis, in turn the result of any one of a variety of infections about the face, sinuses, or ear—part of a spreading infectious process.

A list of syndromes could fill many pages, but note how many should instead be labeled diseases. Marfan's *syndrome*—aortic valve and arch disease, lenticular dislocations, arachnodactyly, high palatal arch, etc—should be called Marfan's *disease*, since it is known to be a disease of connective tissue inherited as a dominant trait with variable expression. In fact, the disease presents with different pictures or formes frustes of the originally described syndrome. Many others are kept on the syndrome list because of ignorance, habit, or conservatism.

This is especially true of chromosome-linked disorders which are now called syndromes but should actually be dubbed diseases. A prolonged QT interval, deafness, and sudden death, now recognized to be a definite genetically linked syndrome, should likewise be labeled a disease after more investigation.

On the other hand, a frequent concurrence of symptoms or clues does not necessarily make a syndrome. Consider the coincidence of baldness and athlete's foot, each in itself a common condition. They are obviously not related.

A syndrome must be recognized or detected just as a cluster is. It may be listed as a problem in the problem list. Or it may help you establish the primary disease which is associated with or causing the syndrome, in which case the disease itself would be listed as the problem. For instance, an aortic aneurysm or carcinoma at the apex of the lung may be the cause of Horner's syndrome.

Key Clue. When various clues do not form a definite cluster, do not seem to relate, and are nonspecific in nature, you may not know where to begin. If so, seek out a *key clue* and track it down. This principal clue may be a symptom, a physical finding, or a paraclinical abnormality; many examples of key clues were presented in Chapter 3.

Select an important or principal clue, such as anemia or jaundice—a clue which can generally lead to a solution by a branching or algorithmic approach. This means that the various causes of the key clue can be categorized and subdivided by performing discerning studies. One test rules out all but one category. A second test rules out all but one subcategory. The end point of this *divide and conquer* strategy is a diagnosis.

For example, the findings of weakness, fatigability, nausea, anorexia, and weight loss are all nonspecific and not suitable for a departure point on an algorithmic search. However, suppose this patient also has an enlarged abdomen that you determine is caused by ascites; this is your key clue, and you can begin your search with the causes of ascites—cirrhosis, nephrosis, metastatic cancer, tuberculosis—and proceed from there.

Pivotal Clue. This is similar to though not synonymous with a key clue. It is the turning point or linchpin about which hypotheses are formed and diagnoses made in very complicated cases like the presentation of a clinicopathologic conference. Such cases are so complex and so replete with important information that mathematical manipulations of multiple clues are impossible, hypothesis generation is premature, and differential diagnoses are too lengthy to manage. In these instances, the clinician derives a pivotal clue by aggregating a set of findings into a *pattern* (7). Since most medical knowledge is stored according to disease, the pivot is an aggregated pattern across which the physician can move from a large group of symptoms and signs to a manageable list of possible diagnoses.

Suppose the complicated, complex case has several hundred bits of information needing processing and aggregation. You must capture the important features which add up to a pivotal point before generating a cause list.

For example, a patient presents with a confusing picture. But from the multitude of clues you can select a few which add up to: a 48-year-old man with diffuse lung disease characterized mainly by a diffusion defect; diabetes insipidus in a 58-year-old woman who is losing weight; a coagulopathy in a 48-year-old woman under treatment for breast cancer; aortic regurgitation in a tall man; or malabsorption in a 60-year-old woman.

Each of these pivotal points represents a pattern that was aggregated from selected clues. The first patient had, among many other items, dyspnea on exertion, a slight cough, linear infiltrates and patchy opacification seen on chest radiography, and a marked decrease in carbon monoxide diffusing capacity. The second patient had polyuria, polydipsia, a urine specific gravity of 1.002, a good response to pitressin, anorexia, and weight loss. And so on for the others.

A wieldy differential diagnosis can be formed in each instance. The diagnostic list is then pruned by utilizing the existing data in Bayes' theorem fashion, and one diagnosis is selected and subsequently validated (7).

Forming a Differential. Whether you start with a cluster of clues, a key clue, a pivotal point, or an initial concept, you must eventually form a *list of possible causes* for the patient's complaints. This differential diagnosis may be generated early (provisional hypotheses) or later after more data are obtained. You may not formulate it until you have all or almost all the information. But no matter when it is formed, it should be as complete as possible. Common causes should probably come first, though some clinicians might prefer to list the more urgent or more curable first. The more complete the list the less apt you are to overlook the correct diagnosis. In any particular case the ultimately diagnosed disease may be neither common, urgent, nor curable.

Usually a differential diagnosis is simple and easy to form; it may include only two or three possibilities. Bloody diarrhea in a 34-year-old woman means ulcerative colitis, regional enteritis, or bacillary dysentery. Often the differential is more lengthy but is easily committed to memory. If the initial concept is left ventricular failure, you have to consider mainly hypertensive heart disease, coronary heart disease, aortic stenosis or aortic regurgitation, mitral regurgitation, and cardiomyopathy. Sometimes the list is more complex and can be recalled by house staff-generated mnemonic lines. You may consult one of numerous textbooks that outline the various causes of key clues or clusters, or you may look up one of the suspected diseases and read the differential diagnosis subhead found in all standard disease-oriented textbooks.

The differential diagnosis may include diseases in only one body system—e.g. neurologic, hematologic, or cardiovascular. But the problem may be such that the cause can lie in any one of many systems, and you may have to sift through all the modules stored in your brain.

One of the great difficulties confronting the medical novice is the formation of a reasonably all-inclusive list of possible explanations for patient presentation. It is easy to overlook common important possibilities unless you have developed a system for forming such a list.

All diseases can be divided into categories. If you go from one category to another and wherever applicable choose a disease that might explain the presenting picture, you will form a suitable list of diagnostic possibilities. A convenient division of all diseases is:

1. Infectious
2. Neoplastic
3. Endocrine-metabolic
4. Neuropsychiatric
5. Special organs (heart, lung, kidney, gastrointestinal)
6. Connective tissue and autoimmune
7. Hematologic
8. Genetic
9. Traumatic
10. Nutritional
11. Iatrogenic and drug-induced.

Suppose you are confronted by a patient with long-standing fever and must formulate a list of possibilities. By going through the previous categories one by one, you select tuberculosis, bacteremia, occult abscess, and enteric fevers from category 1; occult carcinoma from category 2; none from 3 or 4; infective endocarditis, cirrhosis, and regional enteritis from category 5; systemic lupus erythematosus from 6; leukemia, lymphoma, and pernicious anemia from 7; none from categories 8, 9, or 10; and drug-induced fever from 11. Now you have a good working list. Similar broad presentations can be managed in the same way.

Once the differential diagnostic list is formed, you refine and eliminate, then select and prove according to the various other problem-solving methods discussed in this chapter.

Proof by exclusion is a technique that is commonly used once the differential is established. After having listed the possible interpretations of a clinical picture, all are proven impossible and eliminated—except one. Whichever has not been excluded must therefore be the correct answer. But inference by exclusion has limited value because it is difficult to be sure that the original list of possibilities is all-inclusive. However, you are reasonably safe if you consider only the common possible diagnoses. Physicians often use this technique with great success.

A similar but more positive strategy would be to consider all possible diagnoses, then pick the one which seems most likely and prove it conclusively. The others must be kept in mind until excluded by a minimal number of studies. Thus you establish a differential diagnosis, prove one, and eliminate the others.

Suppression of Information. This diagnostic technique is used when a plethora of information is present (8). The patient may give nth-degree details, starting way back when he was 2 years old. Much is extraneous and nonpertinent. The picture may be so smoggy that you cannot see the clues and problems. All the details may indeed be accurate, but they becloud the main issue. You must be able to separate pertinent data from unrelated detail. For instance, you can recognize the main theme of some impressionistic paintings only by squinting, thereby eliminating some of the less prominent brush strokes.

The same mechanism may be invoked if you are listening to a piano concerto and wish to concentrate on the melody of the solo instrument. You must consciously suppress the accompanying orchestral distractions. Similarly, you might listen to an entire symphony without noticing the flute; whereas if you were alerted in advance, you would undoubtedly hear it, excluding all other sounds from your consciousness.

Particular care must be taken with the psychoneurotic patient who often has a large number of positive symptoms and may answer yes to every question. Organic disease may be buried in a maze of affirmative answers, and it takes great skill to separate the psyche from the soma. Here, suppression of nonrelated information is the required problem-solving technique, and a complete data base is mandatory.

The reverse situation may occur when very little information is available. If the patient is unconscious and relatives give meager history, if the patient is an infant,

mute, or senile, or if information is scant for other reasons, you must flesh out a skeleton of facts. Construct the entire tableau from a few clues, just as you visualize an entire image from Picasso's few brush strokes.

Hunch and Intuition. At this point, the diagnostician becomes less than scientific. A "hunch" is a premonition or suspicion—a feeling—that something is so. It is not a stab in the dark or a mere guess. There is more to it than that. Usually it is an educated deduction made almost subconsciously on the basis of a single observation—a bit of seemingly unimportant information mentioned by the patient, a facial expression, perhaps an odor—coupled with a case seen or read about the previous week. A hunch stands somewhere between a guess and intuition in degree of certainty. Hunches can often be wrong, but the more experience and knowledge the physician has, the more apt his hunches are to be right.

Intuition, on the other hand, is often regarded as a mystical process, but it is based on more solid evidence than a hunch is. The dictionary defines intuition as the "direct perception of a truth or fact independent of any reasoning process." Or it is defined as a cognition obtained or conclusion reached without recourse to conscious inference, reasoning, or reflection, as if it were a magical insight or gifted instinct.

I would contend that intuition—medical intuition—is not so abstract as definers would have us believe. It is probably the product of multitudinous messages transmitted across the vast neurochemical network linking memory, thought, knowledge, experience, judgment, and horse sense.

The intuitive process may be a complex, highly intellectual skill that arises from the finest assembly of microcomputers that ever was or ever will be built—the human brain.

One does not intuit a judgment, decision, diagnosis, or treatment by pulling a rabbit out of a hat, no matter how instinctive or spontaneous the action may seem. Instead, such performances result from many *conscious and subconscious* mathematical calculations and psychologic transactions.

Since calculations of this sort may lack precision, intuitive decisions may, of course, sometimes be incorrect.

The "intuitive" decision to perform a test depends on quick evaluations of the operating characteristics of the test, the need for elevating or lowering the disease probability, the cost-risk-benefit factors, time-emergency elements, and the availability and skill of the test performer. And on these bases, the physician may say "do the test." Attaching numbers and percentages to the multivariant aspects of this decision makes the intuitive process more explicit.

Lanthanic Method. This is another verbal concept introduced by Feinstein (5) and refers to the patient without symptoms who sees the physician because of an abnormality detected on a routine examination. The word "lanthanic" comes from the Greek and means "to escape attention." A patient may be symptomatic for one disease and consult the physician for it. Yet he may have a lanthanic disease present too. For instance, there may be an abnormality in the urine, blood, x-ray, ECG, or physical examination. No symptoms—yet possibly serious disease!

Today, when so many routine examinations are being done, when complete chemistry profiles are generated no matter what the reason for a patient's hospitalization, numerous lanthanic situations exist. For instance, a very high serum uric acid warrants a second look at the history for joint pains, kidney stones, or family history of gout. A heart murmur discovered by the school physician deserves a cardiologic investigation. A small infiltrate is noted on an annual chest x-ray. The blood count discloses marked lymphocytosis.

More and more, asymptomatic problems are being encountered in practice. Common examples include albuminuria, glycosuria, pyuria, leukocytosis, anemia, polycythemia, hyperglycemia, hepatomegaly, splenomegaly, hyperglycemia, hypercalcemia, increased alkaline phosphatase, and radiographic or electrocardiographic abnormalities. Several examples of such presentations and their solutions are portrayed in Section

Three. How to solve them? Each presents its own challenge—no symptoms, possibly some physical findings, yet a definite abnormality! The physician must know or look up the various causes of the abnormality and proceed from there, using any or many solving techniques. Usually he eliminates the possibilities one by one and proves the existence of only one. He may remain in doubt, choose to wait and observe, or opt for a consultation as with any problem. The algorithmic method of problem solving (described later in this chapter) is often adaptable in these cases.

Anatomic Approach. Here the patient presents because of a discrete anatomic abnormality which he sees or feels. This might be a rash, and the problem might be solved by simple observation, potassium hydroxide preparation, or biopsy. Often the patient notices a lump or tumor, such as a large thyroid, a lump in the neck or breast, or a protruding mass in the abdomen. Each of these may represent a serious problem which must be solved. The techniques differ and may range from a biopsy for a lump in the breast or neck to a complete survey for a mass in the abdomen. You can see how the range of problem-solving techniques shifts for the patient with a strictly anatomic clue.

A large thyroid needs evaluation for size, shape, consistency, mobility, nodularity, and vascularity; no doubt thyroid function tests and an isotopic or ultrasound scan will be done too. A solitary thyroid adenoma requires scrutiny for hardness, mobility, and size, thyroid function tests, a carefully done scan, and often a needle aspiration or surgery for the final solution.

A breast lump will almost always require an excisional biopsy, regardless of the physical findings. Neck lumps need careful examination, since they may represent congenital rests, cysts, tumors, or metastatic carcinomas. In addition to a meticulous evaluation of the lump itself, a complete physical examination must be done if you suspect it may be a metastatic lesion. Surgical excision with biopsy is often the ultimate procedure.

Masses noted in the abdomen by the patient himself are fairly common presentations. You wonder how long the mass has been there. Does the patient suddenly note a long-present mass because he has lost weight on a self-imposed diet? Is the mass associated with unplanned weight loss? The identification of a mass may be simple or complex. The location, size, shape, tenderness, and consistency are important. Does it move with respiration? Structures which are intraperitoneal and close to the diaphragm do; retroperitoneal masses do not. Thus spleens and livers move considerably, kidneys move only slightly, and retroperitoneal tumors do not move at all.

The differential diagnosis revolves around anomalously shaped or misplaced normal organs, enlarged organs, masses in organs, or separate masses. Regardless of the findings on physical examination, additional studies, scans, and other radiographic procedures must often be done to be sure of the solution to the problem.

This holds true for abdominal masses for which different sets of diagnoses can be postulated depending on where the mass is found. In the right upper quadrant, consider tumors, cysts, or enlargement of the colon, gallbladder, liver and kidney; in the left upper quadrant, investigate the spleen, pancreas, kidney, colon, and stomach; and so forth.

Maneuvers with Clues. The manipulation of clues is not a problem-solving technique in itself but is used in conjunction with most of the techniques already discussed. Even if we generate early hypotheses, form clusters, and recognize patterns and syndromes, additional clues must still be maneuvered into the clinical setting by using a variety of tactics. Most important to remember is that such clues range from simple items in the history to complex diagnostic procedures.

Some clues are used for *screening* purposes. This strategy is employed to reject hypotheses and eliminate diagnostic possibilities. For example, hepatitis B tends to be excluded if there is no history of injections, transfusions, intravenous drug abuse, homosexuality, or occupational hazard. Second-

ary syphilis is "screened out" by a negative serologic test for syphilis since the test is highly sensitive and false negatives are virtually nonexistent in this stage of the disease. Except in unusual circumstances, a negative intermediate strength purified protein derivative skin test virtually excludes pulmonary tuberculosis. For all practical purposes, a normal urinalysis denies kidney disease. Screening is also a demonstration of *proof by exclusion.* Eliminate all possibilities save one!

As noted in previous chapters, additionally acquired clues are used to search and scan—to exclude and confirm. Sensitive clues exclude if negative; specific clues confirm if positive. Sensitive clues confirm if positive only when the clue is also highly specific and false positives are few. By the same logic, specific clues exclude if negative only when the clue is also highly sensitive and false negatives are rare.

Pattern building is a device whereby clues are added until the picture of a disease is constructed. Given an initial cluster and a tentative diagnosis, look for those clues which are found in the suspected disease. If they are present, you have engaged in a case-building strategy *for* the disease; if enough of them are absent, the strategy tends to rule *against* the disease.

Template matching is another tactic. It is similar to but not identical with pattern building. You know the entire clinical picture of the suspected diagnosis, and you know the features of the patient's data base. Try to select and build the clues into an architectural pattern that coincides with the textbook template as closely as possible. If pieces are absent, get the additional data needed to complete the design. The match does not have to be perfect. There may be only a family resemblance. But if too many needed clues are absent and contrary ones are present, a match has not been achieved and the suspected diagnosis may not be valid.

When you are not sure a diagnosis is correct, yet many clues point in that direction, you might say that the *weight of evi-*

dence is in favor of the diagnosis. As more positive clues are found, the weight of evidence increases. Five positives are heavier than three. Also, the more sensitive the clues, the heavier the combined weight. If a highly specific clue is present, no additional weight is needed, and the diagnosis is confirmed.

Note the similarities and slight variations between pattern building, template matching, and weight of evidence. Some authors use these terms interchangeably.

Mathematical Operations. Here too clues are maneuvered in consideration of a preselected hypothesis, cluster, pattern, or syndrome; but the manipulations are mathematical and numbers are used. After estimating the disease probability, a test or clue can revise the probability—upward if positive and downward if negative. This revision of probability is accomplished by Bayes' theorems in a precise mathematical style. All you need to know is the initial P(D), the operating characteristics of the test or clue, and the result of the test.

But when two or more clues must be applied, the Bayesian method becomes impractical and unwieldy. Then rough approximations can be made and precision compromised.

The probability theorems of Bayes, the overlapping diagrams of Venn, and the algebraic notations of Boole all help in making logical deductions but are not in themselves problem-solving methods. Much about their applicability to clinical reasoning was presented in Chapter 5.

Dendrograms. These are tree-like structures which schematically represent a variety of similar problem-solving techniques using branches and branching points (nodes). They are in common use and include such mechanisms as flow charts, algorithms, and decision trees, all of which have a structural resemblance.

Regard the concept of a large diagnostic tree which represents all of medical knowledge radiating from a main trunk in a multiple branching fashion (Fig. 9.1).

Start at the roots with some basic clues

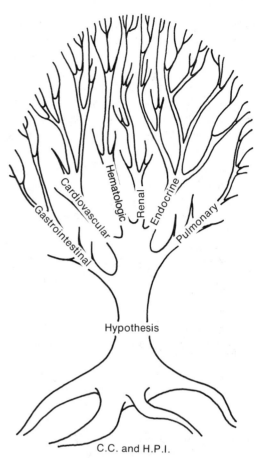

Fig. 9.1. The diagnostic tree. *C.C.,* chief complaint; *H.P.I.,* history of present illness.

gotten from the chief complaint and present illness. Formulate one or two provisional hypotheses as you go up the trunk to the first major bifurcation. Let each large branch represent a disease system, such as cardiovascular or endocrine. Then go up the branch which seems appropriate, gathering pertinent data as you proceed. Each node on a branch represents a further branching point at which a question is asked or data are discovered and a decision is made. Note that nodes can branch in a binary, tertiary, or quaternary fashion. You may not be able to proceed beyond a certain node because of lack of additional data. This point may therefore represent your highest possible resolution of the problem for the moment.

On the other hand, you may have to retreat one or two nodes and go off in another direction if you find you are getting only negative information and seem to be going astray. Ideally, a branch should terminate in an item on your problem list.

For example, the chief complaint and history of present illness have told you that the problem is cardiovascular and probably an instance of left ventricular failure. As you go up the main cardiovascular branch, you come to ensuing nodes, gather more data, and proceed up the correct subbranches: the history is compatible with left ventricular failure; so are the physical findings; the cause of the failure is determined to be cardiomyopathy mainly by exclusion; the final branching process leads to a definition of problem 1, alcoholic cardiomyopathy. The solution is reached by exclusion of other causes of cardiomyopathy plus the presence of features pointing to alcohol.

Many educators and physicians regard all of diagnosis as a huge branching tree. They feel that diagnosis consists of simply tracing one of a large number of pathways through a system of branches. Each of these systems is in reality a flow chart or series of questions with yes or no answers directing the branching process. The physician quickly derives a few important clues (one or several) and departs down one branch of the diagnostic tree. If pursuit is hot, questions continue along that line. But if he finds by a series of negative responses that he is going in the wrong direction, he comes back to a node and follows another branch. After solving the main problem, he completes his data base. In so doing, he forms a problem list by numbering the tree's blooming branches and pruning those that are dead.

You can see, at least in theory, how the diagnostic process may be computerized. This has already been done for some diagnostic problems with varying degrees of success. The branching technique can also be easily converted into traditional flow charts, widely utilized in today's journals.

Decision Path. This is similar to the diagnostic tree first described except that it deals with only one branch and a discrete number of questions bearing yes or no an-

swers (Fig. 9.2). The attending physician often starts down such a path as soon as he hears the chief complaint. He sees how few questions he can ask and still solve the problem. The questions must be discriminating and none can be wasted. It is as if you are trying to solve a riddle with a minimum number of questions. The number of nodes, questions, and branchings will vary with expertise and experience.

Screening and triage too require great skill and must be done with as few questions as possible. Especially when working through an interpreter with people who speak a foreign tongue, time is a factor and decisions must be based on a minimum of questions.

Questions with negative answers may be the ones which lead you to a correct conclusion, and positive answers sometimes lead to dead ends. But the reverse is the usual situation. A decision path may well consist of both positive and negative answers (Fig. 9.2). This figure is only schematic and is not meant to portray the sequence of inquiry in the case which follows.

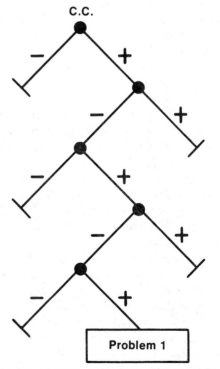

Fig. 9.2. A decision path. *C.C.*, chief complaint.

Consider a 28-year-old man who develops acute monarticular arthritis of the right knee. Pertinent nodes, decisions, and branching points will revolve mainly about the provisional hypotheses of gout and acute suppurative arthritis. Direction of inquiry will be made along the line of: (*a*) urethral discharge; (*b*) previous episodes; (*c*) history of new sexual contact, gout in family, renal stones; (*d*) examination of vital signs, ears, joint, and genitalia; (*e*) serum uric acid; (*f*) Gram's stain of urethral discharge, if present; and (*g*) examination of joint aspirate for bacteria, white blood cells, and urate crystals. These steps should establish a diagnosis.

If a urethral discharge is present or newly acquired, a gonococcal joint is likely, though gout could conceivably coexist. The presence of previous episodes would favor gout though not rule out gonorrhea. A history of new sexual contact obviously hints at gonorrhea, whereas a positive family history and a history of renal stones favor gout. Note that no single clue has completely excluded either possibility because there may be coincidence or coexistence. The vital signs may help but not be convincing, since a high fever is more likely with suppuration. Tophi in the ear would guarantee the existence of gout but would not assert that this hot joint is necessarily *caused* by gout. The examination of the joint may not be helpful since both diseases may appear the same. However, if tissue adjacent to the joint is also inflamed, gout is more suspect. As for the genitalia, confirm the presence or absence of a urethral discharge even when its presence is denied by history. A high serum uric acid level points toward gout, but people with hyperuricemia can develop gonorrhea, and people with gout can have normal serum uric acid levels. If the Gram's stain of the urethral discharge is positive for gramnegative intracellular diplococci, gonorrhea is present in the urethra, and probably though not certainly present in the joint. Sodium urate crystals in the joint fluid diagnose gout; bacteria confirm an infection; the presence of both would be most unusual.

Though the answer to each question in the decision path is a simple yes or no, the implications of a simple answer may be complex as was just noted. Your evaluation of the entire series of answers should give the correct diagnosis. A more extensive presentation of a similar case is detailed in Chapter 22.

What a fascinating puzzle-solving game the physician plays every time he sees a patient!

Algorithms. An algorithm is a printed format that uses a branching pattern to solve problems. Given a chief complaint or key clue, the graphic structure of the algorithm represents a plan for the collection of data. From these data, the user is guided logically through a predetermined branching sequence of steps needed to make a decision. A characteristic feature of the algorithm is that the result of one test or one piece of information allows you to eliminate large chunks of the overall structure and directs you to follow only one path. Thus your line of inquiry is diverted to one pathway as if by a switch at a railway junction point.

The aim is to formalize the diagnostic process, to learn an organized approach to clinical problems, to outline succinctly the tests or studies to be performed, and to understand how the results determine subsequent diagnostic and therapeutic management. Textbooks do not describe clinical sequential data interpretations and their impact on subsequent decisions.

Algorithms substitute symbols, lines, directions, and strategies for detailed language, thereby acting like a Michelin guide that methodically tells you where to stay, where to go, and what to do.

Should it be determined at the first decision point that a patient with anemia has a hypochromic microcytic anemia, you need only pursue the diagnostic plan for that type of anemia, and you may exclude all other lines of inquiry. Follow the track that obtains data referable to blood in the stool and abnormal vaginal bleeding. On the other hand, knowing the type of anemia that exists, you would not steer the course for macrocytic anemias, nor would you seek information referable to malnutrition, malabsorption, gastric acidity, vitamin B_{12} absorption, and B_{12}-folate blood levels.

In time, algorithmic pathways become indelibly imprinted in the minds of good clinicians, and a medical problem immediately conjures up a seemingly instantaneous plan.

The principal values of algorithms are that they teach the student, help the practitioner to think and decide, improve patient care, decrease the cost of medical care, act as consultants, and make chart audit easier. Students read and understand algorithms better and faster than prose. While physicians should be able to collect information properly, act logically, and make appropriate decisions, this is not always the case, and algorithms may be of value there too. There is abundant evidence that common conditions like diabetes, hypertension, and urinary tract infections are improperly handled; algorithmic guidelines might help (9). And in this era of computerized everything, algorithms are ideally structured for computerization and may thus be recalled for any of the aforementioned purposes.

One can hardly pick up a journal or book today without seeing algorithms inside. They are in common usage and are helpful for physicians' assistants, clinical nurses, medical students, physicians, and professionals in all other fields. Books that are completely composed of algorithms have been written.

Figure 9.3 is a symbolic prototypical algorithm. They can be structured with varying complexity. Start at the extreme left with a cluster, key clue, chief complaint, pivotal clue, or hypothesis and retrace the entire algorithm while studying its structure and design. Each *square* represents a node where a test is performed or a bit of information is obtained; on this basis a decision is made to go in one direction or another. Inside each decision node is a number which designates the decision number. Note that decisions are made on the basis of test results (or information query) all along the various paths, and decision levels *1* through *5* are indicated at the *top*. Each decision node leads to multiple pathways, but a decision eliminates the

need to pursue all but one track, thus rapidly narrowing the field of diagnostic possibilities. If decision *1* leads to *A* and eliminates *B* and *C*, diagnoses *6* through *20* are immediately ruled out, and two-thirds of the algorithm may be ignored.

Note too that there are 20 possible diagnostic outcomes in this algorithm (*D1* to *D20* at the extreme *right*). The number of decisions and tests needed to reach an acceptable level of diagnostic certainty varies from two (decisions *1* and *4*) for diagnosis *15*, to five (decisions *1, 4, 12, 22,* and *24*) for diagnosis *20*. The various letter-number combinations (*A1-x, B2, C4y2*) represent the need to designate classes of disease, subclasses, and diagnostic possibilities and their various levels of diagnostic resolution. *A, B,* and *C* represent large classes; *A1, A2,* and *A3* represent subheadings under class *A*; and *A1-x* and *A1-y* signify diagnostic possibilities that exist in subclass *A1*.

It should be apparent that the number of decisions or tests needed to solve a problem varies with the path that you are obliged to follow. At times the algorithm planner feels that an additional test, number *23*, is needed before going from diagnostic level *5* to diagnostic level *6* (*B1-z2* to *D10*). But at other times, such as in proceeding from *B1-z1* to *D9*, this is not deemed necessary.

To construct an algorithm, first identify the nature of the problem to be solved, decide the level of the intended user, and determine the outcomes to be obtained. Then outline the steps needed to reach the desired conclusion, and from there draw the diagram that details the alternative outcomes at each step. Insert the steps that are further needed to raise each alternative outcome to the desired level of diagnostic resolution. You have just constructed the first draft of an algorithmic tree that must now be tested, revised, and refined until users get uniform results (10).

If you fail to see the difference between an algorithm and a decision tree (Chapter 8), you can be forgiven. While the basic dendrogram structures are the same, there are important differences. A decision analysis tree

Decision level

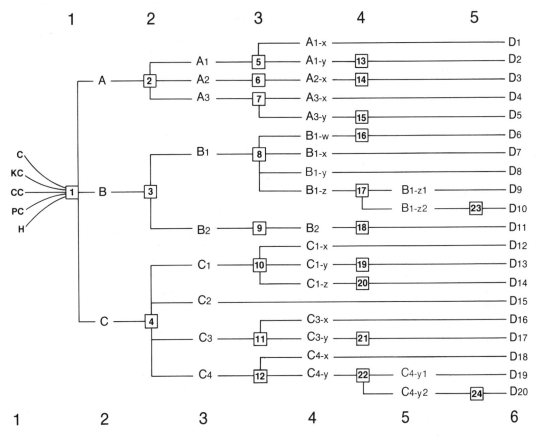

Fig. 9.3. Algorithm. See the text for a detailed explanation.
C, cluster
KC, key clue
CC, chief complaint
PC, pivotal clue
H, hypothesis

Diagnostic level

deals with numbers, percentages, and probabilities; a clinical algorithm does not. Decision analysis tells you whether it is more desirable to do this or that, and what is the probability that this or that is so. Algorithms say, "given this, do that." The former are more precise and more quantitative and are structured to operate under conditions of diagnostic uncertainty. The latter are more directive in seeking a diagnosis, do not require mathematical computations, and are of great help to the clinician (10).

Arguments have been proposed that lessen the value of algorithms. For example, some say they inhibit independent thinking and tend to turn physicians into thoughtless robots; others say they are either too complex or do not apply to individual patients; last, there are those who say that physicians don't think algorithmically and therefore cannot learn from them. There are valid rebuttals to each of these objections. We do not choose sides here.

Flow Charts. Along with algorithms, flow charts with similar construction have become increasingly popular and are used with varying effectiveness in texts, journals, and instruction booklets. Whole books consisting of nothing but flow charts are available. These printed aids guide the reader through a labyrinth of questions with yes or no answers until an end point is reached (Fig. 9.4).

You start with a presenting picture or key clue and go to *question 1.* Yes or no answers lead you along different lines of questioning. By following the *arrows* you should reach a conclusion that may vary from "*go to flow chart 2*" to "*reexamine in 1 month*" to "*consult surgeon*" to "*diagnosis 1.*" Note that the physician has only to supply yes or no answers based on data he has gathered and then go on to the next question, which is governed by whether the answer was yes or no. Questions bearing yes or no answers may be replaced by any information that is dichotomous—negative or positive, normal or abnormal—and the flow chart format still holds.

Note the resemblance of flow charts to algorithms, and of flow charts to protocols (Chapter 26). In flow charts, each information node has two possible answers which are opposites, there is greater complexity, and there may be different varieties of outcomes—not simply a diagnosis or a treatment.

The same pros and cons are true for both flow charts and algorithms. While they may be of help in selected instances, they should not be relied on too heavily. Perhaps their greatest use lies in teaching. Printed flow charts should not be regarded as a problem-solving panacea! They are little more than prefabricated dendrograms which serve as recipes for a mindless cook. They are difficult to write, rigid, may inhibit independent thinking, and are often so intricate as to require a road map and compass. Often you come across a flow chart which is 3 pages long and therefore almost incomprehensible. At other times you may see a full-page flow chart that could be replaced by a short paragraph.

The good physician generates his own flow chart every time he sees a patient and solves a problem. He should not need to follow printed pathways. But for the physician who needs help, the student who seeks

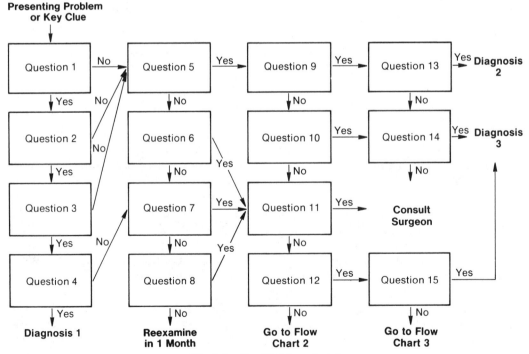

Fig. 9.4. Simplified flow chart 1.

guidance, and the problem which is unusual, they may be of value.

Computers. The various computer roles in medicine are well known. They include data storage, data retrieval, record keeping, laboratory management, complex radiographic imaging procedures, medical economics, problem solving, and decision making. We are concerned here only with those computer capabilities which enable us to solve problems. This implicates computer functions in medical information storage, patient data processing, mathematical manipulations, and artificial intelligence. It is disconcerting to note that the development and implementation of computer applications relating to clinical use and medical teaching have lagged far behind those relating to finances and office management.

Information generated by set theory, Venn diagrams, Boolean algebra, Bayes' theorems, and dendrograms of all sorts can easily be stored in the memory bank of a computer because the structure of these entities is ideal for that purpose. The question is whether or not computerized mathematical and statistical models manipulated by a machine can perform a better job than the human diagnostician. Opinions differ.

On the surface, it would seem that computers have several advantages. The computer system—with data acquisition, data display, instant recall, perfect memory, and computational powers—epitomizes the application of high technology to diagnosis. Furthermore, the increase of medical knowledge has far exceeded the capacity of human cognition (11). So why *not* get help from computers?

But there are undoubtedly roles that the computer *can't* play. It has only one sensory organ that receives electrical messages. It has only one organ of communication—video display or print-out. It cannot initiate independent thought. It cannot write its own sentence. And "it is doubtful that any electromechanical device will ever detect the subtleties of the unique interaction between the doctor and the patient, or respond to the many levels of communication that occur

in the examining room or at the bedside" (11), efforts at simulating high-level natural intelligence notwithstanding.

One thing worries me when I discuss new computer applications in medicine with medical students. They are intrigued with the prospect of obtaining complete diagnoses and treatment at the push of a button. The first question asked is not "how does it work?," but "when will it be ready for use?" I fear that many of them are merely seeking ways to avoid thinking and learning. However, some already have computer backgrounds and their questions may have nobler motivation.

On the other hand, another concern is that the medical profession has been slow to recognize the computer's potential. This is for three reasons (11). First is inertia—the reliance on previously useful but outdated methods. Second is pride and the fear of becoming useless. Third is the lack of faculty leadership in achieving computer literacy among teachers and students as is being done in other professions.

Lusted (12) asks if it is possible to construct an algorithm (i.e. write a computer program) for the entire diagnostic process. He thinks not but goes on to explain that a few well-defined problem areas of medicine can be managed effectively by a computer using Bayesian concepts.

Numerous mini-programs developed over the past 10 years have proven him correct. These include microcosmic systems that work well only when operating within small task domains (13). For example, there are computer programs that provide the drug dosage needed to maintain a therapeutic drug level, given the patient's age, gender, weight, renal function, drug kinetics, etc. Other programs deal with the suggested management of acute renal failure and electrolyte disturbances in specific settings, antimicrobial therapy, diagnosis of thyroid disorders, and the management of abdominal pain. The latter program claims to be at least as accurate as a student or average clinician, but not so accurate as a superb clinician.

A computer protocol for the emergency

room management of chest pain is performing with modest success "at least as well as a physician" (14). This computer-based decision-making program is governed by nine flow chart-derived clinical factors, including age, gender, previous pains, description of pain, its radiation, presence of diaphoresis, effect of manual pressure on the chest, and specific electrocardiographic changes. Its authors suggest that the program is best used to *corroborate* the clinical impression. Such efforts stimulate questions such as "why use computers if human beings suffice?," "where *can* we use computers?," and "where *must* we use people?"

Ubiquitous acronyms describe computer programs for data storage, information access, quick consultations, cancer protocol availability, medical records for traveling patients, and so forth. Included are: GTE Minet, MUMPS, COSTAR, PROMIS, PDQ, MYCIN, CMIT, ONCOCIN, and others. These are described in any reference source on the uses of computers in medicine. But for problem solving and diagnosis, small programs such as CAMPS, a basic diagnostic drill that allegedly teaches students to solve problems, and PIP, which simulates an expert taking a history, are available. Such teaching programs need further evaluation.

As for the *entire macrocosm* of medical diagnosis, Wulff (15) sounds a more negative note. He regards the concept of an "on line" library and consultant as an intriguing vision but doubts it will ever come to be. Noting the limitations of mathematical models based on variable and sometimes incorrect facts, he adopts a pessimistic view. He accepts the computer's function in record keeping and information retrieval but is skeptical of its role in diagnosis.

On the other hand, Pauker et al (16) succeed in demonstrating methods of problem solving by computer which very closely simulate the techniques of the expert clinician. They use programming concepts which resemble the complex theories of clinical cognition. Their program makes the computer act like a human brain in that it generates hypotheses rapidly, tests them, branches, returns, and uses clusters—just like a physician. This represents a tremendous effort to produce *artificial intelligence*, a system that manipulates ideas, clues, and symptoms rather than one that merely stores data and juggles numbers. Pauker and his fellow workers feel that the entire body of medical information, composed of some two million facts and twenty million words, can be stored by a future computer of reasonable cost. They believe that technology will soon be able to cope with all of medicine, that computers know more than any physician possibly can and will be able to solve problems at least as well.

INTERNIST-I is an experimental computer-based program that acts as a diagnostic consultant for the entire field of internal medicine (17). It differs from other diagnostic programs by the size and diversity of its knowledge base. The intellectual core of this system is a huge problem-solving algorithm that operates by symbolic reasoning (artificial intelligence) rather than by strict Bayesian mathematical principles. Entered into the computer are:

1. 500 disease profiles
2. 3550 clues for diseases, which include items from the history, physical examination, laboratory, x-ray, and biopsy
3. 3400 links or interconnections between diseases
4. two bits of information attached to each clue; each bit has an evoking strength rated from 1 to 5 (1 being "rare" and 5 "essentially always"):
   a. Given a clue, how likely is the disease? (predictive value)
   b. Given a disease, how likely is the clue? (sensitivity)
5. all the disease states that can explain a given clue, again with ratings from 1 to 5 as above.

The system's performance was experimentally compared to the performance of clinicians. It scored "favorably" when compared to "average clinicians" but was inferior to "clinical experts" (17). The present consensus is that INTERNIST-I is not yet sufficiently reliable for clinical use. The specific deficiencies that must yet be overcome are: (*a*) its inability to reason temporally or anatomically; (*b*) its inability to deal with multiple problem areas; (*c*) its inability to explain its logic; and (*d*) its limited understanding of pathophysiology.

Much work remains to be done. But should this program or any other ever become successful, it would be an incomparable reference source and an invaluable problem solver. The physician's principal task would be to gather data about the patient and enter it into the system. There the data would be grouped, matched, evaluated, and cerebrated; out would come the diagnosis, treatment, request for specific additional data, and prognosis. Medical education could undergo a *technologic revolution* in that training time might be cut in half, residencies might become obsolete, and medical journals might be drastically revised.

But Camelot may not be upon us, and some healthy pessimism is to be maintained. Computer-rendered decisions are no more reliable than the information in the computer program. It is difficult to conceive of total mathematical accuracy in establishing disease profiles and writing Bayesian formulas for clues and diseases. The innumerable pieces of data entered into this or any program may vary according to source and time. What is fact today may be fancy tomorrow, and what is true in a Boston series may not correspond with results in Phoenix. Constant updating will be necessary, and combinations of disease in the same patient may be a difficult obstacle. Perhaps we are beginning to reflect *too much Bayes and not enough Osler.* In any event, final judgment must be withheld for 10 more years.

Feinstein (5) takes the middle road between the *clinician and computer.* He sees the need for mutual recognition and respect: "A clinician fears that the computer will demolish the 'art' of clinical medicine. The computer can only help remove some of the jargon, mysticism, intuitions, unverified judgments and fallacious science that are now regarded as the clinical 'art.' The computer cannot participate in the true art of medicine. It has none of the subtle sensory perception, intellectual imagination and emotional sensitivity necessary for communicating with people and giving clinical care. It has neither the capacity to design a complete plan of clinical management nor the versatility to execute the plan. There is surely nothing in clinical skill that a computer can replace with its capacities for mechanical coordination, data processing and mnemonic storage."

Twenty years of optimism that computer technology would play an important role in clinical decisions have not yet been justified. There are few if any medical situations in which computers are routinely used. At present there is no *decent* decision-making program nor *any* computer that physicians would use for solving problems on a *regular* basis. It is abundantly clear that computers will never replace physicians, and there is no well-defined monolithic diagnostic process that machines can wisely handle (18).

Conclusions

Numerous problem-solving techniques have been described and examples given. Many are practical methods used daily by the physician. Some are variations on a single theme. Others have only limited value. Most decisions and diagnoses are straightforward and simple and require only a limited number of thought processes.

For the patient whose clues cannot be quickly clustered or in whom a key clue cannot be easily found, it is best to proceed in the traditional way. Gather a complete data base, block by block. Seek out the clues, synthesize them into diagnostic possibilities, then prove your hypotheses. All the cuts of the key must fit before the lock will open. This method is lengthy and thorough, though often necessary.

But for most cases a key clue is easily identified, or the quick formation of a cluster, syndrome, or pattern is possible. Then a hypothesis is rapidly generated and proven via a branching technique. This remains the most commonly used, speediest, and most practical method of problem solving. Another common effective technique would be to form a list of possibilities for a cluster or key clue, then prove one and eliminate the others.

Set theory, Boolean algebra, and Venn diagrams help us think clearly and develop our logic but do not in themselves solve problems. Bayes' theorems are most helpful, since playing the odds, probabilities, and statistics greatly influences our selection of the most likely diagnosis. Algorithms and flow charts offer help in selected instances. Computers have yet to find and prove their rightful place.

Indeed, when it comes to problem solving the brain seems to be divided into two parts which act independently. The left hemisphere operates as a digital device which is scientific, precise, mathematical, and deals with language, logic, and analytic thought. By contrast, the right hemisphere operates more as an analog device which is involved with art, music, recognition, intuition, short-term memory, judgment, and less definable techniques. This is true schizophrenia. When both hemispheres are more fully developed and the corpus callosum makes them work in tandem, problem solving will reach its zenith.

For the moment, one hemisphere prevails: the less precise one. Who but the physician, face to face with the patient, can quantitate headache, angina, or anxiety? Who can best attach relevance to a murmur, an enlarged node, or the degree of pain?

Numbers are of no help here. No two patients are alike. Every problem has unique features which are outside the realm of what has been quantified by computer or formula. Detecting subtle patterns and balancing conflicting evidence needs human judgment. How can a statistical or mathematical approach deal intelligently with those aspects of a problem which make it unique—or with those cases which are complicated by several coexistent problems, certain features of one being inconsistent with the other?

When I asked Mr. Green how severe his headache was (before I knew he had a subdural hematoma), he said, "they're so bad, I'd be on the next plane to the Mayo Clinic if I were able." This symptom can be expressed in digital terms only if you know Mr. Green.

What machine or formula can distinguish chronic obstructive lung disease from left ventricular failure if both have the same clues and exist in the same patient? Which of the two is causing symptoms today? Which next week? The good clinician at the bedside can sometimes tell. The computer cannot!

Elstein (19) puts both sides into proper perspective: the *mathematical-psychologic* vs the *clinical* approach to problem solving. The former reaches diagnostic decisions using formulas, diagrams, statistics, probabilities, flow charts, and computers. The latter invokes bedside logic, the art of diagnosis, *clinical judgment*, and informal qualitative strategies generally employed by the clinician. Elstein gives proper weight to both techniques, recognizing that the science of mechanistic diagnosis is yet in its infancy. At the same time, he rightly urges physicians to be aware of the future potential of these newer diagnostic aids. For the moment it would seem that *"experienced competent practitioners of an art may well know more than formal theories encompass"* (19).

References

1. Elstein AS, Shulman LS, Sprafka SA: *An Analysis of Clinical Reasoning.* Cambridge, MA, Harvard University Press, 1978.
2. Kassirer JP, Gorry GA: Clinical problem solving: a behavioral analysis. *Ann Intern Med* 89:245–255, 1978.
3. Sprafka SA: In Proceedings of Symposium on Problem Solving, University of Vermont, 1981.
4. Cutler P: The formulation of a diagnosis. In Spittell JA Jr (ed): *Clinical Medicine.* Philadelphia, Harper & Row, 1982, vol 1, chap 3, pp 1–17.
5. Feinstein AR: *Clinical Judgment.* Baltimore, Williams & Wilkins, 1967.
6. Murphy EA: *The Logic of Medicine,* ed 2. Baltimore, The Johns Hopkins University Press, 1980.
7. Eddy DM, Clanton CH: The art of diagnosis: solving the clinico-pathological exercise. *N Engl J Med* 306:1263–1268, 1982.
8. Hodgkin K, Knox JDE: *Problem Centered Learning.* New York, Churchill-Livingstone, 1975.

9. Editorial: Algorithms for the clinician. *Lancet* 2:528–529, 1982.
10. Margolis CZ: Uses of clinical algorithms. *JAMA* 249:627–632, 1983.
11. Levinson D: Information, computers, and clinical practice. *JAMA* 249:607–609, 1983.
12. Lusted LB: *Introduction to Medical Decision-Making.* Springfield, IL, Charles C Thomas, 1968.
13. Blois MS: Clinical judgment and computers. *N Engl J Med* 303:192–197, 1980.
14. Goldman L, Weinberg M, Weisberg M, et al: A computer-derived protocol to aid in the diagnosis of emergency room patients with chest pain. *N Engl J Med* 307:588–596, 1982.
15. Wulff HR: *Rational Diagnosis and Treatment,* ed 2. London, Blackwell Scientific Publications, 1981.
16. Pauker SG, Gorry GA, Kassirer JP, et al: Towards the simulation of clinical cognition. *Am J Med* 60:981–986, 1976.
17. Miller RA, Pople HE Jr, Myers JD: INTERNIST-I, an experimental computer-based diagnostic consultant for general internal medicine. *N Engl J Med* 307:468–476, 1982.
18. Barnett GO: The computer and clinical judgment. *N Engl J Med* 307:493–494, 1982.
19. Elstein AS: Clinical judgment: psychological research and medical practice. *Science* 194:696–700, 1976.

Section Two

Data Management: Synthesis and Analysis

Chapter 10. From Patient to Paper

Chapter 11. From Data Base to Problem List

Chapter 12. The Case Presentation

Chapter 13. Data Resolution Skills

Section Two

Introduction

Even though we teach shortcuts in problem solving, the acquisition of a complete data base must be mastered.

Difficult complex problems often require a data base which has been obtained in an orderly, complete, traditional fashion since no shortcuts may seem feasible. Even when the problem is solved by quick methods, the complete data base must be acquired too, so that the prime problem may be confirmed and any additional problems uncovered.

Our aim in this section is to teach by example: how to transcribe an informal conversation into a formal written record; how to selectively elicit, evaluate, and process patient data; how to construct a complete data base; how to formulate and assess a problem list derived from the data base; and how to condense a complete data base into a concise case report or case presentation.

The steps by which information is derived from and about the patient, forged into an orderly record, subjected to internalized cross-examination, and then displayed for critique and peer review are what the *management of medical data* is all about. Therefore the capacities for *synthesis* and *analysis* must be added to the long list of skills needed to be a good physician.

Chapter 10—"From Patient to Paper"—takes you through the patient interview process, demonstrates the logic underlying the intelligent quest for information, and finally exemplifies the way in which all the elicited data are rearranged, reordered, and placed into format. For it is one thing to take a history and another to write it up. It is false to assume that data recording is a natural sequence of data acquisition and requires no special skill.

Also included in this chapter is a section that discusses the errors students commonly make in their relationships with patients and in written record management. The last part of the chapter demonstrates the importance of the first few minutes of the interview through the medium of five separate patients, all of whom present similarly but turn out to have different problems.

Chapter 11—"From Data Base to Problem List"—assumes that the history, physical examination, and basic laboratory data have already been obtained and written up. An introductory section in this chapter describes some graphic aids in keeping records; these tend to make data more interpretable and thereby help solve problems.

The first case presented—"Sample Data Base 1"—is most thorough, in that it includes all information derived from the history, all findings in the physical examination, and all laboratory study results. No attempt was made to eliminate unimportant and irrelevant information. The varied type styles, however, discriminate between pertinent data as opposed to "smog." Important clues are thus extracted and grouped, and a problem list is formed and assessed.

Another complete data base—"Sample Data Base 2"—is presented in the same chapter; but here the reader can select the clues which go into the creation of the problem list and do the assessment himself. He can compare his skills with those of the author by concealing the author's problem list, creating and assessing his own, then looking at the author's.

Chapter 12—"The Case Presentation"—shows the student how to miniaturize a data base for presentation on rounds or for explanation to a confrere or consultant. First, the ABC's of case presentation are explained. Then Sample Data Bases 1 and 2 from Chapter 11 are trimmed and abbreviated by eliminating the nonpertinent data from the written cases. We may assume, though, that all the deleted questions and examinations were already done as in Chapter 11.

Gradually the data base is boiled down to its most significant parts so that it becomes essentially a case presentation. Generally, the medical student writes his cases in the format of Chapter 11—the intern in the format of Chapter 12. The resident and attending physician are even more brief.

In this chapter, the third year student should learn how to present cases on rounds.

These oral presentations must resemble the succinct meaty summaries written by more advanced students (interns and residents).

Chapter 13—"Data Resolution Skills"—explores the talents needed to handle information about the patient. It consists entirely of self-evaluation exercises. Included are selective searches into special data subsets, decisions on precisely what additional information will give a high yield, and the determination of data relevance. Given an opening statement about the patient, form initial hypotheses; then select a limited number of historical, physical examination, and laboratory data that are apt to give you the diagnosis. Given a mini-case, you should be able to state the relative relevance of subsequent individual items of information.

The four chapters in this section detail the important skills required to process and manage medical data—*listen, converse, select, evaluate, relate, organize, record, condense, articulate*, and *explain*. (*P. C.*)

Chapter 10

From Patient to Paper

PAUL CUTLER, M.D.

What follows is a dialogue between patient and physician. Note the conversational quality of the interview. Also especially notice the use of open-ended questions and who does most of the talking. Observe that the physician follows no rigid format yet misses very little, tracks positive clues, goes off on tangents, and then returns to the departure point. If it seems that too many questions are sometimes asked at one time, you are correct. This is done here for the purpose of editorial brevity, but should not be done when taking a history. On occasion *an enclosed box* is inserted during the colloquy; it denotes the physician's interim thoughts and impressions.

At the conclusion of the interview, the physical examination is presented. Try to formulate a problem list based on the history and physical examination alone.

Subsequently you will note the author's version of how this case should be written up. If any information was not obtained in the original interview, this can be ascertained by inspecting the written version. Then go back to the patient and fill in the gaps. The initial problem list, assessment and plan for each problem, test results, and a final problem list follow the written history and physical examination.

A last section of this chapter portrays several short dialogues from which a chief complaint and history of present illness can be derived. Each patient has the same chief complaint, but thereafter the resemblance

ceases. The natures of the underlying illnesses differ.

Patient Interview

(The patient's statements are indented.)

Good morning, Mrs. Smith. I haven't seen you in several years. How are you?
  Well, not so good, doctor.
What's troubling you?
  Lots of things; but mainly I can't eat.
Oh?
  I seem to have lost my appetite.
Tell me more about that!
  It's been going on for 3 or 4 months. First I thought it was just my nerves. You see, I've been depressed about my daughter who just got divorced; and my son isn't making such a good living. But the appetite doesn't get better. In fact, it's gotten worse. It's an effort to eat.
Have you lost weight?
  Oh, yes, my clothes don't seem to fit anymore. My usual weight is 165 pounds, but I'm down to 145. All my life I've been overweight and now it's finally coming off.
You don't want it to?
  Yes, but not this way.
How do you feel otherwise?
  Not really good. I tire easily and have to take a nap each afternoon. You know me, doctor, I usually keep busy from morning to night. But I've been feeling too weak;

in fact, I've stopped my volunteer work at the hospital. And that's not like me.

```
1. Anorexia          depression?
2. Weight loss       cancer?
3. Weakness
```

I know, Mrs. Smith. How old are you now?
58, and I've always been so well!
Well, not really. You remember, I've treated you for several problems. And then when you lived in California you saw a doctor several times.
Oh, yes, I forgot about my blood pressure and blood sugar.
Where do these two situations stand right now?
Well, the blood sugar seems to be under good control with the two pills I take each day. As for the blood pressure, it doesn't bother me so I don't bother it!
If you remember, I started you on both medications about 10 years ago. What happened?
The doctor in California checked me and told me to continue with the blood sugar pills. He said the blood pressure was normal so I stopped the pills for that.
Do you have severe thirst or frequent urination?
No. I check my urine sugars often, and the tape is always yellow.
What about chest pains, trouble with your vision, or leg pains?
None of that, either. I wear glasses but see well. The eye doctor gave me new glasses a year ago and told me my eyes were perfect.
Any headaches, dizziness, shortness of breath, swollen legs, or palpitations?
Never!

```
1. Hypertension—control?
   no complications
2. Diabetes—good control
   no complications
```

Tell me what you do each day.
I'm up at 7 and get my husband off to work with breakfast and a packed lunch.

Eating out is so expensive these days. I pass the morning straightening up the apartment, have a bite of lunch, and then have to nap. Can you imagine that! By 4 I begin supper. Bill gets home at 5, and he's real hungry. After dinner, he helps me with the dishes and we spend the evening watching TV. Then to bed by 11.
Any other activities?
Well, it's church on Sunday. I wouldn't miss it. Our minister gives such good sermons. Occasionally, we visit friends, but I've cut down on that. I really get too tired and I'm embarrassed by not being able to eat. No more dancing, either, and I did so want to learn to rock-and-roll! Oh, well, my knitting will have to do.
Tell me about where you've lived, your education, and your family.
I've lived in Pennsylvania all my life, except for the past 7 years in California. We left and returned when my husband changed his place of employment. He works so hard, I'm worried for him too. Being a construction manager isn't easy, but he's managed to make a good living for all of us these past 35 years. I dropped out of college to marry him—it was wartime, you know. My education stopped, but I do manage to keep reading. I read lots about everything. Between reading, knitting, watching TV, the house, and the kids—that takes care of my time. I told you my children are a great concern to me. I have three. One son is 33 and can't seem to find himself or get a job. My daughter is 31, has two children, and just got a divorce. The 22-year-old fancies himself a musician, plays in local bands on Saturdays, but otherwise just hangs around the house.

```
Patient profile
   depression?
   well adjusted?
   organicity—yes
```

What about your parents, and your sisters or brothers?
My father died suddenly when I was

young. I'm told he had diabetes. Mom died at 80 of cancer—stomach, I think. I have three younger sisters and one brother. They're all well so far. Oh, yes, one sister has high blood pressure, and my brother has a touch of sugar.

Well, I see things aren't completely pleasant for you. Do you take any medications, and what about tea, coffee, alcohol, and cigarettes?

I've never smoked, drink coffee or tea several times a day, have a cocktail or two with my husband on weekends, and take no medications other than my diabetes pills. Oh, yes, I do take an occasional aspirin for knee pains, and a teaspoon of paregoric for loose bowels.

Paregoric?

Just for the past few weeks. My bowels have been a little loose from time to time, so I've taken 1 or 2 teaspoons a day.

What are your bowel movements like?

Usually I have one BM a day. The past few weeks, on certain days, I have two or three. They're slightly loose, and occasionally watery.

What color are they?

I don't notice.

Is this unusual for you?

Oh, yes. If anything, I tend to be on the constipated side. I think the diarrhea is from my nerves, too. Nerves can do anything, can't they?

Well, uh, I guess so. Any trouble swallowing?

No.

Any indigestion, heartburn, gas, belching, abdominal pain, or jaundice?

None of those. I do seem to fill up easily when I eat, but I guess that's my bad appetite.

> Recent diarrhea
>
> Paregoric
>
> Easy satiety

Do you have any other symptoms?

No. Isn't that enough?

Yes, it is. Any difficulty, pain, or frequency of urination?

No.

When did your menstrual periods stop?

They began at 12 and stopped at 50. I've had no periods since then, but I do notice a few drops of blood after intercourse.

Tell me about that.

It's only been the past 6 or 8 months. There's just a little bleeding after my husband and I have sex. It lasts a day or two. I guess my membranes are thin.

No vaginal discharge or pain?

No.

What about your chest? Do you have any cough, do you bring up any phlegm, or do you have shortness of breath?

Well, sometimes I get short of breath.

Tell me about it.

It only happens once in a while. I find I must breathe deeply and can't get enough air.

Does it come on exertion or at rest?

Funny thing! I can walk around the house, and when I felt stronger I could go up steps and go marketing, and it never bothered me. But sometimes just while sitting or watching TV I would notice it. It even made me a little lightheaded, but I found it would go away by itself in a few minutes. Lately I haven't noticed it so much.

Any trouble with your eyes, ears, nose, or mouth?

No.

Let me be more specific. Do you have spots before your eyes, difficulty with vision, inflammation or pain in the eyes, double vision, or tearing?

No. But I do wear glasses.

Is your hearing good? Do you get earaches, ringing in the ears, or discharge from the ears?

No.

How about your mouth and throat? Are your teeth OK?

They're all gone—had them extracted 5 years ago. They were all bad anyway. I wear dentures.

Any trouble with your lips, mouth, tongue, or voice?

No, except for a little hoarseness if I talk to my husband too much. He's almost deaf, you know.

Do you have any pain or stiffness in your joints?

My knees are stiff when I get up in the morning. I've had that for several years. It seems to get better when I'm up and about. Come to think of it, they're a little aching and stiff after I've watched TV for a few hours too.

---

1. Arthritis
2. Postmenopausal bleeding
3. Hyperventilation

What about your breasts? Any pain, swelling, lumps, or discharge from the nipples?

No. I used to have swollen lumpy breasts before my menstrual periods, but that doesn't happen anymore.

Is your sex life satisfactory?

I'd say "yes." We don't do it as much as we used to, but we still enjoy it. Guess we're both getting old. Do you think it causes my bleeding?

We'll have to see. Refresh me on your past health. Any serious illnesses, operations, or accidents?

No illnesses we haven't discussed. No accidents, either, thank God. But you do remember my gallbladder was removed 20 years ago for stones.

Oh, uh, yes. A few more questions and then we can begin our examination. Have you ever had allergies, wheezing, or hives?

No.

How about headaches and dizziness?

I already answered that one.

Any trouble with your skin, hair, or nails?

My hair seems to have gotten thinner in the past 10 years, but they tell me that's natural.

What about chills and fever?

Never.

You've always considered yourself to be in good health, haven't you?

Yes, until recently.

Are you very concerned about your health?

Not really. You've got to get sick sometime!

Well, let's do your physical examination now. Come with me.

The physical examination shows a well-developed, fairly well-nourished woman appearing her stated age, comfortably sitting in a chair and in no distress. Height 62 inches, weight 144 lb, T 36.5 C, BP 188/110 in both arms, R 16. On inspection she appears pale and shows some evidence of weight loss in that her skin folds are loose. No jaundice, rashes, abnormal pigmentation, venous distention, or deformities are present.

The hair is gray and slightly thinned. Her conjunctiva, tongue, and nailbeds are pale, and the palmar creases are not pink. The Chvostek sign is negative. She is edentulous, wears dentures, and has a deviated nasal septum. There are no other abnormalities noted about the head, face, eyes, ears, nose, mouth, and throat, except for the fundi which show a few tiny round punctate hemorrhages and arteriolar narrowing and tortuosity. The thyroid gland is not palpable, and the trachea is in the midline. No abnormal lymph nodes are felt in the neck or anywhere in the body.

The lungs are normal on examination; the diaphragm moves well and equally on both sides. The cardiac apex beat is 11 cm from the midsternal line in the fifth left intercostal space and occupies an area with a diameter of 3 to 4 cm; it feels forceful. An S_4 is heard over the apex. Otherwise there is nothing of note. The breasts show no abnormalities in the sitting and reclining positions. There is no tenderness, rigidity, or mass palpable in the abdomen. The liver is 12 cm on percussion from top to bottom in the right midclavicular line, but this is imprecise because of the breasts; its edge is not palpable.

Rectal examination is normal. The feces are brown and test +3 for occult blood. Speculum examination of the cervix reveals a 1-cm-wide bleeding friable area at 6 o'clock. A Pap smear is taken. Pelvic bimanual examination shows the uterus to be normal in size and position and freely movable. The adnexa are not palpable. Peripheral pulses are normal. No varicose veins are present. Both knees are slightly swollen and Heberden's nodes are noted on the hands.

Orthopaedic and neurologic examinations are normal.

Written Record—Author's Version

Mrs. Smith is a 58-year-old housewife whose history is reliable and accurate and whose chief complaint is "I can't eat" for the past 3 or 4 months.

History of Present Illness. For the past 3 to 4 months, the patient has had anorexia and 19 lb of weight loss. She also tires easily and, unlike her busy routine, has been obliged to stop volunteer hospital work and take a nap each afternoon. She thinks this may well be related to her nerves since she has been depressed about her divorced daughter and two jobless, aimless sons.

Past Medical History. She has had diabetes and hypertension for 10 years. For the diabetes she takes tolbutamide twice daily, frequent checks of her urine show no glucose, and she has no severe thirst or polyuria. She started medication for hypertension 10 years ago but was subsequently told her blood pressure was normal so she stopped. She has no symptoms attributable to hypertension or its complications, such as headache, dizziness, visual disturbance, dyspnea on exertion, swollen legs, or palpitations. She takes an occasional aspirin for headache and paregoric for loose bowels. The gallbladder was removed 20 years ago.

Patient Profile. Mrs. Smith is an intelligent, somewhat anxious and depressed woman who seems to show no more than a normal concern for her symptoms and possible illnesses. Her diabetes and hypertension hardly seem to matter. She does think a lot of her trouble is due to nerves but isn't sure. She is a sturdy, considerate, kind woman who cares for her husband and seems well adjusted, adaptable, and in control. One gets the feeling that her problems are organic in spite of anxiety and depression. She has lived in Pennsylvania all her life except for the past 7 years when she had been in California; the move was because of her husband's change in job site. He is a construction foreman who has always provided well and is now getting old and deaf.

Mrs. Smith dropped out of college to get married during wartime and although her formal education stopped she has kept busy reading, doing charity work, and watching TV. She knits, likes to dance, although she fatigues too much for that now, attends church regularly, and seems to have good psychosocial and sexual relationships with her husband. She gets to bed by 11, is up at 7, makes breakfast and lunch for her husband, naps in the afternoon, makes dinner, and she and her husband clean up together. She does not smoke, drinks two to three cups of coffee or tea daily, and has one or two cocktails with her husband on weekends.

Family History. Her father died suddenly when he was young, and he had diabetes. Her mother died at 80 of cancer, possibly of the stomach. She has three younger sisters and one brother; one sister has hypertension and her brother has diabetes.

Systems Review.
1. *General.* There have been no chills or fever and she considers herself in good health until recently.
2. *Head.* There are no headaches or dizziness.
3. *Skin, Hair, Nails.* There has been thinning of the hair for 10 years, but the nails and skin show no abnormalities.
4. *Eyes, Ears, Nose, Throat.* She wears glasses and has no spots before the eyes, visual difficulty, inflammation or eye pain, double vision, or tearing. She has good hearing and no tinnitus or aural discharge. She has no teeth and wears dentures. There are no symptoms referable to the lips, mouth, tongue, or voice. She gets a little hoarse sometimes but attributes this to her husband's deafness.
5. *Pulmonary.* She has no cough or expectoration. She gets short of breath sometimes (i.e. "can't get enough air"), but this does not occur on ex-

ertion and usually happens when she is watching TV or is at rest. It sometimes makes her lightheaded but goes away in a few minutes.

6. *Cardiovascular.* Covered under Past Medical History.
7. *Breasts.* No pain, lumps, swelling, or discharge.
8. *Allergy.* She has had no allergies, wheezing, or hives.
9. *Gastrointestinal.* Though she is usually constipated, she has had diarrhea for the past 3 weeks. This consists of two to three bowel movements a day, which are slightly loose and occasionally watery. She doesn't observe whether the stool is black or bloody. There is no dysphagia, indigestion, heartburn, gas, belching, abdominal pain, or jaundice. She does seem to have early satiety.
10. *Genitourinary.* There has been no pain, frequency, or difficulty with urination. Her menses began at age 12 and ended at 50. For the past 6 to 8 months there has been postcoital bleeding lasting a day or two each time, but no vaginal discharge or pain.
11. *Musculoskeletal.* The knees are stiff and aching on getting up in the morning and after sitting a while.

The physical examination has been detailed in the protocol. *In summary,* however, the physical examination shows a 58-year-old white woman who looks drawn and pale. The blood pressure is 188/110, and she demonstrates pallor, particularly in the palmar creases, weight loss, no teeth, a deviated nasal septum, diabetic and grade I hypertensive changes in the fundi, an enlarged heart with a diffuse, forceful apical beat, an S_4, 3+ occult blood in the stool, a cervical lesion, swollen knees, and Heberden's nodes.

Problem List.

1. Weakness, weight loss, anorexia, anemia

2. Easy satiety
3. Diarrhea
4. Hypertension
5. Left ventricular hypertrophy
6. Diabetes
7. Anxiety and depression
8. Cervical lesion
9. Hyperventilation syndrome
10. Hypertrophic osteoarthritis
11. No teeth
12. Postcholecystectomy

Assessment of Problem List (and Plan). Problem 1 consists of weakness, weight loss, anorexia, and anemia. This is the most urgent problem in this case and is the cause for her presentation to the physician. The first three symptoms could be compatible with a large variety of organic problems as well as depression. However, the presence of anemia makes one think more in terms of an organic lesion. These four clues direct your attention to a malignancy, especially in a patient this age. But the possibility of uremia, tuberculosis, or a hematologic disorder must be considered. Studies to be done would include a complete blood count to assess the degree and type of anemia, repeat stool examinations for occult blood to confirm the original finding, a chest x-ray, sigmoidoscopy, barium enema, and a gastrointestinal series. A gastrointestinal malignancy must be strongly considered in a woman this age who presents this way.

As for problems 2 and 3, these suggest that the site of her disease process is in the gastrointestinal tract and could relate to either carcinoma of the stomach or carcinoma of the colon.

Hypertension is noted by her history, blood pressure reading, and changes in the fundi. It needs treatment. Left ventricular hypertrophy is listed as a separate problem, although it is merely an extension of problem 4. It is evidenced by the enlargement of the heart, the strong apical impulse, and the fourth heart sound. She does not appear to be in left ventricular failure.

Her sixth problem, diabetes, seems to be

under good control, as shown by the history, the lack of symptoms, and the test results which she obtains. However, further evaluation necessitates repeated blood glucose determinations and urine glucose tests.

The anxiety and depression exist for obvious reasons, and these must be dealt with at some future date.

Problem 8, a cervical lesion, is probably a serious one. Postmenopausal bleeding must always be considered with gravity. The lesion that was noted could be malignant, but at this point we can only call it a cervical lesion and may label it as carcinoma of the cervix only when and if a Pap smear or biopsy is conclusive.

The hyperventilation syndrome is clearly demonstrated by the fact that she is noted to sigh and take deep breaths during the interview, by that fact that her shortness of breath occurs at rest and not particularly on exertion, and by the typical description and its association at times with dizziness and a feeling of faintness. This is caused by the respiratory alkalosis which she herself creates. Problem 10 is based on the history of joint stiffness plus the findings of swelling of the joints and Heberden's nodes.

Studies.

1. Urinalysis is normal except for 3+ albuminuria.
2. Complete blood count shows 3 million red blood cells/mm³, 6 g Hb/100 ml, white blood cells and platelets normal, and hypochromic microcytic red blood cells.
3. Stools are +2, +3, negative, +3 for occult blood.
4. Eighteen-test blood chemical profile is normal except for 136 mg of glucose/dl. The sodium, potassium, chloride, bicarbonate, urea nitrogen, protein, albumin, calcium, phosphorus, cholesterol, uric acid, creatinine, total bilirubin, alkaline phosphatase, creatine phosphokinase, lactate dehydrogenase, and glutamic-oxaloacetic transaminase are all normal.

5. Chest x-ray is normal except for mild to moderate left ventricular enlargement.
6. Pap smear of cervical lesion shows clumps of *cancer cells* (grade 5).
7. ECG shows mild left ventricular hypertrophy and strain.
8. Proctosigmoidoscopy is normal.
9. Barium enema reveals a *polypoid irregular lesion of the cecum.*
10. Upper gastrointestinal x-ray series is normal.

Final Problem List. Problems 1, 2, and 3 can now be combined into one problem—carcinoma of the cecum. Problem 8 can be elevated to a diagnostic resolution—carcinoma of the cervix. A new problem has been detected and it must be given a new number—13. Albuminuria. This may be a separate problem related to kidney disease of undisclosed origin or it may result from diabetes.

Reassessment. The ECG and chest x-ray confirm the previous impressions. It should be noted that Mrs. Smith's anemia is caused by the cecal carcinoma and not by cancer of the cervix. The amount of blood loss from the cervical lesion would be minimal in this instance. However, large quantities of blood can be lost in the stool over a long period of time and not be apparent to the patient. Her shortness of breath is not related to congestive heart failure even though she has an enlarged heart. She does not have basal rales or any other evidence of heart failure. By her own description, she has the hyperventilation syndrome.

Until recently such a patient would have immediate intestinal surgery, followed perhaps a bit later by treatment for the cervical cancer. But newer technology enables a search for metastases, which, if present, might preclude unnecessary and noncurative surgery. You would probably order a γ-glutamyltransferase, computed tomographic scans of lung and liver, and a radionuclide bone scan in order to rule out metastases before deciding on surgery. Others would not search so intensively.

Epilogue. The preceding sections of this chapter dealt with data acquisition, data synthesis, and data analysis. These are the processes a physician utilizes with each patient he sees. Fortunately, most cases are much simpler than Mrs. Smith's. But, in any event, these are the skills a student must acquire and master.

Mistakes Students Make

There is a consistency in the types of errors that many students make when they handle medical data. An instructor who teaches medical students from year to year notices the same mistakes being made by a predictable percentage of the class

The reader should carefully note the following wrongdoings and try to avoid them.

Errors revolve mainly around the style of history taking, the writing of the chief complaint and history of present illness, the use of the English language, and the formulation and assessment of the problem list. Since communicative skills are so much a part of the problem-solving process, failings to communicate by spoken or written word are also included here.

What was written in the previous sections of this chapter is what the medical student and house officer must do daily in patient workups. The errors described in the following paragraphs relate mainly to the management of the previously discussed case, though the same types of errors are probably encountered in any case. The many do's and don't's of data collection were detailed in Chapter 2. But a discussion of specific errors encountered over the past few years with students who have had to tangle with the saga of Mrs. Smith might serve as a warning beacon for future students who deal with other Mrs. Smiths.

The following problems were commonly seen in more than 1000 workups by students given the audiotaped and printed interview of Mrs. Smith. The students were asked to write the history in a traditional format, consider the physical examination results given them, and then write a problem list,

assess it, and request further diagnostic studies as needed. Each student's writeup was read and the faults and errors compiled. They follow.

Errors in the History. The chief complaint was very often too long, contained additional symptoms that rightfully belonged in the history of present illness, and the time element was frequently not mentioned.

Many faults could be found in the history of present illness. At times it was not orderly from a temporal or pathophysiologic standpoint. Too often, the reader could not determine whether the illness was constant, progressive, rapidly deteriorating, or remittent. There was a tendency to put more into the history of present illness than belonged there; for example, the concomitant diabetes, hypertension, and hyperventilation had no role in the present illness, though they were often included.

The systems review omitted many systems, and rather than describe the presence or absence of symptoms in each system, the student might use perfunctory and unacceptable terms such as "cardiovascular system normal" or "cardiovascular system negative."

Patient profiles were often rigid and too brief and did not convey a feeling of who the patient was, what she did, what she ate, how she related to her illness, and the various other items that give you the feeling that you know the patient as a person.

The past medical history at times did not suffice, for it did not elaborate on the patient's other illnesses that did not relate to the main problem. For example, if diabetes exists, we want to know for how long, how it was discovered, what was and is the treatment, whether there are any symptoms, what is the present state of control, and what complications exist. It is not enough to state that "the patient has diabetes." The same comments could be made regarding her hypertension.

Errors in Style of Writing. Incorrect spelling, punctuation, and grammar and poor sentence structure are not acceptable from graduate students. A telegraphic style using short phrases connected by dots and dashes does not belong in a medical record. Use sentences. Unknown or impromptu abbreviations are to be deplored. If abbreviations are used, make sure they are commonly understood. Your hospital may print a list of accepted abbreviations. But remember that MS can mean morphine sulfate, mitral stenosis, or multiple sclerosis.

There are other caveats for those who write patient histories. Avoid the frequent use of "patient denies, admits, complains"—the prosecuting attorney syndrome. Are you accusing the patient of something? Along these lines, do not begin almost every sentence with "the patient." Carefully consider what you write or say because the chart is subject to review by other hospital personnel, your peers, your superiors, the patient, and the patient's attorney.

And last, use scientific terminology wherever appropriate—thrombus for clot, convulsions for fits, and hypertension for high blood pressure.

Errors in the Problem List. Most serious errors lie here. Often the list is too short and omits problems which coexist. At other times, the list is too long and consists of an enumeration of all symptoms and abnormal physical signs; no serious attempt is made to cluster the clues into cohesive groups. However, the most common error lies in the inability of the student to raise the level of problems to the resolution possible with the data on hand. Often the level is too high or too low for the existing information.

The latter issue often boils down to the degree of certainty with which the student is comfortable before committing himself to a definite diagnosis. Some will not label a definite diagnosis until there is a positive biopsy or bacterial identification. Others will do so when they are *reasonably* sure. Either approach is correct, and neither can be criticized. However, while some students are aggressive in their approach, others are a bit too timid.

In the case of Mrs. Smith, on the basis of

the history and physical examination, you could only group the clues and suspect but not label the problem as being gastrointestinal cancer. Further proof is needed. Also, the cervical lesion should be labeled as such—not as vaginal bleeding or cancer. On the other hand, you could confidently list left ventricular hypertrophy as a problem on the basis of the hypertension, the diffuse displaced apex beat, and the S_4; x-ray and electrocardiographic proof are not needed. Hypertrophic osteoarthritis could be labeled simply on the basis of the history and the few physical findings—no need for x-rays.

Given a previously healthy patient with cough, expectoration, fever, chills, pleuritic chest pains, and signs of right lower lobe consolidation, you could safely state that problem 1 is lobar pneumonia. Some might prefer to wait for a chest x-ray, sputum culture, and ventilation-perfusion scan, but this would probably signify excessive caution.

There is no place for "probable" or "possible" in the problem list. These modifiers are often used when the data synthesizer lacks confidence and is uncertain. Question marks, equivocation, and differential diagnosis belong in the asssessment, not in the problem list.

Errors in Assessment and Plan. Often this portion of the record is too brief and poorly done. Yet this is where the data synthesizer-analyzer lets you know if he knows what he is talking about.

The student may not list all the clues that led him to label a problem as such. For example, if essential hypertension is listed as a problem, the facts that the blood pressure is high and the fundi are abnormal may not be mentioned. If congestive heart failure is a problem, the student may not list in his assessment that there are basal rales and an S_3.

Refer to Chapter 2 and read what an assessment and plan should include. Too frequently, the student doesn't let you know which problems are the most urgent, doesn't give a differential diagnosis for a cluster of clues, and doesn't explain the underlying pathophysiologic processes that account for the clinical picture or relate different problems.

As for the *plan*, the greatest misdemeanor is the ordering of excessive, unnecessary, and invasive diagnostic procedures coupled with the failure to order simple high-yield tests like a blood count and urinalysis. Mrs. Smith often received all types of scans but no blood count or stool study for occult blood. Arthrocentesis, arthroscopy, and x-rays were ordered for her arthritis; all she needed was a little reassurance and an occasional analgesic. Students sometimes order everything in the book rather than only what is necessary.

The First Few Minutes

It is in the initial portion of the interview that the student or physician acquires the chief complaint (CC) and history of present illness (HPI). Refer to Chapter 2 under the subhead "Two Minutes In." This is where the wheels begin to turn, where initial statements are formed, where hypotheses are initiated and where the interviewer first starts to organize his thoughts and decide what additional information he needs. This too is where the "star trek" through the universe of pathophysiology begins and the courses of illness are plotted.

The following mini-interviews are typical ones between patient and physician. *Each patient has a similar chief complaint*, but note how the history of each illness characterizes the underlying pathophysiologic process. After each short interview, the CC and HPI are written as they should be, provisional hypotheses are formed, and the additional data deemed helpful are cited.

The *reader might profit* by trying to write his own CC and HPI immediately after reading each interview and then compare it to the author's rendition. These are all examples where the problem is solved or almost solved after talking for 2 minutes. Note the line of questions determined by the initial

impressions. (*The patient's portion of the dialogue is indented.*)

Dyspnea on Exertion. Mr. Nelson is a 58-year-old accountant.

How are you, Mr. Nelson?
> Not so good, doctor. These past few weeks I've been feeling short of breath.

Short of breath?
> Yes. I get winded when I walk fast or go up a flight of steps.

Is this unusual for you?
> It sure is. I'm usually quite active, and until a month ago I was playing singles tennis. But I stopped because it was making me too short of breath. I've also noticed I tire easily at the same time. The whole thing seems to be getting worse.

In what way?
> Well, for the past few nights I've even been short of breath at night. I feel more comfortable when I sleep on three pillows, but even then I sometimes wake up and have to sit on a chair by the window to breathe better. Cough a bit during the night, too. So you can see I'm not sleeping well.

Do you smoke?
> No.

Bring up any phlegm?
> No.

Are your legs ever swollen?
> No.

Palpitations or skipped heartbeats?
> Once in a while.

Ever had chest pain or high blood pressure?
> Yes, both.

CC. Mr. Nelson is a 58-year-old accountant who complains of dyspnea on exertion for 1 month.

HPI. The patient was well until 1 month ago. Since then he has noticed progressively worsening dyspnea and fatigue on exertion. For the past few nights he has had orthopnea, cough, and difficulty in sleeping. He does not smoke and has no expectoration and no leg edema, but he does have palpitations. He has had chest pains and hypertension.

Discussion. Mr. Nelson has left ventricular failure. The cause can probably be derived by further questions about his hypertension and chest pains. Pulmonary disease is not likely to be at the root of his complaints; there are no symptoms specifically related to lung disease. Note that the course of the illness is that of gradual progression and worsening. On examination, look for hypertension, ophthalmoscopic evidence thereof, distended cervical veins, basal rales, enlarged heart with associated murmurs and gallops, enlarged liver, and leg edema. A chest x-ray and ECG should complete the picture.

Dyspnea at Rest. Mrs. Williams is a 46-year-old homemaker.

Hello, Mrs. Williams. You seem upset.
  You would be too, if you couldn't breathe.
Couldn't breathe?
  Yes, I can't catch my breath.
Tell me about it.
  I've had it for 4 days. Just can't breathe right and I feel like I'm suffocating (takes intermittent deep breaths). I get numb and giddy and feel like fainting.
When do you have it?
  On and off—all the time. Even get it watching TV, but also had it when doing my housework. I've had it for a few years, but never this bad. Usually I'm OK.
Ever had heart trouble?
  No—unless this is it.
Lung trouble?
  No.
Is it worse on walking up steps?
  Not really.
How may pillows do you sleep on?
  One.
Legs swell?
  No.
Any cough?
  No.
Cigarettes?
  Never.
Been upset lately?
  Not that I know of.
How old are you now?
  46.

What's with your husband?
  Oh, he's fine. Works regular. We're getting along well.
Your children?
  That's another story.

CC. Mrs. Williams is a 46-year-old homemaker who has had difficulty with breathing for 4 days.

HPI. The patient has been troubled by intermittent episodes of suffocation and not being able to catch her breath for a few years. During these episodes she gets numb, giddy, and feels faint. They are not particularly related to exertion and seem to be worse now. She has no history of heart or lung trouble, doesn't smoke, and has no orthopnea, leg swelling, or cough. Relations with her husband seem good, but there are problems involving her children.

Discussion. Note particularly that the "dyspnea" is not exertional. This immediately suggests a functional problem like the hyperventilation syndrome. The symptoms of respiratory alkalosis result from episodic overbreathing. Therefore the clinical picture is chronic and intermittent but not progressive. More information about the patient profile and her family problems is needed. Normal findings in the heart and lungs plus a duplication of symptoms by command hyperventilation helps prove the clinical impression. A normal chest x-ray and ECG offer further confirmation.

Sudden Dyspnea. Mrs. Green is a 36-year-old executive who is being seen in the emergency room.

What happened, Mrs. Green?
  I've been terribly short of breath for the past 2 hours. (patient visibly breathing rapidly)
Ever had this before?
  No! Never!
Do you know of any heart or lung trouble?
  No.
Have you any other symptoms?
  Yes. I have a vague heavy feeling in my chest and I feel just awful.
Any cough or chest pain?
  No. Can't you do something?

I'll try, Mrs. Green. Have you been sick lately?

No, but I was in an auto accident a month ago.

Were you hurt?

Just a little. I banged my right leg and it was swollen and achy for a week. But I think it's OK now.

CC. Mrs. Green is a 36-year-old executive who has had dyspnea and a heavy feeling over the chest for 2 hours.

HPI. This patient has been in good health. One month ago she was in an automobile accident resulting in a swollen, aching right leg for 1 week. For the past 2 hours she has had the sudden onset of severe shortness of breath associated with a vague heavy feeling in the chest.

Discussion. Sudden severe dyspnea following traumatic thrombophlebitis in an otherwise healthy young woman sounds very much like a pulmonary embolus. No further questions seem necessary. Examination should center around the vital signs, heart and lungs, and legs. The absence of edema, calf tenderness, or a Homans' sign in no way rules out deep venous thrombosis; nor does a normal heart and lung examination! The pulse and respirations should be rapid. A chest x-ray will likely be normal. The ECG may show suggestive abnormalities in up to 30% of cases. Arterial blood gases may offer some help. But the ventilation-perfusion radionuclide scan will be diagnostic with a high degree of certainty.

The fact that leg vein thrombosis preceded this acute event does not guarantee a relationship. Even though unlikely, myocardial infarction must be excluded.

Short-Duration Worsening Dyspnea. Mrs. Connors is a 52-year-old nurse.

What brings you here, Mrs. Connors?

For the past week I've been getting more and more short of breath. I hardly noticed it at first. But then after a day or two it became more definite. I found that I was getting short of breath on helping a patient to the bathroom or on going up only one flight of steps. Over the past few days it's gotten worse. I get short of breath on taking only a few steps. In fact, I think I'm even short of breath doing nothing. Like now!

Yes, you do look a little short of breath. Does anything else bother you?

No, not really. I haven't been coughing. I have no pain. And until a week ago I felt quite well. My sleep hasn't been too good the past few nights, though. Maybe I'm just worried.

Do you have any illnesses that you know of? Diabetes? Hypertension? Heart or lung disease?

None of those. I did have my left breast removed almost 2 years ago and received cobalt therapy afterwards. But my checkups since then have all been good, even the one done a month ago.

CC. Mrs. Connors is a 52-year-old nurse who complains of worsening shortness of breath for 1 week.

HPI. For 1 week she has had gradual onset, progressively worsening dyspnea, first on exertion, and more recently even at rest. There are no symptoms other than difficulty in sleeping for the past few nights. The left breast was removed 2 years ago; cobalt therapy followed. She says her checkups for cancer since then have been satisfactory.

Discussion. You are strongly tempted to relate the breast cancer to her dyspnea and you are probably correct. Pleural effusion resulting from metastasis is very likely. Note the subacute and rapidly progressive dyspnea. At first Mrs. Connors could hardly notice it. Then it clearly got worse and progressed from dyspnea on exertion to dyspnea on slight exertion to dyspnea even at rest.

A large pleural effusion is likely. This should be easily discernible on physical examination. It is likely to be on the left side (but not necessarily). There should be flatness, absent breath sounds, and absent fremitus, with a possible tracheal shift to the other side. The chest x-ray should be conclusive, as should a pleural aspiration for tumor cell study. If the chest x-ray is normal, look elsewhere for the cause of dyspnea. Cardiac dyspnea would not be so rapidly progressive, nor would it be likely to occur in an otherwise healthy person. However, she could be another Mrs. Green.

Dyspnea and Cough. Mr. Jones is a 64-year-old carpenter.

What brings you here, Mr. Jones?
   This cough of mine's getting lots worse, and I've been short of breath.
Tell me about it.
   Well, you known this little chest problem I've had for years—cough and phlegm—it's getting me down. The past few days it's been so bad I've coughed up some blood.
Blood?
   Yes. My sputum is usually greenish-gray, but I've noticed a few specks of blood recently. Yesterday I coughed up a spoonful.
What have you done about your smoking?
   Haven't been able to stop that, Doc. Still smoke two or three packs a day. Been doing it these past 50 years, you know.
Refresh me on your cough. How long have you had it?
   For at least 20 years. Didn't bother me too much though—mostly in the morning and just after I light up. Phlegm has been about the same except when I had those attacks of acute bronchitis you treated me for. Oh, yes, I have noticed some shortness of breath the past year or two when I move a little too fast, but I blamed that on my weight. Never coughed any blood, though.
How have you felt generally? You don't look like you've gained weight.
   Not really good. Appetite has been off the past few months. Lost about 15 or 20 pounds. I seem to tire easily, too.

CC. Mr. Jones is a 64-year-old carpenter who complains of chronic worsening cough, dyspnea on exertion, and recent hemoptysis.

HPI. For 20 years he has had a chronic cough with greenish-gray expectoration in the morning and on lighting up; this has transitorily worsened during several attacks of acute bronchitis. For the past year or two there has been some dyspnea on exertion which the patient blames on his weight. Over the past few months, Mr. Jones has lost 15 to 20 pounds, and he has had anorexia and easy fatigability. The cough has worsened in the past few days, and he has noticed flecks and once a teaspoonful of blood in the sputum. He has smoked two to three packs of cigarettes daily for 50 years.

Discussion. The sequence of events and the course of the illness point toward severe chronic obstructive pulmonary disease with a strong possibility of superimposed lung cancer. The HPI tells the whole story—a +4 cigarette habit, years of cough with expectoration, subsequent dyspnea, more recently a downhill course terminating in severe coughing and hemoptysis. You can almost see the hilar mass, the hyperaerated lungs, the coarse bronchial markings, and the low diaphragms without taking a chest x-ray.

Your examination of the neck and chest will be thorough. Search for clubbing, Virchow's node, tracheal shift, localized wheeze, or other pulmonary abnormalities. The chest x-ray should be conclusive. Cancer is not a certainty, and you may wind up with only chronic obstructive pulmonary disease, bronchiectasis, or even tuberculosis. But our bets are on the initial impression. Sputum studies and fiberoptic bronchoscopy may provide the decisive clue.

Aphorism. The following truth is now self-evident: Two minutes of meaningful conversation direct you to the correct diagnosis nine times out of ten.

Chapter 11

From Data Base to Problem List

PAUL CUTLER, M.D.

Some Aids First

Refer to the introduction to Section Two where the purposes of Chapter 11 are given. The aim is to provide the reader with further assistance in writing the data base and in making the transition to problem list, assessment, and plan.

Two detailed patients will be presented. These presentations include the orderly written data base, problem list, assessment, and plan. By following the boxed instructions preceding each case, you should become more adept at doing patient workups.

While the collection of data, the processing of data, and the formation of problem lists were discussed in Chapter 2 (and should now be reviewed), the nuts and bolts of actually performing these operations on particular patients follow.

First, it might be a good idea to clarify and point out a few more items.

The exact written format for a history and physical examination should be noted. This is not the Webster's unabridged format. The "correct" format may vary from one reference source to another, and it may vary according to the professional person's preference.

Fortunately, most cases are not so complicated as those that follow, and they require less writing and less thought. Also be aware that you may first see some patients after they have already been in the hospital for several or more days. In doing such a workup, you must be clear about what transpired prior to and since the hospital admission. This warrants the inclusion of the hospital course in the writeup. Outpatients and hospital patients must be similarly managed, though outpatients are usually less polypathic and less effort is required in studying them.

In recording data referable to the physical examination, several aids should be mentioned. Sketches of the eye, neck, chest, or abdomen are often helpful. It is easy to diagram an ocular or fundal abnormality, an area of suspected disease in the chest, the location and extent of a breast mass, the outline of the liver or spleen, or an abdominal mass. To paraphrase the Chinese proverb, a drawing is better than many sentences.

Many students never do learn how to describe abnormalities of the *chest examination*. This is best done by a simple initial sentence that describes the contour, symmetry, respiratory rate, expansion, diaphragmatic excursion, and tracheal position. The next sentence should mention the abnormalities of fremitus, percussion, and auscultation on a *regional* rather than an *procedural* basis whenever possible.

Suppose you see a patient with right lower lobe pneumonia. The description of the chest findings would probably be as follows: "The chest contour is normal and symmetrical, the trachea is in the midline, the left hemidiaphragm moves well but the right is not measurable, the right hemithorax has a slight lag, and there are 24 respirations/ minute. Increased tactile and vocal fremitus, dullness, bronchial breath sounds, egophony, whispered pectoriloquy, and numerous fine moist end-inspiratory rales are noted over the right lower lobe (posteriorly)."

Sometimes the findings cannot be so neatly described and you must resort to a procedural basis of inspection, palpation, percussion, and auscultation—mentioning the abnormalities wherever they are noted with each modality of examination.

Descriptions of physical findings must be complete. It is not enough to say that a patient has a systolic murmur. You must include the shape, duration, pitch, timing, location, intensity, and radiation.

Last, in recording or describing a patient's hospital course, *flow charts* can be of great value. Take the patient who is admitted in diabetic ketoacidosis. Numerous laboratory tests are done daily. A chart that clearly depicts the blood glucose, urine glucose and acetone, blood gases, electrolytes, urea nitrogen, fluid intake and output, insulin doses, etc—all tabulated according to date and times of day—is much more comprehensible than a recitation of chemistries found on each day. Trends can be easily noted.

Sample Data Base 1

Information relevant to the formation of this patient's problem list is *italicized*. Read the history, physical examination, baseline studies, problem list, assessment, and plan. Note carefully how the italicized data are incorporated into the assessment of the problem list.

History

Identification Data. Mr. Calvin Travis, 715 Jefferson Drive, Lockwood, MO, telephone 655-6322, is a 58-year-old white man.

Information. History is obtained from the patient who is mentally clear and a good historian. His responses seem accurate, reliable, and complete.

Chief Complaint. *"Shortness of breath and smothering feelings for the past 10 nights."*

Patient Profile. The patient was born in Lockwood, MO, and has lived here all his life. Other than a 5-year period starting in 1940 when he served in the Army, first in North Africa and then in Italy, he has remained in this area (except for short vacation trips). He is married, completed a high school education, and is the owner and operator of a cigar and tobacco shop. His hobbies are reading and playing poker.

He has been following the general guidelines of an 1800-calorie *American Diabetic Association diet* for the past 17 years. He has smoked one to two packs of cigarettes daily (inhales the smoke) since he was 16 years old. Except for an occasional beer, he does not drink alcoholic beverages. He has one cup of black coffee every morning with breakfast.

Present Illness. During the past *6 months*, the patient has been unable to walk even short distances because he becomes *easily "winded" and tired*. He felt that the entire situation was due to "too many cigarettes" and "old age." For 10 nights prior to admission, he suffered an increasing number of *paroxysms of coughing*, awakening him from sleep. There was an associated feeling of *breathlessness and "smothering" necessitating that he sit upright in bed* for 20 to 30 minutes before obtaining relief. He learned that he could decrease the frequency of these episodes by sleeping in a sitting position *propped up in bed on three to four pillows.* There has been no hemoptysis, fever, or palpitations. While he has had an annoying *morning cough* with some white mucoid *expectoration for 5 to 10 years*, it has been much *worse during the past 6 months.* The sputum has not changed color.

It is noteworthy that *6 years ago* the patient was hospitalized with severe chest pain, and a diagnosis of *acute myocardial infarction* was made. He recovered without complications and gradually returned to normal activities. About *2 years ago,* however, he began experiencing occasional *episodes of retrosternal "squeezing" pain* which usually *radiated* into the *neck* and the *left shoulder* and were associated with a deep aching along the *medial aspect of the left arm down to the wrist.* The attacks almost invariably appeared *during physical exertion* and were relieved in a minute or two with rest. The last episode occurred 3 weeks prior to admission and was similar to the others.

Past Medical History. The patient considers himself to have been in the best of health, despite the history of myocardial infarction and occasional chest pain with exertion, until 6 months ago, when his "wind started giving out."

Previous Examinations. Army physical examinations for enlistment in 1940 and for separation in 1945 revealed no significant abnormalities. During a population *screening survey in 1960*, he was found to have *sugar in his urine.* He was subsequently evaluated by a physician (patient does not recall his name) who ordered a glucose tolerance test. After this procedure, the physician told him he had *"mild adult diabetes"* and started him on an 1800-calorie American Diabetic Association *diet.*

Hospitalization. In June 1971 he was admitted to Lockwood General Hospital, Lockwood, MO, with acute myocardial infarction (see "Present Illness"). There have been no other hospitalizations.

Past Illnesses and Injuries. In childhood (preschool age), the patient suffered mumps, whooping cough, and measles, from which he recovered without complications or sequelae. He does not recall having chickenpox. At age 14 he sustained a fracture of the right forearm which was treated with closed reduction. He made complete recovery without residual deformity or limitation of motion. In 1960, he was found to have "adult-onset" diabetes (see "Previous Examinations"). He lost approximately 10 lb and has remained stable since following the diet. In 1971, while hospitalized for acute myocardial infarction, his blood sugars were in the "high normal" range. The status of his diabetes has not been checked since then.

Drug Reactions. None.
Medications. None
Systems Review.

1. *General Health.* Except for present illness, patient's health has always been good and he has been relatively asymptomatic during his lifetime.

2. *Skin, Nails, and Hair.* No changes in pigmentation or texture of skin. There has been no eruption, pruritus, easy bruising, bleeding, hair loss, or nail change.

3. *Head.* Patient has occasional mild nonthrobbing temporal or frontal headaches about five or six times a year, readily relieved by aspirin. There have been no episodes of lightheadedness and no history of head trauma.

4. *Eyes.* At age 45 he began wearing bifocal lenses for "astigmatism." His most recent evaluation 2 years ago led to a change in his correction. He has no problems with visual acuity when he wears his glasses. There has never been blindness, diplopia, scotomata, flashes of light, halos around lights, photophobia, excessive tearing, or pain centered in the eyes.

5. *Ears.* No suggestion of deafness. No pain or vertigo. Occasional transient short-lasting episodes of high-pitched tinnitus in either ear.

6. *Nose, Throat, Mouth, and Teeth.* There has never been chronic nasal drainage or obstruction, recurrent epistaxis, or hoarseness. Except for a few carious teeth that have been filled, dental history is negative.

7. *Pulmonary.* (See "Present Illness.")

8. *Cardiovascular.* (See "Present Illness.") There is no history of hypertension having been detected or any history suggestive of rheumatic fever. There has been no intermittent claudication.

9. *Breasts.* No lumps, pain, or discharge from nipples.

10. *Allergic.* No history of "hay fever," urticaria, or eczema. No wheezing or dyspnea except as noted in present illness.

11. *Gastrointestinal.* Occasional episodes of "heartburn" and epigastric discomfort (distinctly different from retrosternal pain of

present illness) following eating of spicy food. These symptoms occur once or twice a month and are readily relieved by Tums. No difficulty in swallowing; no regurgitation, nausea, vomiting, hematemesis, or tarry, bloody, or clay-colored stools. Patient recalls slight jaundice of skin, yellow "eyeballs," anorexia, and dark urine that stained his shorts brown in 1942 while serving with the Army in North Africa. He did not seek or receive medical attention for these complaints, and the entire picture cleared within 10 to 14 days; there has been no recurrence. He had had no abdominal cramping, colic, diarrhea, or other changes in bowel habits.

12. *Endocrine.* Patient was found to have diabetes in 1960 (see "Past Medical History"). There *has never been any polyphagia, polyuria, polydipsia, or excessive weight loss.* There has been no change in hat or shoe size for the past 30 years. The patient has no goiter, intolerance to either heat or cold, changes in secondary sex characteristics, or any diminution of libido.

13. *Genitourinary.* He has no dysuria, frequency, urgency, incontinence, oliguria, polyuria, nocturia, hematuria, urethral discharge, burning on urination, passage of stones, or venereal disease.

14. *Musculoskeletal.* Fracture of right arm at age 14 (see "Past Medical History"). Otherwise, no trauma, weakness, or joint symptoms.

15. *Lymph Nodes.* No history of enlargement or inflammation.

16. *Nervous System.* No history suggestive of cranial nerve involvement. He has never noted any motor weakness, paralysis, incoordination, or sensory symptoms. At age 12 he was "knocked out" for a moment or two after falling off a horse but recovered quickly. There were no residual effects. He has never suffered fainting spells or seizures.

17. *Psychiatric.* The patient has no moodiness, depression, or anxiety. There was nothing in the patient's responses to suggest obsessions, delusions, illusions, or hallucinations.

Family History. His *father died at 62* of a *"heart attack."* His *mother*, 79, suffers with

Parkinsonism and *diabetes* which is controlled by diet and oral medications. One brother, 52, and one sister, 48, are both living and well. His wife is 54 and well. One son, 30, has "mild high blood pressure." There is no history of bleeding disorders, anemia, epilepsy, allergy, gout, cancer, or mental illness.

Physical Examination

1. *General Appearance and Inspection.* The patient is a *mesomorphic*, slightly *obese*, white male who appears to be somewhat older than his stated age of 58. He is moderately *dyspneic sitting up* in bed, but not cyanotic. He is alert, intelligent, cooperative, and speaks clearly and coherently. There is no evidence of pallor, jaundice, abnormal pigmentation, rashes, petechiae, ecchymoses, or angiomata. No venous distentions or deformities are noted.

2. *Vital Signs.* He is 68 inches tall and weights 187 lb. Temperature measured rectally is 37.6 C. The *pulse* is regular, full, and equal on both sides; the rate is *116/minute.* Respiratory rate is 24/minute with regular rhythm. *Inspiration is deep and expiration seems longer than inspiration.* Blood pressure with the patient sitting upright in bed is 128/80/72 in the right arm and 120/80/74 in the left.

3. *Head and Face.* The head is symmetrical, of normal size and shape, and without exostoses, masses, deformities, defects, or signs of injury. There are no bruits. The scalp is normal with no evidence of inflammation. The hair is black with slight graying and is of normal consistency, texture, and distribution. There is no enlargement or tenderness of the parotid glands.

4. *Eyes.* There is no exophthalmos, enophthalmos, strabismus, or nystagmus. The extraocular muscles function normally. Both visual acuity and visual fields are normal bilaterally by gross testing. The conjunctivae and sclerae are normal in color, they are not icteric or injected, and there are no petechiae. The lacrimal sacs and punctae are normal, and there is no discharge or

excessive lacrimation. The eyelids are not edematous or inflamed and there is no ptosis, lid-lag, or edema. The corneae are clear bilaterally and there is no scarring, ulceration, or vascularization. The pupils are round, equal in size, and react equally well to light and accommodation. The consensual reflex is present and equal bilaterally. The anterior chambers and vitreous are clear. Ophthalmoscopic examination reveals normal retinas without evidence of hemorrhages, exudates, detachment, unusual pigmentation, or neoplasms. The arterioles are slight narrowed and there is occasional arteriovenous nicking. The optic discs have distinct borders and are not atrophied or edematous. The maculae are normal bilaterally. The ocular tension is equal bilaterally and of normal degree as determined by finger palpation, though tonometry was not done.

5. *Ears.* There is no mastoid tenderness and no tophi are present. The external canals are clear and normal bilaterally. The tympanic membranes are intact without evidence of inflammation. Auditory acuity is grossly normal (watch ticking heard 20 cm away bilaterally), and both air and bone conduction are normal by the Weber and Rinne tests.

6. *Nose.* The nares are open and equal in size. The mucous membrane appears normal and is not edematous or inflamed. There is no discharge or blood. The septum is deviated slightly to the right but there is no obstruction of the passageways. No ulcerations, neoplasms, or perforations are present.

7. *Mouth and Throat.* The lips show no pallor or cyanosis and there are no fissures or ulcerations. The tongue is normal in size and is "geographic," but it shows no ulcerations, mass, or atrophy. The gums are completely normal and, except for a few minor caries, the teeth are in excellent condition. The tonsils are atrophic. There are no ulcerations, growths, exudates, or inflammations in the buccal cavity, palate, or throat. Vocal cord examination was deferred in view of the patient's dyspnea and discomfort.

8. *Neck.* The neck is supple and there is no tenderness or limitation of motion. There are no masses. The *neck veins* are distended *4 cm above the clavicles* bilaterally with the patient sitting up at about 45°. No pulsations are perceptible. The carotid arteries are palpable and equal bilaterally and there are no associated thrills or bruits. The trachea is in the midline. The thyroid gland is symmetrical and firm, but it is not hard, nodular, tender, or enlarged. The submaxillary glands are not enlarged or tender.

9. *Lymph Nodes.* There is no enlargement or tenderness of any of the lymph nodes in the neck, axillae, or groins.

10. *Chest and Lungs.* The chest is symmetrical and moves with no respiratory lag. The anteroposterior diameter appears to be slightly enlarged, and there are no deformities. *Respirations are slightly labored and rapid, and expiration is prolonged.* Vocal fremitus is equal and normal bilaterally. The percussion note over the entire chest is resonant to slightly hyperresonant. There is no dullness (except for the cardiac area) and no flatness. *The diaphragms move slightly* (1 cm on the right and 2 cm on the left) with deep inspiration. Breath sounds are vesicular. There are a few transient *inspiratory and expiratory wheezes all over the chest* and *fine late inspiratory rales in both lower lung fields* posteriorly and in the axillae. Tactile fremitus is normal.

11. *Heart.* Upon inspection, a definite *apical impulse* is visible in the *fifth and sixth left intercostal spaces at the anterior axillary line.* There are no palpable thrills, but a *diffuse forceful apical impulse* is easily palpable in the area discribed. Also present is a distinct *double apical impulse, the first one being of greater intensity, followed closely by a more subtle one.* The *cardiac border* is definitely *shifted to the left* as determined by percussion. Dullness is present to the left anterior axillary line in the fifth and sixth left intercostal spaces and to a point halfway between the midclavicular and anterior axillary line in the fourth left intercostal space. The cardiac rhythm is primarily regular but a *premature beat* followed by a compensatory pause is occasionally heard. The rate is 116/minute. The second heart sound is

physiologically split and the *pulmonic component is slightly louder than the aortic. A medium-pitched grade 2/6 ejection murmur is heard across the base of the heart*. It does not radiate into the neck, back, or axilla. At the apex, a distinct low-pitched sound is heard in early diastole with the bell of the stethoscope; it is thought to be a *third heart sound*. No ejection sound, opening snap, or fourth heart sound is present.

12. *Breasts*. Normal male, symmetrical breasts with no masses and no discharge from the nipples.

13. *Abdomen*. There is no superficial vein distention or umbilical hernia. The abdomen is soft, flat, and not tender. There is no organomegaly and no masses are palpable. There is no tympany to percussion and no shifting dullness or fluid wave. No pulsations are felt and no bruits are heard. Peristaltic sounds are present and normal.

14. *Genitalia*. Normal circumcised male. No urethral discharge. There are no herniae, tenderness, or masses. The left testicle is atrophic and soft.

15. *Rectum*. Small nonthrombosed, non-tender *external hemorrhoids* are noted at 6 o'clock. There are no fissures. There is good sphincter tone with no tenderness or masses. Stool on the examining glove is brown and negative for occult blood. The prostate gland is slightly and diffusely enlarged. It is firm but not hard, not tender, and not nodular. No masses are present.

16. *Extremities*. There are no deformities. The nails are normal in color and consistency. The radial, ulnar, femoral, popliteal, and posterior tibial pulses are of good intensity and equal bilaterally. *The left dorsalis pedis pulsation is absent*, though the right is present (3+). There are no significant color or skin changes, no varicosities, and no edema.

Baseline Laboratory Data

1. Hematocrit 45%, hemoglobin 15 g/dl; red blood cell count 5 million/mm^3, white blood count 5700/mm^3 with 72% neutrophils and 28% lymphocytes.

2. Urinalysis: specific gravity 1.021, *glucose 1+, albumin 3+*; microscopy shows no cells or casts.

3. *Glucose 175 mg/dl*; urea nitrogen 21 mg/dl; creatinine 1.1 mg/dl; sodium 142 mEq/liter; potassium 4.0 mEq/liter; chloride 100 mEq/liter.

4. *ECG: old inferior myocardial infarction, left ventricular hypertrophy.*

5. *X-ray chest: moderately severe cardiomegaly; markedly increased bronchovascular markings both bases, particularly on right side, basal pulmonary congestion, and low diaphragms.*

Problem List

1. Atherosclerotic heart disease with old myocardial infarction.
2. Angina pectoris secondary to diagnosis 1.
3. Left ventricular failure secondary to diagnosis 1.
4. Diabetes mellitus, adult onset.
5. Chronic obstructive pulmonary disease.
6. Peripheral vascular disease, left foot.
7. External hemorrhoids.
8. Albuminuria.

Assessment and Plan for Each Problem

1. This is clearly established on the basis of the history and ECG. No further studies are indicated.

2. The history over the past 2 years is typical for angina pectoris. He probably has multivessel disease, and one or two coronary arteries have become sufficiently narrowed to cause further ischemia. It seems fairly stable, needs no urgent attention, and may even improve if problems 3 and 5 can be treated and improved. If not, drug therapy or angiographic study may be in order later.

3. This is the principal problem needing attention at the moment. It is clearly documented by the 6-month history of dyspnea and fatigue on exertion, recent orthopnea and night cough, and the physical findings that go with failure. These include the enlarged heart, loud P_2, S_3, fine rales, chest x-ray, and ECG. Mild distention of the neck veins indicates that right ventricular failure is just beginning. The basal ejection murmur

may be related to disease or dilatation in and around the aortic valve and is not a cause of the main heart problem. No further studies are indicated. Treatment with rest, salt restriction, digitalis, and diuretics should start promptly.

4. Detection in the past, reconfirmed borderline glucoses, the 175-mg value on admission, and glycosuria indicate that mild adult-onset diabetes is present. A few additional glucose determinations and the urines checked four times daily will show if dietary treatment alone is sufficient.

5. This has been listed as a separate problem because of the history of excessive smoking, the chronic cough and expectoration, prolonged expiration, wheezes, and relatively immobile low diaphragms. The wheezes could be from the failure alone. Blood gases should be done now and after recovery from failure; pulmonary function tests should be done later too. Cigarettes should be stopped and additional bronchodilator medication may be needed later.

6. Peripheral vascular disease is listed because of the absent dorsalis pedis pulse in one foot and the history of diabetes. No symptoms exist so far and no further studies or treatment are indicated.

7. Asymptomatic external hemorrhoids are listed as a problem only because their presence should be kept in mind. Bed rest, change in diet, and medications may all cause constipation and make the hemorrhoids troublesome later on.

8. Albuminuria is an abnormal chemical finding which is not explained by any of the above problems. It should be rechecked. Heart failure is not the cause, since only overt right ventricular failure will cause it. It probably results from diabetic glomerulosclerosis. No action is indicated.

Comment. Other positive aspects of the history are not deemed worthy of inclusion in the present problem list. He had a fracture as a youngster (fell off a horse and had transitory unconsciousness) and had hepatitis while in the Army years ago. There are no sequelae or evidence of liver disease or brain damage.

Other positive historical events—such as the wearing of bifocals, rare tinnitus, a few caries, occasional indigestion, and headaches—are within the normal limits of occurrence and are not considered to be problems.

The family history of coronary disease and diabetes is, however, quite significant. His son's high blood pressure does not appear to have relevance.

Minimal fundi abnormalities, mild prostatic hypertrophy, slight increase in the anteroposterior diameter of the chest, and slight hyperresonance of the chest could all be significantly abnormal findings, especially in view of some of the problems. But the findings are only slightly or questionably abnormal, so they were not included in the assessment.

Sample Data Base 2

> *Reader:* Do not look at problem list or assessment until you have formed your own. This represents an excellent and profitable exercise only if the reader does as requested. *You learn to do only by doing it yourself.* Sample Data Base 1 showed you how the author does it. Now try your hand.

History

Identification Data. Mrs. William Hayes, 8139 Treasure Drive, Apt. 239, San Antonio, TX, telephone 828-5094, is a 62-year-old white woman.

Information. The patient has given the entire history and she has a good memory; the information obtained seems reliable and accurate.

Chief Complaint. Pain, swelling, and stiffness of both knees for 8 years, much worse in the past week.

Patient Profile. Mrs. Hayes was born and has lived in San Antonio all her life. She visited Houston and Dallas on several occasions, and visited Mexico once with her parents as a child. Otherwise she has traveled nowhere. Prior to marriage she was a secretary but has been a housewife since then. She lives alone in a small apartment, her husband having died 2 years ago. Financial support is derived from Social Security and her son. She has one son and three daughters, aged 40, 37, 36, and 30, respectively, and all live in different distant cities. Her education ended on completion of high school. She does not smoke or drink alcohol, but does drink three to four cups of coffee in the evening while watching television. Most of her day is spent in tidying the apartment, reading, and reminiscing. Occasionally a friend visits her. She eats at least three meals a day and consumes plenty of meat, vegetables, fruit, cereals, pastries, and bread. Chili and spaghetti are her favorite foods.

Present Illness. For 10 years she has noticed deformities of the finger joints in both hands, though they are rarely painful. She is, however, conscious of her "ugly hands." Over the past 8 years she has had difficulty with both knees. They have gradually gotten stiff, somewhat swollen, deformed, and painful. The right knee gives her more trouble than the left. On awakening or getting out of a chair the stiffness is worse, but it seems to improve after a few minutes of activity. However, when she is on her feet for any appreciable period of time, the knees start to hurt again and she is obliged to rest. At times one or the other knee becomes more swollen, painful, and slightly warm. She has consulted several physicians in the past 8 years, had x-rays and blood tests, and was told she had an old-age "wear-and-tear" type of arthritis for which very little could be done. For the past week the knees have been particularly painful and yesterday she noted slight warmth and tenderness of the right one. This brought her to the physician again.

Past Medical History. In spite of having had a number of other illnesses in the past, the patient considers herself to be in reasonably good health now except for her arthritis. She has not had a complete physical examination in several years. She has been examined many times for various other problems and has had six previous hospitaliza-

tions, four for the delivery of children. As an 18-year-old girl, she was hospitalized for 6 months for pulmonary tuberculosis and was discharged "cured."

From the time of her second pregnancy she has been troubled by gradually worsening varicose veins in both legs. In fact, 8 years ago, 4 days after a cholecystectomy for stones, she had an episode of thrombophlebitis of the left leg; the leg was swollen and warm but got better on bed rest. Occasionally the leg still swells.

She has been obese for many years, but has gained an additional 20 lb since the death of her husband. She blames this on being depressed, having nothing to do, and eating more, especially in the evenings.

There have been no injuries and her six hospitalizations have been described. She has no drug allergies or sensitivities that she knows of, and she takes no medication except an occasional aspirin for her knees.

Systems Review.

1. *General Health.* She feels healthy except for her arthritis and depression.

2. *Skin, Nails, and Hair.* Patient has noticed dryness of the hair and skin in the past few years. Much of her hair has fallen out and she attributes this to old age. No pigmentation or easy bruising has been noticed.

3. *Head.* She has no headaches, dizziness, or history of head injury.

4. *Eyes.* She has worn glasses for 15 years and gets them changed every 2 to 4 years. She can read well, has no visual difficulties, spots before the eyes, double vision, or flashes of light. On several occasions over the years, she has had redness, discomfort, and tearing of both eyes, which cleared in a few days with eye drops.

5. *Ears.* Hearing is "normal," and there has never been ear pain, running ears, or ringing in the ears.

6. *Nose, Throat, Mouth, and Teeth.* She wears dentures because all her teeth were extracted 6 years ago "to cure her arthritis." There are no nosebleeds, nasal obstruction, or postnasal drip. She thinks she may have noticed a slight coarsening and hoarseness

of her voice in the past few years but is not sure of this since she is alone a lot and does not talk much.

7. *Pulmonary.* There is no cough, expectoration, hemoptysis, dyspnea, or wheezing. Cough was present many years ago when she had active tuberculosis.

8. *Cardiovascular.* She has never had chest pains, dyspnea on exertion, or orthopnea. Occasionally she gets a transitory flutter in her chest. The left leg sometimes swells but not the right.

9. *Breasts.* No lumps, pain, discharge, or nipple retraction.

10. *Allergic.* No history of asthma, hay fever, eczema, or hives.

11. *Gastrointestinal.* There is no difficulty in swallowing, the appetite is good; she has occasional heartburn for which she takes Alka-Seltzer but has no other form of indigestion or abdominal pain. For many years she has had recurrent periods of constipation which seem to clear spontaneously. There is no blood noted in the stool, the stools are not black, and she does not have cramping.

12. *Endocrine.* There is no history of diabetes and the patient has polyphagia but no polyuria or thirst. She feels equally comfortable in summer and winter and stopped having menstrual periods at the age of 44. She has no interest in men and is reluctant to discuss libido.

13. *Genitourinary.* Occasionally there are brief periods of dysuria and urgency but no frequency or burning on urination. On coughing or straining, she loses some urine from her bladder, wetting her undergarments. At times she notices a protrusion from her vagina, especially when straining to have a bowel movement.

14. *Musculoskeletal and Extremities.* Veins, phlebitis, and arthritis were already discussed. She has no other aches or pains anywhere.

15. *Lymph Nodes.* None ever noticed.

16. *Nervous System.* No symptoms to suggest cranial nerve involvement, sensory or motor loss, or lack of coordination. There are no seizures or fits or fainting spells.

17. *Psychiatric.* She has been very depressed since her husband's death, though she always was a "moody person." She sleeps poorly, awakens four or five times per night, feels she has nothing to live for, and is extremely lonely. However, there are no hallucinations, delusions, or obsessions. She has a few female friends her age who occasionally visit and then she feels better. Suicide has not entered her mind.

Family History. Her father died at 42 of pulmonary tuberculosis. He was ill for several years before being hospitalized. Her mother died at 73 of a "heart condition." She has one brother in California from whom she has not heard in 15 years. As far as she knows, all her children are well. There are no familial disorders, such as high blood pressure, anemia, bleeding disorders, epilepsy, allergy, gout, or mental illness. She thinks her mother's heart condition may be familial, since two uncles also died of heart disease.

Physical Examination

1. *General Appearance and Inspection.* The patient is markedly obese, is sitting up in bed, and does not appear to be in any acute or chronic distress. She is alert, intelligent, cooperative, and gives a lucid history. There is no evidence of rashes, pallor, jaundice, plethora, or cyanosis. Distended tortuous veins are noted on both lower extremities, and the left leg appears swollen and edematous. Her face has coarse features but there is no clear-cut evidence of an endocrine facies. She appears her stated age.

2. *Vital Signs.* Height 64 inches, weight 205 lb, BP 136/84 (both arms), R 12, P 56, T 36.2 C. The pulse is full, regular, and equal in both arms. Respirations are regular and duration of inspiration equals duration of expiration.

3. *Head and Face.* The head has a normal contour and has no deformities, lumps, or bumps. No bruits are heard over the eyeballs. The scalp appears normal but the hair is a bit coarse, thinned, and mostly gray.

4. *Eyes.* The eyes are symmetrical and do not protrude; the eyebrows are as sparse as the hair. Extraocular motions are normal

and there is no nystagmus. Gross testing shows normal visual fields and normal visual acuity with glasses. The pupils are round, equal, and react well to light, accommodation, and consensual reflex. The lacrimal apparatus looks normal, there is no tearing, and the lids, conjunctiva, and sclera are also normal. Ophthalmoscopy reveals clear vitreous with normal discs and blood vessels and no hemorrhages or exudates. Ocular tension is normal by tonometry.

5. *Ears.* Both pinnae and external auditory canals are normal. The eardrums are grayish-pink and not inflamed. Gross tests for auditory acuity are normal in both ears. Weber and Rinne tests were therefore not done. No tophi are noted.

6. *Nose.* Both nares, the meati, and the septum are normal. No discharge is noted and the mucous membranes are normally pink.

7. *Mouth and Throat.* The lips, tongue, and gums appear normal. She has full-mouth dentures. The tonsils are tiny; the inner aspect of the cheeks, palate, and uvula are normal. Mirror laryngoscopy shows normal vocal cords that move well.

8. *Neck.* Motion is normal. No masses are seen or felt. Veins are not noted in the neck and there are no abnormal pulsations or bruits. Obesity precludes a good examination, but the thyroid is not palpable nor could the trachea or lymph nodes be felt.

9. *Lymph Nodes.* None are palpable in the neck, axillae, groins, or epitrochlear areas.

10. *Chest and Lungs.* Chest motion is normal and symmetrical, respirations are not labored, tactile and vocal fremitus are everywhere diminished, percussion note is everywhere hyporesonant, breath sounds are vesicular but distant, and no rales are heard. It is difficult to assess diaphragmatic motion.

11. *Heart.* The apical impulse is neither visible nor palpable. Heart sounds are distant, though distinctly audible. S_1 and S_2 are normal, and there is no S_3 or S_4 heard. S_2 is physiologically split, but the split appears a bit wider than normal (0.04 to 0.05 second). No murmurs, friction rubs, clicks, or thrills

are detected. The heart rhythm is regular though there is a sinus bradycardia of 56.

12. *Breasts.* These are pendulous, but the nipples and areolae are normal, there is no discharge, and a meticulous examination discloses no lumps.

13. *Abdomen.* The veins are not distended, a huge fatty apron is present, and no organomegaly, masses, or ascites is detected. An occasional peristaltic sound is heard. No herniae are noted. A right upper quadrant vertical scar is present.

14. *Genitalia.* This examination is done with difficulty because of knee pain. The external genitalia are normal and the vaginal mucosa is atrophic. The cervix looks pale but not diseased. No mucus, pus, or blood is noted. On withdrawing the speculum, a moderate-sized rectocele and cystourethrocele are seen. Bimanual examination discloses a uterus which is enlarged to the size of a 3-month pregnancy, firm, irregular, and somewhat nodular.

15. *Rectum.* The anus, anal sphincter, and rectal examination are normal. No masses or tenderness are noted. The stool on the examining finger is brown and tests negative for blood. The uterine mass is felt on rectal examination too.

16. *Extremities.* Numerous varicosities are seen on both legs in the distribution of the lesser and greater saphenous veins. The left leg is slightly edematous. Homans' sign is negative and there is no calf tenderness. Good arterial pulses are felt in all the appropriate locations in both legs. Both knees are slightly swollen and deformed, though nontender and not acutely inflamed. They are a bit warm to the touch and pain is elicited on trying to flex them. The distal interphalangeal joints of both hands are deformed and demonstrate Heberden's nodes, and some of the terminal phalanges are deviated.

17. *Neurologic Examination.* Cranial nerves, sensation, reflexes, motor power, and equilibrium are all within normal limits.

Baseline Laboratory Data

1. Hematocrit 42%; hemoglobin 12.5 g/dl; red blood cell count 4,200,000/mm³;

white blood cell count 7,800/mm^3, normal differential.

2. Urinalysis—specific gravity 1.020; negative for glucose, albumin, white blood cells, red blood cells, and casts; occasional epithelial cells noted.

3. Glucose 92 mg/dl; urea nitrogen 18 mg/dl; creatinine 0.8 mg/dl; electrolytes normal.

4. Sedimentation rate 12 mm/hour; uric acid 4.0 mg/dl; rheumatoid factor negative.

5. ECG: right bundle branch block; sinus bradycardia.

6. X-ray chest: heart size and configuration normal; bones and diaphragm normal; lungs normal except for evidence of fibrocalcific lesions in both apices.

7. X-ray knees: the joint spaces are markedly narrowed, and periarticular lipping and increased bone density are notable.

8. Urine culture negative.

Comment. Additional history was obtained from two of the patient's friends. They have noted a change in her facial appearance but feel it occurred gradually and may simply be related to her age. There are no pictures available for comparison. The friends too have noted the change in timbre of her voice. Some of the alterations in physical findings plus some of the negative findings could be related to the severe obesity. As noted, a satisfactory neck, chest, and abdominal examination could not be obtained.

NOW—Formulate your own problem list, select the clues that go with each problem, and assess the need for further diagnostic studies related to each problem. You may try your hand at management too. *THEN*—look at the author's problem list and assessment which follow.

Problem List

1. Hypertrophic osteoarthritis—knees and fingers
2. Exogenous obesity
3. Depression
4. Varicose veins
5. Old thrombophlebitis left leg
6. Old healed pulmonary tuberculosis
7. Uterine fibroids, rectocele, cystourethrocele
8. Right bundle branch block
9. Status postcholecystectomy
10. Coarse scant hair and eyebrows, dry skin, bradycardia, hoarseness.

Assessment and Plan for Each Problem

1. The long history of knee trouble, Heberden's nodes, stiffness lasting only a few minutes on resumption of activity, with pain on continued activity, all point to the diagnosis. So do the normal white blood cell count, erythrocyte sedimentation rate, rheumatoid factor, uric acid, the age, and the obesity. Even in osteoarthritis, a knee occasionally becomes slightly inflamed, though usually the joints exhibit none of the evidences of severe acute inflammation. If doubt exists, arthrocentesis will reveal nonturbid fluid with a low cell count and normal viscosity. Management will consist of rest, warm compresses, physiotherapy, and antiinflammatory agents.

2. Obesity is no doubt contributing to problem 1. It appears to be nonendocrine in origin. She obviously consumes too much food, impelled at least in part by her loneliness and depression. Inactivity caused by problem 1 contributes to her obesity. Dietary measures are in order.

3. Depression no doubt results from her life situation—her husband's death, her children far away, and nothing much to do. Treatment should begin immediately. Occupational therapy and psychotherapeutic counseling are in order. This should help both problems 1 and 2.

4. Varicose veins are common, especially in women who have borne many children. No treatment is indicated.

5. The old phlebitis seems incontestable by the history of a recurrently swollen leg. No further treatment is indicated here either. Elastic stockings would probably be ineffective, not tolerated, and possibly harmful.

6. The tuberculosis is old and healed

according to the x-ray, lack of symptoms, and normal erythrocyte sedimentation rate. Family contact is notable. No further studies or treatment are indicated.

7. A definite gynecologic problem exists. The recurrent episodes of dysuria and urgency are probably related, though there is no evidence of urinary tract infection now. Stress incontinence and protrusion from the vagina are usually troublesome to patients. A gynecologic consultation is indicated, since surgery may be advisable in the near future.

8. The abnormal ECG is a surprise. There are no clues to suggest heart disease, except for the widely split S_2 which goes along with the right bundle branch block. Its significance is not clear. It may represent subclinical coronary artery disease or beginning degeneration of the conduction system. The family history of heart disease could go with either. No further studies or treatment are indicated at this time. Repeat ECGs are in order.

9. Nothing is indicated.

10. The combination of findings suggests the possibility of hypothyroidism. The voice change, hair and skin changes, possible altered facies, and bradycardia are on the plus side. Lack of intolerance to cold and the presence of normal reflexes are pertinent negatives. So far a definite diagnosis cannot be made and the problem needs further resolution with thyroid function tests.

Chapter 12

The Case Presentation

PAUL CUTLER, M.D.

The Medes and Persians

While some claim there are no hard and fast rules for case presentations, this is really not so. To bantamize a complete patient data base, whether for oral expression on teaching rounds, for display on a written record, or even for the purpose of a consultation, we should follow rigid precepts—almost as strict as the rules of the Medes and Persians. Yet beginners usually get little coaching in this skill.

The oral presentation of a case on rounds should always be made in an abbreviated format—whether by student, intern, or resident. On busy ward rounds, it is most difficult to endure a half-hour case presentation by a third-year student or intern. A case presentation should consist of sifted, selected, and processed data and must be delivered in a lucid, brief, precise manner. It ought to include only the important positive findings and a few pertinent negatives. Listening to the bedside presentation of a new patient, one can tell if the presenter knows his patient's problems and can properly process and organize data. Even the most complicated case should take no longer than 5 minutes. If the story is lengthy, the student is not confident of his skill in separating the wheat from the chaff, tends therefore to present too much material, and supersaturates his listeners.

Attending physicians differ in the way they want cases presented. If this is the student's first attempt, a detailed complete data base is indicated since the attending physi-

cian wants to know if the student can perform a complete history, do a thorough physical examination, and order and interpret laboratory data.

But once he is satisfied in this regard, abbreviated presentations are not only acceptable but desirable. In fact, the shorter the presentation becomes, the more thought and organization must go into it. When the story rambles on and on, you know the presenter cannot organize the clues, his thoughts, and the patient's problems. A crisp several-minute "all meat" presentation, however, denotes skill, knowledge, organization, and understanding.

A patient may be presented by one of two methods:

1. traditional
2. problem-oriented.

In utilizing the first method, the presenter follows the routine of data gathering, having previously eliminated the negative or irrelevant material. First a few words about the patient, then the chief complaint and history of present illness, followed by what's relevant (positive or pertinent negative) in the past medical history, systems review, family history, patient profile, physical examination, and laboratory data. He then presents the problem list derived from all this sifted data, assesses it, and gives his plan for each problem.

The second way—the one I prefer—is one in which the case is presented in a more problem-oriented fashion from the start. First a few words about the patient and his chief complaint. Then embark directly on the separate problems in order of their importance or cause and effect. As each problem is enumerated, state its supporting data, its priority in management, and your proposed method for its direction. In short, tell what the patient's problems are; then explain the data that substantiate each problem and what you plan to do about it; last, restate the problems. This is what the good lecturer does—tell them what you're going to tell them; then tell it; then tell them what you've told them. It's simple. It's clear. It's sufficient.

Both systems start with the same opening sentence which includes the name, age, gender, race, occupation, chief complaint, duration of chief complaint, and number of hospitalizations for the problem. The chief complaint need not be in the patient's own words; it may be preferable to use the presenter's interpretation.

Examples of opening sentences are as follows: "This is the fourth hospital admission of Mr. William Collins, a 56-year-old white carpenter whose chief complaint is severe chest pain for 2 hours." Or you could say: "Mrs. Ann Yardley is a 36-year-old beautician who is being seen here for the first time because of profuse vaginal bleeding for 2 days."

At this point *the traditional method* elaborates on the chief complaint in the history of present illness, then touches on a summation of the patient profile. A sentence or two follows with the relevant and pertinently negative portions of the past medical history, family history, and systems review. For example, you might say that "the systems review and family history are noncontributory" or "the systems review and family history are noteworthy only in that . . . ."

The physical examination begins with an opening statement on the patient's general appearance and proceeds rapidly to the vital signs. For example: "This moderately obese man is breathing rapidly, seems to be in great distress, is in a cold sweat, and clutches his entire chest; the blood pressure is 90/60 mm Hg, pulse is 128 and thready, respirations are 28/minute, and the temperature is

36 C." Then advance quickly through all the abnormal and pertinent negative findings from head to toe. Blanket statements such as "there is no evidence of . . ."; or "the rest of the examination is normal (except for) . . ."; or "examination from the waist down including the neurologic and orthopaedic systems is normal" are quite acceptable.

Do not read all the test results. Relate only the significant ones. But be prepared to state the findings on all tests and studies if requested to do so. It is important to realize that different presenters can vary in their formulations of the problem list yet each be equally satisfactory.

The *problem-oriented method* jumps from the opening sentence directly to the problem list and its assessment and plan.

There are pros and cons for each method. The traditional style may be more interesting for the listener and develops the case in a story-like manner. It provides the fun of gamesmanship. Also it stimulates the listener to form his own ideas as the presentation proceeds and forces him to pay close attention. On the other hand, the presenter is delivering preselected and processed information in such a way that you are induced to concur with him as he leads you through a tunnel toward a predetermined light. He tells you only the data he deems important to reach his own conclusions. This tends to suppress independent thinking and opposing views.

The problem-oriented presentation is clear, straightforward, and also predigested and preabsorbed. When delivered, it too tends to suppress the listener's logic because the conclusions and their explanations are already set forth. However, it may be the method of choice when multiple problems exist, for otherwise the delivery becomes too complicated and difficult to follow.

When the actual presentation is to be made, there are other strict rules and guidelines to follow. First you must notify the patient and have his consent. Then decide whether the initial discussion should be in front of or away from the patient; this determination depends on many common-sense factors. At least part of the presentation should be at the bedside, and total "blackboard rounds" are to be deplored. You should carefully prepare, rehearse, and even tape your presentation before its delivery. Generally, the history takes 3 minutes, the examination 1 minute, and the problem list and its evaluation and plan another 2 minutes. It is a good idea to have in hand the chart, the x-rays, other data results, previous records, and this morning's still unreported blood culture result. Never discuss difficulties in data collection or possible laboratory errors in front of the patient.

Since case presentations are so indicative of a trainee's capacity to process data and solve problems, some commonly made errors should be mentioned (1). It is shocking to learn that frequently omitted items are: the reason the patient sought care; the reason for admission to the hospital; the medications being taken; and aspects of the physical examination germane to the problem. Such deficiencies invariably lead to confusion and large numbers of questions and interruptions.

The following four abbreviated data bases—A, B, C, D—can either be written on the chart as such (if a short writeup is preferred) or they may be presented orally on teaching rounds.

Data bases A and B represent, respectively, the traditional and problem-oriented abridged versions of the first patient (Mr. Travis) discussed in Chapter 11. Data bases C and D represent, respectively, the traditional and problem-oriented abridged versions of the second patient (Mrs. Green) discussed in Chapter 11.

Abbreviated Data Base (A)
(Traditional Style)

> This is Sample Data Base 1 (Chapter 11) presented in an abbreviated form. It includes positives and pertinent negatives and has been miniaturized in the traditional manner.

Mr. Calvin Travis is a 58-year-old white male who is a good historian and complains of nocturnal dyspnea for the past 10 days.

He had an acute myocardial infarction 6 years ago, has had angina on exertion for the past 2 years, dyspnea and fatigue on exertion for 6 months, and orthopnea, night cough, and paroxysmal nocturnal dyspnea for 10 days.

He has been a heavy smoker for many years and has had a morning cough with expectoration for 5 to 10 years which has been worse in the past 6 months. For 17 years he has had asymptomatic diabetes mellitus, allegedly controlled on diet alone.

Physical examination reveals a mesomorphic, slightly obese, moderately dyspneic man sitting up in bed. T 37.6 C, P 116, BP 128/80/72 in both arms, R 24 with deep inspirations and slightly prolonged expirations. The fundi show mild arteriolar narrowing and occasional arteriovenous nicking. The neck veins are distended 4 cm above the clavicle at 45°. The chest shows a slightly increased anteroposterior diameter, respirations are somewhat labored, expiration is prolonged, and diaphragmatic motion is poor (1 to 2 cm). There are a few fine inspiratory and expiratory wheezes heard all over, fine moist late inspiratory rales at both bases and in the axillae, and slight diffuse hyperresonance with normal fremitus and breath sounds.

The apex is seen and felt at the anterior axillary line in the fifth and sixth intercostal spaces, is forceful, and there is a palpable and audible S_3. An occasional premature ventricular contraction is noted. P_2 is louder than A_2, and a grade 2/6 systolic ejection murmur is present at the base.

The liver is not enlarged (10 cm from top to bottom in the midclavicular line), though it is palpable 3 cm below the costal margin; there is no abdominal distention or ankle edema. External hemorrhoids are noted, the prostate is slightly enlarged, and the left dorsalis pedis pulse is absent.

Laboratory studies show 1+ glycosuria, 3+ albuminuria, serum glucose 175 mg/dl; the complete blood count and other chemistries are normal. The ECG shows an old inferior myocardial infarction plus left ventricular hypertrophy; the chest x-ray discloses a moderately enlarged heart, increased bronchovascular markings at both bases, a low diaphragm, and bilateral pulmonary congestion.

Note. This concludes the abbreviated data base. It must be assumed that this is a distillate of a complete data base which has been obtained in a routine fashion. The problem list and assessment are the same as in Sample Data Base 1 (Chapter 11). This case could easily have been presented exactly as it is written.

Abbreviated Data Base (B)
(Problem-Oriented Style)

> Another way to write up a data base and present a patient in a concise manner is to use a problem-oriented approach from the beginning. Thus, if we consider the same patient discussed in Chapter 11, the summation could be done by grouping related data with each problem from the start.

Mr. Calvin Travis is a 58-year-old white male who is a good historian and complains of nocturnal dyspnea for the past 10 days. He has the following problems:

1. *Atherosclerotic heart disease* with old myocardial infarction. This is established on the basis of history (1973) and an ECG which shows an old inferior myocardial infarction. His father had coronary disease.

2. *Angina pectoris* for 2 years. He has typical retrosternal squeezing pain radiating into the neck, left shoulder, and medial aspect of the left arm. It is brought on by exertion, relieved by rest, and seems stable.

3. *Left ventricular failure,* secondary to problem 1. This is substantiated by a 6-month history of dyspnea and fatigue on exertion followed by more recent night cough, orthopnea, and paroxysmal nocturnal dyspnea. The heart is noticeably enlarged both on percussion and by locating the apex beat at the anterior axillary line. The beat is forceful, there is a palpable and

audible S_3, P_2 is louder than A_2, and fine moist rales are present at the bases. A grade 2/6 ejection type murmur is heard at the base of the heart. The neck veins show a slightly increased pressure. The liver is not enlarged and there is no edema. The ECG shows left ventricular hypertrophy in addition to the old infarction, and the chest x-ray shows moderate cardiac enlargement and pulmonary congestion. It is this problem which made him seek medical aid.

4. *Diabetes mellitus* for 17 years. This was discovered on routine examination and never gave symptoms or required treatment other than diet. Allegedly he is well controlled. Plus-one glycosuria and a blood glucose of 175 mg/dl are noted on admission. His mother has diabetes.

5. *Chronic obstructive lung disease* (5 to 10 years). He smokes excessively, has a long-standing chronic cough with expectoration, faint wheezes on inspiration and expiration, and a relatively immobile diaphragm on physical examination. Chest x-ray shows increased basal bronchovascular markings and a low diaphragm.

6. *Peripheral vascular disease.* This is asymptomatic and is suggested only by the absence of the left dorsalis pedis pulse.

7. *External hemorrhoids.* These too are asymptomatic and are detected on physical examination.

8. *Albuminuria.* This abnormality is found on routine urinalysis. It may result from diabetic glomerulosclerosis, but the cause is uncertain.

Assessment. Problems 1, 2, and 3 are chronologically and etiologically related. Problem 3, left ventricular failure, needs immediate treatment and is the most pressing issue. Salt restriction, diuretics, rest, and digitalization are indicated. Problem 4 will be treated with an 1800-calorie diabetic diet, and the blood and urine glucoses will be studied before a decision on need for further therapy is made. Problem 5 needs only cessation of smoking. Problems 6, 7, and 8 need no management for the present.

In summary, Mr. Travis has the following problems: 1-2-3-4-5-6-7-8 (restate them).

Before proceeding to abbreviated data bases C and D, the reader should review Sample Data Base 2 in Chapter 11 and try to compose his own case presentation. Do it in both formats and decide which one you prefer. Then compare your work with the author's versions. Note that the following case is that of an outpatient.

Abbreviated Data Base (C)
(Traditional Style)

Mrs. William Hayes is a 62-year-old white female with a reliable history who complains of pain, swelling, and stiffness of both knees for 8 years, much worse in the past week.

For 10 years she has had deformities of the distal interphalangeal joints of both hands. Over the past 8 years her knees have gotten stiff, swollen, deformed, and painful, the right worse than the left. The stiffness is worse on awakening and after sitting, improves with activity, then the knees become stiff and painful again. At times, one or the other knee becomes worse and slightly warm. Previous physicians told her she had old-age "wear-and-tear" arthritis. For the past week there has been much pain and yesterday the right knee became warm and tender.

Past history reveals "cured" tuberculosis as an 18-year-old, four children, worsening varicose veins, a cholecystectomy 8 years ago followed by left-sided thrombophlebitis, long-standing obesity, depression, and further weight gain since the death of her husband.

Systems review is notable for loss of hair, dryness of hair and skin, coarseness of voice, occasional swelling of the left leg, stress incontinence, and protrusion from the vagina when straining; she sleeps poorly and is very lonely. She has no intolerance to heat or cold and no cough, expectoration, sweats, or hemoptysis.

Family history is possibly significant in that her father died of tuberculosis and there

is much heart disease in the family. The patient profile seems noncontributory, except for obesity, loneliness, and depression.

Physical examination. The patient is not acutely ill and in no apparent pain. She is obese, has severe varicose veins in both lower extremities, and the left leg appears swollen; her facial features are coarse. The vital signs are normal except for a pulse of 56 beats/minute and a weight of 205 lb. The eyebrows and hair are sparse. The S_2 is widely split, there is a right upper quadrant scar, cystocele and rectocele are present, and the uterus is irregularly enlarged to the size of a 3 months' pregnancy. Both knees are swollen, deformed, slightly warm, and painful on flexion; Homans' sign is negative, and there is no calf tenderness. Heberden's nodes are noted in the distal interphalangeal joints of both hands.

Laboratory studies including erythrocyte sedimentation rate, uric acid, and rheumatoid factor are negative or normal. The ECG displays right bundle branch block and sinus bradycardia. The chest x-ray demonstrates fibrocalcific lesions in both apices. X-rays of the knees reveal changes typical of hypertrophic osteoarthritis.

The problem list is then stated. It is the same as in Sample Data Base 2, Chapter 11. The assessment and plan may be abridged.

Abbreviated Data Base (D)
(Problem-Oriented Style)

Mrs. William Hayes is a 62-year-old white female with a reliable history who complains of pain, swelling, and stiffness of both knees for 8 years, much worse in the past week. She has the following problems:

1. *Hypertrophic osteoarthritis.* She has had Heberden's nodes for 10 years, and stiff, painful, swollen, deformed knees for 8 years which periodically worsen. They are especially bad when she gets up in the morning or after sitting for a while, improve with a little activity, then become stiff and painful again. She was told she has a "wear-and-tear" arthritis that comes with old age, and for the past week her knees have been warm,

tender, and more painful. At present both are swollen, deformed, slightly warm, and painful on flexion.

2. *Exogenous obesity.* She weighs 205 lb and is 64 inches tall; she has always been obese, but has been especially so since her husband's death. She eats more and has gained an additional 20 lb.

3. *Depression.* This has been present since her husband's death.

4. *Varicose veins.* She has four children, and during her second pregnancy she developed varicose veins which have gotten progressively worse.

5. *Thrombophlebitis left leg.* This occurred subsequent to a cholecystectomy. Her leg still swells on occasion but is otherwise not troublesome nor does it show evidence of active inflammation. Homans' sign is negative and the calf is not tender.

6. *Old healed pulmonary tuberculosis.* This was noted by chest x-ray and was extensively treated at age 18. She has no symp-toms now. Her father died of tuberculosis at 42.

7. *Uterine fibroids, cystocele, and recto-cele.* These are noted on physical examination and may be associated with her recurrent brief periods of dysuria and urgency.

8. *Right bundle branch block.* This incidental finding explains the widely split S_2 but there are no other signs or symptoms of heart disease.

9. *Status postcholecystectomy.*

10. Coarse scant hair and eyebrows, dry skin, bradycardia, and hoarseness (to be investigated for hypothyroidism).

Her management will consist of a reducing diet, antiinflammatory agents for arthritis, physiotherapy and exercises, and superficial psychotherapy. Thyroid function tests will be requested.

Reference

1. Klos M, Reuler JB, Nardone DA, et al: An evaluation of trainee performance in the case presentation. *J Med Educ* 58:432–433, 1983.

Chapter 13

Data Resolution Skills

PAUL CUTLER, M.D.

Considerable material in reference to data processing and data evaluation has already been presented. Chapter 2 and the Introduction to Section Two dwelled in detail on the ways in which the medical person gathers, interprets, classifies, and manages patient information.

It is not an easy matter to decide whether two clues relate, whether a bit of information is relevant, or whether a finding should be ignored. To be an effective medical sleuth, you must be able to categorize every single item concerning the patient. For this you need good data resolution skills.

Such talents include knowing how to put things together; knowing the signs and symptoms of diseases; knowing the additional high-yield data needed to solve knotty problems; knowing the clues that exclude or confirm a diagnosis; and knowing the subsets of data to be investigated for many common complaints.

For example, you might need to know whether a single clue is evidence for, evidence against, or neither for nor against a suspected diagnosis. Also you might want to know if an additional piece of information is relevant, possibly relevant, or irrelevant to the chief complaint. Perhaps it is a pertinent negative clue. On the other hand, it may indicate the existence of a problem other than the principal one.

When you receive information about a patient, you must quickly decide what to do with it and where to categorize it.

This chapter aims to sharpen your skills in this regard.

The methods to be employed are: (*a*) the selection of data subsets for eight mini-cases; (*b*) the performance of relevance exercises involving three common medical presentations; and (*c*) the decoding of three problem sets.

In all instances, the reader will be asked to furnish the answers, then find the author's answers in the pages that follow, and compare skills. Don't be surprised, disappointed, or chagrined if you disagree with the author. *You* might be the correct one. At least the exercises will encourage you to think!

The numerous cases to be discussed in Section Three give hundreds of examples of data evaluation. However, in the present chapter we present many small exercises that are designed to acquaint the reader with some special skills needed to process data, to improve these skills, and to prepare him for the more complex and detailed cases that follow in the next section.

Make sure you try your hand at the following exercises before seeking the author's answers. Course instructors may conceive additional mini-cases and ask their students to select special data subsets for each one. This type of exercise is particularly effective when students prepare such cases in small groups and then exchange their ideas in larger groups under instructor supervision.

Selecting Data Subsets

In the following exercises, only the initial statement is given. This includes the age, gender, and chief complaint. The reader should then select a few likely diagnoses that could explain the initial statement. Following this, choose a few (three to seven) bits of historical information that might offer the most help. Then list three to seven items in the physical examination that will further narrow the field. And last, mention one to four tests or procedures that are most likely to clinch the diagnosis. Request only data that will be very productive, and do not ask for useless information. Such exercises make you very selective in your search for clues and demand that you know exactly what you are looking for and how to find it. *The author's answers follow the eight initial statements.*

Case 1. A 48-year-old woman with swollen legs for 2 weeks.
  (a) List the differential diagnosis.
  (b) Ask three to seven questions.
  (c) Examine three to seven parts.
  (d) Which one to four tests will help most?

Case 2. A 52-year-old woman who has noticed a mass in the left upper quadrant for 1 week. Do (a), (b), (c), and (d).

Case 3. A 36-year-old woman who has just had a first grand mal seizure. Do (a), (b), (c), and (d).

Case 4. A 60-year-old man who has had cough and expectoration for 6 weeks. Do (a), (b), (c), and (d).

Case 5. A 46-year-old woman who has noticed an enlarged thyroid gland for 6 weeks. Do (a), (b), (c), and (d).

Case 6. A 68-year-old man with markedly diminished vision in the right eye. Do (a), (b), (c), and (d).

Case 7. A 58-year-old woman with a 2-week discharge from the left nipple. Do (a), (b), (c), and (d).

Case 8. A 12-year-old boy notices a lump in his right groin. Do (a), (b), (c), and (d).

Answers to Case Data Subsets

Case 1. (a) The differential diagnosis must include: 1. right ventricular failure and its various causes; 2. cirrhosis of the liver; 3. nephrotic syndrome; 4. venous or lymphatic obstruction.

(b) Productive questions will determine the presence or absence of: 1. dyspnea on exertion; 2. heart disease or murmurs; 3. heavy alcohol ingestion; 4. previous hepatitis; 5. kidney disease; 6. vein trouble.

(c) Examination should search for: 1. cardiac enlargement or murmurs; 2. other evidence for right ventricular failure (elevated neck vein pressure, large tender liver, diffuse lung disease); 3. large, nontender liver and other stigmata of chronic liver disease; 4. an obstructing intrapelvic tumor; 5. evidence of venous thrombosis (calf tenderness and positive Homans' sign).

(d) Helpful studies include: 1. chest x-ray for enlarged heart, pulmonary congestion, or chronic pulmonary disease that might cause right ventricular failure; 2. liver function tests (serum albumin, transaminase, alkaline phosphatase, and bilirubin); 3. urinalysis for proteinuria; 4. venogram only if doubt exists.

It is important to note that the above list can be radically reduced if the answer to a question or the result of an examination leads you in one direction rather than another. For example, if this patient were a known severe alcoholic and had an enlarged liver, ascites, and palmar erythema, there would be no need for additional questions, examinations, and tests—except for completing the data base.

Or if the answers led you in the direction of heart failure, much less additional information would be needed. If there were no symptoms or signs of heart disease, this possibility could be excluded with a high degree of certainty. On the other hand, if the history and examination were fruitless, heavy albuminuria and hypoalbuminemia would label the nephrotic syndrome but not the precise pathologic lesion of the renal disease causing it.

But given a normal heart, liver, and kidneys, the pelvic examinaton and a variety of studies for deep vein patency are indicated.

The algorithmic principle by which we build on pieces of positive data to direct our further line of inquiry is a method commonly used by the problem solver.

Case 2. (a) Possible causes are: 1. splenomegaly (lymphoma, leukemia, etc); 2. pancreatic pseudocyst; 3. kidney cyst, tumor, or hydronephrosis; 4. leiomyosarcoma of stomach; 5. carcinoma of colon.

(b) High-yield questions revolve around: 1. how and when the mass was first noted (weight loss?); 2. general strength, fatigue, appetite; 3. present or recent severe abdominal pain suggesting pancreatitis; 4. gallstone or alcohol history that may predispose to pancreatitis; 5. bowel symptoms of colon cancer (blood in stools, constipation, narrow stools); 6. urinary tract symptoms; 7. easy satiety, hematemesis, or black stools that might correlate with a stomach mass.

(c) 1. Locate, delineate, and characterize the mass, noting tenderness and mobility with respiration; 2. search for enlarged lymph nodes; 3. detect anemia.

(d) 1. Stools for occult blood; 2. complete blood count for anemia and leukocyte abnormalities; 3. urinalysis for renal disease; 4. x-ray studies may be helpful and necessary; depending upon where previous data lead, you may need a plain abdominal film, an intravenous pyelogram, a barium enema, a gastrointestinal series, and/or a computed tomographic (CT) scan. A chest x-ray may detect metastases or hilar adenopathy.

Here too you may be immediately detoured into one line of diagnostic logic by a single clue. If the mass is thought to be spleen, the patient is pale, and diffuse lymphadenopathy is present, a complete blood count alone may conclude the search.

On the other hand, if the mass seems to arise in the kidney, and all of (b) and (c) are fruitless, a CT scan or sonogram might be the thing to do.

Again, you must learn to flow along logical diagnostic pathways and protocols.

Case 3. (a) 1. Idiopathic epilepsy; 2. drug withdrawal or overdose; 3. brain tumor; 4. insulinoma; 5. meningitis.

(b) In the history, look for: 1. exact description of the preictal, ictal, and postictal state; 2. precise drug and alcohol history; 3. headaches, visual disturbances, or other neurologic symptoms that suggest an expanding intracranial lesion; 4. fever; 5. preceding trauma.

(c) 1. Neurologic examination, including fundi; 2. temperature, nuchal rigidity, Kernig's and Brudzinski's signs for meningitis; 3. evidence of head trauma; 4. track marks on arms.

(d) 1. Toxic drug screen; 2. electroencephalogram; 3. blood glucose after 24-hour fast; 4. insulin immunoassay; 5. lumbar puncture; 6. x-ray skull and CT brain scan.

Most information and studies are not needed if a positive lead is gotten early. Track marks from stimulant drugs obviate the need for further information. Fever and nuchal rigidity mandate a lumbar puncture but little else. If there is suspicion of a brain tumor, even in the absence of any other positive clues, a dye-enhanced CT scan is the road to take.

But do not be trapped by fuzzy logic. The fact that a sister has epilepsy does not exclude the patient's having meningitis. Diagnoses must be buttressed by harder evidence.

Case 4. (a) To be considered are: 1. lung cancer; 2. tuberculosis; 3. chronic bronchitis; 4. chronic obstructive pulmonary disease; 5. other parenchymal lung diseases.

(b) Historical data germane to the case include: 1. smoking history; 2. chronic exposure to toxic industrial pollutants; 3. occupational history; 4. recent respiratory infection that did not clear; 5. wheeze or dyspnea; 6. exposure to a tuberculous individual; 7. description of sputum.

(c) Examine for: 1. clubbing of fingers, suggestive of cancer; 2. detailed chest examination for rales, wheezes, consolidation, localized areas of disease, diaphragmatic excursion, and expiratory duration; 3. supraclavicular hard lymph nodes.

(d) Essential studies include: 1. chest x-ray; 2. sputum examination for acid-fast bacilli and tumor cells; 3. fiberoptic bronchoscopy with the same intents and possible biopsy; 4. pulmonary function tests for diagnosis 4.

The diagnosis should be easily evident. If all in (c) and (d) are negative, suspect chronic bronchitis. Eschew conclusions like cancer on the feeble evidence of smoking. Don't be caught in a spider's web between tuberculosis and cancer unless biopsy or bacteriologic proof is established. Evidence for serious disease must be robust. And detours that reach diagnoses quickly and eliminate the need for studies apply here as in other cases.

Case 5. (a) Diagnostic considerations include: 1. simple goiter; 2. adenomatous thyroid hyperplasia (toxic or nontoxic); 3. subacute thyroiditis; 4. Hashimoto's disease (with or without hypothyroidism); 5. carcinoma.

(b) Questions to be asked center about: 1. growth of thyroid; 2. existence of pain, fever, or "sore throat"; 3. evidence of toxicity (heat intolerance, sweats, good appetite, weight loss, nervousness); 4. clues for hypofunction (cold intolerance, sluggishness, skin changes, weight gain).

(c) Examine the: 1. thyroid for consistency, size, tenderness, and nodularity; 2. eyes for exophthalmos (and other signs), hands for fine tremor, skin for warmth and dampness, hair for fine silkiness; 3. facial features, hair, eyebrows, and skin for evidence of hypothyroidism; 4. pulse and blood pressure for indications of thyroid hypofunction or hyperfunction; 5. reflexes for quick or slow responses.

(d) From the supermarket of tests, you need choose only the triiodothyronine resin uptake (T_3RU), thyroxine (T_4), and the thyroid-stimulating hormone (TSH) measurements to determine thyroid function. If medullary carcinoma is suspected, order a calcitonin radioimmunoassay, and a serum calcium and 24-hour urine catecholamines for possible Sipple's syndrome (associated parathyroid adenoma and pheochromocytoma). Thyroid aspiration biopsy must be considered too. High titers of antithyroglobulin antibodies confirm suspected Hashimoto's disease, and a very rapid sedimentation rate coincides with subacute thyroiditis.

Thyroid palpation and patient inspection are paramount in diagnosis here. Cancer is usually a single mass, rarely diffuse. It would be a tour de force performance to find a type II multiple endocrine adenomatosis. If medullary carcinoma is suspected, look for other endocrine abnormalities too. An enlarged thyroid without endocrine dysfunction most commonly signifies benign diffuse (possibly nodular) hyperplasia, simple goiter, or Hashimoto's disease. In all cases, a feel of the thyroid gland directs you to the correct line of inquisition.

Case 6. (a) One bit of information must precede all others, for it divides the tentative hypotheses into two separate groups. Did the poor vision come on slowly or rapidly? For if the onset were slow and the progression over months to years, you consider cataract, glaucoma, refractive error, retinitis pigmentosa, macular degeneration, etc. But if the vision diminished acutely over a time frame of seconds to days, you are in another ball park. The latter situation occurred in this case. Therefore consider: 1. retinal artery thrombosis or embolus; 2. retinal vein thrombosis; 3. retinal detachment; 4. cerebrovascular accident; 5. retinal or vitreous hemorrhage; 6. acute angle closure glaucoma; 7. optic neuritis (papillitis, retrobulbar).

(b) Other helpful historical hints are: 1. preceding flashing sensations in retinal detachment; 2. pain in acute glaucoma; 3. history of previous vascular episodes; 4. other neurologic symptoms denoting a more widespread intracerebral vascular accident; 5. the presence of diabetes or hypertension; 6. painful eye movements as seen in optic neuritis.

(c) Examination should be diagnostic. You may find: 1. high intraocular tension in a red eye if acute glaucoma exists; 2. characteristic ophthalmoscopic evidence of retinal artery occlusion, retinal vein thrombosis, detachment, or vitreous hemorrhage; 3. carotid artery bruit and diminished internal carotid pulsation if platelet aggregates have embolized to the retinal artery; 4. thickened tender temporal arteries if the retinal artery disease is part of the generalized arteritis of polymyalgia rheumatica; 5. visual field studies that determine for certain whether the loss of vision is clearly in one eye or in one half of each eye (homonymous hemianopsia); in the latter instance the lesion would be intracerebral.

(d) Studies will offer little of value. Request an erythrocyte sedimentation rate if arteritis is suspected. Study for a coagulopathy if venous thrombosis has occurred. Visualize the carotid arteries with ultrasound if warranted.

The crucial clues here are the rapidity of onset, presence or absence of pain, and visualization of the fundi. Since vision is poor, pupillary light reflexes will be sluggish, and the fundi will be easily seen. Optic neuritis is a diagnosis of exclusion and is unlikely at this age. Migraine can present with hemianoptic prodromes. While a presentation such as this is usually an ocular problem, it is important to recognize that it may be a local manifestation of a generalized disease.

Case 7. (a) The possibilities are many; they include breast lesions, such as intraductal papilloma, carcinoma, and fibrocystic disease, as well as a large number of endocrine problems. In the latter category belong prolactinomas, hypothalamic-pituitary disorders, hypothyroidism, the taking of specific drugs, and the cessation of oral contraceptives.

(b) The type of discharge and involvement of one or both breasts are decisive bits of information. Inquire about or look at the discharge. If it is watery, it may mean nothing. If it is *milky and bilateral*, the cause is endocrine. And if it is *bloody and unilateral*, the cause is neoplastic. Since this patient is 58, we need not inquire about oral contraceptives or menses, but do ask about reserpine, phenothiazines, and α-methyldopa—known lactogenics.

(c) Physical examination is directed primarily at the breast. Feel for fibrocystic disease. Search carefully for a breast lump, inspect the skin for dimpling or retraction, and meticulously feel the nipple and subareolar tissue. Then inspect the patient for stigmata of hypothyroidism or pituitary adenoma.

(d) Tests to be done depend on the direction you are taking. If neoplastic disease is your prime choice because the discharge is unilateral and bloody, order mammography or high-resolution mammography. Ductography may help and open biopsy may be

indicated. But if the discharge is bilateral and milky, and the above-mentioned obvious causes have been excluded, a search for intracranial or intrasellar tumor is indicated. This may necessitate a CT scan or microtomograms of the sella for a prolactinoma. Serum prolactin levels are neither sensitive nor specific.

This is really a simple problem. The answers to two questions send you off on one quest or another.

Case 8. (a) This could be a lymph node, an undescended testicle, or a hernia. It sounds simple.

(b) How long has it been there? Does it hurt? Does it come and go? Does it go away on lying down and reappear when straining?

(c) Examine, locate, elicit, and describe the "lump." Is there a testicle in the right scrotum? See if the lump disappears on lying down and reappears on standing or straining. Put your finger in the inguinal canal and have the boy cough. Search for other lymph nodes and splenomegaly.

(d) No studies should be necessary. If the possibility of a lymph node disorder exists, a blood count and biopsy may be indicated.

Most patients seen in the office or outpatient department are diagnosed as easily as the one just presented. A few questions, one or two places to examine, and the answer is apparent. Quite often there is an unlikely possibility to be excluded when certainty is needed.

Performing Relevance Exercises

Initial statements about three different patients will be presented. Following each statement, a large number of individual bits of acquired information will be given. Decide whether each item **per se**, as it relates to the initial statement, is:

(a) relevant
(b) possibly relevant
(c) pertinent negative
(d) irrelevant
(e) a separate problem.

This is an exercise in data evaluation.

After you have written your own answers and justified them, compare your thoughts with the author's logic on pages 212–217. Also compare your logic with the author's defense of each judgment. You may not be in agreement. If you can rationally relate a clue that the author could not, *you* may be correct. Give each item much thought and be able to justify your answer. *More than one answer may be applicable.* Information derived from the history and physical examination will be stressed.

Patient with Anemia. *This is a 66-year-old woman with weakness and diffuse pallor for 6 months.* Evaluate the following pieces of data using the (a)-(b)-(c)-(d)-(e) scale just described (*see p. 212 for answers*):

1. smokes ten cigarettes daily
2. drinks eight cups of coffee daily
3. 20-lb weight loss in last 3 months
4. no weight loss
5. poor appetite
6. good appetite
7. considerable indigestion
8. nonbleeding hemorrhoids
9. bleeding hemorrhoids
10. loose bowels for 2 months
11. black stools noted occasionally
12. menopause at age 48
13. no vaginal bleeding
14. spleen palpable
15. chronic worsening cough
16. hemoglobin 6 g/dl; red blood cell count 3 million/mm^3
17. slight jaundice present
18. trachea in midline
19. thyroid not palpable
20. urinalysis normal
21. aortic area systolic grade 2 ejection murmur
22. patient of Swedish extraction
23. patient comes from California
24. patient is black American
25. does housework
26. conjunctiva pale
27. hematocrit 35%; red blood cell count 2.5 million/mm^3
28. eats two trays of ice cubes daily
29. severe backaches for 1 month
30. backaches for 5 years
31. very obese
32. stools positive for occult blood
33. stools negative for occult blood
34. vaginal bleeding for 2 years
35. vaginal bleeding after examination
36. cholecystectomy 10 years ago
37. frequent nosebleeds and bleeding gums
38. lethargy and mental confusion
39. mastectomy 1 year ago
40. tongue pale but otherwise normal
41. tongue red and sore
42. blood pressure 130/80
43. blood pressure 200/120
44. sparse coarse hair
45. albuminuria +4
46. physical examination normal except for pallor
47. fundi normal
48. glycosuria +2
49. leg paresthesias
50. no lymph nodes palpable

Patient with Chest Pain. This is a *52-year-old man who has had severe substernal* pain for 3 hours. Determine the relevance of the following bits of information using the same (a)-(b)-(c)-(d)-(e) scale as in the previous case (*see p. 214 for answers*):

1. pain radiates to right arm
2. never had pain before
3. had same pain many times before, brought on by exertion
4. has had similar shorter pains, but never on exertion
5. chronic headaches
6. recurrent nosebleeds
7. father died at 48
8. mother has diabetes
9. plays tennis daily
10. had dental extraction 2 months ago
11. also has nausea and vomiting
12. attends church regularly
13. on no dietary restrictions
14. smokes two packs cigarettes daily
15. has had hypertension for 15 years
16. drinks 12 beers daily
17. is an attorney

18. fundi normal
19. blood pressure 180/100
20. blood pressure 80/60
21. blood pressure 130/80
22. blood pressure equal in both arms
23. blood pressure differs by 50 mm Hg in the arms
24. cold and clammy
25. skin warm and dry
26. recent 24-hour bus trip
27. inguinal hernias for 10 years
28. jaundice present
29. liver enlarged
30. S_4 present
31. mitral systolic grade 3 murmur radiating to axilla
32. rales both bases
33. atrophic left testicle
34. temperature normal
35. temperature 38.5 C
36. pericardial friction rub on admission
37. pericardial friction rub not present on admission
38. legs swollen
39. aortic diastolic murmur present
40. prostate gland 2+ enlarged
41. tender calves
42. appears dyspneic
43. blood pressure 140/30 both arms
44. no pulse in left dorsalis pedis artery
45. varicose veins present
46. chest x-ray normal
47. stat creatine kinase-MB isomer normal
48. initial ECG normal
49. initial ECG abnormal
50. ECG normal on 3 successive days

Patient with Jaundice. *A 46-year-old woman has had clearly visible jaundice and dark urine for 10 days.* Determine the relevance of the following data using the same (a)-(b)-(c)-(d)-(e) scale as in the two previous cases (*see p. 216 for answers*):

1. bowel operation 3 years ago
2. bowel operation 3 months ago
3. favorite food is seafood
4. is a nurse
5. works in a restaurant kitchen
6. recently returned from North Africa
7. drinks coffee twice daily
8. father died of heart attack
9. has itching of skin
10. gets weekly injections for "no pep"
11. takes aspirin for headaches
12. takes α-methyldopa for hypertension
13. takes isoniazid for recently discovered positive purified protein derivative skin test
14. has no pain
15. has diffuse abdominal pains
16. has had recurrent severe right upper quadrant pains
17. nausea for 2 weeks
18. nausea for 2 months
19. nausea for 2 years
20. takes no narcotic injections
21. feels well
22. feels sick
23. occasional ringing in the ears
24. is being treated for diabetes
25. stools black
26. stools brown
27. stools clay-colored
28. has lump in breast
29. drinks alcohol "socially"
30. doesn't smoke
31. does smoke
32. stopped smoking 2 weeks ago
33. poor appetite for 2 weeks
34. poor appetite and weight loss for 2 months
35. eyeballs yellow
36. has seasonal hay fever
37. liver not palpable
38. liver enlarged and tender
39. liver enlarged and nodular
40. spleen not palpable
41. abdomen not distended
42. abdomen distended
43. no large veins on abdomen
44. no spider angiomata
45. neck veins flat at 45°
46. palmar erythema present
47. tender mass in right upper quadrant
48. mass in right lower quadrant
49. varicose veins present
50. menses normal; pelvic examination normal

Answers to Data Evaluation Exercises

Patient With Anemia. *A 66-year-old woman with weakness and anemia for 6 months* presents a common problem. You immediately consider a constellation of common causes. These include primarily: malignancy somewhere, primary anemia, secondary anemia due to blood loss, diffuse granulomatous disease, and uremia from chronic renal failure.

You seek additional data to confirm or negate the tentative hypotheses. While each separate item is considered here by itself, generally a bit of information is not evaluated in a vacuum. Its interpretation often hinges on previously collected data. For pedagogic reasons this exercise deals only with single clues by themselves.

1. **(d).**
2. **(d).**
3. **(a).** This signifies underlying serious disease like cancer or lymphoma.
4. **(c).** This tends to deny malignancy.
5. **(a), (b).** This probably denotes serious disease, although anorexia is nonspecific.
6. **(c).** A good appetite speaks against serious disease.
7. **(b).** This might be related to a gastrointestinal ulcer or neoplasm that is chronically bleeding.
8. **(d).** This is not related unless it be the "sentinel pile" of colon cancer.
9. **(a), (b), (e).** This is possibly a separate problem, though it could be the cause of her anemia.
10. **(b), (e).** This could signify colon cancer or malabsorption syndrome (not listed as a hypothesis), or it could be a separate problem.
11. **(b).** Truly black stools usually mean melena (blood in the stool) and testify to repeated episodes of gastrointestinal bleeding from a source above the mid-transverse colon.
12. **(d).**

13. **(c).** This indicates there is no blood loss from the genital tract.
14. **(a).** A palpable spleen is an enlarged speen, and, found together with anemia, the hypotheses of lymphoma or leukemia are strengthened.
15. **(a) or (b).** Chronic pulmonary tuberculosis is possible though it does not present primarily as an anemia.
16. **(a).** The anemia is hypochromic and suggests chronic blood loss.
17. **(a), (b).** Jaundice and anemia suggest hemolysis, or cancer with metastases to the liver.
18. **(d).**
19. **(d).**
20. **(c).** Uremia from renal failure almost invariably causes severe urine abnormalities (casts, albumin, etc).
21. **(a), (e).** The murmur could be a flow murmur resulting from chronic anemia, or it may be a separate problem.
22. **(b), (d).** Pernicious anemia is more common in Scandinavians, but Swedes have other causes for anemia too, so it may well be irrelevant.
23. **(d).**
24. **(d).** "Ethnic anemias" are not apt to appear at this age.
25. **(c).** Although weak and pale, she is still able to do housework.
26. **(a).** This merely confirms the visible pallor.
27. **(a).** The anemia is macrocytic, and pernicious anemia, folic acid deficiency, etc are suspect.
28. **(b).** Pagophagia is not uncommonly seen as a *result* of chronic iron deficiency anemia.
29. **(b).** This suggests a malignancy with spinal metastases.
30. **(e).** It is unlikely that backaches and anemia would be related for 5 years; myeloma or metastases would most likely have caused death before then.
31. **(c), (d), (e).** It is either unrelated, a separate problem, or may be considered a pertinent negative in that the patient seems not to have a disease that causes both weight loss and anemia.

32. **(b).** This very important finding, especially if persistent, suggests that the anemia results from chronic gastrointestinal blood loss

33. **(c).** This negative finding is against chronic gastrointestinal blood loss, unless the lesion bleeds intermittently and you are testing only between bleeding episodes (an unlikely event).

34. **(a), (b), (e).** This very significant abnormality may well be the cause of the patient's anemia, but don't be lulled into complacency. There could be two unrelated problems here.

35. **(d).** Bleeding was probably caused by the examination, especially if no lesion was visualized.

36. **(d).**

37. **(a), (b).** This combination is highly suggestive of a bleeding disorder which, in turn, indicates a problem of red blood cell and platelet production (leukemia, myeloma, or marrow failure or replacement).

38. **(a), (b), (e).** Severe anemia can cause cerebral anoxia and mental symptoms. Pernicious anemia is notorious in this regard. This could be a separate problem resulting from one of many possible causes in somebody this age (Chapter 30).

39. **(b).** The possibility of breast cancer metastases to the bone marrow must at least be considered.

40. **(a), (c).** This confirms evident pallor but is against primary anemias like pernicious anemia.

41. **(a), (b).** This suggests pernicious anemia, though it could also be a glossitis resulting from concomitant vitamin deficiencies (B or folic acid).

42. **(c), (d).** This is probably irrelevant, though it may be considered a pertinent negative if renal failure is a diagnostic consideration.

43. **(b), (e).** If uremia is the cause of the anemia, hypertension may well be part of the renal disease complex; on the other hand, it may be a separate problem.

44. **(b).** This finding suggests hypothyroidism (not one of the originally proposed diagnoses).

45. **(b).** Severe renal disease and uremia become possibilities; as always, this too could be a separate problem.

46. **(c).** This includes many highly pertinent negatives. The *absence* of splenomegaly, lymphadenopathy, evidence of weight loss, a rectal lesion, abnormal fundi, neurologic abnormalities, and uremic breath are all points against some of the speculative diagnoses.

47. **(c).** This normal finding is against severe chronic hypertension associated with chronic renal disease and also against primary anemias where fundal abnormalities are common.

48. **(e).** This is probably a separate problem and unrelated to the anemia. Long-standing diabetes with its associated renal failure is a long shot.

49. **(b), (e).** These are very possibly associated with the posterolateral sclerosis of pernicious anemia, though such paresthesias have many other causes and could represent another problem, especially at this age.

50. **(c).** This finding makes chronic lymphatic leukemia unlikely and also signifies the absence of metastatic cervical lymphadenopathy.

Again, note that each bit of information is evaluated in its own context. Usually, however, we deal with entire clusters of data which tend to reinforce each other. For example, the presence of clues 3, 5, 7, 11, 16, 26, 28, 32, and 40 all together weigh very heavily in favor of gastrointestinal cancer. But clues 4, 6, 14, 17, 22, 26, 27, 33, 38, and 41 would be almost conclusive for pernicious anemia.

In fact, only three or four of these clues in a patient would heighten your suspicion. And as each new clue is added you are building a weight of evidence for the diagnosis. With the appearance of each positive clue you increase the likelihood ratio of $D:\bar{D}$. (Recall that D signifies a suspected disease, and $\overline{D}$ represents the absence of the suspected disease or the presence of another disease).

Patient with Chest Pain. In a *52-year-old man with severe substernal pain for 3 hours,* the first and foremost consideration is acute myocardial infarction. But also included in the differential diagnosis are acute pericarditis, dissecting aneurysm, and pulmonary embolus. Esophageal pain (spasm or esophagitis) and acute cholecystitis are more remote speculations.

1. **(a)**. While atypical for coronary chest pain radiation, it is highly specific when it occurs.
2. **(a), (c)**. Usually coronary artery thrombosis is preceded by one or more shorter episodes of pain. No previous pain suggests possible other causes.
3. **(a)**. This sounds very much like angina pectoris terminating in myocardial infarction.
4. **(a), (b)**. While not typical for angina pectoris, this may represent variant angina which may also terminate in a myocardial infarction.
5. **(d)**. There is no relationship. If you stretch hard, you might relate analgesic use to gastric hyperacidity and esophageal reflux.
6. **(d)**. Even if there is associated hypertension, which can predispose to myocardial infarction or aortic dissection, nosebleeds are probably not related to hypertension.
7. **(b)**. Early paternal death might signify hereditary coronary artery disease.
8. **(b)**. Parental diabetes may indicate subclinical diabetes in the son or an increased incidence of coronary artery disease even in the absence of diabetes.
9. **(c), (d)**. This is arguable. Playing daily tennis implies great exercise capacity without the production of angina. These implications may not be accurate. You might reasonably expect the patient to have had some prior angina on exertion if he were presently having a myocardial infarction. On the other hand, the absence of symptoms suggests this is not

an infarction, and it could be regarded as a pertinent negative.

10. **(d)**. This is irrelevant unless we have discovered a "zebra" who has aortic valve endocarditis with coronary embolization.
11. **(a), (b)**. Nausea and vomiting can occur with any severe visceral pain, but acute cholecystitis increases in likelihood.
12. **(d)**.
13. **(d)**. However, he may have diabetes, obesity, or hyperlipidemia but may not have received or heeded medical advice.
14. **(b)**. This is a definite risk factor for coronary artery disease.
15. **(b)**. This too is a risk factor for coronary artery disease, but it also contributes to aortic dissection.
16. **(e)**.
17. **(d)**. This is irrelevant unless you subscribe to the theory that "high-pressure work" causes coronary disease or hypertension.
18. **(c)**. This is a point against sustained severe hypertension.
19. **(b)**. Not only is hypertension a risk factor for two possibilities, but the fact that it is still elevated bears diagnostic, prognostic, and therapeutic implications.
20. **(a)**. Hypotension with a low pulse pressure indicates a potentially catastrophic illness (infarction or dissection).
21. **(b), (c)**. This may represent a drop from a previously high pressure, or it may signify normal pressure and tend to discount but certainly not exclude infarction or dissection. Check both arms!
22. **(c)**. This is against aortic dissection.
23. **(a)**. This is strongly suggestive of aortic dissection and signifies partial occlusion of blood supply to one arm (unless this differential preexisted).
24. **(a)**. This finding bespeaks a severe illness like infarction or dissection (or even pancreatitis).
25. **(c)**. This is against a catastrophic illness, but pulmonary embolization, myocardial infarction, and dissecting aneurysm may exist even though evidence of critical illness (shock, hypotension, clammy skin) is lacking.

26. **(b), (d).** This is probably irrelevant, though prolonged leg dependency predisposes to venous thromboembolism.
27. **(e).**
28. **(b), (e).** None of the mentioned hypotheses cause jaundice early. Acute cholecystitis with complications, pancreatitis (not hypothesized), and pulmonary embolism (with infarction) can all produce varying degrees of jaundice, but not within 3 hours.
29. **(e).**
30. **(a), (b).** This is a sensitive clue in myocardial infarction.
31. **(a), (b).** If not present before, it suggests infarction with papillary muscle dysfunction and mitral regurgitation.
32. **(a), (b).** This indicates probable myocardial infarction with left ventricular failure, unless the rales have been long present from smoking, chronic bronchitis, etc.
33. **(d).**
34. **(c).** This is a pertinent negative for pericarditis and cholecystitis but is consistent with other diagnostic possibilities.
35. **(a), (c).** Fever on admission suggests pericarditis or cholecystitis but is against other predications. Fever occurs 12 to 24 hours later in myocardial infarction and often not at all in pulmonary infarction or aortic dissection.
36. **(a).** This indicates pericarditis. The friction rub of myocardial infarction occurs 1 or more days later.
37. **(c).** This finding is against pericarditis, though the clue does not have high sensitivity.
38. **(b).** Swelling may point to leg vein thrombosis with pulmonary embolization; otherwise it is not related to the other possibilities.
39. **(a), (b), (e).** This can be seen with retrograde dissection causing aortic valve malfunction and regurgitation, but it may represent a preexisting valvular problem that is associated with decreased coronary blood flow, ventricular hypertrophy, relative coronary insufficiency, etc.
40. **(e).**
41. **(b).** Most calves are tender if squeezed, but you must consider thromboembolism again (even though this is a low sensitivity, low specificity clue).
42. **(a).** Dyspnea argues for pulmonary embolism or myocardial infarction with left ventricular failure.
43. **(a), (e).** The wide pulse pressure hints at aortic regurgitation which may be an old problem or, if new, may represent retrograde aortic dissection.
44. **(b), (e).** This represents peripheral vascular disease, a close cousin of coronary artery disease.
45. **(d), (e).** These are not related; emboli rarely come from varicose veins.
46. **(c).** There is no aortic widening, no evidence of congestive failure, or no evidence of pulmonary embolus; but more technologic procedures may be needed to exclude the former and latter possibilities.
47. **(d).** This neither excludes nor confirms a myocardial infarction; more hours are needed before this enzyme increases.
48. **(c).** Electrocardiographic abnormalities are at most 50% sensitive for pulmonary embolism; while the sensitivity is higher if myocardial infarction pain has existed for 3 hours it is not uncommon to wait longer before electrocardiographic evidence of infarction is apparent. So keep looking.
49. **(a), (b), (e).** The abnormalities may have existed for a long time, but if new, myocardial infarction or pulmonary embolus is suspect (the changes may or may not permit you to distinguish one from the other).
50. **(c).** Under these circumstances, myocardial infarction is not likely, though small areas of necrosis may occur without electrocardiographic but with enzyme confirmation. Consider other possibilities more strongly.

If we were to consider clusters of clues rather than individual ones, the presence of clues 3, 7, 8, 14, 15, 20, 24, 30, 32, 42, and 49 virtually guarantees the diagnosis of acute myocardial infarction. Dissecting aneurysm is highly likely if clues 2, 15, 19, 23, 48, and 50 are present. And if findings 26, 38, 41, and 42 are present, the diagnostic pointer swings toward a pulmonary embolus. If only some of the mentioned clues exist, the respective diagnoses are less likely. Additionally, if only a few clues are positive, if there is considerable overlap of clues between two diagnoses, or if some clues are *unexpectedly* positive or negative, further information is needed. This may necessitate more data from the history and physical examination or additional diagnostic tests and procedures.

   Patient with Jaundice. The brief clinical picture suggests the possibilities of: hepatitis, obstruction from stone or cancer (biliary tract or pancreas), metastatic carcinoma to liver, and cirrhosis

1. **(b).** Surgery for possible colon cancer could result in liver metastases 3 years later.
2. **(b).** Recent surgery relates to early liver metastases or to viral hepatitis (if transfusions were given).
3. **(b), (d).** This is probably not related, but inquire further about eating raw seafood (clams) from polluted waters. Hepatitis may result.
4. **(b).** Hepatitis is an occupational hazard of nursing.
5. **(d).** This fact is only a questionable risk for the patient but a definite risk for the diner if the patient has hepatitis.
6. **(b).** Hepatitis is rampant there.
7. **(d).**
8. **(d).**
9. **(a).** Cholestasis with retention of bile salts causes itching.
10. **(b), (d).** Injections can transmit hepatitis, but this is less likely with the use of disposable syringes; "no pep" may be a symptom of underlying serious disease resulting in jaundice.
11. **(d), (e).**
12. **(b).** This drug can cause hepatitis.
13. **(b).** This drug also can cause hepatitis.
14. **(c).** Absence of pain is strongly against common duct stone and favors other

considerations, such as cirrhosis, pancreatic cancer, and hepatitis—although the latter two often also have abdominal pain.
15. **(b).** This suggests diffuse abdominal carcinomatosis.
16. **(b).** This implies cholelithiasis with recurrent cystic duct obstruction and a common bile duct stone.
17. **(b).** This points to recent onset of hepatitis.
18. **(a).** This argues for a longer illness such as upper gastrointestinal tract carcinoma with liver metastases.
19. **(d), (e).** This is hardly consistent with a present illness of jaundice.
20. **(c).** This argues against needle-spread hepatitis.
21. **(c).** This suggests that widespread cancer is not present; it also tends to negate hepatitis, whose victims usually feel sick. It does not rule out an early small obstructing cancer.
22. **(a).** Patients with acute hepatitis and metastatic cancer usually feel sick.
23. **(e).**
24. **(b), (d), (e).** Diabetes is probably another problem and is irrelevant; but remember that pancreatic cancer can present as diabetes, and that oral hypoglycemic agents only rarely cause jaundice.
25. **(b).** Black stools suggest a bleeding gastrointestinal malignancy with associated liver metastases.
26. **(c).** Brown stools deny melena and complete biliary duct obstruction.
27. **(a).** This finding typifies complete obstructive jaundice (stone or cancer or severe hepatitis at its summit).
28. **(b), (e).** The lump may be a separate problem, or it may be the cause of liver metastases.
29. **(b).** "Social drinking" often means heavy alcohol intake and may therefore hint at cirrhosis.
30. **(d).**
31. **(e).** This is irrelevant unless the patient has lung cancer with metastases.
32. **(b).** Abrupt cessation of smoking may

be related to a sudden distaste for cigarettes, often an early symptom of viral hepatitis.

33. **(b)**. Recent anorexia is often the first symptom of hepatitis.
34. **(a)**. This sinister combination argues for widespread cancer.
35. **(a)**. This confirms the chief complaint.
36. **(e)**.
37. **(c)**. In hepatitis the liver is usually enlarged and tender; in cirrhosis it is usually enlarged; in metastatic cancer it may be enlarged and nodular. But in any of these cases it may *not* be palpable. Bear in mind that liver size as judged by palpation is neither highly sensitive nor specific.
38. **(a)**. This speaks for viral hepatitis.
39. **(a)**. This indicates metastatic cancer or posthepatitic cirrhosis; the nodules of alcoholic cirrhosis are small and usually not felt.
40. **(c)**. The spleen may be enlarged yet not palpable; if palpable and therefore much enlarged, cirrhosis with portal hypertension must be considered. This negative clue is probably not very pertinent here.
41. **(c)**. This argues against cirrhosis with ascites.
42. **(b)**. While there are many causes for abdominal distention, in this case ascites from cirrhosis and metastatic cancer are considerations.
43. **(c)**. This is against cirrhosis with portal hypertension.
44. **(c)**. This is against alcoholic cirrhosis; spider nevi are uncommon in posthepatitic cirrhosis.
45. **(d)**. This is a normal finding.
46. **(b)**. This suggests cirrhosis, though it is nonspecific; remember that cirrhosis can exist and cancer be superimposed.
47. **(a)**. This speaks for cholelithiasis with a cystic duct stone obstructing the gallbladder and perhaps another in the common bile duct.
48. **(a)**. This picture is suggestive of cecal carcinoma with liver metastases.
49. **(e)**.
50. **(d)**.

Again, if the order of data accumulation were such that findings 4, 17, 22, 33, and 38 were elicited in rapid sequence, hepatitis would be the leading contender. On the other hand, in the event that findings 15, 22, 25, 34, and 39 were present, metastatic cancer would be most likely. This is how clues are aggregated to form likely diagnoses which, in turn, are confirmed by additional information.

Comment. The three patients just discussed—one with anemia, one with chest pain, and one with jaundice—will be presented in Section Three in a more typical way. There, findings will be evaluated in chunks or in the light of previously acquired data. So rather than regard bits of information separately, the patient problem will be approached in a more realistic style. It is felt that the elementary exercises just experienced are good preparation for real-life patient confrontations.

Decoding Problem Sets

Here is another way to improve your data management skills. The same set of clues occurring in dissimilar population subsets can have vastly different diagnostic and therapeutic implications.

Consider first the problem of *headache, confusion, stiff neck, and fever* in a:

1. 2-year-old child who has been sick for 3 days
2. 53-year-old healthy woman who became suddenly sick 24 hours ago
3. 48-year-old man being treated for Hodgkin's disease
4. 19-year-old recent Army recruit
5. 32-year-old woman with known polycystic kidney disease
6. 26-year-old male sewer worker
7. 38-year-old horse rancher in Texas
8. 52-year-old man 5 days postcraniotomy
9. 8-year-old child with running left ear
10. 4-year-old child recovering from measles
11. 18-year-old girl with sore throat and diffuse lymphadenopathy

12. 16-year-old boy with a lengthy preceding upper respiratory infection and who lives in a mouse-infested home

Clearly we are dealing with three possible diseases, each of which has diverse etiologic agents. Yet all can present in the same way. *Meningitis, encephalitis, and subarachnoid hemorrhage are under consideration.* But each of the 12 "initial statements" has certain features that seem to set it apart from the others by virtue of age, occupation, and clinical background. Be cautious! Things are not always what they seem, and one type of meningitis may exist even when you suspect another. However, based on the information given, venture an educated guess of the diagnosis and the specific etiologic agent. Whatever you think, a lumbar puncture will probably be needed in almost all cases.

The diagnoses that initially occur to the author are:

1. *Haemophilus influenzae* type B meningitis—common at this age
2. subarachnoid hemorrhage from berry aneurysm
3. *Enterobacter, Pseudomonas,* or *Listeria* meningitis—patient is immunosuppressed
4. meningococcal meningitis
5. subarachnoid hemorrhage—aneurysms are common in polycystic renal disease
6. leptospirosis—contact with excreta of infected rodents
7. equine encephalitis—even though uncommon
8. *Staphylococcus aureus* meningitis
9. pneumococcal meningitis
10. encephalitis
11. infectious mononucleosis—Epstein-Barr virus
12. lymphocytic choriomeningitis—RNA virion

When given certain hints, we are immediately directed toward a specific microbial diagnosis, but this type of logic, while perhaps most often correct, can lead you astray. The sewer worker can have meningococcal meningitis. The boy living in the mouse-infested home may contract a bacterial meningitis. The suspected subarachnoid hemorrhage may be meningitis and vice versa. And the horse rancher is statistically more apt to have a bacterial meningitis than equine encephalitis, in spite of his occupation.

Now ponder another cluster—*flank pain, fever, and dysuria*—in a:

1. recently married young woman
2. 68-year-old man with 3 years of worsening nocturia and frequency of urination
3. 2-year-old girl
4. Vietnam veteran with paraplegia
5. 36-year-old football player immobilized for months with a body cast
6. 28-year-old woman who is 6 months pregnant
7. 38-year-old executive taking large quantities of milk and absorbable alkali for chronic indigestion
8. 52-year-old woman with bone pains, constipation, and known bilateral renal calculi

The small amount of critical clinical information given in each circumstance enables you to predict the diagnosis and underlying pathophysiology with reasonable accuracy. Additional particulars are needed to confirm your impression and guide your treatment in each case. Urinary tract infections (acute cystitis and acute pyelonephritis) exist in all, but the causes vary:

1. possibly related to excessive sexual activity
2. enlarged prostate gland with obstruction and retention
3. ureterovesical reflux or other congenital defect
4. neurogenic bladder or nephrolithiasis (immobilization)
5. renal calculi resulting from prolonged immobilization
6. ureterectasis and pyelectasis of pregnancy
7. calculi caused by excessive intake of milk and alkali for possible duodenal ulcer

8. calculi in a patient with probable hyper-parathyroidism (stones may predispose the patient to infection)

In each instance you must analyze the presentation. See if the age, gender, occupation, geography, or other demographic features influence your impression. Occasionally an additionally stated clue will help you draw a conclusion, and you must therefore seek more data to confirm or reject your hypothesis.

A third problem set to examine is the patient with *fever, malaise, anemia,* and a *heart murmur.* Suppose it occurs in a:

1. 42-year-old woman who had mitral valve replacement 2 months ago
2. 28-year-old woman with a papular rash, diffuse lymphadenopathy, and mild polyarthritis
3. 21-year-old male heroin addict
4. 64-year-old woman with a sore tongue and leg paresthesias
5. 5-year-old child with a large spleen
6. 46-year-old woman with a long-standing mitral diastolic rumble
7. 52-year-old man with large glands in the neck and left axilla
8. 68-year-old man with weakness, weight loss, and indigestion for several months
9. 16-year-old Haitian girl with chronic cough and expectoration
10. 4-year-old underdeveloped cyanotic child

Although all four clues in the stated cluster may be present in each of the ten presentations, in some cases one clue may not be prominent. For example, the fever may be low grade or the murmur slight. Sometimes the murmur may be secondary to the ane-mia and not to the disease. In fact, the murmur may represent an added problem. You must be able to deal with the varied degrees of expression of a clue, with the fact that a clue may not be part of the pathophysiologic cluster, and even with a discrepant clue.

The initial hypothesis in each presentation follows:

1. infective endocarditis on a valve prosthesis
2. sarcoidosis or systemic lupus erythematosus
3. infective endocarditis—*S. aureus* likely
4. pernicious anemia—fever is usually mild, and the murmur is secondary to the chronic anemia
5. acute leukemia—the murmur is secondary to anemia, fever, and/or high flow state
6. infective endocarditis—*Streptococcus viridans* is likely to be imposed on a stenotic mitral valve; atrial myxoma is another consideration
7. lymphoma is likely—the murmur is not explained
8. gastrointestinal carcinoma with liver metastasis—murmur not clearly explainable
9. pulmonary tuberculosis—the murmur may represent another problem
10. infective endocarditis—superimposed on a serious congenital heart defect

It is a simple matter to originate many other problem sets revolving about such clusters as: cough, expectoration, and chest pain; enlarged liver and jaundice; polyuria and polydipsia; and so forth. Then postulate the various brief clinical settings in which such groups of clues may occur, and you have organized *a lively medical rap session.*

Section Three

Problem Solving in Action

Chapter 14. Hematologic Problems

Chapter 15. Endocrine Problems

Chapter 16. Cardiovascular Problems

Chapter 17. Pulmonary Problems

Chapter 18. Gastrointestinal Problems

Chapter 19. Renal Problems

Chapter 20. Electrolyte Problems

Chapter 21. Gynecologic Problems

Chapter 22. Musculoskeletal Problems

Chapter 23. Neurologic Problems

Chapter 24. Multisystem Problems

Section Three

Introduction

Now we turn our attention to problem solving in action with a detailed analysis of 65 common patient presentations, using the techniques described in Section One.

These cases have been carefully selected and planned so that they comprise a *core of presentations* as well as a *core of knowledge.* A single mode of patient presentation requires the consideration of many diseases for its resolution. "Swollen abdomen" needs a knowledge of cardiac, renal, hepatic, and malignant diseases. To solve "dyspnea on exertion" you must know about anemia, as well as cardiac and pulmonary failure.

Perhaps we are being presumptuous in speaking of "cores," since the term is not clearly definable and no two teachers or clinicians agree on which are the principal problems encountered in medicine. In fact, the delineation of a core of medicine has defied curriculum planners for years. The words "nucleus," "essentials," and "basics" beg the question.

The dictionary defines core as "the central part of the fleshy fruit containing the seeds"; or "the central, innermost or most essential part of anything." I prefer to define a "core of presentations" as "the common ways in which patients present to the physician." On the other hand, a *core of knowledge* is the information needed about commonly seen and important diseases. This core must be stored in the brain ready for instant recall, in contrast to the fleshy part of the fruit which can be gotten from notes, books, references, or persons.

Why the Need for a Core? Five hundred years ago a renaissance man could know all of medicine, architecture, and astronomy—along with a panoply of other arts and sciences. Fifty years ago a physician could know all of medicine. But today, with medical literature proliferating exponentially, the knowledge base doubles every 5 to 10 years and former feats are no longer possible. The memorization of a 2000-page textbook of medicine is an exercise in futility. It is hard to do, it is not patient-oriented, medicine keeps changing, and texts are partially obsolete even when first published. Moreover, the half-life for brain-stored knowledge is only a few years at best, and, in addition, the average brain cannot possibly store enough information to solve all problems.

Interpretation of "core" will vary with the subset of health care provider and receiver. Primary care physicians who manage heart disease need to know about coronary disease, heart failure, aortic and mitral valve diseases, hypertension, and a few arrhythmias. That should take care of 90 to 95% of cardiac patients seen. The rest can be researched or referred for consultation. Renal failure, stones, hematuria, and infection account for the bulk of renal problems encountered; go to the references for the rest. And so on for each group of diseases.

If you work in a veterans' hospital, a knowledge of coronary disease, hypertension, heart failure, alcoholism, cirrhosis, chronic obstructive lung disease, diabetes, and ulcer should suffice for a high percentage of patients.

Anxiety, depression, obesity, hypertension, diabetes, minor gastrointestinal disturbances, and simple diseases of the skin, eye, ear, nose, and throat will account for 70 to 90% of adult patients seen in office practice. In "free clinics," psychosocial problems (venereal disease, contraception, and drug abuse) predominate. For the specialist, the spectra are totally different.

Now for the Medical Student! Once teacher and student have accepted the fact that it is impossible to learn all of medicine in 4 years, the question is "how much?" Shall the student learn only about the patients he sees? Only what is common? That which teaches and exemplifies basic pathophysiology? Hospital problems? Mainly ambulatory care? Enough to pass? Certainly there is no need to learn all 18 causes of splenomegaly or the 10 causes of eosinophilia. Yet he should definitely be expected to know the pathophysiology and clinical manifestations of congestive heart failure and diabetes mellitus. The third-year clerk in medicine goes through 12 to 14 weeks of fear and anxiety, not knowing what is expected of him at this stage.

Therefore we propose that he learn common presentations, common diseases, problem-solving techniques, and where to get more information. Then he is ready for *front-line medicine*, since most patient presentations are simply and easily solved; only a few need more detailed information, which can usually be gleaned on the job. Those patients who are assigned directly to the student should be known and understood to the *n*th detail—their disease processes, rationale for studies and treatment, current status, and therapy.

The contents of this section should serve as a good nucleus. Additional reading, patient care, teaching rounds, and work rounds are the outer rings which complete the atomic structure. Put another way, if the material presented in this book is learned, the reader will know the bulk of common clinical presentations, much about frequently seen diseases, how to process data, and how to solve problems.

In this section, all of medicine is divided into 11 modules—renal, endocrine, pulmonary, neurologic, etc—and a number of patients are presented for problem solving in each one. If we eliminate the rare "once in a practice" diseases, patients with problems

related to these modules present to the physician in a finite number of ways.

For instance, in cardiology, patients present in only seven or eight ways. In pulmonary disease, there may be six or seven modes of presentation to the physician, each of which can be caused by a varying number of diseases. In each module we have tried to include as many logic discussions (problem-solving sessions) as there are common modes of presentation. This is easily done in some divisions of disease, but it is more difficult in others where there can be very many presentations. In the latter instance the most common, and sometimes those with the most teaching potential, were sought.

Certain modules, such as dermatology, ophthalmology, and otolaryngology, have not been included, since many more pages would be needed and since problem solving in these fields (with a few exceptions) usually does not require the detailed analysis and synthesis used elsewhere. In these three specialties, straightforward anatomic approaches are often used, and what you diagnose is usually what you see.

Infectious disease, immunologic disease, and oncologic disease have been included in the various other modules, so they were not given separate chapters. Each of these three overlaps into all the other disease systems.

The last chapter in this section consists of case studies which cross modular boundaries, which involve multisystem diseases, or whose pathophysiology may originate in any one of several systems.

Individual logic sessions are presented in a "think along with me" manner, whereby data and logic are alternately interspersed. This method was chosen because it simulates what goes on in the physician's mind as he gathers each new bit of information and, furthermore, because it is easier to understand serialized reasoning than a lengthy discussion following a complete case presentation. The reader can block out the intermittent logic and compare his own data interpretation with that of the author.

By the iterative process of following the data-logic sequence portrayed in each case, and by then identifying the strategems used, you can begin to solve problems in much the same way.

An examination with detailed answers follows most of the logic sessions. This is designed not only to test comprehension of concepts in the case discussions, but also to enlarge on the information base and teach additional material that could not be covered in the data and logic already presented. Try to supply your own answers before reading those of the author.

If you refer to this book's "Introduction," many pages are devoted to "How to Use This Book." There the reader is strongly urged to participate in the self-evaluation exercises scattered throughout Section Three and to read more about each case.

This book is patient presentation-oriented rather than disease-oriented, and since it deals mainly with problem solving, each case discussion dwells only lightly on basic physical diagnosis and pathophysiology (which the reader should already know). If he does not, possibly unfamiliar items like S_3, blood gases, and T_3RU can be relearned in lecture notes or standard textbooks. To get the most out of each case discussion, a review of such items is recommended.

At the conclusion of *the first case study in each module,* you will note a list of subjects that should be reviewed or learned in order to acquire a knowledge base sufficient for this problem in all of its ramifications ("Problem-Based Learning"). But for other cases, the reader should devise his own list of related material to be reviewed in a standard textbook of medicine and in a specialty book. If more information is needed for a case presentation or for more detailed study, several recent review articles on the subject should be selected from the *Index Medicus.* For symptoms and signs that you may not recall, or about which you may need to know more, refer to a medical dictionary or a textbook of physical diagnosis.

In addition, a *"Suggested Readings"* list follows every logic session. Each list is designed to furnish references which elaborate on the didactic information discussed in the case study. Following most references there is a brief notation of their contents and why they were chosen; in others, the title is self-explanatory.

Generally, a reading list is composed of one or two *subspecialty* textbook references, a reference of historical or classic significance, and a number of other readings that bear on interesting facets and subheadings of the major subject, plus articles that are especially tuned to recent diagnostic advances and new concepts. Almost all references are from the 1980s, some as current as 1985. But for a brief didactic overview of each subject, you may wish first to consult your favorite textbook of surgery or medicine. There are three or four of each. Take your pick. Then proceed into the "Suggested Readings" list as deeply as you wish or must.

Rare diseases are usually not detailed in the logic sessions or are perhaps only mentioned in passing. Further information on such diseases may be found in standard textbooks. Complete descriptions and details of the common diseases are not included either; here, too, textbooks and cited references may be utilized for additional information.

Different techniques of problem solving are used for each case presentation. Most case discussions include a "Comment" in which the particular problem-solving methods, decision points, and pathways of logic used in that case are noted. The reader may try his hand at identifying the techniques used in each case before reading the editor's commentary.

One Last Word of Caution! The reader should not get the impression that all problems are solved as neatly and smoothly as those described here. Some sick hospitalized patients defy accurate diagnosis for long periods of time in spite of and even because of diagnostic measures. These patients are usually polypathic, replete with complications, and often made more undiagnosable by iatrogenic problems. The solution may come only with an autopsy—or perhaps not even then. (*P. C.*)

Chapter 14

Hematologic Problems

While the examination of the stained blood smear is usually the keystone of problem solving in the patient with a blood disease, the history, physical examination, and a profusion of other laboratory tests play an important role too. Many aspects of the patient profile and family history are especially significant, for the key clue may be found in the patient's occupation, race, habits, medications, nutrition, environment, or the presence of a similar illness in his family.

Exposure to marrow toxins in the environment or at work is probably more common than realized; this may include food additives, paint solvents, and insecticides. House painting used to carry the risk of lead poisoning, also seen in battery workers; and marrow depression caused by benzene-like solvents is well known. High blood lead levels and lead intoxication in ghetto children result at least in part from eating old varieties of lead-containing paint that peel from the walls. Cases of aplastic anemia for which a cause is never found may follow undetected exposures to as yet unrecognized marrow depressants.

As for race, Mediterranean anemia in those from the eastern basin, sickle cell anemia in blacks, and pernicious anemia in Scandinavians are well-recognized relationships. Family history may offer the key clue; hemoglobinopathies, congenital hemolytic jaundice, hereditary telangiectasia, and familial polyposis may each account for anemia as well as a host of other related clinical manifestations. The patient who tells you

his siblings or parent are also anemic may have one of these inherited diseases.

A careful history of drug ingestion is critical. The list of drugs which can cause depression of one or all three cellular components of marrow could fill a page. But the ones to be regarded with particular concern are the anticonvulsants, gold, chloromycetin, sulfonamides, propylthiouracil, and quinidine; these are all in common usage. Peculiar eating habits should alert you to the possibility of iron deficiency anemia; the ingestion of large quantities of ice, clay, or starch (a condition referred to as pica), once thought to be the cause of this form of anemia, is now considered to be its result. And, last, diet may also play an important part in deciding on the cause for an anemia. Taking a nutritional history that seeks iron, B_{12}, or folic acid deficiency due to inadequate intake demands that the history taker know the foods wherein those elements are found. Iron is present in spinach, beef, milk, eggs, chicken, and liver; B_{12} is found in glandular organs, muscle, eggs, cheese, and milk; folic acid is contained in green vegetables and organs like liver and kidney.

The presenting pictures of patients with blood diseases are multiple, but only a handful are commonly seen. First, there is the patient who has no symptoms but is found to have anemia, polycythemia, or a white blood cell abnormality during a routine examination or in the course of an unrelated illness. Next, perhaps the most common symptomatic presentation is that of anemia—weakness and easy fatigability—a picture that can be caused by many diseases and pathophysiologic mechanisms. Acute and chronic anemias present differently, and it is important to realize that anemias are most apt to be manifestations of some underlying disease, such as carcinoma of the colon or duodenal ulcer. "Anemia" is a finding, not a diagnosis, and is not commonly a disease in and of itself. Repeated infections may reflect neutropenia or a γ-globulin disorder. Then there is the common complaint of "I bruise easily"; it needs careful evaluation. A sizable percentage of women have this symptom; it usually turns out to be of no consequence. But spontaneous bruising, with a history of prolonged bleeding after tooth extractions or after minor injuries, may indeed signify a serious coagulopathy. In this instance a good history is usually more reliable than many laboratory tests.

Other less common presentations must be mentioned. The patient notices enlarged lymph nodes or a left upper quadrant mass which may be an enlarged spleen. Bone pains from myeloma, leukemia, or lymphoma may bring other patients to your office. Chronic leg ulcers, hemolytic crises, postural syncope, sore tongue, neurologic symptoms, and dysphagia may each be the initial problem. But be especially careful of the patient who has latent coronary disease, peripheral vascular disease, chronic obstructive pulmonary disease, cerebral ischemia, or heart failure, whose symptoms of angina, claudication, dyspnea, or lightheadedness may surface because of a gradually developing anemia. His complaint may be referable to the underlying chronic disease, not to the anemia or to the disease causing the anemia.

The subset of the physical examination concerned with blood diseases includes evidence of pallor; jaundice; smooth and/or red tongue; large lymph nodes; splenomegaly; hemorrhages in the fundi, skin, and mucous membranes; tender bones; manifestations of high cardiac output; and neurologic evidence of posterior and lateral column disease.

The following are some common clusters and their usual causes. Anemia, bone pains, and uremia often signify multiple myeloma; anemia and jaundice suggest hemolytic anemia or metastatic cancer; anemia and weight loss often result from malignancy; anemia and bruises mean aplastic anemia or leukemia; anemia plus splenomegaly points to leukemia, lymphoma, or hemolytic anemia; anemia plus gallstones hints at hemolytic anemia; and anemia, jaundice, and severe abdominal pain suggest a hemolytic crisis.

New technology has made it possible to determine the size and nature of histopathologic abnormalities that may exist in the liver and spleen. This can be helpful in hematologic diagnosis.

Controversy persists in the staging of lymphomas. Some experts still resort to exploratory laparotomy and lymphangiography, while others are content with scanning techniques. With the better understanding of lymphocyte populations, the nosology of lymphomas is undergoing revision.

Classic blood studies have not changed appreciably in the past decade. Exceptions are the *plasma ferritin concentration* that is used to reflect total body iron stores accurately, and the *mean corpuscular volume* (MCV) that is now thought to be the most significant index for classifying anemias. In fact, the MCV and the *reticulocyte index* are the two important determinants in the algorithmic pursuit of an anemia's cause.

Anemias that have been caused by new technology and new fads must be mentioned. The mechanical damage of red blood cells by aortic and mitral prosthetic heart valves can result in hemolytic anemia. Some joggers and marathon runners have also been found to develop a mechanical hemolytic state. And hosts of new anticancer drugs have caused a profusion of blood diseases. These diseases include those resulting from depression of one or more marrow elements and also some that result from abnormal marrow stimulation and the production of leukemias. (*P. C.*)

Case 1
Weakness and Joint Pains
DAVID A. SEARS, M.D.

DATA A 46-year-old woman comes to your office complaining of increasing fatigability and a "tired and weak" feeling for the past 3 or 4 months. She has had rheumatoid arthritis (RA) for 8 years and her joint symptoms have been controlled by 12 to 16 tablets of aspirin/day.

LOGIC Symptoms of weakness and fatigue are so common and nonspecific that, taken alone, they provide little guidance. More details are needed. Is the patient tired immediately on arising in the morning, or does fatigue increase throughout the day? Fatigue on arising is often psychoneurotic in origin, while fatigue coming on after some work or activity tends to be organic. Have her activities actually changed as a result of the symptoms? For example, does she still clean house, work at her job, and pursue her hobbies? One must ask questions to distinguish between weakness, shortness of breath, and tiredness, which are different symptoms with varied implications, but which may be used interchangeably by patients describing how they feel. In the present patient, with a known chronic disease of fluctuating severity, you need information about the activity of her RA.

DATA The patient says she has had no severe pain, tenderness, redness, swelling, or heat in her joints for 2 years while on regular doses of aspirin. She has some mild morning stiffness in her metacarpophalangeal and proximal interphalangeal joints and occasional soreness in the wrists, elbows, and knees. In answer to your step-by-step questions about her level of daily function, she indicates that she has continued to carry on most of her activities as a housewife and mother but with less energy and endurance than in the past. She finds she must stop and rest during her household chores, and by the end of the day she is exhausted. What limits her is fatigue more than true muscular weakness or shortness of breath. You are unable to detect any significant changes in her environmental or living situation. Her husband and two children, ages 17 and 13, are in good health and she describes no tension in her relationships with them or others. She denies crying spells or feeling "blue" and has had no anorexia, weight loss, or insomnia.

LOGIC At this point you have no positive indications of emotional causes for her symptoms and no evidence of increased activity of her arthritis, though these cannot yet be ruled out as causes for her symptoms. You simply need more information and proceed to complete your data base.

DATA Past history reveals no additional pertinent information. System review is negative except for the following. For several years she has noted some mild postprandial nausea and eructations after eating fried or greasy foods and therefore avoids them. Six months ago she had a 1-hour episode of dull right upper quadrant pain. In addition, she sometimes experiences midepigastric and substernal burning pain relieved by an antacid. She denies other abdominal pain, vomiting, jaundice, and black or tarry stools. There has been occasional urinary frequency and nocturia once or twice a night. For the past year her menstrual periods have been irregular. They have occurred at shorter or longer intervals than previously, and many have been prolonged with heavier than normal flow. She has had occasional hot flushes and assumed that she might be entering the menopause. Family history reveals that she is of Italian extraction and that one sister was mildly anemic and was told she had Mediterranean anemia.

On physical examination, the patient is a slightly obese white woman whose vital signs are: pulse 76, regular; BP 115/70; respirations 14/minute; T 37 C. Slight pallor of the skin, tongue, and palms is noted. The skin otherwise, head and neck, heart and lungs, and pelvic and rectal examinations are normal. There is no stool in the rectum for guaiac testing. No lymph nodes are palpable. The abdomen is mildly obese but there is no tenderness, masses, or organomegaly. Slight swelling of the proximal interphalangeal joints gives her fingers a fusiform appearance, and there is some thenar and hypothenar atrophy but no ulnar deviation or subluxation. The wrists and knees too are slightly swollen but there is no restriction of joint motion. Neurologic examination is normal, peripheral pulses are normal and equal, and there is no ankle edema.

LOGIC   You decide to obtain routine laboratory studies to complete your data base: blood count, urinalysis, chest x-ray, ECG, and also an erythrocyte sedimentation rate as a nonspecific test of activity for rheumatoid disease. You also schedule an oral cholecystogram because of fatty food intolerance, the episode of abdominal pain, and your suspicion of gallbladder disease. While you prefer ultrasound for this purpose, the sonographer is on vacation. The cause of her presenting symptoms is not at all apparent thus far, though her slight pallor is leading you toward an organic cause.

DATA   Laboratory results are: hematocrit 28%; hemoglobin 7.0 g/dl; red blood cell (RBC) count 4.0 million/mm^3; MCV 70 μ^3; mean corpuscular hemoglobin 17.5 pg; mean corpuscular hemoglobin concentration 25%; white blood cell (WBC) count 11,200/mm^3 with 2% bands, 76% segmented neutrophils, 18% lymphocytes, and 4% monocytes. Platelets are described as "adequate." The urinalysis shows specific gravity 1.016, pH 5, glucose and protein negative, and microscopic examination of the spun sediment reveals six to eight WBCs/high power field and no RBCs or casts. The sedimentation rate (Westergren method) is 62 mm/hour.

The chest x-ray and ECG are normal; oral cholecystogram fails to visualize the gallbladder on the first try, but with a double dose of contrast material two radiolucent stones can be seen. When the anemia is established, you immediately examine the blood smear and order a reticulocyte count. The blood smear shows moderate anisocytosis of red cells with predominant microcytosis and also mild to moderate hypochromia. No abnormal WBCs are seen, and platelets appear to be present in increased numbers. The reticulocyte count is 2.2%.

LOGIC   Your suspicion of gallbladder disease is confirmed, and this may explain at least some of the gastrointestinal (GI) symptoms. The sedimentation rate is moderately elevated, but you are unsure if this is due to her RA, which by history and physical examination seems inactive. The urinary symptoms, low-grade pyuria, and slight leukocytosis warrant a search for urinary tract infection and you order a urine culture.

The anemia is one of underproduction of red cells, as indicated by the calculated reticulocyte index of less than 1 ($2.2 \times 28/45 \times 1/1.85$). The 28/45 fraction corrects for the degree of anemia, and the 1.85 value represents the number of days needed for a reticulocyte to mature into an RBC. These modifications of the reticulocyte count result in a reticulocyte index which measures marrow productivity.

When this index is regarded along with the RBC morphology determined from red cell indices and your personal examination of the blood smear, the anemia can be classified as that of abnormal cytoplasmic maturation (defective hemoglobinization). This immediately suggests a problem in iron metabolism, and your differential diagnosis would include true iron deficiency, the anemia of chronic disorders, sideroblastic anemia, thalassemia minor, and lead poisoning. Let us consider each of these.

Iron Deficiency Anemia. With rare exceptions this is due to blood loss. Menstruating women are often in a precarious state of iron balance and this patient has a history of heavy menses. The GI tract is the other common site of blood loss and must be considered even when another etiology may be present as in this patient. In addition, this lady takes large doses of aspirin and could very well have hemorrhagic gastritis as a result. Examination of stools for occult blood and measurement of the serum iron and total iron-binding capacity are in order. A determination of serum ferritin may be considered in place of or in addition to the measurement of serum iron and iron-binding capacity. The association of unusual appetites (pica) with iron deficiency is sufficiently common to warrant some additional specific questions.

Anemia of Chronic Disorders. This is very common, perhaps the most frequent cause of anemia in hospitalized patients. This patient has a disease (RA) that is often associated with this type of anemia.

Sideroblastic Anemia. This may occur as a hereditary or idiopathic acquired disorder or secondary to other diseases (such as RA). Since it is a disease of excessive iron loading, the serum iron will distinguish it from the above disorders.

Thalassemia Minor. Though world-wide in distribution, it is particularly common in individuals of Mediterranean ancestry. Your patient is of Italian extraction, and there is a history of the disorder in the family. The blood smear does not show target cells or basophilic stippling to suggest thalassemia minor but, with the history, determination of hemoglobins A_2 and F is warranted.

Lead Poisoning. The patient has no history of exposure. She has no gingival lead line. The blood smear shows no basophilic stippling. This diagnosis seems unlikely and need not be pursued further.

The combination of gallstones and anemia makes you briefly consider a hemolytic type of anemia. But this becomes most unlikely when you consider the facts that the reticulocyte index is less than 1 and the anemia has many features suggesting iron deficiency.

DATA Additional history indicates that she does not eat clay or starch, but she likes to chew on ice cubes; for the past 5 to 6 months she has consumed the contents of one or two refrigerator trays of ice daily. Further laboratory data are as follows: urine culture negative; serum iron 39 μg/dl; serum total iron-binding capacity 300 μg/dl; hemoglobin F 1.5% (normal <2%); hemoglobin A_2 3.0% (normal <4.0%). The patient fails to bring in stool specimens as requested.

LOGIC Sideroblastic anemia is excluded by the low serum iron and β-thalassemia minor by the normal levels of A_2 and F hemoglobin; α-thalassemia minor is not ruled out but would not explain the low serum iron. True iron deficiency is strongly suspected on the basis of the low serum iron and normal binding capacity which combine to give a calculated saturation of 10%. The history of pagophagia (ice pica) is also consistent with and seen as a result of iron deficiency. However, she has a chronic inflammatory disease (RA) often associated with the anemia of chronic disorders, and that form of anemia cannot be absolutely differentiated from iron deficiency by the data thus far available. Determination of tissue iron stores will distinguish iron deficiency from the anemia of chronic disorders since storage iron is absent in the former and present in the latter. Iron stores may be assessed indirectly be measurement of the serum ferritin level. It is usually normal or elevated in the anemia of chronic disorders and low in true iron deficiency. Iron stores may be assessed directly by an iron stain of aspirated bone marrow.

DATA The serum ferritin level is 6 ng/ml (normal is usually >10 ng/ml in women).

LOGIC The diagnosis of iron deficiency is established, and therapy with oral ferrous sulfate can begin. However, occult GI bleeding has not been excluded. It must be sought even though there are other explanations for her iron deficiency (menorrhagia and aspirin gastritis).

DATA The patient brings in samples from three stools and two are found to have a 2+

positive test for occult blood. Sigmoidoscopy and an upper GI x-ray series are negative, but the barium enema shows a definite filling defect in the cecum. The patient is taken to surgery and a carcinoma of the cecum is resected.

LOGIC   Statistical probability would suggest that this patient's iron deficiency was due to her menorrhagia or to aspirin-induced gastritis, and the cecal carcinoma was an unexpected finding. However, this patient illustrates the importance of ruling out the serious diagnosis of GI malignancy in a patient with iron deficiency. The elevated sedimentation rate and mild leukocytosis were probably due to the tumor. Carcinoma of the cecum has a notoriously silent onset, often with only intermittent bleeding and iron deficiency anemia, as in this patient. It causes obstruction less commonly than do tumors of the descending or sigmoid colon. It is uncertain whether her presenting complaint of easy fatigue can be attributed directly to her moderate degree of anemia since many people tolerate this much anemia with no symptoms. Her future course will settle the issue.

Several loose ends remain to be tied. You might question why the surgeon did not remove the diseased gallbladder at the same time. His judgment was against doing two major procedures, although many might disagree. This matter will need management in the future. The urine culture was negative, but in view of her previous history of frequency it should be repeated if symptoms recur.

Since several possible causes for iron deficiency anemia were not ruled out in this patient, we have only assumed that carcinoma of the colon was the cause. It may not be so. Should the anemia recur, endoscopy for aspirin gastritis may have to be done. Furthermore, the alleged menopause with increased blood loss is worrisome. Usually menses are diminished. This too could be a source of continuing blood loss, and needs observation and possible dilation and curettage to make sure an endometrial carcinoma is not present.

QUESTIONS

1. If the evaluation of this patient had led to a diagnosis of anemia of chronic disorders due to active RA rather than iron deficiency, the correct therapy would have been:
   (a) parenteral rather than oral iron
   (b) transfusion
   (c) more vigorous treatment of the arthritis
   (d) a multivitamin preparation containing iron, pyridoxine, and folic acid.

2. Aspirin may predispose to GI blood loss for each of the following reasons except:
   (a) a direct effect on gastric mucosa
   (b) interference with platelet function
   (c) inhibition of hepatic synthesis of plasma clotting factors
   (d) production of thrombocytopenia.

3. Assume your patient's barium enema had not disclosed a carcinoma of the cecum. Your next step would have been to:
   (a) treat with oral iron and observe
   (b) do fiberoptic gastroscopy
   (c) start steroids for arthritis
   (d) do a dilation and curettage.

4. Who of the following is/are particularly prone to have iron deficiency:
   (a) a 6-month-old baby who has been fed only milk
   (b) an adolescent girl
   (c) a man with a prosthetic aortic valve which has become partially loosened leading to hemodynamic abnormalities and traumatic hemolysis of red cells
   (d) a man with multiple telangiectases on his face and body.

ANSWERS

1. **(c) is correct.** With control of the underlying disease (RA), the anemia will correct itself. A major mechanism responsible for the anemia of chronic disorders is inability to mobilize reticuloendothelial iron for red cell production. Thus, iron therapy, either by mouth or by injection, is not effective. Transfusion would not be warranted for this patient and would be of transient, if any, benefit for her symptoms. Use of "shotgun" hematinics is never appropriate. Specific diagnosis is the key to therapy for anemia.

2. **(d) is correct.** Aspirin does not produce thrombocytopenia. It does cause gastritis and predisposes to peptic ulcer. Even small doses inhibit the platelet release reaction and, therefore, platelet aggregation and primary hemostasis. (c) is probably rarely of clinical significance, but in very large doses aspirin may have a coumadin-like action and suppress the vitamin K-dependent clotting factors.

3. **(b) is correct.** In the presence of iron deficiency anemia and occult blood in the stool, your

next step would be to consider and rule out hemorrhagic aspirin gastritis, or some other bleeding lesion from the stomach or duodenum. Its finding would necessitate a change in therapy. (d) might be a reasonable answer at this stage, but blood in the stool makes (b) more appropriate. Treatment with iron may be in order, but a cause for the GI bleeding must be discovered if possible. The arthritis seems quiescent and well controlled, so steroids would be a poor choice, especially if there is already demonstrated GI bleeding from an unknown source.

4. **All are correct.** Unsupplemented milk is a poor source of iron, and rapidly growing infants have a large requirement. The adolescent girl has the combined increased iron requirements imposed by rapid growth and menstruation (and may have a deficient diet as well). Chronic intravascular hemolysis may lead to iron deficiency due to loss of iron as hemosiderin and ferritin in the urine. In Osler's disease, the telangiectases are often in the GI tract, too, and may bleed recurrently.

COMMENT This case study emphasizes the importance of finding the precise cause for anemia before beginning treatment. Furthermore, the study is notable for the number of problem-solving techniques used by the author.

First he found a key clue—anemia; the other clues, fatigue and weakness, were too nonspecific to use as a departure point. This was a difficult problem because there were many distracting possibilities, each of which could have caused the anemia but did not. These included RA, aspirin ingestion, indigestion and abdominal pain from a bleeding upper GI lesion, irregular menses, and Mediterranean anemia. Instead, because of unexplained occult blood in the stools and the high incidence of cancer in this age group, the author pressed on to find carcinoma of the colon. This was the probable cause for the anemia, but we are left with another possibility yet to be reckoned with—abnormal vaginal bleeding.

Obviously, some clues were therefore misleading or false positive insofar as the anemia was concerned (e.g. arthritis, family history, indigestion, aspirin). Other positive clues led to the correct diagnoses. Pertinent negative clues demonstrated the inactivity of her arthritis. Principles of cause and effect were considered in the relationship of pica and iron deficiency anemia.

Having established the presence of a problem in iron metabolism, a list of possibilities was constructed, several likely hypotheses were chosen, all but one were excluded, and that one was eventually proven. (*P. C.*)

PROBLEM-BASED LEARNING To get the most out of this seemingly complicated presentation, much reading must be done. There are many facets to this patient's illness about which the reader may need to be reinformed. A thorough study of this case should cover:

1. classification of all anemias by both the RBC indices and the reticulocyte index
2. ability to calculate reticulocyte indices and RBC indices given the necessary data
3. symptoms and signs of various common anemias
4. understanding of the relationship between RA and anemia, and how to determine the activity of arthritis
5. relationship between aspirin ingestion and anemia
6. comprehension of the clinical picture of gallbladder disease
7. knowledge of the clinical features of thalassemia, anemia of chronic disorders, and sideroblastic anemia
8. kinetics of iron deficiency anemia and its relation to chronic blood loss
9. detection of and workup for chronic GI blood loss
10. clinical features of carcinoma of the colon
11. familiarity with the laboratory aspects of an anemia study with special attention to occult blood in the stool, reticulocyte index, RBC indices, and the serum iron, total iron-binding capacity, and ferritin.

It should be clear that a complete study and comprehension of just this one case entails the mastery of a large body of information that goes beyond hematology into the GI tract, the genitourinary tract, and the diseases of joints. Ten or 20 cases like this and you know a lot of medicine.

Suggested Readings

1. Hillman RS, Rinch CA: *Red Cell Manual*, ed 4. Philadelphia, Davis, 1974.
   This excellent manual gives a clear and concise explanation of the physiologic classification of the anemias and the proper approach to diagnosis using the reticulocyte index.
2. Dallman PR, Yip R, Johnson C: Prevalence and causes of anemia in the United States, 1976–1980. *Am J Clin Nutr* 39:437–445, 1984.
   Special attention is given to the two most common causes—iron deficiency and inflammatory disease.
3. Sears DA, George JN: Anemia without reticulocytosis. In Lichtman MA (ed): *Hematology for Practitioners*. Boston, Little, Brown, 1978, pp 21–49.
   A brief, fully referenced review of anemias due to decreased red cell production.
4. Crosby WH (ed): *Iron*. New York, Medcom, 1972.
   A short, readable, well-illustrated monograph covering many aspects of iron metabolism and iron deficiency.
5. Lee GR: The anemia of chronic disease. *Semin Hematol* 20:61–80, 1983.

The mechanisms for anemia in cancer, infection, and inflammation are explored.

6. *Semin Hematol* 19:1–67, 1982.
   An entire issue of this journal (five articles) is devoted to iron deficiency and iron overload.

7. Rowley PT: The diagnosis of beta-thalassemia trait: a review. *Am J Hematol* 1:129–137, 1976.
8. Hansen TM, Hansen NE, Birgens HS, et al: Serum ferritin and iron deficiency in rheumatoid arthritis. *Scand J Rheumatol* 12:353–359, 1983.

Case 2
Bleeding Gums and Bruising

SHIRLEY P. LEVINE, M.D.

DATA A 23-year-old woman comes to the emergency room complaining of bruises over the body and bleeding gums for the preceding 36 hours.

LOGIC The combination of bruising and oral mucosal bleeding suggests a widespread coagulopathy rather than a local process such as trauma or pyorrhea. A careful history is the most valuable diagnostic aid at this point.

DATA The patient has never had easy bruisability, epistaxis, gum bleeding, or bleeding into the joints. Menarche was at age 13 and menses have been normal. The last menstrual period was 16 days prior to admission and was normal in amount and duration. The patient had several dental extractions at age 17 and oozed for 12 to 18 hours thereafter. There has not been excessive bleeding with minor trauma. She has not had surgery or pregnancies. Family history is negative for bleeding disorders.

LOGIC These negative clues strongly suggest an acquired bleeding abnormality. It is important to establish any prior bleeding history and to evaluate carefully the hemostatic response to previous trauma or surgical procedures. You may be worried about her bleeding following dental extraction, but this was only slightly prolonged. Oozing lasting longer than 24 hours, or fresh bleeding occurring after a few days would arouse suspicion of abnormal hemostasis. There-

fore the recent onset of bruising and mucosal bleeding, the absence of any abnormal postoperative bleeding, and the negative family history make a congenital disorder unlikely. The differential diagnosis at this point is broad and includes:

1. Abnormalities of plasma coagulation—i.e. deficiencies of clotting factors or the presence of circulating inhibitors
2. Abnormalities of blood vessels and abnormalities of platelet number or function
3. A combination of both.

DATA On physical examination the patient is a well-developed young woman without pallor or jaundice. Vital signs are normal. Ophthalmoscopic examination is unremarkable. There is oozing of the gingivae with several small hemorrhagic bullae on the buccal mucosa. There is an ecchymosis and oozing in the right antecubital area secondary to a venipuncture, and there are several ecchymoses and multiple petechiae on both lower extremities. There is no palpable adenopathy or splenomegaly. The remainder of the physical examination is normal.

LOGIC Purpuric bleeding (ecchymoses and petechiae) is characteristic of abnormalities of the platelets or blood vessels. Ecchymoses can occur in apparently healthy individuals. They appear without trauma and account for a lifelong history of "easy bruisability." They are especially common as isolated small ecchymoses over the hips and thighs of women ("devil's pinches"). The ecchymoses and petechiae on the extremities can also be seen with vascular abnormalities (allergic vasculitis, meningococcemia, or scurvy). Thrombocytosis, with platelet counts greater than 1 million/mm^3, can be associated with an increased tendency to bleeding, but petechiae would be uncommon. Acquired defects of platelet function rarely cause a profound coagulopathy. In the case of dysproteinemias or uremia, the acquired defects are of insidious onset and are associated with other symptoms of the underlying disease process. The hemorrhagic bullae are nearly specific for thrombocytopenic purpura.

DATA The physician in the triage area had immediately ordered a complete blood count, prothrombin time (PT), and partial thromboplastin time (PTT). Results were as follows: PT 13.2/12.0-sec control; PTT 37.5/32.0-sec control; hematocrit 38%; hemoglobin 12.5 g/dl; red blood cell count 4.2 million/mm^3; white blood count 6700/mm^3; differential normal; platelet count 8000/mm^3.

Review of the peripheral smear confirmed the thrombocytopenia, revealing several large platelets or megathrombocytes. The other blood studies were normal.

LOGIC The normal PT and PTT make a combined clotting factor/platelet disorder unlikely. Liver disease can cause a prolongation of the PT and PTT due to decreased production of clotting factors and thrombocytopenia due to hypersplenism. Disseminated intravascular coagulation (DIC) is the other common cause of multifactorial bleeding and would also usually produce a prolongation of the PT and PTT as well as thrombocytopenia—all due to consumption.

The differential diagnosis of her thrombocytopenia at this point includes:

1. Decreased platelet production due to

ineffective thrombopoiesis, marrow injury, or invasion
2. Increased peripheral platelet destruction, utilization, or pooling
   a. Autoimmune thrombocytopenic purpura as in systemic lupus erythematosus (SLE), drug reactions, or idiopathic thrombocytopenic purpura (ITP)
   b. Peripheral platelet consumption as in DIC or thrombotic thrombocytopenic purpura (TTP)
   c. Platelet pooling due to hypersplenism.

We can eliminate ineffective thrombopoiesis (B$_{12}$ and folate deficiencies) and marrow aplasia because of the normal hematocrit and white blood cell count; pooling due to hypersplenism is unlikely in the absence of a palpable spleen. Even if the patient did have a large spleen (palpable or not), hypersplenism only rarely causes severe thrombocytopenia and clinical bleeding.

It is possible to see thrombocytopenia as the presenting sign of marrow invasion, but, again, this level of thrombocytopenia would be unusual without a concomitant decrease in hematocrit or white blood cell count. That leaves marrow megakaryocyte injury or peripheral destruction/consumption as the best possibility. A bone marrow examination to determine megakaryocyte number should be the next step in the evaluation.

DATA On further questioning, the patient states that she has not been exposed to chemicals or prescription drugs except for birth control pills. She has taken a variety of pills from the local health food store but believes that they contain only vitamins. She has an occasional social drink and smokes one-half to one pack of cigarettes per day.

A sternal bone marrow aspiration was performed and demonstrated normal cellularity, an increased number of megakaryocytes, normal myeloid and erythroid maturation, and no abnormal cells.

LOGIC Even before the bone marrow examination, it was unlikely that this patient had thrombocytopenia due to a decrease in megakaryocytes. She had had no chemical or drug exposure and admitted to only occasional ethanol ingestion. Thrombocytopenia due to bone marrow suppression occurs commonly in alcoholics, but rarely is it this severe.

Few platelets in the blood with many platelet precursors in the marrow tells you that platelets are being excessively destroyed or consumed. You must now evaluate the patient for thrombocytopenia due to increased peripheral consumption or destruction. The lack of clinical evidence for one of the many causes of DIC and the lack of PT/PTT prolongation make you feel that consumption is unlikely. You may still, however, want to obtain a fibrinogen level, thrombin time, and fibrin split product titer to rule it out completely. TTP should be briefly considered. The peak incidence for TTP is from 10 to 40 years of age, and 60% of cases are in female patients. It is characterized by microangiopathic hemolytic anemia, thrombocytopenia, and a fluctuating neurologic state (triad)—and fever and renal failure (pentad)—in most patients. Microangiopathic hemolytic anemia is invariably present at the time of diagnosis of TTP, but you may want to order a reticulocyte count and blood urea nitrogen to dismiss this diagnosis completely.

It is most likely that the patient has antibody-mediated thrombocytopenic purpura. This can be due to drugs (the most common being quinidine), SLE, lymphoproliferative disorders, or it can be idiopathic. You quickly eliminate drugs or lymphoproliferative disorders because of the negative history and lack of lymphocytosis or lymphadenopathy.

DATA   On further questioning, the patient did admit to occasional joint pains but denied swelling or erythema of the involved joints. She was thought to have viral pericarditis at age 21 but has had no further episodes of chest pain. She has no alopecia, butterfly rash, arthritis, or other clues suggestive of collagen vascular disease.

You recheck her urinalysis, which was

said to be normal by the triage doctor, and find that it has two to three white blood cells/high-power field and is otherwise also normal. You order an antinuclear antibody test and lupus erythematosus cell preparation.

LOGIC   This patient had a classic presentation of acute ITP. You may have immediately suspected this diagnosis because ITP is said to be more common than all of the secondary types of thrombocytopenia and has a higher incidence in females than males. But because of the number of other disease processes which can produce thrombocytopenia, you had to take a careful history, perform a complete physical examination, and rely on a variety of laboratory studies. It would have been helpful if there were reliable routine methods to detect platelet antibodies, but these methods are still laborious enough to be restricted to specialized research laboratories.

If the collagen vascular disease workup is negative, the patient will be presumed to have ITP. However, she may develop classic SLE, Hodgkin's disease, or a lymphoproliferative disorder in the future. The thrombocytopenia can precede other manifestations of these diseases, occasionally by several years.

More than 90% of children with acute ITP have a spontaneous remission, but remission is rare enough in adults to warrant prompt steroid therapy. If there is no response to steroids during the initial hospitalization, splenectomy may be indicated.

QUESTIONS
1. If this patient had presented with mucosal bleeding and a lifelong history of easy bruisability, the diagnosis would most likely be:
   (a) von Willebrand's disease
   (b) hemophilia A
   (c) antithrombin III deficiency
   (d) hemophilia B.
2. If you were trying to differentiate coagulopathies on the basis of bleeding characteristics, which of the following would make you favor a deficiency of clotting factors?
   (a) petechiae
   (b) hemarthroses
   (c) multiple superficial ecchymoses
   (d) significant bleeding from superficial cuts.

3. If the patient had been anemic, leukopenic, and less severely thrombocytopenic, you would have had to consider the following diagnosis(es):
   (a) SLE
   (b) folate deficiency
   (c) aleukemic leukemia
   (d) chloramphenicol ingestion.
4. If this patient had not had petechiae on initial examination, and screening studies had demonstrated only a prolonged PTT, what laboratory study would you have ordered next?
   (a) fibrinogen level
   (b) thrombin time
   (c) inhibitor assay (mixing her plasma with normal plasma 1:1 before repeating PTT)
   (d) fibrin split products titer.
5. If this patient were also jaundiced and the gastroenterologists asked you to prepare her for a percutaneous liver biopsy, what would you recommend?
   (a) give several units of fresh frozen plasma and proceed cautiously
   (b) order 6 to 8 units of platelet concentrates and hold them for transfusion if problems occur
   (c) give the patient 10 to 12 units of platelet concentrates and proceed with biopsy
   (d) advise them that percutaneous liver biopsy is contraindicated in this situation because you cannot correct her hemostatic defect and make the procedure safe.

ANSWERS

1. **(a) is correct.** Von Willebrand's disease is an autosomal dominant coagulopathy characterized by both a deficiency in factor VIII and abnormal platelet function. In contrast to hemophilia A and B, spontaneous soft tissue bleeding and hemarthroses are rare. Spontaneous mucous membrane bleeding, including epistaxis, menorrhagia, and gastrointestinal bleeding, is common.

   Both hemophilia A and B are sex-linked coagulopathies. Although they have occasionally been reported in females born to a hemophilic father and carrier mother, this is rare. Antithrombin III deficiency is an uncommon inherited disorder characterized by repeated episodes of thrombosis, not bleeding. Antithrombin III is one of the major plasma inhibitors of activated clotting factors and leads to a hypercoagulable state when deficient in amount.

2. **(b) is correct.** Hemarthroses (spontaneous bleeding into joints) are characteristic of the clotting factor deficiency states but are rare in the disorders of platelets or vessels. On the other hand, petechiae, persistent and often profuse bleeding from superficial cuts and scratches, and multiple small superficial ecchymoses are characteristic of platelet and blood vessel abnormalities. Other characteristics which would make you think of a clotting factor deficiency are deep dissecting hematomas, large and solitary superficial ecchymoses, and delayed or prolonged bleeding following procedures like dental extractions.

3. **All are correct.** Pancytopenia can occur in each of the disorders listed. SLE commonly has depression of one or more cell lines due to autoimmune peripheral destruction. Deficiencies of folate (and B_{12}) result in ineffective hematopoiesis of all three cell lines due to a generalized disturbance of DNA metabolism. Aleukemic leukemia is leukemia presenting as a peripheral pancytopenia without circulating peripheral blasts. Marrow aspiration, however, confirms the presence of leukemia—either the acute myelocytic, monocytic, or lymphocytic variety. If there had been a history of chloramphenicol administration, the presence of pancytopenia would make you worry about a developing aplastic anemia.

4. **(c) is correct.** Without petechiae, you would have seriously had to consider an acquired clotting factor deficiency, not a disorder of platelets and blood vessels. When the initial screening studies reveal only a prolonged PTT, the most likely acquired disorder would be a circulating inhibitor to one of the clotting factors in the intrinsic system. The presence of an inhibitor is demonstrated by a lack of correction of the PTT when the patient's plasma is mixed 1:1 with normal plasma.

5. **(d) is correct.** A patient with severe thrombocytopenia due to peripheral destruction would probably not increase her platelet count with platelet concentrate infusions. These platelets would have the same decreased survival (often a $T_{1/2}$ of only several hours). Patients rarely suffer spontaneous bleeding until their platelet counts are below 20,000/mm³. But even platelet counts in the 60,000 to 80,000/mm³ range can lead to an increase in bleeding complications when patients undergo invasive procedures. Fresh frozen plasma would not have been indicated because the patient has normal levels of plasma clotting factors. Likewise, this would not help the bleeding due to thrombocytopenia.

COMMENT. Coagulopathy is the key clue in this case. Data collection built a pattern of bleeding that could be explained only by an acquired thrombocytopenia, which then became the next key clue. The possible causes for thrombocytopenia were listed, all except one were eliminated by an exclusion process, and that one was then proven by additional data.

Being female makes this patient more likely to

have TTP and ITP; her being female and young makes you lean more toward SLE. To disprove DIC, no cause could be demonstrated nor could any effects of DIC be found ($C{\rightarrow}E_1{\rightarrow}E_2$) (Fig. 4.6). ITP is statistically the most common cause of thrombocytopenia.

This is a straightforward example of problem solving. The author proceeded in a logical orderly way, returned for more historical data as needed, developed a complete differential diagnosis, and then relied heavily on pertinent negative and positive clues to solve the problem—that is, to nearly solve the problem. The results of the last few studies and additional time will take you to the end of this branch where the exact answer lies. (*P. C.*)

Suggested Readings

1. Wintrobe MM, Lee GR, Boggs DR, et al (eds): *Clinical Hematology*, ed 8. Philadelphia, Lea & Febiger, 1981, pp 1045–1157.

   Particularly pertinent are Chapter 45, dealing with "The Diagnostic Approach to the Bleeding Disorders," and Chapter 47, "Thrombocytopenia."

2. Colman RW, Hirsh J, Marder VJ, et al: *Hemostasis & Thrombosis.* Philadelphia, Lippincott, 1982.

   This recently published textbook will become the standard reference for physicians interested in coagulation disorders. Chapter 20 (pp 274–342) is a comprehensive review of "Platelet Immunology" with 561 references pertinent to all phases of immunologic destruction of platelets.

3. Harrington WJ, Minnich V, Hollingsworth JW, et al: Demonstration of a thrombocytopenic factor in the blood of patients with thrombocytopenic purpura. *J Lab Clin Med* 38:1–10, 1951.

   This is the classic paper on immune thrombocytopenia. The authors themselves were the non-thrombocytopenic recipients who were transfused, which makes this one of the unique experimental papers in medical literature.

4. McMillan R: Chronic idiopathic thrombocytopenic purpura. *N Engl J Med* 304:1135–1147, 1981.

   All about the quantitative defects in ITP.

5. Huebsch LB, Harker LA: Disorders of platelet function; mechanisms, diagnoses, and management. *West J Med* 134:109–127, 1981.

   Presents the qualitative platelet defects of function as they relate to von Willebrand's disease, thrombasthenia, drugs, alcohol, etc.

Case 3
Lethargy and Confusion
DAVID A. SEARS, M.D.

DATA   A 78-year-old woman of Italian ancestry is brought to the emergency room by her family because of increasing lethargy and mental confusion. She can provide little medical history, but her daughter reports a gradual decline in her mother's previous good health over the past 3 to 6 months. During this period she spent much of her time sitting in a chair or napping and evidenced occasional memory lapses which the family attributed to old age. An episode of urinary incontinence led them to bring her to the hospital.

LOGIC   These are nonspecific chronic symptoms that suggest deterioration of cerebral function. In a woman her age you consider principally arteriosclerotic cerebrovascular disease but also a host of other causes, such as anemia, uremia, diabetes, cancer, liver disease, cardiac or respiratory disease, and depression.

DATA   Further history from the daughter reveals that the patient has stumbled and fallen two or three times when she has arisen at night to go to the bathroom, but not at other times. Her appetite has been poor, her eating habits erratic, and she has lost 10 lb. She has always abstained from alcohol and tobacco and takes no medications. There is no past history of renal disease, and she has had no polydypsia or polyuria. There have been no significant changes in her living situation. No additional history is immediately available.

LOGIC   The weight loss is worrisome, and you consider the possibility of malignant disease with intracranial metastases to explain the changes in mental function. Falling at night suggests that she depends on her vision to maintain balance. This could simply be "old age." But you should also suspect a defect in one of the other systems that control balance—that is, cerebellar function, proprioception, and the vestibular apparatus. In any case, this history suggests that you will want to check certain portions of the neurologic examination carefully. The absence of past renal disease speaks against uremia but does not rule it out. Diabetes causing the clinical pattern of weight loss and confusion is most unlikely in the absence of severe thirst and frequent urination. No alcohol intake tends to eliminate liver disease.

DATA On physical examination the patient is a slightly confused and agitated, elderly, gray-haired woman. Vital signs are normal. The pulse and blood pressure are not significantly altered when she changes from a supine to sitting posture. Her skin is generally pale and palmar creases are white. You think that the skin and sclerae may be slightly icteric, but you are not sure. The breath is not uremic, fruity, or musty. She has a large ecchymosis on the right thigh from a recent fall.

LOGIC These few simple observations serve to focus your thinking. The normal vital signs speak against cerebral anoxia due primarily to a cardiac or pulmonary cause. The pallor suggests anemia, and the stability of her blood pressure and pulse with changes in posture is against hypovolemia. Thus, if she is anemic it is most likely chronic. The questionable icterus will be important in considering the cause of anemia if present and, of course, raises the possibility of liver disease. In evaluating her ecchymosis, try to decide if it is excessive for the amount of trauma. If it is, you think of thrombocytopenia or coagulation factor deficiencies. Normal odor of the breath is against uremia, diabetic ketoacidosis, and hepatic failure.

DATA The remainder of the physical examination reveals normal retinae, no palpable lymph nodes, normal lungs, a soft nontender abdomen with normal bowel sounds and no masses, and normal extremities. The tongue is red and devoid of papillae. A grade 2/6 nonradiating systolic ejection type murmur is heard at the base of the heart, and a strong apical impulse is felt 1 to 2 cm outside the midclavicular line in the fifth intercostal space. Heart sounds are normal, and the rhythm is regular. The liver edge is felt 2 cm below the right costal margin in the midclavicular line, but its vertical height at this point is 9 cm by percussion. With the patient in the right lateral decubitus position, the tip of the spleen is felt at the left costal margin in deep inspiration. Rectal examination is normal, and the finger specimen of stool is negative for occult blood.

Neurologic examination shows intact cranial nerves, normal reflexes, and no pathologic reflexes. She is oriented to place and person but not to time, has impaired recent memory, and peforms serial sevens poorly. Light touch and pinprick are normally perceived, but vibratory sensation is lost from the iliac crests down; position sense is abnormal in both big toes. The Romberg test is positive with the eyes shut. Stereognosis, rapidly alternating movements, and finger-to-nose test are normal, and there is no nystagmus.

LOGIC You continue to suspect anemia in this patient, and the finding of a palpable spleen is important. It indicates an enlarged spleen and the enlargement must be explained. On the other hand, although her liver is palpable it is not enlarged. The vertical height is thought by some to be crucial in deciding about liver size. The absence of lymphadenopathy indicates that her splenomegaly does not seem to be part of a general process affecting lymphoid organs. Diseases like malignant lymphomas may affect the spleen alone but more commonly involve lymph nodes as well.

Examination of the stool specimen for occult blood is an important part of the evaluation of the anemic patient. While one negative test does not rule out gastrointestinal blood loss as a cause of anemia, it makes it less likely. Your neurologic examination indicates cerebral dysfunction and posterior column disease, but there is no evidence of disease of the lateral columns, cerebellum, or vestibular apparatus. The cluster of anemia, posterior column disease, and atrophic glossitis in an elderly person suggests the diagnosis of pernicious anemia (PA).

DATA A tube of blood is sent to the lab for blood counts, and the Coulter counter print-out reads as follows: white blood cell count 4100/mm³, hematocrit 20%, hemoglobin 6.4 g/dl, red blood cell count 1.6 million/mm³, mean corpuscular volume 125 μ^3, mean corpuscular hemoglobin 40 pg, mean corpuscular hemoglobin concentration 32%. The technician has written in a differential white blood cell count of 48% segmented neutrophils, 44% lymphocytes, 5% monocytes, and 3% eosinophils, and has checked the box by platelets that says "decreased." Urinalysis and blood chemistry measurements (6-test chemistry profile) are normal.

LOGIC Your suspicion of anemia has been confirmed, and attention should now be directed at defining it by mechanism and morphology. For the former, a reticulocyte count will be most useful and should be ordered immediately. For the latter, consider the red cell indices and examine the blood smear. The high mean corpuscular volume indicates macrocytosis. The mean corpuscular hemoglobin concentration shows normal cellular hemoglobin concentration. Both are mean values and do not tell you anything about the degree of variation in cell size and shape. Because of the laboratory's notation about decreased platelets and the patient's questionable icterus, you order a platelet count, serum bilirubin, and liver function tests. An ECG and chest x-ray are also done.

DATA The additional data are as follows: reticulocyte count 4.2%, platelet count 82,000/mm³, serum bilirubin 0.3 mg/dl conjugated, 2.8 mg/dl total, serum glutamic-oxaloacetic transaminase 17 mIU/ml, lactate dehydrogenase 975 mIU/ml (normal < 220), alkaline phosphatase 78 mIU/ml (normal < 125). ECG is normal, and the chest x-ray shows minimal cardiomegaly. On the blood smear there is marked anisocytosis of the red cells with predominance of macrocytes, many of which are oval in shape; some microcytes are seen too. The latter account for a moderate degree of poikilocytosis, as they are irregular and distorted in shape. No immature white cells are seen, but many of the segmented neutrophils have nuclei with four or five lobes, and an occasional "poly" with a six- or seven-lobed nucleus is seen. Platelets appear slightly decreased in number but normal in morphology.

LOGIC When the reticulocyte count is corrected for the patient's anemia and for the consequent early release and prolonged circulation of reticulocytes, you arrive at a reticulocyte index of 1.0. Thus, red cell production has not increased in response to the severe anemia. Impaired red cell production and the abnormalities noted on the blood smear strongly suggest megaloblastic anemia. The term megaloblastic refers to morphologic features of precursor cells in the bone marrow, and examination of aspirated marrow is an appropriate next step.

DATA The bone marrow shows marked megaloblastic changes in nucleated red cells and white cell precursors.

LOGIC The patient has now been proven to have megaloblastic anemia. The ineffective erythropoiesis (death of red cell precursors before leaving the marrow) associated with megaloblastic anemia explains the patient's unconjugated hyperbilirubinemia (due to hemoglobin catabolism) and the very high lactate dehydrogenase (released from destroyed red cell precursors). The mild leukopenia and thrombocytopenia are also characteristic of megaloblastic anemia, and splenomegaly is significant. The heart murmur and slight cardiomegaly may be due to the severe chronic anemia per se.

Except for rare circumstances, megaloblastic anemia is due to B_{12} or folic acid deficiency. These two causes cannot be distinguished by blood counts or morphology of blood or marrow, but the clinical setting in which each occurs is often different and provides clues as to which vitamin is lacking. B_{12} deficiency is almost never due to dietary lack. It results from impaired absorption caused by atrophic gastritis with failure of intrinsic factor secretion (pernicious anemia) or malabsorption due to intestinal disease or surgery. Folic acid deficiency, on the other hand, is usually related to inadequate diet and less often to malabsorption. Alcoholic patients are often folate deficient. In addition, lack of B_{12} may produce a wide variety of neurologic abnormalities, while lack of folic acid rarely or never does.

DATA   Further history from the patient and her daughter reveals that although she had been eating poorly, she did have some meat every day and usually ate a green salad at lunch. The stools were described as loose on occasion but not light-colored, foamy, frothy, greasy, or unusually foul smelling.

LOGIC   The clinical picture strongly suggests classical pernicious anemia. There is no evidence of dietary folic acid deficiency or malabsorption. She has atrophic glossitis, which commonly accompanies the atrophic gastritis of PA, and posterior column disease is one of the common neurologic abnormalities associated with PA. Her cerebral dysfunction may also be a direct result of B_{12} deficiency ("megaloblastic madness") and may account for the weight loss which occurs in only 5% of PA patients. The classical triad of weakness, sore tongue, and paresthesias is present in only a minority of patients. Because PA necessitates lifelong therapy with parenteral B_{12}, confirmation of the diagnosis is important. Several studies may be done:

1. Gastric analysis after pentagastrin stimulation.
2. Serum B_{12} assay.
3. Schilling test for B_{12} absorption. It is important to recognize that the large parenteral dose of B_{12} given as part of the test will render a therapeutic trial impossible and that collection of an accurate 24-hour urine specimen may be difficult in an elderly, confused patient.

4. A therapeutic trial. A proper trial requires two or three baseline observations of the hematocrit and reticulocyte count, daily administration of physiologic doses of the vitamin to be tested, and measurement of the reticulocyte count every other day. A rise in count, usually peaking by 7 to 14 days, signifies a positive test.

DATA   On testing, the patient is found to have histamine-fast achlorhydria, and the diagnosis of pernicious anemia is made. Blood is sent for serum B_{12} assay, but the result will not be available for several days. Treatment with parenteral B_{12} is begun.

QUESTIONS

1. Megaloblastic anemia due to folic acid deficiency may be associated with each of the following except:
   (a) pregnancy
   (b) gastric carcinoma
   (c) Dilantin therapy
   (d) severe hemolytic disease.
2. In addition to classical PA, B_{12} deficiency may result from each of the following except:
   (a) subtotal gastrectomy
   (b) fish tapeworm (*Diphyllobothrium latum*) infestation
   (c) strict vegetarianism for 3 months
   (d) intestinal "blind loop" syndromes.
3. If this patient had had a resection of her terminal ileum 5 years earlier for regional ileitis, the most likely cause of her megaloblastic anemia would have been:
   (a) B_{12} deficiency
   (b) folic acid deficiency
   (c) B_{12} and folic acid deficiency
   (d) iron deficiency.
4. Which of the following is/are associated with pernicious anemia?
   (a) antibodies to gastric parietal cells
   (b) antibodies to intrinsic factor
   (c) antithyroid antibodies
   (d) all of the above.
5. Which of the following abnormalities will be reversed by B_{12} therapy in this patient?
   (a) anemia, leukopenia, and thrombocytopenia

(b) neurologic abnormalities
(c) achlorhydria
(d) all of the above.

ANSWERS

1. **(b) is correct.** Gastric carcinoma occurs with increased frequency in patients with PA, not in those with folate deficiency. Demands on folic acid stores are increased by fetal requirements in pregnancy and by increased cell turnover as occurs with active hemolysis, so folate deficiency may occur in each of these states. Anticonvulsant drugs, particularly Dilantin, may produce folate deficiency by still uncertain mechanisms.

2. **(c) is correct.** Individuals who avoid not only meat but also eggs and milk ("vegans") may develop dietary B_{12} deficiency, but much longer periods of time (years) would be required because of the larger stores of B_{12} in the liver. Even though subtotal gastrectomy leaves some intrinsic factor-producing cells, there is a significant incidence of B_{12} deficiency after removal of most of the stomach. The intestinal fish tapeworm may compete with its host for ingested B_{12} and prevent absorption of the vitamin. Although this rarely occurs outside Finland, there are recent reports of fish tapeworm infestation in the vicinity of the Great Lakes. Changes in the bacterial flora of the small bowel due to stasis or altered circulation of intestinal contents (as may occur in "blind loops") can produce B_{12} deficiency by a similar mechanism in which overgrowing bacteria compete with the host for available B_{12}.

3. **(a) is correct.** B_{12} (linked to intrinsic factor) is bound by receptors and absorbed in the terminal ileum. Because of body B_{12} stores, deficiency may not appear until several years after absorption of food B_{12} stops. Folic acid is absorbed in the proximal small bowel. Iron deficiency does not produce megaloblastic anemia.

4. **(d) is correct.** While it is not clear what pathogenic role the antibodies against parietal cells and intrinsic factor play in PA, they are found in a high percentage of patients. Antibodies against intrinsic factor are fairly specific for PA, while anti-parietal cell antibodies are found in other groups of patients as well. Hypothyroid patients may share some of the autoimmune manifestations of patients with PA, and the two diseases coexist with a frequency that is greater than chance would dictate.

5. **(a) is correct, and (b) may be correct.** The hematologic abnormalities are completely corrected by B_{12} therapy. The neurologic abnormalities of B_{12} deficiency may be irreversible, partially reversible, or completely reversible over long periods of treatment. It is important to remember that neurologic manifestations in B_{12} deficiency are extremely variable. They may be the presenting complaint in a patient with little or no anemia, or they may be entirely absent. The achlorhydria will persist because it is part of the basic pathologic defect of PA—atrophic gastritis.

COMMENT At first, the nonspecificity of symptoms causes you to consider a wide variety of possibilities. As more data are gathered, many diagnoses are ruled out. A cluster of anemia, mental changes, posterior column disease, and atropic glossitis is found, suggesting PA. But anemia becomes the key clue. A few well-chosen studies establish the presence of a megaloblastic anemia; further data and logic result in a diagnosis of PA rather than folate deficiency.

The presence of weight loss and anorexia is a distracter since these are uncommon in PA. Common clues, such as fever, sore tongue, and paresthesias, are lacking, showing that not all classical findings need be present. Palpable splenomegaly is present in fewer than half the patients. Mild neurologic signs may occur in as many as 30% of these patients, though it used to be more common when the disease was diagnosed later.

Probability theory is especially applicable here. The odds are that an elderly lady with megaloblastic anemia who eats adequately, does not drink alcohol, and does not have malabsorption has PA rather than folic acid deficiency. Treatment was initiated on the basis of a strongly presumptive diagnosis, to be confirmed by the not yet reported serum B_{12} level. *(P. C.)*

Suggested Readings

1. Beck WS: Megaloblastic anemias. In Wyngaarden JB, Smith LH Jr (eds): *Cecil Textbook of Medicine*, ed 16. Philadelphia, Saunders, 1982, pp 853–860.
   A clear, current, and concise review of B_{12} and folate metabolism and deficiencies.
2. Wintrobe MM, Lee GR, Boggs DR et al (eds): *Clinical Hematology*, ed 8. Philadelphia, Lea & Febiger, 1981, chap 21, pp 559–604.
   An excellent reference textbook of hematology and a good place to start in looking up any hematologic subject. This chapter covers megaloblastic and other macrocytic anemias.
3. Kass L: *Pernicious Anemia*. Philadelphia, Saunders, 1976.
   This 247-page monograph includes good illustrations of blood and marrow morphology and also reviews the fascinating history of PA.
4. Sullivan LW: Vitamin B_{12} metabolism and megaloblastic anemia. *Semin Hematol* 7:6–22, 1970.
5. Streiff RR: Folic acid deficiency anemia. *Semin Hematol* 7:23–30, 1970.
   The clinical features of folate deficiency are covered in only seven pages.

6. Castle WB, Ham TH: Observations on the etiologic relationship of achylia gastrica to pernicious anemia. *JAMA* 251:514–521, 1984.
   A landmark article first published in 1936 and reprinted in 1984 because of its great impact on medical practice.
7. Lindenbaum J: Status of laboratory testing in the diagnosis of megaloblastic anemia. *Blood* 61:624–627, 1983.
   A concise excellent review of several valuable tests.
8. Hillman RS, Steinberg SE: The effects of alcohol on folate metabolism. *Annu Rev Med* 33:345–354, 1982.
   How alcoholism induces folic acid deficiency.

Case 4
Backache, Weakness, Nosebleeds

JAMES N. GEORGE, M.D.

DATA A nosebleed which had been persistent for more than a day brings this 60-year-old woman to the office. She has noticed intermittent brief nosebleeds for about 1 month, and 1 week earlier an episode of bleeding lasted through the entire day. Epistaxis is a new problem for this patient. She has not noticed any other symptoms suggesting a problem with hemostasis except for a large bruise and hematoma of her left thigh which followed minimal trauma.

The patient has been a healthy, active woman all her life with no previous hospitalizations. However, for the past 4 months she has felt progressively more fatigued, and during the past 2 months she has been unable to do her housework. The only specific symptoms she noted were constipation and backache of the mid- and lower spine.

LOGIC Symptoms of excessive bleeding are not specific. Epistaxis can result from many underlying causes: vascular abnormalities such as telangiectases, increased blood pressure, or a hemostatic abnormality. The recent onset of this problem indicates that it is an acquired, not a congenital, abnormality, making a vascular problem unlikely. Her other symptoms suggest the possibility of a chronic, progressive disease. Weakness, backache, and constipation are all common and nonspecific symptoms. The history that the fatigue was severe enough to change her life style (inability to do housework) makes this a significant problem.

DATA Examination reveals a temperature of 37 C, pulse 90, blood pressure 130/70, and respirations of 18/minute. She appears chronically ill but alert and well oriented. Her neck is supple. The conjunctivae, nasal and oral mucous membranes, and tympanic membranes are pale; the eyegrounds demonstrate venous engorgement and a large left retinal hemorrhage. Examination of the chest is normal. There is an area of tenderness over the lower thoracic spine and another area of tenderness over the midlumbar spine. Heart sounds are regular; no friction rub, murmurs, or gallop rhythm sounds are heard. There are no petechiae or bruises other than the left thigh hematoma, no breast masses, and no lymphadenopathy or hepatosplenomegaly. The neurologic examination is normal.

LOGIC The physical examination rules out hypertension as a predisposing cause for the epistaxis. The presence of the left thigh hematoma and the retinal hemorrhage suggest a hemostatic defect. The retinal vein engorgement is probably related to the retinal hemorrhage and may indicate increased blood volume or increased blood viscosity. The localized areas of tenderness over the thoracic and lumbar vertebrae are a serious concern. Although this could be caused by benign osteoporosis, such discrete and localized painful areas raise the question of a malignant disease.

DATA   Initial laboratory data in the office were: hematocrit 27%, reticulocyte count 3%, white blood cell count 5000/mm^3 with a normal differential. The blood smear revealed normal red blood cell morphology but significant rouleaux formation; white cell morphology was normal, and the platelets were reduced to an average of four per oil field. No abnormally large platelets were seen, and one nucleated red cell was noted. Urinalysis: clear, yellow, specific gravity 1.010, no glucose or protein (by Clinistix), and no cells or bacteria in the sediment.

Chest x-ray showed a lytic lesion in the left clavicle and a compression fracture of the tenth thoracic vertebra. Lumbar spine films revealed a compression fracture of L3. The patient was admitted to the hospital for further evaluation.

LOGIC   These initial data indicated the presence of a disease which may have accounted for the 4 months of chronic progressive symptoms. The anemia was due to marrow failure because the reticulocyte count corrected for the degree of anemia (reticulocyte index) was only 0.9. Also the presence of thrombocytopenia indicated marrow failure.

The other major and alarming abnormality was the presence of vertebral compression fractures and an osteolytic lesion of the clavicle. These bone changes were most likely due to a widespread malignant disease, and the associated hematopoietic abnormalities suggest marrow replacement. Metastatic carcinoma may cause this, and now the normal breast examination assumes new importance. Leukemias and lymphomas do not usually cause osteolytic lesions. Multiple myeloma, a malignant proliferation of plasma cells, is probably the most common cause of widespread osteolytic lesions with bone marrow failure at this age.

Now the back pain may be explained. The anemia, which probably developed gradually, may be less responsible for the fatigue than the underlying chronic disease. The platelet count, estimated from the blood smear to be over 50,000/mm^3, would not be expected to cause significant nosebleeds. The constipation remains unexplained. Because of these abnormalities, blood chemistry measurements and routine coagulation studies were ordered.

DATA   During the next day in the hospital the patient improved with local nose packs for the epistaxis. The laboratory reports showed further abnormalities: erythrocyte sedimentation rate 120 mm/hour, serum creatinine 4.2 mg/dl, total serum protein 9.3 g/dl, serum albumin 2.7 g/dl, serum calcium 11.2 mg/dl, partial thromboplastin time 43 seconds (control 31 seconds), prothrombin time 13 seconds (control 11.5 seconds), and thrombin time 18 seconds (control 10 seconds). It was noted that the clot in the tube collected for serum failed to retract.

LOGIC   Now that the patient's epistaxis was controlled, primary attention was focused on her chronic disease. At this time multiple myeloma was the presumptive diagnosis for many reasons. (*a*) Very high serum globulin could be the myeloma paraprotein. (*b*) Increased globulin in myeloma typically causes marked rouleaux formation of red cells in the peripheral blood smear and an extremely high erythrocyte sedimentation rate. (*c*) Paraproteins can interfere with blood coagulation, most commonly by inhibiting fibrin polymerization. This abnormality is most apparent in the thrombin time and clot retraction. (*d*) Occasionally immunoglobulin (Ig) paraproteins of the non-IgM type can cause plasma hyperviscosity and increased blood volume. A physical sign of this phenomenon is engorgement of the retinal veins and sometimes even "sausage linking" of the veins due to intense rouleaux formation and sluggish circulation. (*e*) Myeloma can be associated with the renal failure indicated in this patient by the high creatinine. This is usually related to renal excretion of the immunoglobulin light chains (Bence Jones protein) resulting from unbalanced immunoglobulin synthesis. The absence of proteinuria on the routine initial urinalysis may only be due to the insensitivity of the routine Clinistix to Bence Jones protein. (*f*) The osteolytic bone lesions are characteristic of multiple myeloma; and (*g*) can be associated with hypercalcemia. Hypercalcemia could account for her constipation. Also, the hypercalcemia can itself cause renal damage. Of interest is that the related disease of macroglobulinemia, with an IgM paraprotein and malignant cells having more the appearance of lymphocytes than plasma cells, is not associated with osteolytic lesions. (*h*) Anemia due to decreased red cell production is characteristic of myeloma, and granulocytopenia and thrombocytopenia are also common. To confirm the diagnosis of multiple myeloma, the studies described below were done.

DATA Further characterization of the hyperglobulinemia was obtained by routine serum protein electrophoresis, serum immunoelectrophoresis, and quantitative serum immunoglobulins by radioimmunodiffusion. Also a random urine sample was tested for Bence Jones protein and a 24-hour urine specimen was collected for total protein measurement, routine protein electrophoresis, and immunoelectrophoresis.

These studies demonstrated a tall narrow "*spike*" of protein in the globulin region of the protein electrophoresis. Immunoelectrophoresis defined this paraprotein as an IgG immunoglobulin with only κ light chains. The homogeneity of the light chains suggested a monoclonal origin of the paraprotein. Quantitative analysis of the immunoglobulins demonstrated: IgG 5300 mg/dl, IgA 47 mg/dl, and IgM 23 mg/dl. The urine test for Bence Jones protein was positive, and the analysis of the 24-hour urine demonstrated 1.4 g of protein which migrated in the globulin region and were identified as κ immunoglobulin light chains. Serum viscosity was 3.8 times the viscosity of water (normal less than 1.8).

Additional x-rays demonstrated multiple osteolytic lesions of the skull. A sternal bone marrow aspiration was performed. Cellularity appeared normal, but megakaryocytes were decreased. On the low-power examination a marked increase in plasma cells, readily identifiable by their deep blue cytoplasm, was immediately apparent. Both erythropoiesis and myelopoiesis appeared morphologically normal under oil immersion, but the percentage of plasma cells was increased to 37% (normal less than 5%). Many of the plasma cells were large with immature-appearing nuclei.

LOGIC These data explained the patient's chronic symptoms and provided an explanation for her presenting symptom of epistaxis; the picture is classic for multiple myeloma. The occurrence of an IgG paraprotein is most common, since myeloma proteins occur with the same relative frequency as the concentration of immunoglobulins in normal serum (i.e. IgG > IgA > IgM $\gg$ IgD $\gg$ IgE). Similarly, κ light chains are more common both in normal IgG immunoglobulins and IgG myeloma paraproteins. A decreased concentration of the other major serum immunoglobulins, IgA and IgM, is common in myeloma. Also, it is presumed that the patient is deficient in normal functional IgG. The urine Bence Jones protein is merely the excreted excess κ light chains synthesized by the neoplastic plasma cells but not assembled into a complete IgG molecule.

These immunoglobulin abnormalities are the hallmark of multiple myeloma, and it is extremely difficult to make this diagnosis without such an abnormality. Seventy-five percent of patients will have a globulin spike on serum protein electrophoresis, and a third of these patients plus almost all of the remainder will have Bence Jones proteinuria. This patient's serum viscosity was abnormal due to the paraprotein but not high enough to cause symptoms. However, whole blood viscosity was abnormal as shown by rouleaux formation.

The marrow aspirate was typical of multiple myeloma. But, as the name of the disease implies, there may be nonuniform distribution of malignant plasma cells. Therefore different results may be obtained by marrow aspiration from different sites.

Benign monoclonal serum immunoglobulin paraproteins occur with increasing frequency with advancing age. These conditions are distinguished from multiple myeloma by the absence of Bence Jones proteinuria, skeletal lesions, and marrow replacement by plasma cells. The disease associated with an IgM paraprotein (macroglobulinemia) is clinically distinct from multiple myeloma with its paraproteins IgG, IgA, IgD, or IgE. The major problem with macroglobulinemia is hyperviscosity, osteolytic lesions are rare, and the malignant cell resembles a lymphocyte more than a plasma cell.

Approximately one-fourth of patients with multiple myeloma will have no serum paraprotein spike on standard electrophoresis. These patients synthesize only the immunoglobulin light chain, which is rapidly cleared from the plasma and appears in the urine as Bence Jones proteinuria. Their clinical disease is the same as other patients with multiple myeloma.

QUESTIONS

1. Which one of the following statements about a serum monoclonal immunoglobulin is false?
   (a) It appears as a narrow peak in the β- or γ-globulin region of the protein electrophoresis.
   (b) It may appear in otherwise normal persons.
   (c) It contains only one heavy chain type.
   (d) It contains both κ and λ light chains.
2. Which one of the following is least likely to be found in a patient with newly diagnosed multiple myeloma?
   (a) splenomegaly
   (b) hypercalcemia
   (c) renal insufficiency
   (d) abnormal plasma coagulation studies.
3. Which one of the following statements is false? Bence Jones proteinuria:
   (a) is related to renal failure in multiple myeloma and is therefore a poor prognostic sign
   (b) can be diagnosed by specific heat precipitation properties
   (c) consists of immunoglobulin light chains
   (d) is ruled out by a negative standard Clinistix test for proteinuria.
4. A "broad-based" polyclonal increase in γ-globulin may occur in all of the following diseases except:
   (a) multiple myeloma

(b) tuberculosis
(c) osteomyelitis
(c) decubitus ulcers.

ANSWERS

1. **(d) is the false statement.** The definition of a monoclonal paraprotein is that it is homogeneous by all criteria, consisting of only a single heavy chain and light chain type. The homogeneity of a monoclonal immunoglobulin is also the explanation for statements (a) and (c) being true.
   Monoclonal immunoglobulins of low concentration, not associated with any clinical signs of multiple myeloma, occur with increasing frequency with increasing age. Estimates of the incidence have been as high as 1% of the normal population in their sixth decade increasing to 5% in their ninth decade.
2. **(a) is correct.** Although plasma cells are derived from B lymphocytes, the tumors of malignant cells occur almost exclusively in the bone marrow, and lymphadenopathy and splenomegaly are not seen. Hypercalcemia is a common sequela of bone destruction, and renal insufficiency is a common sequela of Bence Jones proteinuria. Abnormal plasma coagulation is usually related to interference with fibrin polymerization by the myeloma paraprotein.
3. **(d) is the false statement.** The standard urine test by Clinistix is sensitive only to albumin, not immunoglobulin fragments. Other standard clinical tests of proteinuria, such as drop-testing with 20% sulfosalicylic acid, will detect Bence Jones proteins. The classic method of diagnosis of Bence Jones proteinuria is the precipitation of immunoglobulin light chains at 56 C and their solubility when the temperature is increased to 100 C. This distinguishes Bence Jones proteinuria from the more common albuminuria, since albumin is soluble at 56 C but precipitates as the temperature approaches 100 C. Bence Jones proteins have been identified as immunoglobulin light chains. These are filtered by the renal glomerulus but are toxic to renal tubules, and are therefore associated with the development of renal failure and a poor prognosis in patients with multiple myeloma.
4. **(a) is correct.** The development of the abnormal monoclonal paraprotein in myeloma is associated with a decreased concentration of normal immunoglobulins. Therefore the β- and γ-globulin regions of the protein electrophoresis adjacent to the narrow paraprotein spike are usually flat. A broad-based hyperglobulinemia is typical of normal polyclonal antibody response to a severe chronic infec-

tious disease, such as tuberculosis, osteomyelitis, or decubitus ulcers.

COMMENT Multiple myeloma has clinical manifestations in many organ systems and therefore the presenting symptoms can vary. In this patient the distressing problem of persistent epistaxis caused her to seek medical help.

A downhill course, back pains, and renal failure can be seen in other diseases too (metastatic cancer, lymphoma, coincidental renal disease). But nosebleeds, anemia, and lytic bone lesions weighted the evidence heavily for myeloma, especially in a 60-year-old woman. Protein studies and bone marrow examination made the diagnosis certain. Cause and effect were thoroughly explored in relating the pathophysiology to the clinical picture. The sensitivity and specificity of monoclonal spikes, marrow aspirate abnormalities, and lytic bone lesions were included in the logic.

A good physician noting anemia, bone pain, renal failure, and a previous downhill course would immediately study the serum and urine proteins, bone marrow, and skull and vertebral films. The problem would be solved in 24 to 48 hours. (*P. C.*)

Suggested Readings

1. Boldt DH: Clinical and laboratory approach to the patient with serum protein abnormality. In Stein JH (ed): *Internal Medicine*, Boston, Little, Brown, 1983.
    This chapter is an excellent summary of current laboratory analyses of serum and urinary paraproteins and their clinical significance.
2. Kyle RA: Multiple myeloma: a review of 869 cases. *Mayo Clinic Proc* 50:29–40, 1975.
    A thorough analysis of the enormous Mayo Clinic experience.
3. Kyle RA: Monoclonal gammopathy of undetermined significance. Natural history in 241 cases. *Am J Med* 64:814–826, 1978.
    This study reports a large experience with a common laboratory observation. The long follow-up emphasizes the benign nature of this problem in most people.
4. Bloch KJ: Plasma cell dyscrasias and cryoglobulin. *JAMA* 248:2670–2676, 1982.
    Multiple myeloma, paraprotein disorders, and chain diseases are covered in seven packed pages.
5. Kyle RA, Greipp PR: "Idiopathic" Bence Jones proteinuria. *N Engl J Med* 306:564–567, 1982.
    A long-term follow-up; only some patients develop serious disease.
6. Case records of the Massachusetts General Hospital. Weekly clinicopathologic exercises. Case 17—1984. Pulmonary infiltrates in a 74-year-old man with multiple lytic defects. *N Engl J Med* 310:1103–1112, 1984.
    This case casts much light on the diagnostic process.
7. Fritz E, Ludwig H, Kundi M: Prognostic relevance of cellular morphology in multiple myeloma. *Blood* 63:1072–1079, 1984.
    This fine work from Vienna predicts longevity by detailed histologic cell features.
8. Cohen DJ, Sherman WH, Osserman EG, et al: Acute renal failure in patients with multiple myeloma. *Am J Med* 76:247–256, 1984.
    Details the varied causes of renal failure in this disease.
9. Kyle RA: "Benign" monoclonal gammopathy. A misnomer? *JAMA* 251:1849–1854, 1984.

Case 5
Cough, Fever, then Fatigue
DAVID A. SEARS, M.D.

DATA A 24-year-old black man is admitted to the hospital because of increasing fatigue following a respiratory infection. He felt well until 5 days ago when he developed nasal stuffiness, sore throat, and dry cough. Three days later his cough became productive of thick yellow sputum, the temperature rose to 39.4 C, and he began to note sharp pain in the left posterior thorax with deep inspiration. His physician made a clinical diagnosis of pneumonia and prescribed tetracycline and three to four aspirin tablets daily for fever. Cough and fever abated, but he felt progressively weaker and was therefore hospitalized.

LOGIC Thus far, the history sounds most compatible with a viral upper respiratory infection followed by the development of pneumonia. However, the latter diagnosis must be confirmed and the etiology established. Increasing weakness raises the possibility of a complication of the respiratory infection.

DATA Past history reveals that the patient had been healthy all his life. He had been told that he had "yellow jaundice" as a newborn but that he had not required transfusion or other specific therapy. The review of systems is entirely negative except for the fact that he has noted his urine to be dark brown for the past 1 or 2 days. Family history is negative or unobtainable. His parents are dead and his only sibling, a sister, is in good health.

LOGIC The history of jaundice as a newborn is difficult to evaluate. Isoimmune hemolytic disease of the newborn or prematurity would be the most likely causes. The history of dark urine is important. Since urine in the febrile, dehydrated patient is concentrated and often appears darker than usual, it is important to ascertain its color by careful questioning and direct observation. Among the causes of dark urine are ingested foods or drugs (beets, phenolphthalein), bilirubin, red blood cells, hemoglobin, myoglobin, porphyrins, and melanin. The cause in this patient is not yet apparent.

DATA On physical examination he appears acutely ill. Nail beds and mucous membranes are not cyanotic but appear slightly pale. His pulse is 95/minute, BP 120/70 without postural changes, respirations 18/minute, and temperature 37.3 C. The sclerae are slightly icteric and the pharynx is slightly reddened without exudate. Respiratory movements of the thorax are asymmetrical with splinting on the left. There is dullness to percussion, breath sounds are bronchovesicular, and many fine to medium moist rales are heard over the left lung posteriorly. The heart is not enlarged to percussion and the apex beat is normally located, but the precordium is active with a forceful left ventricular impulse. The heart sounds are normal, and there is a grade ⅙ systolic ejection murmur heard best along the left sternal border. The abdomen is soft and nontender, and the liver and

spleen are not palpable. The remainder of the examination—including the rectum, nervous system, and extremities—is normal.

LOGIC The physical examination is consistent with the expected pneumonia and does not give evidence of complications, such as pleural effusion, empyema, pericarditis, endocarditis, or meningitis. Scleral icterus may rarely occur in pneumonia due to lysis of red cells in the pneumonic lesion, but it is much more likely to reflect a complication like focal hepatic necrosis, underlying liver disease, or hemolysis. Taken together with the dark urine in this patient, you may consider liver disease with bilirubinuria or hemolysis with hemoglobinuria. Laboratory studies are important at this point.

DATA Results are as follows: hematocrit 25% (the plasma in the microhematocrit tube appears pink); reticulocytes 15%; white blood cell count 14,500/mm^3 with 81% segmented neutrophils, 12% bands, 2% metamyelocytes, and 5% lymphocytes. The blood smear reveals generally normochromic and normocytic red cells, but there is moderate poikilocytosis with occasional fragmented cells and microspherocytes. No true sickled cells are seen. There are many large polychromatophilic red cells and a rare nucleated red cell. Platelets are slightly increased. A sickle cell preparation is positive. The urine is clear and mahogany brown in color, specific gravity 1.025, pH 5.0, protein 1+, and glucose, ketones, and bilirubin are negative. Dipstick test for occult blood is positive. The spun sediment contains amorphous debris but no cells or casts. Stool is guaiac-negative. Sputum is thick and yellow; Gram stain reveals occasional white blood cells and a few gram-positive diplococci. It is cultured. Chest x-ray: a homogeneous density involves much of the left lower lung field; no pleural fluid is seen; the heart is of normal size and configuration. The blood urea nitrogen, glucose, electrolytes, serum glutamic-oxaloacetic transaminase, serum glutamic-pyruvic transaminase, and alkaline phosphatase are normal. Total serum bilirubin is 5.2 mg/dl—4.7 mg unconjugated and 0.5 mg conjugated.

LOGIC A good deal of light has been shed on the patient's problems. The reticulocyte index of 4.5 (15 × 25/45 × 1/1.85) indicates good marrow production of red cells. Therefore the mechanism of the anemia is either acute blood loss or hemolysis, and the clinical picture clearly indicates the latter. The blood smear suggests red cell fragmentation but does not indicate a specific cause for the hemolytic process. The mild leukocytosis and granulocyte immaturity are compatible with acute hemolysis and/or the patient's pneumonia. The dark color of the urine is due to heme pigment as shown by the dipstick test for occult blood. It could be red cells, free hemoglobin, or myoglobin. However, red cells were not seen in the sediment, and the urine specific gravity was not low enough to suggest osmotic lysis of red cells. The myoglobin molecule is only one-fourth the size of hemoglobin and is rapidly cleared from the plasma by filtration in the kidney. Therefore, in the absence of renal failure, myoglobin does not accumulate in the plasma and produce visible pigment. We can conclude that the urinary pigment is hemoglobin (or more likely methemoglobin, its oxidized form, which is brown in color) and that hemoglobin is also responsible for the pink color of the plasma. Thus, the patient has intravascular hemolysis with hemoglobinemia and hemoglobinuria. The unconjugated hyperbilirubinemia is also due to his hemolysis.

DATA The tentative diagnosis of partially treated probably pneumococcal pneumonia is made and parenteral penicillin is started. Attention is turned to further evaluation of his hemolytic anemia.

LOGIC The differential diagnosis includes both congenital and acquired disorders and can be fairly lengthy at this point. Among the more common ailments to be considered are the following:

Congenital

1. Sickle cell disease or other hemoglobinopathy: The history of good health and the absence of sickled forms on the blood smear make homozygous sickle cell disease unlikely. The history and absence of target cells make doubly heterozygous states like sickle cell-C disease and sickle cell-thalassemia unlikely as well. Sickle trait is most likely. Hemoglobin electrophoresis should be ordered for further evaluation of the hemoglobinopathy.
2. Red cell glucose 6-phosphate dehydrogenase (G-6-PD) deficiency: This is a good possibility. A special stain of his red cells for Heinz bodies may be helpful as well as a G-6-PD assay on his red cells.
3. Hereditary spherocytosis: The absence of family history, lack of splenomegaly, and acute nature of the hemolysis are against this diagnosis.

Acquired

1. Drug-related immune hemolysis: Of the drugs given, only penicillin is associated with immune hemolysis; but his hemolysis preceded that therapy.
2. Idiopathic autoimmune hemolytic anemia: This cannot be excluded, and a Coombs' test should be done.
3. Cold agglutinin hemolysis due to *Mycoplasma pneumoniae* infection. While the patient's pneumonia is not characteristic of *Mycoplasma* infection, its cause is not yet established, and this possibility should be considered. A Coombs' test for complement on the red cell surface, serum cold agglutinin titer, and complement fixation test for *M. pneumoniae* should be obtained.

DATA Additional studies are done as follows: hemoglobin electrophoresis shows 62% A and 38% S hemoglobin. Methyl violet staining reveals Heinz bodies in a few of the patient's red cells. A screening test for red cell G-6-PD gives equivocal results, and an assay shows 5.8 IU of G-6-PD/g of hemoglobin (normal 5.5 to 10.0). The direct Coombs' test is negative for both γ-globulin and complement on the red cell. The serum cold agglutinin titer is 1:4. The complement fixation test for *Mycoplasma* will not be available for several days. Serum heme pigment level is 35 mg/dl (normal < 5), and methemalbumin is present. Haptoglobin is absent.

LOGIC The elevated serum heme pigment, methemalbuminemia, and absent haptoglobin merely confirm the intravascular hemolysis which has already been appreciated by other simpler observations. The negative Coombs' test virtually excludes immune hemolysis, and the normal serum cold agglutinin titer rules out hemolysis secondary to *M. pneumoniae* infection. The hemoglobin electrophoresis and sickle prep allow the diagnosis of sickle cell trait to be made with certainty. This abnormality has no apparent relationship to the patient's hemolysis or pneumonia.

The finding of Heinz bodies in the patient's red cells is a crucial observation. Heinz bodies represent membrane-bound hemoglobin, denatured and precipitated due to oxidative damage. Increased susceptibility to this oxidative change can result from an inherited defect in the reductive mechanisms of the red cell (by far the most common of which is G-6-PD deficiency) or from an inherited unstable hemoglobin. The presence of these rigid intracellular precipitates predisposes the red cell to fragmentation injury or destruction in the splenic microcirculation. Since G-6-PD deficiency occurs in about 10% of black men in the United States, this is by far the most likely diagnosis in the present patient. The low normal enzyme level by assay does not militate against this diagnosis. The enzyme level is higher in younger red cells, and a deficient individual with a marked reticulocytosis (i.e. a young population of red cells) may have a level in the normal range. The oxidative challenge that precipitates hemolysis in a patient with G-6-PD deficiency is often a drug but may be an acute illness as in this patient. Neither tetracycline nor aspirin in the doses taken by this patient precipitates hemolysis in the

G-6-PD deficiency common to black men in this country.

DATA The patient's sputum culture is negative, probably due to the prior antibiotic therapy. Serologic testing of acute and convalescent sera shows no evidence of *Mycoplasma* infection. He responds to penicillin therapy with clearing of the pneumonia which is assumed to have been pneumococcal. Hemolysis ceases, and the hematocrit slowly returns to normal. A G-6-PD assay on his red cells months later shows a level about 10% of normal. The neonatal jaundice may have been due to his G-6-PD deficiency with hemolysis precipitated by an acute illness or oxidative drug (such as vitamin K).

QUESTIONS

1. The patient's sister:
   (a) cannot have inherited the gene for G-6-PD deficiency
   (b) may have inherited the gene for G-6-PD deficiency from her father
   (c) has a 50% chance of carrying the gene for G-6-PD deficiency and, if affected, may be susceptible to hemolysis induced by oxidant drugs
   (d) has a 50% chance of carrying the gene for G-6-PD deficiency but, even if affected, is not susceptible to hemolysis induced by oxidant drugs.
2. Although hemoglobin was demonstrated in this patient's urine, his pigmenturia could have been due to:
   (a) hemosiderinuria
   (b) urobilinogenuria
   (c) bilirubinuria
   (d) none of the above.
3. Sickle cell trait is characterized by:
   (a) the absence of clinical illness, normal blood counts, and normal blood smear
   (b) rare episodes of pain in the extremities due to the hemoglobinopathy
   (c) normal hematocrit, slightly elevated reticulocyte counts, and slightly shortened red cell survival
   (d) hemolytic episodes during severe exertion.
4. A positive direct Coombs' test may be seen in each of the following except:
   (a) hemolysis due to a cold agglutinin appearing after *M. pneumoniae* infection
   (b) an Rh-negative (D−) woman who has borne an Rh-positive (D+) baby

(c) a patient receiving large doses of penicillin who develops hemolysis due to anti-penicillin antibodies

(d) a patient with systemic lupus erythematosus who develops hemolytic anemia.

5. Hereditary spherocytosis is characterized by each of the following except:

(a) splenomegaly

(b) red cells on the blood smear with reduced diameter and absent central pallor

(c) return to normality of red cell shape following splenectomy

(d) red cells with increased osmotic fragility.

ANSWERS

1. **(c) is correct.** G-6-PD deficiency is transmitted as an X-linked recessive trait. Therefore the patient inherited it from his mother, a presumed heterozygote, and his sister would have a 50% chance of being a heterozygote as well. Though female heterozygotes on the average have higher enzyme levels than the male hemizygotes because of their second (normal) X chromosome, the Lyon hypothesis of random inactivation of the X chromosome predicts that some female heterozygotes will have very low enzyme levels. Furthermore, clinical experience has shown that heterozygous women may have hemolytic episodes, and the diagnosis must be considered in women as well as in men.

2. **(d) is correct.** The patient could have hemosiderin in his urine due to uptake of filtered hemoglobin by tubular cells and conversion of the iron to this insoluble storage compound. Usually more prolonged hemolysis is required to produce detectable urinary hemosiderin which is identified by staining the sediment with Prussian blue. However, hemosiderin does not discolor the urine. Urobilinogen, arising from bacterial degradation of bilirubin in the gut, is increased in the urine in hemolysis, but it also does not discolor the urine. Bilirubin may produce a yellow to brown color in the urine, but only conjugated (direct-reacting) bilirubin is excreted by the kidney. This patient's increased bilirubin was unconjugated (indirect) and would not appear in the urine.

3. **(a) is correct.** Painful crises do not occur in sickle cell trait as implied in answer (b). Red cell survival is normal, and hemolysis is not precipitated by exertion, illness, or other common stresses.

4. **(b) is correct.** Such a woman might have a positive indirect Coombs' test due to anti-D antibodies in her serum but would not have a positive direct Coombs' test (i.e. antibodies on her D-negative red cells). A positive direct Coombs' test occurs in cold agglutinin hemol-

ysis, usually due to the presence of complement on the red cell surface which has been fixed there by the cold-reactive IgM antibody. Penicillin-related immune hemolysis occurs when penicillin, present in high concentration, binds to the red cell surface and reacts there with anti-penicillin IgG antibodies. The red cell is damaged even though the antibody is not directed against red cell antigens. If penicillin is present, a positive direct Coombs' test may be seen. Obviously the Coombs' test will not be positive if administration of penicillin has been stopped and the drug is cleared from the circulation. Autoimmune hemolytic anemia may complicate systemic lupus erythematosus, and the anti-red cell autoantibody is detected by the direct Coombs' test.

5. **(c) is correct.** While splenectomy virtually cures the hemolytic process so that red cell life span returns to near normal, the inherited abnormality of red cell shape persists. Mild splenomegaly is characteristic of hereditary spherocytosis. Spherocytes in hereditary spherocytosis are microspherocytes and appear on the blood smear as described in (b). Because of their decreased surface area:volume ratio, hereditary spherocytes have a limited ability to swell in hypotonic solution and therefore characteristically have increased osmotic fragility.

COMMENTS   It was evident in this case too that the patient had another disease process coincident with or caused by the pneumonia.

Any one of several key clues could have led to the correct diagnosis using a branching process. You could start with either dark urine, anemia, or icterus. An analysis of the urine would have pointed directly to hemoglobinuria. Myoglobinuria is ruled out by special tests or by the absence of pigment in the serum. Had you begun with anemia, the high reticulocyte index in the absence of obvious hemorrhage would lead to the same conclusion. Bilirubin fractionation would have indicated hemolysis had you started with jaundice as the key clue.

From that point, it was simply a matter of pinpointing the cause for the hemolysis. This too was easily accomplished by a branching process or decision tree. The results of the Coombs' test, *Mycoplasma* complement fixation, hemoglobin electrophoresis, and G-6-PD measurement led in one direction or another. In essence, the author followed a self-constructed flow chart.   *(P. C.)*

Suggested Readings

1. Wintrobe MM, Lee GR, Boggs DR, et al (eds): *Clinical Hematology*, ed 8. Philadelphia, Lea & Febiger, 1981, chap 29, pp 734–754.

This chapter provides a good discussion of general considerations about hemolytic anemia. The individual disorders are covered in subsequent chapters.

2. Beutler E: Glucose -6-phosphate dehydrogenase deficiency. In Stanbury JB, Wyngaarden JB, Fredrickson DS, et al (eds): *The Metabolic Basis of Inherited Disease*, ed 5. New York, McGraw-Hill, 1983, pp 1629–1653.
   Beautiful diagrams and photographs portray the latest words on this genetic problem.

3. Winslow RM, Anderson WF: The hemoglobinopathies. In Stanbury JB, Wyngaarden JB, Frederickson DS, et al (eds): *The Metabolic Basis of Inherited Disease*, ed 5. New York, McGraw-Hill, 1983, pp 1666–1710.
   An in-depth excellent presentation of all the disorders of hemoglobin composition.

4. Steinberg MH, Hebbel RP: Clinical diversity of sickle cell anemia. *Am J Hematol* 14:405–416, 1983.
   Shows how genetic subtypes have different manifestations.

5. Beutler E: Sickle cell anemia and related disorders. In Williams WJ, Beutler E, Erslev AJ, et al (eds): *Hematology*, ed 3. New York, McGraw-Hill, 1983, pp 583–609.
   A good textbook summary of the hemoglobinopathies.

6. Charache S: Treatment of sickle cell anemia. *Annu Rev Med* 32:195–206, 1981.
   A brief sensible review of the subject.

7. Sears DA: The morbidity of sickle cell trait: a review of the literature. *Am J Med* 64:1021–1036, 1978.

8. Weed RI: Hereditary spherocytosis. A review. *Arch Intern Med* 135:1316–1323, 1975.
   An excellent review of what is known about this basic red cell defect and the role of the spleen in this disorder.

9. Swisher SN: Autoimmune hemolytic disorders. *Semin Hematol* 13:247–353, 1976.
   This whole issue is given to eight papers on the clinical, serologic, and experimental aspects of autoimmune hemolytic diseases.

Case 6
Elevated Hematocrit
ROGER M. LYONS, M.D.

DATA A 55-year-old white male oil rig worker was admitted to the hospital for an elective herniorrhaphy. The preoperative workup revealed a hematocrit (Hct) of 56 and surgery was delayed.

LOGIC In considering a patient with an elevated Hct you must first distinguish between a transient and a persistent increase in Hct above the upper limit of normal (52% for a man and 47% for a woman). Even with the limited information given above it is clear that the patient is not severely ill as is usually the case in patients who are dehydrated with a transient increase in Hct (e.g. diarrhea, diabetic ketoacidosis, heat prostration, and severe burns).

DATA Six months prior to this admission he was told that he had "too much blood," and a review of his records revealed elevated Hct levels recorded on two separate occasions over the previous year.

LOGIC In view of this information, both a transient elevation in Hct and a laboratory error can be excluded. Here is a pathophysiologic classification of patients with persistently elevated Hct levels:

1. Polycythemia rubra vera (P. vera)
2. Polycythemia secondary to physiologically appropriate excessive erythropoietin production associated with hypoxia: e.g. pulmonary disease, high altitude, cyanotic heart disease, hemoglobinopathy with high oxygen affinity, and carboxyhemoglobinemia
3. Polycythemia secondary to physiologically inappropriate production of erythropoietin by a tumor or renal cyst
4. Relative (spurious) polycythemia.

Relative polycythemia is separated from P. vera and the secondary polycythemias by the fact that the elevated Hct in relative polycythemia does not indicate a true increase in body red cell mass. The plasma volume is decreased, so that the red blood cell count is only relatively increased. It is important to note that relative or spurious polycythemia is the most common cause of an elevated Hct in the general population in this country.

Normally the red cell mass is hormonally controlled by a negative feedback loop. A persistent fall in arterial oxygen saturation results in the production of erythropoietin, a glycoprotein that is made almost entirely by the kidney in adult humans. Erythropoietin acts on the red blood cell precursors in the marrow, resulting in an increase in red cell production, red cell mass, and oxygen-carrying capacity of the blood. If the red cell mass increases to abnormally high levels, the viscosity of the blood increases, resulting in decreased blood flow and paradoxical tissue hypoxia, particularly in the central nervous system. This sequence is physiologically appropriate for chronic hypoxia.

On the other hand, certain tumors can elaborate an erythropoietin-like substance which does the same thing. This is not physiologically appropriate and can be caused by seemingly unrelated tumors like cerebellar hemangioblastoma, renal carcinoma or cyst, hepatoma, and unusual uterine tumors.

P. vera is not associated with increased erythropoietin levels. In this case an abnormal clone of red blood cell precursors appears to be exquisitely sensitive to stimulation by erythropoietin, and red cell production continues despite a very low level of erythropoietin.

With the information available, none of these possibilities can be excluded. If the patient were a woman rather than a man, relative polycythemia would be unlikely since that condition rarely occurs in women. The patient's age is not helpful since the mean age of onset of P. vera is 60 years and that of relative polycythemia is 52 years.

DATA On further questioning the patient admitted to a 30 pack-year cigarette history. He had a chronic morning cough productive of small amounts of brown sputum, but he had no shortness of breath. He had been a heavy drinker but had not had any alcohol intake for more than 5 years. Recently he spent a 2-week vacation in Mexico but had not been at high altitude. He gave no family history of blood problems, but there was a significant family history of hypertension. He had previously been diagnosed as having mild hypertension but had not taken the medication prescribed. There were no night sweats, bleeding, weight loss, or pruritus.

LOGIC The history of smoking suggests the possibility of carboxyhemoglobinemia as the result of carbon monoxide in cigarette smoke. Carbon monoxide binds to hemoglobin and prevents the latter from binding oxygen; the half-life of the carbon monoxide-hemoglobin complex is about 4 hours. Tissue hypoxia may result, and this stimulates erythropoietin production with a resultant increase in the Hct. Approximately 45% of smokers have been noted to have an elevated carboxyhemoglobin level and 3% have an elevated Hct.

The absence of a family history of blood problems suggests that a hemoglobinopathy is unlikely, but this possibility cannot be completely ruled out. Time spent at high altitude can be ruled out as a cause for the increased Hct. However, it is interesting to note that hypoxia due to low atmospheric pressure causes an almost immediate increase in erythropoietin concentration with resultant reticulocytosis at 3 to 5 days and then a slow increase in the Hct. Many months may pass before the Hct reaches a new stable level. The rise in the Hct is roughly proportional to the altitude.

DATA The initial part of the physical examination revealed a moderately obese man in no acute distress. His vital signs were normal with the exception of a blood pressure of 130/95. On inspection he had a ruddy complexion but was not cyanotic.

LOGIC The general appearance and the absence of weight loss suggest that he does not have a widespread malignancy. However, both localized hypernephromas and hepatomas have been associated with ectopic erythropoietin production, and the incidence of hepatoma is increased in patients with alcoholic liver disease. These are rare and thus unlikely but are not ruled out. The patient's ruddy complexion is consistent with his elevated Hct, hyperviscosity, and resultant inadequate oxygenation of circulating hemoglobin. One must be careful not to overinterpret the complexion since people who spend much of their time outdoors, as this man does, frequently have ruddy complexions.

DATA   Further examination revealed dilatation of his conjunctival blood vessels and retinal veins. His heart and lungs were normal. The liver was not tender but was palpable 3 cm below the right costal margin with a total vertical span of 15 cm. The tip of the spleen was clearly palpable 1 cm below the left costal margin on deep inspiration. No other abdominal masses could be felt. He did not have calf tenderness, pedal edema, or adenopathy. Neurologic examination, including gait and coordination, was completely normal. Stool guaiac test was negative.

LOGIC   The dilatation of conjunctival and retinal vessels suggests an increased blood volume and hyperviscosity of the blood as is seen in polycythemia, but which may also be seen in association with the hyperviscosity of paraproteinemia or occasionally in patients who have CO_2 retention. The lack of significant cardiac or pulmonary abnormalities suggests that cyanotic heart disease or severe pulmonary disease is unlikely.

The abdominal examination in a patient with an elevated Hct is of critical importance. Hepatomegaly in this man is consistent with his drinking history, but the lack of gynecomastia, spider hemangiomas, palmar erythema, and testicular atrophy suggests that he does not have extensive alcohol-induced hepatic damage. Splenomegaly could be present on the basis of hepatic cirrhosis and portal hypertension, but, as just indicated, he probably does not have

severe liver disease. Hepatomegaly is present in 30 to 50% and splenomegaly in 75% of patients with P. vera. Splenomegaly is a major point in the differential diagnosis of an elevated Hct since it is not likely to be present in either secondary or relative polycythemia. The normal neurologic examination is strong evidence for the absence of a cerebellar hemangioblastoma, a third type of tumor that has been associated with ectopic erythropoietin production.

DATA   The Hct was 55% and 56% on two separate occasions. The white blood cell count was 14,000/mm^3 with a normal differential, and the platelet count was 550,000/mm^3. The blood smear did not show rouleaux formation, and the red blood cell morphology suggested mild microcytic hypochromic changes. An 18-test chemistry profile was normal except for a uric acid of 9.5 mg/dl. Prothrombin time and partial thromboplastin time were normal as was a serum protein electrophoresis.

LOGIC   An elevated white blood cell and platelet count are strongly suggestive of P. vera. This is one of the myeloproliferative disorders which are presumed to be manifestations of disease of the hematopoietic stem cell. In these disorders (P. vera, chronic granulocytic leukemia, essential thrombocytosis, myelofibrosis, Di Guglielmo's syndrome, and acute granulocytic leukemia), erythrocytic, granulocytic, monocytic, and megakaryocytic cell lines proliferate en masse (to a variable degree in each disorder) rather than individually.

The hypochromic microcytic red cells suggest iron deficiency which almost universally accompanies P. vera. This is usually due to increased gastrointestinal blood loss. There is a defect in hemostasis in P. vera on two bases. First, local vessel dilatation from hyperviscosity and tissue anoxia results in a defect in the vascular phase of hemostasis with an inability of the vessels to contract normally when injured. Second, platelet function is frequently defective, especially at high platelet counts (e.g. 1 million/mm^3).

The incidence of peptic ulcer disease is increased in P. vera, most likely because of the increased basophil count and blood histamine levels that have been observed in this disease; this results in increased gastric acid production.

Despite the strong suggestion at this point that the patient might have P. vera, the diagnosis has not been definitely established and therapy would be inappropriate. The Hct is only a relative number reflecting the ratio of red blood cell mass to plasma volume. Thus a decrease in plasma volume in association with a normal red cell mass (as in relative polycythemia) might be present. It is not until the Hct is more than 60 that one can be sure that the red cell mass is increased enough to make a diagnosis of either P. vera or secondary polycythemia. We have not ruled out the possibility of hypoxia (i.e. physiologically appropriate secondary polycythemia) as the cause of this man's problem.

Frequently patients with chronic hypoxic pulmonary disease will have a normal Hct despite a persistently decreased arterial oxygen saturation. All causes of anemia should be considered in a patient with a normal Hct who is hypoxic and should be polycythemic. Chronic infection as seen in many patients with bronchitis or bronchiectasis could result in the observed Hct. In addition, many patients with chronic pulmonary disease have an increased plasma volume and an increase in red cell mass appropriate for their hypoxia. The resultant Hct would be normal.

DATA   Arterial blood was drawn and the pO_2 was 85 mm Hg with a saturation of 96%. The ^{51}Cr red cell mass was 40 ml/kg (normal is <36 ml/kg for a male), and the plasma volume measured as the ^{125}I albumin space was normal. A leukocyte alkaline phosphatase score was 130 (normal is 20 to 100) and the vitamin B_{12} level was 1100 pg/ml (normal is 200 to 900). Serum iron was 30 μg/dl and the total iron-binding capacity was 400 μg/dl with a low saturation of 7.5%.

LOGIC   The diagnosis of polycythemia rubra vera is established on the basis of an elevated red cell mass, and polycythemia due to hypoxia is excluded on the basis of the normal arterial oxygen saturation (i.e. >92%). In association with splenomegaly, these findings are adequate criteria for the diagnosis of P. vera. If splenomegaly were absent, two of the following (all present in this patient) would have been necessary to confirm a diagnosis of P. vera:

1. thrombocytosis >400,000/mm³
2. leukocytosis >12,000/mm³ in the absence of fever or infection
3. leukocyte alkaline phosphatase score >100 in the absence of fever or infection
4. vitamin B_{12} >900 pg/ml or unbound B_{12}-binding capacity of >2200 pg/ml.

The increased B_{12}-binding capacity and B_{12} level reflect either increased turnover of granulocytes (which contain B_{12}-binding protein) or the production of an abnormal B_{12}-binding protein. The etiology of the increased leukocyte alkaline phosphatase is unknown.

If adequate criteria to diagnose P. vera were not present, the other major causes of secondary polycythemia would have been evaluated as follows:

1. renal cyst or tumor—intravenous pyelogram; in spite of new diagnostic procedures, the intravenous pyelogram is still deemed best by most clinicians. Computed tomography is so sensitive that it detects small meaningless cysts in many patients, and ultrasound is not so sensitive as the intravenous pyelogram for hypernephroma.
2. carboxyhemoglobinemia—carboxyhemoglobin level
3. hemoglobinopathy with increased oxygen-binding affinity—$P_{50}O_2$: a decrease in $P_{50}O_2$ (the oxygen tension at half-maximal saturation of hemoglobin with O_2) indicates an abnormal hemoglobin with increased oxygen binding

4. hepatoma—liver-spleen scan; a variety of scanning procedures is available

As a last resort, measurements of erythropoietin can be obtained from some research laboratories to evaluate the presence of excessive erythropoietin production. The usefulness of the commercially available radioimmunoassay for erythropoietin has not yet been established. A diagnosis of relative polycythemia (normal red cell mass and decreased plasma volume) does not necessarily indicate a benign prognosis since these patients have an increased incidence of hypertension and thromboembolic disease with a shorter life span than the general population.

DATA　The patient had two units of blood removed per week until his Hct was below 47; it was maintained at this level by phlebotomy for 4 months. At that time he was readmitted to the hospital and underwent herniorrhaphy without complications.

LOGIC　Hemorrhage and thrombosis are common complications in a surgical patient with uncontrolled P. vera. The complication rate is immediately lowered by phlebotomy to a Hct of <47 but does not return to normal until the patient has been under adequate control for approximately 4 months.

DATA　The patient was followed on a regular basis and his Hct maintained at approximately 47 by phlebotomy. The elevated uric acid was controlled with allopurinol. However, his platelet count continued to rise until it was persistently over 1.5 million/mm³. He began to complain of easy bruisability and distressing pruritus, especially after bathing. The pruritus did not respond well to antihistamines or cholestyramine. However, after his platelet count had been lowered to less than 1 million/mm³ with hydroxyurea, his pruritus decreased in severity.

LOGIC　P. vera is associated with increased cellular production and turnover giving rise

to hyperuricemia, hepatomegaly, and splenomegaly. The etiology of the pruritus is unclear, but it is associated with the increased cellular turnover (not only with an increased platelet count).

Occasionally as the disease progresses it may transform into another myeloproliferative disorder. Myelofibrosis develops in 10 to 20% of patients with P. vera. The increased risk of developing acute leukemia is influenced by the type of treatment given; this complication occurs in 11% of those receiving an alkylating agent like chlorambucil, but in only 3.8% of patients treated with radioactive phosphorus. Despite complications the prognosis with good care is excellent; median survival is 9 to 16 years.

COMMENT　This problem is readily solved by a flow chart approach (Fig. 14.1). We are dealing with one key clue which has a limited number of causes and specific tests to prove each one. The use of two tests (red blood cell mass and oxygen saturation) determines which branch of the diagnostic tree to follow. Additional clues guide you further (depending on their positivity or negativity) until a solution is reached.

In general, patients with P. vera need not have studies beyond the arterial oxygen saturation, and the diagnosis is then confirmed by the total clinical picture. But 10% of patients with P. vera will have an arterial oxygen saturation between 88 and 92%. Here the diagnosis is made if other criteria are present, and diseases causing a low pO_2 are excluded.

You must cope with other bits of imperfect information too. Since most patients with hemoglobinopathy or carboxyhemoglobinemia may have normal oxygen saturation, test for those conditions whenever polycythemia exists. The *dotted line* in Figure 14.1 indicates the paradox involving the latter two hemoglobin disorders; while the measured arterial oxygen saturation is usually normal, functional tissue hypoxia is present and the polycythemia is erythropoietin-produced.

When a reliable erythropoietin radioimmunoassay becomes generally available it will be of great help. However, it must be remembered that, as with any other radioimmunoassay, biologically inactive material may be measured and biologically active "erythropoietin-like" material may not be measured. The erythropoietin assay in P. vera is lower than in the secondary polycythemias of *groups 2* and *3* of Figure 14.1 where it is generally high. (*P. C.*)

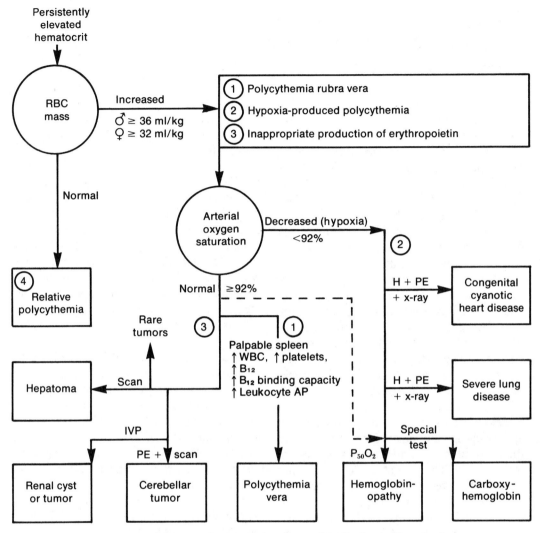

Fig. 14.1. Flow chart for the solution of a persistently elevated hematocrit.

Suggested Readings

1. Berlin NI (ed): Polycythemia. *Semin Hematol* 12:4, 1975; 13:1, 1976.
   Comprehensive review of all information concerning polycythemia known to 1975. These 13 papers are the basis of all modern reviews of polycythemia.
2. Wintrobe MM, Lee GR, Boggs DR et al (eds): *Clinical Hematology*, ed 8. Philadelphia, Lea & Febiger, 1981.
   Chapter 42 contains an excellent review of erythrocytosis, its differential diagnosis and effects. Chapter 65 reviews P. vera in detail with emphasis on its clinical features.

3. Golde DW, Hocking WG, Koeffler HP, et al: Polycythemia: mechanisms and management. *Ann Intern Med* 95:71–87, 1981.
   Excellent update of the pathophysiology of polycythemia. The sections on erythropoietin and the clonal origins of P. vera provide new insights into this disease.
4. Erslev AJ, Caro J: Pure erythrocytosis according to erythropoietin titers. *Am J Med* 76:57–61, 1984.
5. Adamson JW: The polycythemias: diagnosis and treatment. *Hosp Pract* 12:49–57, 1983.
6. Harrison BD: Secondary polycythaemia: its causes, effects, and treatment. *Br J Dis Chest* 76:313–340, 1982.

Case 7
Jaundice, Weakness, Pallor

JAMES N. GEORGE, M.D.

DATA A 19-year-old boy came to your office because of increasing weakness and fatigue. He had been very healthy and active all his life until 4 months ago when his family physician diagnosed hepatitis. At that time he had anorexia, nausea, vomiting, and jaundice, preceded by several days of fever and chills. There had been no known exposure to needles and no known contact with a source of infectious hepatitis. He was in bed at home with this illness and his doctor had treated him with prochlorperazine for his nausea and vomiting. After 3 weeks of bed rest he was not jaundiced, but he continued his prochlorperazine almost daily for nausea and anorexia. He never regained enough strength to return to his job as a truck mechanic, and in the past few weeks had become even more tired.

On physical examination, the patient was a very muscular young man who did not appear chronically ill. Pallor was evident in the skin and mucous membranes. Vital signs were normal. The skin and sclerae were not icteric. His liver was palpable at the right costal margin but not enlarged or tender to percussion. When the patient lay on his right side, the spleen was palpable 3 cm below the left costal margin on inspiration. The remainder of the examination was normal.

LOGIC At this time there were not enough data to make a diagnosis. The history was consistent with the previous doctor's diagnosis of hepatitis. Because of the general principle of relating all symptoms to one diagnosis, if possible, it was reasonable to suspect that the illness was a continuing activity of his hepatitis. The liver was not enlarged or tender, but it was possible that hepatitis had progressed to cirrhosis. Splenomegaly could be due to cirrhosis with resulting portal hypertension, but there were no other physical signs of portal hypertension or cirrhosis: ascites, distended periumbilical

veins, spider angiomata, etc. It did seem certain that serious illness was present. Routine blood counts and urinalysis were performed in the office.

DATA Laboratory data were as follows: hematocrit 12% and white blood cell count 300/mm^3. Examination of the blood smear demonstrated normochromic red blood cells with moderate anisocytosis and poikilocytosis. Red cell volume appeared normal. All white blood cells seen were small, mature lymphocytes. Platelets were moderately decreased, averaging three per oil field. Urinalysis was normal.

LOGIC These abnormalities clearly demonstrated that the illness had been present for some weeks or months, since the patient was able to tolerate severe anemia. The absence of fever or infection with such severe leukopenia was surprising. These data clearly explained the presenting symptoms, but finding the cause of the abnormal blood counts became urgent.

1. Aplastic anemia, consistent with this degree of pancytopenia, may occur following hepatitis. To confirm this, a bone marrow aspiration and biopsy are required. Significantly, the patient had no exposure to certain drugs or organic chemicals which may cause aplastic anemia. Many drugs have a reported association, but chloramphenicol, phenylbutazone, hydantoins, sulfonamides, gold, and benzene appear to carry a greater risk of marrow toxicity than most other agents. Although splenomegaly is not present in aplastic anemia, the spleen may be enlarged if chronic liver disease is present.

2. Phenothiazines, such as prochlorperazine, are common causes of leukopenia; but they do not cause anemia, thrombocytopenia, and splenomegaly.

3. Megaloblastic disease due to a deficiency of vitamin B$_{12}$ or folic acid can cause

severe pancytopenia, and occasionally splenomegaly. Although pernicious anemia (B_{12} deficiency) is unusual at this age, the long period of anorexia may have led to folic acid deficiency. However, there is nothing to suggest this from examination of the peripheral blood smear: the absence of oval macrocytes, striking poikilocytosis, and neutrophils would be unusual. The spleen may be palpable in 20% of patients with pernicious anemia.

4. Severe granulocytopenia and splenomegaly can also occur on an autoimmune basis. A well-recognized cluster of granulocytopenia, splenomegaly, and rheumatoid arthritis is referred to as Felty's syndrome; however, an associated autoimmune disease is not always present. The marrow responds normally and becomes hyperplastic to compensate for peripheral cell destruction. Thrombocytopenia may also occur, but severe anemia is inconsistent. Furthermore, there is no arthritis present.

5. Acute leukemia must be suspected as a cause of extremely severe anemia and leukopenia, especially when accompanied by splenomegaly. Although approximately one-fourth of patients with acute leukemia initially have leukopenia, it is unusual not to find myeloblasts or lymphoblasts when the peripheral blood smear is searched. Chronic myelocytic leukemia and chronic lymphocytic leukemia are always associated with leukocytosis and are not a consideration.

DATA Because of these severe abnormalities, the patient was admitted to the hospital. A sternal bone marrow aspiration was attempted that afternoon, but no marrow was obtained. An attempt to aspirate bone marrow from the iliac crest was also unsuccessful.

LOGIC The fact that a skilled physician cannot aspirate bone marrow is very significant. Three possibilities exist: (*a*) the marrow is severely aplastic with only fat present, (*b*) the marrow is packed with leukemic or tumor cells in association with fibrosis, or (*c*) the marrow is entirely replaced by dense reticulin and collagen fibrosis.

The inability to aspirate bone marrow together with the history and physical examination allow the following diagnostic considerations:

1. Aplastic anemia is consistent with the inability to aspirate bone marrow but does not explain the splenomegaly.

2. Leukopenia due to phenothiazine toxicity should not cause total marrow aplasia or fibrosis, and marrow should be easily aspirated.

3. Megaloblastic disease is associated with a very cellular marrow which is easily aspirated.

4. Autoimmune neutropenia is also associated with a cellular marrow which is easily aspirated.

5. Acute leukemia commonly presents with a densely infiltrated marrow which cannot be aspirated.

6. Myelofibrosis with myeloid metaplasia of the spleen is consistent with inability to aspirate bone marrow and also consistent with the history and physical examination. But it rarely occurs in young people; 60 is the average age of onset.

Therefore acute leukemia was thought to be the most likely diagnosis, and it was probable that the previous hepatitis was entirely coincidental. The absence of enlarged nodes is consistent with a diagnosis of acute leukemia of either lymphoblastic or myeloblastic origin, since about half of patients presenting with these diseases have no palpable lymphadenopathy.

DATA Transfusion with three units of packed red cells was given. The following morning the results of blood chemistry determinations were reported as all normal except for a serum uric acid of 10.3 mg/dl.

LOGIC Transfusion was indicated not just because of the severe anemia but also because there was no apparent quickly reversible cause for the anemia. If, for example, severely megaloblastic hematopoiesis had been found by marrow aspiration, then rapid recovery would be expected after appropriate treatment with the deficient vitamin (B_{12} or folic acid).

The observation of an elevated serum uric acid could be related to a disease such as acute leukemia with accelerated cell destruction and release of nucleic acid urate precursors. This strengthens the suspicion of acute leukemia vs aplastic anemia.

DATA That morning a needle biopsy of the iliac crest bone marrow was done. Wright's-Giemsa stains of the touch imprints of the biopsy, available immediately, provided a definite diagnosis 2 days before the permanent histologic sections of the bone marrow could be available. The imprints demonstrated a nearly solid sheet of uniform mononuclear cells with multiple nucleoli, fine nuclear chromatin, and scant cytoplasm. These cells were primitive blast cells, precursors of either lymphocytes or granulocytes. No other normal marrow cells were seen—no megakaryocytes, no erythroid precursor cells, no intermediate granulocyte precursors.

LOGIC The accumulation of immature cells which are unable to differentiate but continue to divide and eventually replace normal hematopoietic tissue makes the diagnosis of acute leukemia. It was assumed that the previous hepatitis was entirely coincidental. The conventional Wright's-Giemsa stain may not definitely distinguish lymphoblasts from myeloblasts (the latter being the precursor cell of granulocytes and monocytes), and this distinction is important for therapy and prognosis. Special studies were performed later that day.

DATA Careful examination of the marrow biopsy imprint revealed no Auer rods in the cytoplasm of the blast cells and no development of granules to suggest promyelocytes. Either of these findings would be diagnostic of acute myeloblastic leukemia. A peroxidase reaction, to demonstrate cytoplasmic granules with peroxidase activity which are not apparent in the Wright's stain, was negative. This result made the diagnosis of acute myeloblastic leukemia unlikely. A periodic acid-Schiff's reaction to detect cytoplasmic glycogen granules demonstrated large blocks

of periodic acid-Schiff-positive material in some of the blasts, identifying these cells as lymphoblasts and diagnosing the disease as acute lymphoblastic leukemia. The diagnosis was made within a day of the patient's presentation to the office, the nature of the illness was discussed with the patient and his family, and therapy was begun.

Two weeks after beginning chemotherapy with vincristine and prednisone, the patient had a hematocrit of 32%, platelet count of 288,000/mm^3, and a white blood cell count of 5,250/mm^3 with 74% neutrophils. This remission continued for 15 months. Lymphoblasts were then noted on the peripheral blood smear and were increased in the marrow. Chemotherapy was changed and he has remained completely well for 33 months, now 4 years after his original diagnosis. He is married and continues his work as a truck mechanic.

QUESTIONS

1. A 34-year-old asymptomatic man is discovered to have an enlarged spleen at the time of routine physical examination. His hematocrit is 42% and his white blood cell count is 42,000/mm^3. Examination of the peripheral blood smear demonstrates normal red blood cell morphology and normal numbers of platelets. The white cell differential is: segmented neutrophils 36%, band neutrophils 12%, metamyelocytes 10%, myelocytes 14%, promyelocytes 4%, myeloblasts 3%, basophils 5%, eosinophils 4%, lymphocytes 8%, and monocytes 4%. A special stain of the peripheral blood demonstrates absent leukocyte alkaline phosphatase. You immediately suspect:
   (a) acute granulocytic leukemia
   (b) chronic granulocytic leukemia
   (c) polycythemia vera
   (d) neutrophilic leukemoid reaction.
2. All of the following drugs have been postulated to have a causative role in certain cases of acute leukemia except:
   (a) aspirin
   (b) chloramphenicol
   (c) phenylbutazone
   (d) benzene.
3. Which of the following statements about acute lymphocytic leukemia is correct?
   (a) usually occurs in the elderly
   (b) a complete remission (normal peripheral blood and bone marrow) is commonly (more than 85% of patients) achieved with chemotherapy

(c) always presents with a high white blood cell count

(d) commonly presents as the terminal phase of chronic lymphocytic leukemia.

4. Which of the following abnormalities causes the greatest risk of death in a patient with acute leukemia?
   (a) anemia
   (b) granulocytopenia
   (c) hyperuricemia
   (d) leukocytosis.

5. A 62-year-old man notes a mass in the left side of his abdomen. On examination it moves with respiration and feels like spleen. Enlarged lymph nodes are found in the neck, axillae, both groins, and epitrochlear areas. His tonsils are markedly enlarged. He does not appear anemic. The diagnosis is most readily and dependably made by:
   (a) lymph node biopsy
   (b) antinuclear antibody determination
   (c) complete blood count
   (d) computed tomographic scan of liver and spleen.

ANSWERS

1. **(b) is correct.** In contrast to acute leukemia, chronic granulocytic (or myelocytic) leukemia always presents with a high white blood cell count. The peripheral white blood cell differential is approximately the same as in normal bone marrow, suggesting a fundamental defect in marrow release. The histochemical stain demonstrating absent alkaline phosphatase activity in the neutrophils is an empirical but important observation which helps to distinguish this disease from a normal reactive leukocytosis. But the clinical setting and persistence of leukocytosis in chronic granulocytic leukemia make the distinction more definite. The normal appearing granulocyte maturation seen on the peripheral blood smear rules out acute leukemia, a disease in which the primitive cells (blasts) are unable to differentiate and mature. Polycythemia vera is a disease closely related to chronic granulocytic leukemia, but diagnostic critieria include an increased red cell mass (not present when hematocrit is 42%).

2. **(a) is correct.** Acute leukemia can follow marrow injury and aplasia, and all of these compounds except aspirin have been implicated in the etiology of aplastic anemia and acute myeloblastic leukemia. A more dramatic example of this phenomenon was the increased incidence of acute leukemia among the Japanese exposed to atomic bomb radiation.

3. **(b) is correct,** as shown by many studies. The peak age incidence of acute leukemia is less than 10 years. Approximately half of patients

present with normal or low total white blood cell counts. Acute lymphocytic leukemia is an entirely different disease from chronic lymphocytic leukemia and there is never a transition between these diseases. Chronic lymphocytic leukemia is an immunologic disease primarily affecting older adults in which B lymphocytes cannot differentiate into immunologically competent cells, and accumulate in the circulation.

4. **(b) is correct,** since granulocytopenia is the most difficult abnormality to correct by transfusion and the risk of fatal infection is great. Extreme leukocytosis due to blasts is also a threat since these large and rigid cells have difficulty passing through the microcirculation. Clinical studies have suggested that a blast concentration in the peripheral blood of over $100,000/mm^3$ is commonly associated with leukothrombi and infarction of lung and brain. Appropriate chemotherapy can reduce this leukocytosis within 24 to 48 hours. Hyperuricemia can cause acute renal failure but should be well controlled by maintaining a good output of alkaline urine and treatment with allopurinol (a xanthine oxidase inhibitor). Anemia should never cause death.

5. **(c) is correct.** This is a typical presentation for chronic lymphocytic leukemia. The blood count will likely show a marked leukocytosis (e.g. 100,000 white blood cells/mm^3, 99% mature lymphocytes), but there may be no anemia, thrombocytopenia, or symptoms early. Biopsy is a surgical procedure and may not be diagnostic unless this is a lymphoma. (b) and (d) offer nothing useful.

Suggested Readings

1. Boggs DR, Wintrobe MM, Cartwright GE: The acute leukemias: analysis of 322 cases and a review of the literature. *Medicine* 41:163–225, 1962.
   A thorough analysis of acute leukemia prior to modern chemotherapy; therefore the natural history of these diseases is well described.
2. Cline MJ, Golde DW, Billing RJ, et al: Acute leukemia: biology and treatment (proceeding of a UCLA conference). *Ann Intern Med* 91:758–773, 1979.
   This is a thorough review of still current diagnostic procedures, classification of disease, treatment, and prognosis.
3. Swirsky DM, Li YS, Mathews JG, et al: 8;21 translocation in acute granulocytic leukemia: cytological, cytochemical, and clinical features. *Br J Hematol* 56:199–213, 1984.
   Introduces the reader to some of the complexities of chromosomal aberrations associated with leukemias.
4. Lawler SD: Significance of chromosomal abnormalities in leukemia. *Semin Hematol* 19:257–272, 1982.
   Genetic defects are related to many types of

leukemias; the Philadelphia story is expanded.
5. Cork A: Chromosomal abnormalities in leukemia. *Am J Med Technol* 49:321–334, 1983.
    Gene translocations and abnormal clones are related to myeloproliferative and lymphoproliferative disorders.
6. Koeffler HP, Golde DW: Chronic myelogenous leukemia—new concepts. *N Engl J Med* 304:1201–1209, 1981.
    Clinical features and clonal evolution are detailed.
7. Degnan T, Weiselberg L, Schulman P, et al: Dysmyelopoietic syndrome: current concepts. *Am J Med* 76:122–128, 1984.
    Covers the spectrum of faulty stem cell development associated with cytopenias; the intersection between leukemia and pancytopenia is especially important today as environmental toxins, radiation, and cancer chemotherapeutic agents may relate to this syndrome.
8. Camitta BM, Storb R, Thomas ED: Aplastic anemia (2 parts). *N Engl J Med* 306:645–652, 712–718, 1982.
    The roles of drugs, irradiation, and infection are highlighted; the second section deals mainly with treatment.

Case 8
Neck Lumps

CHARLES A. COLTMAN, JR., M.D.

DATA A 17-year-old girl sought medical attention because she noticed lumps in the left side of her neck. She had been in excellent health until 2 years ago when she had similar neck lumps. That illness was associated with fever, sore throat, and malaise from which she recovered in 2 weeks. On the basis of examination and blood tests, a physician had diagnosed infectious mononucleosis (IM). At the present time the patient has none of the symptoms which were associated with her previous neck lumps.

LOGIC The earlier illness sounds like IM and you make a note to contact the previous physician and confirm that impression; you expect she had atypical lymphocytes and a positive heterophil antibody test. Even so, the current lumps are not likely to be recurrent IM and probably represent something new.

A problem of this sort could be solved by the traditional complete history, physical examination, and laboratory tests. But who could proceed without first feeling the lumps, verifying what they are, seeing if there are others, and asking parallel questions?

First, what are the lumps? Are they lymph nodes, tumors, cysts, or congenital rem-

nants? Localized lymph node swelling can be caused by viral diseases, upper respiratory infections, recent immunizations, tooth abscesses, catscratch disease, metastatic cancer, lymphoma, tuberculosis, or an infection anywhere which is draining into regional lymph nodes. Generalized lymphadenopathy, on the other hand, suggests lymphoma, leukemia, sarcoidosis, systemic lupus erythematosus (SLE), brucellosis, IM, syphilis, lipoidoses, Graves' disease, and the use of hydantoins for epilepsy.

DATA There is a 3 × 3-cm firm, nontender, freely movable nodule in the left neck just above the sternoclavicular joint, and several smaller nodes to the left along the clavicle. At the same time you examine the rest of the head and neck and check the vital signs. All else is normal. There is no fever, no icterus, the thyroid gland is normal, the trachea is not deviated, and there are no signs of hyperthyroidism.

LOGIC You are clearly dealing with large pathologic nodes. An inflamed branchial cleft cyst or aberrant thyroid can be dismissed. Absence of tenderness is against acute inflammation or rapid growth. A rubbery consistency, mobility, and the discreteness of nodes suggests Hodgkin's disease. Later on, Hodgkin's and tuberculous glands become matted together. Metastatic cancer is unlikely at her age.

The next important points to determine are whether the lymphadenopathy is local or generalized and whether the spleen (the largest of lymphoid organs) is enlarged.

DATA A firm nontender 2 × 2-cm node is felt high in the left axilla. The chest, heart, breasts, and lungs are normal, though there seems to be some increase in splenic dullness in the midaxillary line. This finding is confirmed by a spleen which is palpable 2 cm below the left costal margin on deep inspiration. The liver has a 10-cm vertical span by percussion. No other lymph nodes are palpable. Indirect nasopharyngoscopy and indirect laryngoscopy show these areas to be normal and free of tumor. The rest of the examination, including the rectopelvic and neurologic portions, is entirely normal.

LOGIC The association of large lymph nodes in two areas (supraclavicular and axillary) with enlargement of the spleen raises the serious question of lymphoma in your mind. But other diseases associated with generalized lymphadenopathy are all still possible.

Lipoidoses are noted at a very young age. Metastatic cancer is unlikely. Primary sites have not been found, though at this age melanoma must be carefully sought and ruled out. There is no rash or arthritis to go with SLE. Anemia, bruises, and petechiae are not present—points against leukemia. A few questions are indicated to detect constitutional symptoms or symptoms related to specific diseases that could cause adenopathy. These questions were all asked while doing the examination.

DATA She has no cat, has never drunk unpasteurized cow's or goat's milk, denies any recent illness, did receive immunizations for a trip to Europe 8 months ago, has had no weakness, anorexia, weight loss, fever, chills, night sweats, or pruritus, never had arthritis, and takes no medication. She

recalls taking some sort of medicine with each acute illness as a child because she had suffered a convulsion in infancy, but she has not taken any in recent years. There is no history of frequent recurrent infections.

LOGIC Hydantoin anticonvulsants are associated with lymphoid hyperplasia, pseudolymphoma, and lymphoma, but their administration so long ago makes the relationship most unlikely. Animal-related diseases are ruled out, and her immunizations are too remote. Three additional important decision points have been passed. The absence of anemia, coagulopathy, and recurrent infections tells you that the bone marrow is not being replaced even though we may be dealing with a lymphoma or leukemia. Furthermore, you have determined there are no constitutional manifestations of a lymphoma and that even if this disease is present it is in an early stage. Last, you have essentially ruled out diseases associated with generalized lymphadenopathy, such as SLE, secondary syphilis, and sarcoidosis, since there are no other manifestations. Laboratory studies are indicated, though a biopsy must ultimately be done.

DATA Thyroxine (T_4) and triiodothyronine resin uptake (T_3RU) are normal. Blood studies show hemoglobin 11.0 gm/dl, hematocrit 33%, red blood cell count 4.5 million/mm^3, mean corpuscular volume 73 μ^3, mean corpuscular hemoglobin 24 pg, white blood cell count 6,200/mm^3, differential normal, platelet count 186,000/mm^3. The smear shows red blood cell hypochromia. Chest x-ray demonstrates a normal posteroanterior view, but encroachment on the retrosternal clear space is noted on the lateral view. Liver function tests are normal, but the alkaline phosphatase is slightly increased (10% above normal). The Venereal Disease Research Laboratory test is negative. Protein electrophoresis, serum calcium, and antinuclear antibody test are normal or negative.

LOGIC The patient has a mild hypochromic microcytic anemia by indices and smear. In a 17-year-old, the most common cause is iron lack due to heavy menses. Platelets are slightly low, but you realize that platelets have a tendency to pool in a large spleen. Leukemia is virtually ruled out. The normal posteroanterior chest x-ray, serum calcium, and proteins are strong evidence against sarcoidosis. SLE can now be eliminated by the absence of commonly associated clinical features. But the suggestion of involvement of the anterior mediastinum as reflected in the retrosternal mass makes lymphoma an increasingly likely diagnosis in a patient with three other lymphatic sites involved. Remember that the thymus and substernal thyroid are in this location too. The elevation of alkaline phosphatase is slight and may be inconsequential, though it raises the question of liver or bone involvement. More studies are needed to prepare for surgical biopsy of the large node.

DATA   Urinalysis, blood urea nitrogen, creatinine, prothrombin time, and partial thromboplastin time are all normal. Computed tomography of the chest confirms the presence of anterior mediastinal adenopathy.

LOGIC   You call the surgeon to examine the node with you so that there is no confusion as to which one is to be removed. You want the largest supraclavicular node to be sampled. Then you call the pathologist to do a touch preparation of the lymph node by pressing the cut surface immediately to a microscope slide and making multiple impressions. The tissue will be fixed and sectioned.

DATA   These studies are all done following removal of the node. The following day you and the pathologist review the tissue. The touch prep, stained by Wright's stain, shows normal lymphocytes and not much else. The fixed tissue shows bands of collagen, a nodular pattern, and rare classical Reed-Sternberg cells.

LOGIC   The pathologist calls this typical nodular sclerosing Hodgkin's disease. The most important question that remains is

how extensive is the disease, since this influences the prognosis. Are the anemia and slight thrombocytopenia a reflection of bone marrow involvement? Is the elevated alkaline phosphatase a result of liver involvement? Is the enlarged spleen due to Hodgkin's disease? Could there be lymph node involvement below the diaphragm?

DATA   A bone marrow biopsy shows no evidence of Hodgkin's disease, but the metarubricytes are small and show delayed hemoglobinization. An iron stain shows no stainable iron. A percutaneous liver biopsy shows normal liver. The patient undergoes a lymphogram and it is negative.

LOGIC   Computed tomography is useful to detect enlarged lymph nodes at any site in the abdomen. Lymphography, however, is particularly useful in staging Hodgkin's disease. It visualizes the retroperitoneal nodes, most commonly involved in Hodgkin's disease, and it can detect lymph nodes which are not only enlarged, but of abnormal structure. In addition, it is useful in directing the surgeon to the diseased nodes, the removal of which can be confirmed by a scout film of the abdomen in the operating room. Finally, if abnormal nodes are visualized, their response to therapy can be followed by periodic scout films of the abdomen to visualize changes in the conformation and size of the retained contrast material.

We now have a patient who has four lymphatic areas involved, including the supraclavicular, axillary, and mediastinal nodes and the spleen. She has a clinical stage (CS) III_sA, meaning that she has disease above and below the diaphragm (III), that she has clinical involvement of the spleen (s), and that she has no systemic symptoms (A). We know that in patients with splenic enlargement in Hodgkin's disease, about one-third do not have Hodgkin's disease in the spleen when it is removed and examined. Similarly, if the spleen is normal in size, one-third have Hodgkin's on pathologic examination. Furthermore, the lymphogram does not visualize upper abdominal, splenic, porta hepatis, or mesenteric nodes. Finally, splenic involvement with Hodgkin's disease enhances the likelihood of liver involvement, in spite of a negative percutaneous biopsy. You would like the patient to have as little therapy as possible because of the risk of complications and a second malignancy. You ask the surgeon to do a staging laparotomy.

DATA   The patient is taken to the operating room and, through a midline incision, the liver is biopsied, the spleen is removed, and multiple lymph nodes are biopsied. She is returned to her room without event. The pathologist slices the spleen in 2-mm-thick slices and finds no gross Hodgkin's disease. All abdominal tissue is negative. The spleen shows follicular hyperplasia.

LOGIC   You know that the enlarged spleen is not due to Hodgkin's disease. She has disease above the diaphragm only (stage II) and has no symptoms (A). There are three sites above the diaphragm involved, so the notation would be (II$_3$). We thus have a patient with CS III$_S$A who after further tissue was obtained was found to have a different, less extensive pathologic stage (PS), IIA. The convention is to use a subscript to note all additional tissue biopsied such as liver ($_H$), spleen ($_S$), nodes ($_N$), and marrow ($_M$), and a (+) or (−) to indicate whether Hodgkin's disease was found on biopsy. Thus, the complete clinical and pathologic staging notation of this patient would be: CS III$_S$A PS II$_3$A$_{M- S- H- N+}$.

It should be emphasized that staging laparotomy is indicated *only* when it is likely that the outcome would influence the choice of therapy. The splenomegaly suggested the presence of upper abdominal disease which may have changed the patient's therapy from radiotherapy alone to combined radiotherapy and chemotherapy.

QUESTIONS

1. Lumps in the left groin bring a healthy 28-year-old man to your office. On examination, the lumps are firm, nontender, pathologic lymph nodes. Furthermore, he has a 1-inch scar on his left foot where a "small tumor" was removed 6 months ago in a nearby town. Severe "athlete's foot" is also present. The first and most helpful thing to do is:
   (a) biopsy a node
   (b) special test on urine
   (c) liver scan
   (d) get pathologic report on "small tumor."
2. In reference to Hodgkin's disease, only one of the following statements is true:
   (a) Mediastinal, splenic, mesenteric, or paraaortic nodes may be involved.
   (b) Mediastinal node involvement suggests intraabdominal node disease.
   (c) The bone marrow is involved in 20% of patients with Hodgkin's disease.
   (d) Anemia may result from marrow involvement, hypersplenism, or hemolysis.
3. Hodgkin's disease can present in many ways. Which of the following presentations is/are possible?
   (a) episodic fever and sweats
   (b) superior vena cava obstruction
   (c) generalized pruritus
   (d) hilar adenopathy on routine x-ray.
4. All of the following symptoms of Hodgkin's disease are associated with a poor prognosis or B symptoms except:
   (a) unexplained loss of more than 10% of body weight in the 6 months prior to evaluation
   (b) unexplained fever above 38 C
   (c) pruritus
   (d) night sweats.

ANSWERS

1. **(d) is correct**. Melanoma sounds likely and a simple telephone call may solve the problem. The urine can be tested for melanin, but this is not commonly positive. A liver scan may disclose large hepatic metastases—common in melanoma. A node biopsy will give a positive diagnosis. Fungal infections can cause large nodes from repeated episodes of cellulitis. All the answers are correct, but (d) is simple, easily done, and may be most productive.
2. **(d) is correct**. The anemia may have one or more of several causes. Mesenteric node involvement is uncommon in Hodgkin's disease. It is common in non-Hodgkin's lymphoma and should raise suspicion about the histologic classification of the original lymph node biopsy if discovered at staging laparotomy. The other nodes mentioned are commonly involved. Abdominal node involvement is suggested by the presence of nodes in the supraclavicular and axillary areas, not in the mediastinum. This relates to the anatomic proximity of the celiac nodes and thoracic

duct. Only 5% of patients with Hodgkin's disease have bone marrow involvement, in contrast to non-Hodgkin's lymphoma where the incidence is 40 to 50% in the nodular forms.
3. **All are correct.** Each can be the initial manifestation or presentation. Large nodes high in the mediastinum can obstruct the vena cava and cause distention of veins and swelling of the neck, arms, and face. Itching is common in younger women. The fever is called Pel-Ebstein fever.
4. **(c) is correct.** Prior to the Ann Arbor Symposium on the staging of Hodgkin's disease in 1971, pruritus was considered to be an adverse systemic symptom. Data were presented at that symposium which refuted this position, and it was deleted from the list of items associated with B symptoms. An open mind should be maintained on the subject, as some investigators still consider it a bad symptom.

COMMENT   Pursuit of a diagnosis here is ideally suited to an algorithmic approach whereby a decision path or flow chart is utilized. Numerous questions and tests can be avoided and diagnostic possibilities quickly eliminated, depending on the direction taken at key branching points. The following decisions must be made: (*a*) Are the lumps caused by enlarged lymph nodes? (*b*) Are they local or disseminated? (*c*) Is the spleen palpable? (*d*) Is there evidence of bone marrow involvement and constitutional symptoms, and are there clues for other diseases causing lymphadenopathy? "Yes" or "no" answers direct you to a terminal branch.

Age and sex enter the picture. Most patients with enlarged glands will have malignancy, infection, or connective tissue disease; the likelihood of each will vary with age and gender.

Likelihoods were listed and excluded one by one. At the same time, a pattern for lymphoma was gradually woven and proven with the decisive clue—a biopsy. A previous episode of swollen glands (IM) and the former taking of medication for convulsions were misleading clues. The specificity, sensitivity, and importance of liver and spleen size were carefully considered. And last, the need for a team approach by three physicians was demonstrated.   (*P. C.*)

Suggested Readings

1. Kaplan HS: *Hodgkin's Disease, "A Commonwealth Fund Book,"* ed 2. Cambridge, Harvard University Press, 1980.
   The second edition of the most impressive monograph on Hodgkin's disease ever published.
2. Bloomfield CD, Jones SE, Peterson BA (eds): Proceedings of the symposium on contemporary issues in Hodgkin's disease: biology, staging and treatment. *Cancer Treat Rep* 66:601–1071, 1982.
   The most recent comprehensive review of Hodgkin's disease. A compendium of 48 papers on the childhood and adult disease.
3. Lester EP, Ultmann JE: Hodgkin's disease, In Williams WJ, Beutler E, Erslev AJ, et al (eds): *Hematology*, ed 3. New York, McGraw-Hill, 1983, pp 1012–1035.
   A complete excellent textbook coverage of the disease.
4. Tan CT, Chan KW: Hodgkin's disease. *Pediatr Ann* 12: 306–321, 1983.
   Includes the clinical picture, workup, staging procedures, treatment, and prognosis.
5. Wedelin C, Björkholm M, Biberfeld P, et al: Prognostic factors in Hodgkin's disease with special reference to age. *Cancer* 53:1202–1208, 1984.
   Results of a Swedish study of 182 patients.
6. Slap GB, Brooks JSJ, Schwartz JS: When to perform biopsies of enlarged peripheral lymph nodes in young patients. *JAMA* 252:1321–1326, 1984.
   Stepwise discriminant analysis proves to be 97% accurate in making this important decision.

SELF-EVALUATION EXERCISES FOR CHAP-TER 14

(Answers appear after the last question.)

1. Assume the patient in Case 1 has stools that are negative for occult blood and she has no cecal carcinoma. However, her knees, elbows, wrists, and fingers are stiff, painful, and swollen. The sedimentation rate is very rapid, and her temperature is 38.4 C. In terms of high, normal, or low, predict the values for her:
   (a) mean corpuscular volume
   (b) serum iron
   (c) serum iron-binding capacity
   (d) serum ferritin
   (e) hemoglobins F and A_2
   (f) reticulocyte index.

2. (a) Which is the principal test that distinguishes this anemia from that of chronic blood loss?
   (b) Which is the most sensitive test?

3. You see an anemic 56-year-old male patient whose examination and history are otherwise normal. Given the following values, calculate his:
   (a) mean corpuscular volume
   (b) mean corpuscular hemoglobin
   (c) mean corpuscular hemoglobin concentration: hemoglobin 6.3 g/dl, hematocrit 21%, and red blood cell count 3 million/mm^3.
   (d) Next estimate whether his serum iron, iron-binding capacity, and ferritin will be high, normal, or low.
   (e) What is the next appropriate study to do?
   (f) If the results of (e) are positive and the nutritional history is normal, what should be done next?
   (g) What would a bone marrow examination reveal?

4. (a) Calculate the reticulocyte index in an anemic patient whose reticulocyte count is 10/100 red blood cells and whose hematocrit is 20%. Assume a normal red blood cell maturation rate.
   (b) Is the bone marrow hypoproliferative, normally proliferative, or hyperproliferative?
   (c) If the reticulocyte count were 20% in the same patient, what would you seek in the blood smear?

5. A 65-year-old man complains of weakness, easy fatigability, and sore tongue. He is pale and has a smooth red tongue and a palpable spleen. Neurologic examination is normal. The blood studies show hemoglobin 8.0 g/dl, hematocrit 24%, and red blood count 2.0 million/mm^3.
   (a) Calculate the mean corpuscular hemoglobin, mean corpuscular volume, and mean corpuscular hemoglobin concentration.
   (b) What type of anemia is this?
   (c) What is the likely diagnosis?
   (d) What do you expect the white blood cell count to show?
   (e) What do you expect to find in the bone marrow?

6. A patient with Hodgkin's disease has enlarged nodes in the neck and mediastinum, and an enlarged liver and spleen, but no symptoms. A neck node, liver biopsy, and spleen biopsy show evidences of Hodgkin's disease. The bone marrow aspirate is normal. Write the clinical and pathologic stages.

Answers:

1. (a) decreased or normal
   (b) decreased
   (c) decreased
   (d) increased or normal
   (e) normal
   (f) low.

2. (a) serum ferritin
   (b) bone marrow for stainable iron.

3. (a) 70 μ^3
   (b) 21 pg
   (c) 30%
   (d) low iron, high iron-binding capacity, low ferritin
   (e) stools for occult blood
   (f) proctosigmoidoscopy, barium enema, and upper gastrointestinal x-rays
   (g) no stainable iron.

4. (a) $10 \times 20/45 \times 1/1.85 = 2.2$
   (b) normally proliferative
   (c) poikilocytosis, anisocytosis, normoblasts, Heinz bodies.

5. (a) mean corpuscular hemoglobin = 40 pg; mean corpuscular volume = 120 μ^3; mean corpuscular hemoglobin concentration = 33%
   (b) macrocytic normochromic
   (c) pernicious anemia
   (d) leukopenia, shift to right, many polylobed (six to seven) polymorphonuclear leukocytes
   (e) high percentage of megaloblasts.

6. CS III_{SH} PS III_2 $A_{M- S+ H+ N+}$.

Chapter 15

Endocrine Problems

Only 30 years ago, endocrinology was still in its infancy, and diseases of the endocrine glands were poorly understood. Today the situation is much improved, thanks largely to the ability to measure blood hormone levels by radioimmunoassay.

Endocrine diseases were simple. There was either hyperfunction or hypofunction of the pituitary, adrenal, thyroid, gonad, or parathyroid glands. To a great degree this is still true. Hyperfunction is caused by tumor, hyperplasia, or stimulation; and hypofunction results from replacement, destruction, or atrophy. But now we recognize feedback mechanisms, many of which are the basis for testing a gland's function. The pituitary gland, once thought to be the king and supervisor of all endocrine glands, is now known to be somewhat subjugated by feedback mechanisms and to be governed by a power behind the throne—the hypothalamus. Numerous new hormones and endocrine glands are now recognized: glucagon, releasing hormones from the hypothalamus, the juxtaglomerular apparatus, gastrin-producing cells in the islets and gastrointestinal mucosa, the thymus, pineal gland, prostaglandins, and somatostatin.

Since there are so many different glands and diseases, each with its own set of symptoms, physical signs, and diagnostic measures, very little overlap exists and one endocrine disease cannot easily be confused with another. But endocrine diseases are often confused with diseases of other systems because of overlapping symptoms or clusters. You must remember too that, if the pituitary gland is diseased, multiple endocrine hypofunction can exist. Furthermore, multiple endocrine adenomatosis with hyperfunction unrelated to the pituitary gland can occur.

As for problem solving, pinpointing the diseased organ should be simple. There are many well-known clusters and key clues. For example, tachycardia, tremor, exophthalmos, and thyromegaly equal hyperthyroidism; no menses since childbirth points to Sheehan's syndrome; weakness, pigmentation, and hypotension suggest Addison's disease. But remember that such diagnostic clusters are not infallible.

Clues that alert you to the possibility of an endocrine disease include hypertension, hyperglycemia, nervousness, amenorrhea, loss of libido, polyuria-polydipsia, altered growth pattern, and changes in facies and body build, hair distribution, sweat pattern, and tolerance to heat or cold. Weakness and loss of vigor are common.

Pattern recognition is simple only if you have the possible disease in mind. Hyperthyroidism, myxedema, acromegaly, and Cushing's disease can be spotted on the sidewalk or in mental institutions if you specifically look for them. Sometimes the manifestations are so prominent you notice the disease even if you are not seeking it. One look at the face and you know the diagnosis.

This is an area where Sherlock Holmes would be at his best. Questions such as "do you change your dentures more frequently than you used to?" "have your hat and shoe sizes gotten larger?" "do you argue with your husband over whether the windows should be open or closed—or the air-conditioner on or off?" "may I see your former photograph?"—can furnish the single clue that solves the mystery.

However, in spite of all that has been said, endocrine disease is often overlooked. There are several reasons: (*a*) the physician is not thinking of it; (*b*) the early symptoms are often vague and nonspecific—e.g. weakness, nervousness, anorexia; and (*c*) the onset is often subtle and not noticed by the patient. Thyroid disorders, in particular, are often overlooked in the elderly for these reasons.

Don't neglect the possibility of an endocrine disease if the patient's complaints seem neuropsychiatric in origin. For most endocrine abnormalities can present with symptoms suggesting either depression, confusion, anxiety, personality changes, organic brain syndrome, etc. Consider the clinical pictures of Addison's disease, Cushing's disease, hyperparathyroidism, hypoparathyroidism, hyperthyroidism, hypothyroidism, hypoglycemia, hypomagnesemia, pheochromocytoma, and hypo- and hyperosmolar states. Note that each may have neuropsychiatric manifestations as a major or minor portion of the history.

On the other hand, patients are often labeled and treated for endocrine diseases they do not have. Many are given thyroid extract for obesity; antithyroid drugs for nervousness, tremor, and weight loss; and estrogens for perspiration, weakness, and hot flushes. Adequate confirmation may not have been obtained, and treatment was started by presumption. Anxiety may be the issue.

New technology has given rise to quantum leaps in the diagnosis of endocrine diseases. For example, high-resolution ultrasound helps evaluate the details of solitary thyroid adenomas, tells you if the nodule is cystic, solid, or mixed, and may then discover other tiny nodules that make the original nodule less apt to be malignant. This study can be augmented or substituted by needle aspiration biopsy. The relative value of each procedure is discussed in Case 9.

Imaging the thyroid gland with radioactive technetium pertechnetate ($^{99m}TcO_4$) may be a helpful tool in differentiating thyroid disorders. This form of nuclear thyroidology may surpass the radioactive iodine uptake in that the uptake is determined in 6 minutes, and morphology may be delineated in 20 minutes. In addition, the test's cost and radiation are less. Both the thyroid and salivary glands trap the isotope, and the thyroid gland is labeled as "hypotrapping, hypertrapping, or normal trapping" in comparison with the scintillation of the salivary glands. The algorithmic pursuit in the diagnosis of a suspected thyroid disorder may begin with this initial branching point.

Reflect too on the use of ultrasound to detect ovarian hormone-secreting tumors and computed tomographic scans to detect adrenal tumors, hyperplasia, and carcinomas, as well as the demonstration of pituitary and parasellar tumors. Recall that finding an adrenal tumor can be a mixed blessing since so many are functionless.

But perhaps the most rapid strides in the study and diagnosis of endocrine disorders have been catalyzed by peptide radioimmunoassays. Measurable hormones include insulin, gastrin, secretin, prolactin, adrenocorticotropic hormone (ACTH), thyroid-stimulating hormone (TSH), luteinizing hormone (LH), follicle-stimulating hormone (FSH), human growth hormone (HGH), vasopressin (ADH), and parathyroid hormone (PTH). Some old standbys, such as triiodothyronine (T_3), thyroxine (T_4), and cortisol are quantified by traditional methods. Numerous enzymes that are not related to endocrine disorders are also measured by radioimmunoassay. These include prostatic acid phosphatase, pepsinogens, lactate dehydrogenase (LDH), creatine kinase (CK) and its important isomer (CK-MB), trypsin, etc.

It is easy to grasp the significance of such a procedure as an aid in diagnosis, a guide to patient care, and a probe into the stratosphere of biochemical research.

Here are a few words about the relative frequency of endocrine disorders. Almost universal is the menopause—not really a disease. Amenorrhea is often encountered too, but in the young adult woman it is likely to be due to pregnancy. Diabetes mellitus is actually the most common endocrinopathy; the average physician sees several to many cases each day. Thyroid diseases are not infrequent; about 10 to 20 new cases of hyperthyroidism and hypothyroidism may be seen each year. Male hypogonadism resulting from pituitary insufficiency or from primary gonadal hypofunction is rela-tively common too; it manifests itself as incomplete sexual maturation or infertility. Hyperparathyroidism is not unusual; however, the diagnosis nowadays most often results from asymptomatic hypercalcemia discovered on routine testing. On the other hand, diseases of the adrenal and pituitary glands are uncommon and may at most be encountered only a few times per year. Other endocrine diseases are rarities.   (*P. C.*)

Case 9
A Thyroid Nodule
CARLOS PESTANA, M.D., Ph.D.

DATA A 29-year-old man undergoes a physical examination for the purpose of taking flying lessons. A nodule is found in his thyroid. The patient comes to you, his regular physician, for further advice.

LOGIC Here is an asymptomatic patient who has something discovered by someone else in a routine physical examination. Your first task is to confirm the presence of the physical finding.

DATA With the patient suitably disrobed, standing in front of you in a good light, you can see no asymmetry or abnormality in his neck. He is a rather thin young man, and you can actually see his sternomastoid muscles, the pulsation of his carotids, and the prominence of his thyroid cartilage. You ask him to swallow, and as he does so, you suddenly see it: His larynx goes up, and a round lump about 2 cm in diameter comes up from behind the right sternoclavicular joint. It lifts the sternomastoid muscle and also bulges medial to it, just lateral to the trachea, then moves down again and out of view. You palpate the area, and there is no question in your mind. A 2 × 2-cm round, smooth, fleshy-feeling mass is present at the base of the neck, to the right of the midline. It moves up and down with swallowing, is not tender, and has no pulsations. You cannot feel the rest of the thyroid gland.

LOGIC You have answered your first question. In fact, you have answered two. He does have a lump in his thyroid, as suggested by the location and the fact that it moves up and down with swallowing; but you have also determined that this is a single nodule, as opposed to enlargement of the whole thyroid gland. Had his whole gland been enlarged, cancer would not be a likely consideration. Instead you would be concerned with the possibilities of Graves' disease, multinodular goiter, compensatory overgrowth because of hypofunction, or thyroiditis. An assessment of thyroid function and autoimmune inflammation would then be indicated. But with a distinct nodule, the main concern is cancer. Thyroid function must be evaluated here too since a benign nodule can be thyrotoxic. Let us complete the history and physical examination before considering further tests.

DATA There is no chief complaint or present illness, so the entire history is a review of systems; but we stress some questions which are particularly pertinent to his problem. He could have a toxic adenoma, and thus have symptoms of hyperthyroidism. Has he lost weight in spite of increased appetite? Any diarrhea? Does he have palpitations? Has he noticed intolerance to heat? Has anyone noticed that he is jumpy, fidgety, or on the move all the time? Any changes in emotional stability? The answers are all negative.

We are also concerned about cancer of the thyroid, but there are few symptoms specifically referable to this disease. These cancers are usually painless, silent, and unobtrusive until they become huge. We ask him about hoarseness, and he denies it. He has no difficulty swallowing. It would be nice to know how long the mass has been there and its rate of growth, but he did not even know of its existence until now. We ask a few specific questions regarding the past medical history and family history. Has he ever had radiation treatments to the head and neck area? This is a well-known carcinogenic event for the thyroid. Has anyone in his family had cancer of the thyroid? (One type, medullary carcinoma, often occurs in families.) The answers are no.

In the general physical examination we continue to stress the pertinent areas. His eyes look normal: no staring gaze, no lid lag, no exophthalmos. He can focus on a close object without one of his eyes wandering off. The skin, hair, and nails are normal; his pulse rate is 78/minute and regular. We ask him to stick out his tongue; when a 3 × 5-inch card is placed over his outstretched hands no tremors are detected. The neck is carefully examined for possible lymph node metastasis along the jugular chain, but none is found. The rest of the physical examination is unremarkable.

LOGIC   It does not look as though he has a toxic adenoma; we are left with the question of cancer vs a benign lump. Further studies of his thyroid function will help define the issue only in a roundabout way. Most thyroid cancers are not functional, and the ones that are—the medullary type—produce thyrocalcitonin, not thyroxine. But on the other hand, it is rare for cancer to occur in a hyperthyroid patient; and, more specifically, a hyperfunctioning nodule is almost never cancer. If we could show that he has a toxic adenoma, we could deal with that and stop worrying about cancer. Furthermore, if we get to the point of surgical exploration, we must be certain that unsuspected hyperthyroidism does not exist. It could be lethal to do an operation in a hyperthyroid patient without appropriate preparation. Let us get laboratory confirmation that he is euthyroid.

What shall we order? In routine evaluation of patients the thyroid status will be correctly reflected in more than 95% of patients by measuring the thyroxine (T_4).

DATA   His T_4 level is 7.5 μg/dl. The normal values range from 4.5 to 12.

LOGIC   He is euthyroid. Well, almost! He could be hyperthyroid and not show it if he were one of those rare cases of triiodothyronine (T_3) hyperthyroidism, so if you are insecure in your clinical judgment, you measure both T_4 and T_3. Furthermore, he could be hyperthyroid but have a low amount of thyroid-binding globulin, thus giving a false low T_4. If you insist on ruling out this pos-

sibility, your test would be a T_3 resin uptake (T_3RU), and now your diagnostic accuracy would exceed 99%. However, in this particular case the T_4 alone should suffice. Doing all three—T_4, T_3, and T_3RU—might border on defensive medicine.

Now we have a euthyroid patient with a thyroid nodule. Is it a cancer? Only your pathologist can tell you for sure. Since the mass is palpable and not too far from the skin, the thought of a needle biopsy might cross your mind. Such an approach is common in Europe and is favored by some in the United States, but most physicians in this country do not recommend it because it is difficult for the pathologist to rule out cancer, particularly of the follicular type, on such a specimen.

Needle aspiration cytology may be a better test, but even when performed by very experienced cytologists it is not 100% accurate in ruling out thyroid cancer. According to the present state of the art, if there are clinical grounds to suspect malignancy an open surgical biopsy is preferable. On the other hand, should the clinical constellation suggest that cancer is unlikely, needle aspiration cytology could be done to conclude the investigation. As experience with this technique is gained, the day may come when we no longer need to gather further "soft" data but can go directly to needle aspiration.

Since in the United States, in 1985, adequate confidence may not be secured by aspiration, should we schedule the patient for surgery? Not yet. Let's get that clinical constellation that pushes us into either an aggressive or a conservative workup. If most thyroid nodules were malignant and most thyroid cancers were rapidly lethal, the presence of the nodule would be enough indication for surgery. But even at large referral centers, where the sickest patients tend to congregate, only about 5 to 10% of all thyroid nodules are found to be malignant. Furthermore, most thyroid cancers are either papillary or follicular, which are very slow growing and take many years to kill the patient. So a more selective approach to who needs surgery can be taken.

We know of several factors that increase

the likelihood of cancer: young age (older patients are more likely to have benign lumps), male sex, a single nodule as opposed to several nodules, and a cold nodule on radioactive iodine scan (in some series as high as 50% of cold nodules are cancer).

In this case, the presence of a single nodule in a young male patient would be enough to persuade many surgeons to do the biopsy, but others might hesitate. We should have one more bit of evidence to help make the decision. If the patient had a thyroid scan that showed normal function of the nodule, the surgeons would be less reluctant to adopt a *"wait and see"* attitude, or to allow a trial of suppressive thyroid hormone administration which might shrink a benign lump. If he had a cold nodule, shown by sonogram to be solid rather than cystic, even the most conservative physician would be prodded to do something more than watch and wait. Let's get the test!

DATA   A thyroid scan with radioactive iodine shows a normal left lobe, isthmus, and upper pole of the right lobe. The lower pole, where the mass is, shows no uptake of iodine. The radiologist reads the scan as showing a cold nodule.

LOGIC   About 20% of cold nodules are cysts, of which approximately 10% are malignant. A cystic mass would thus be less worrisome, and we might be satisfied with aspiration and cytology. A sonogram is in order. We also order needle aspiration cytology.

DATA   The sonogram reports a solid mass. The needle aspiration reports follicular cells, no malignancy.

LOGIC   We discount the needle aspiration results for the reasons outlined above. We requested it primarily to help our pathologist learn so that some day in the future he may be more helpful to us. We also would have found it useful if malignancy had been detected, so we could plan on a bigger operation right from the start. The rest of the findings indicate the need for a surgical bi-

opsy. The patient is an otherwise healthy young man, so the preoperative workup does not need to be extensive.

DATA   A chest x-ray is normal. Hemoglobin is 14 g; white blood cell count is 5500/mm^3; urinalysis is unremarkable. A sample of blood is drawn and stored to be sent for thyrocalcitonin levels only if the tumor should prove to be a medullary cancer. This test is expensive and must be sent to a specialized center to be done. However, if medullary cancer is found, serial calcitonin levels may alert you to tumor recurrence.

A right subtotal thyroid lobectomy is done under general anesthesia. A frozen section diagnoses benign thyroid adenoma. Four days later, at the time when sutures are removed and the patient is ready to go home, the final pathologic diagnosis is still benign, but now somewhat embellished to read *"fetal adenoma."*

LOGIC   The story has a happy ending. The pathologist confirms the clinical impression of a benign adenoma, and no further surgery is needed. Had it been a carcinoma, further pathologic classification would have been necessary since the operative management is different for each of the four types of thyroid cancer.

QUESTIONS

1. A palpable mass in the neck is most likely to arise from the thyroid gland if:
    (a) it is located in the midline, at about the level of the hyoid bone, and moves up and down with swallowing
    (b) it is located at the base of the neck, or a few centimeters from the midline, and moves up and down with swallowing
    (c) it is located in the lateral aspect of the neck, in the vicinity of the sternomastoid muscle, and does not move with swallowing
    (d) it has a history of repeated episodes of inflammation, drainage of pus, and reappearance of the mass.
2. Diffuse enlargement of the thyroid gland can be found in all of the following except:
    (a) Graves' disease
    (b) simple goiter
    (c) Hashimoto's thyroiditis
    (d) papillary cancer.

3. Which of the following thyroid nodules is most likely to be malignant?
   (a) a hot nodule in a middle-aged woman
   (b) a nodule that is slightly larger than several others in the same gland
   (c) a nodule known to have remained the same size for 2 years, which suddenly becomes tender and twice its size
   (d) a cold nodule in a young man.

ANSWERS

1. **(b) is correct.** More often than not, thyroid masses are off the midline because they arise from either lobe, but they could be at the midline if arising from the isthmus. (a) describes the location of a thyroglossal duct cyst. Only rarely will a mass arising from an elongated pyramidal lobe be found in that location. (c) suggests a mass originating from lymph nodes along the jugular chain—either inflammatory, primary neoplastic, or metastatic. Beware if a biopsy from that site is read as "normal thyroid." The thyroid gland is never at the lateral neck during embryological formation and migration, and thus there is no such thing as "lateral aberrant thyroid." Such a case is sooner or later proven to be metastasis from a thyroid cancer. (d) suggests a congenital cystic mass (thyroglossal duct cyst or branchial cleft cyst) with repeated infection.

2. **(d) is correct.** Cancers of the thyroid do not produce diffuse enlargement, except a far-advanced anaplastic tumor which can reach a very large size. Papillary cancer would typically be a single palpable nodule even though pathologically it is often multicentric and seldom large. In fact, at times there are palpable metastases in the neck nodes before the primary lesion can be detected. Diffuse thyroid enlargement occurs in (a), (b), and (c). Simple goiter is not so simple; it can result from diverse causes such as iodine deficiency or the taking of lithium.

3. **(d) is correct.** This answer gives the most suspicious combination of factors. (a) and (b) are variations of the opposite situation: being female, capture of iodine, middle age, and multiplicity of nodules are all factors that lower your level of suspicion. (c) describes a situation that is seen when bleeding occurs inside a thyroid nodule, most often an adenoma. Of course, bleeding can also occur in a carcinoma, and the fact that the nodule has been inactive for 2 years does not rule out cancer. Papillary and follicular carcinomas grow very slowly.

COMMENT To solve this problem, the author first used an anatomic approach. He confirmed the presence of the nodule and established its location in the thyroid gland. Rather than collect a complete data base, he immediately branched into a subset of data to determine if the nodule was malignant or causing hyperthyroidism. The latter was quickly ruled out by the absence of very commonly occurring signs and symptoms. For how could the patient be toxic in the absence of symptoms, tremor, tachycardia, and eye signs? In choosing thyroid function studies, the author was very aware of the specificity and sensitivity of tests. He was selective too—ordering only what was necessary. Then he invoked Bayes' theorems in considering the likelihood of a thyroid nodule's being malignant and further evaluated these odds in terms of sex, age, iodine uptake, tenderness, and pain.

Actually, a dendrogram with three decision points solved this problem:

1. Confirm anatomy
2. Assess thyroid function
3. Evaluate thyroid isotope scan.

The rest of the information was helpful but not crucial. (*P. C.*)

PROBLEM-BASED LEARNING To get the most from this case study, learn all about:
1. thyroid nodules and their causes
2. thyroid enlargements
3. thyroid carcinoma, the pathologic types and their clinical pictures
4. substernal thyroids
5. how to examine the thyroid gland by palpation and auscultation
6. the determination of thyroid function by the clinical picture and by tests
7. the relation between radiation and subsequent thyroid neoplasia
8. other endocrine adenomas associated with medullary thyroid cancer
9. the latest information on needle aspiration cytology, ultrasound, and computed tomographic scans of the thyroid gland
10. the role of radioactive iodine in thyroid studies
11. Hashimoto's thyroiditis
12. "simple" goiter.

Suggested Readings

1. Witt TR, Meng RL, Economu SG, et al: The approach to the irradiated thyroid. *Surg Clin North Am* 59:45–63, 1979.
   A vexing problem for the clinician is the very late occurrence of cancer of the thyroid in persons who received radiation to the head and neck during infancy. This is a comprehensive good look at the present status of that problem.

2. (a) Hastings KW, Burrow GN, Spaulding S, et al: Current therapy of thyroid nodules. *Surg Clin North Am* 54:277–288, 1974.
(b) ReMine WH, McConahey WM: Management of thyroid nodules. *Surg Clin North Am* 57:523–532, 1977.
   The Lahey Clinic and The Mayo Clinic have been two of the referral centers with a special interest and expertise in thyroid surgery. These two papers—one from each institution—nicely and concisely summarize the indications for surgery in a patient with a thyroid nodule.
3. Larsen PR: Tests of thyroid function. *Med Clin North Am* 59:1063–1074, 1975.
   This reference provides information on thyroid function tests and is especially helpful in deciding which tests to order in cases such as the one just discussed.
4. Löwhagen T, Granberg PO, Lundell G, et al: Aspiration biopsy cytology in tumors of the thyroid gland suspected to be malignant. *Surg Clin North Am* 59:3–18, 1979.
5. Prinz RA, O'Morchoe PJ, Barbato AL, et al: Fine needle aspiration biopsy of thyroid nodules. *Ann Surg* 198:70–73, 1983.
6. Rosen IB, Walfish PG, Miskin M: The ultrasound of thyroid masses. *Surg Clin North Am* 59:19–34, 1979.
7. Ramacciotti CE, Pretorius HT, Chu EW, et al: Diagnostic accuracy and use of aspiration biopsy in the management of thyroid nodules. *Arch Intern Med* 144:1169–1173, 1984.
   Two newer diagnostic modalities have been added to our armamentarium in the evaluation of thyroid nodules—aspiration cytology and ultrasound. Their proponents give their experience and recommendations. Keep in mind that these are the experts, with the best results. Less experienced cytologists or sonographers will not help you as much. A good example of that discrepancy is given by the two references on needle aspiration. Löwhagen, from Sweden, is probably the world's foremost expert. Prinz, from Chicago, in a report that is 4 years more recent, cannot yet match the Swedish results. The last and most recent article describes 90% accuracy for needle aspiration, yet raises the worrisome issue of false negative results and concludes that diagnostic protocols must vary from case to case.
8. Van Herle AJ, Rich P, Britt-Marie EL, et al: The thyroid nodule. *Ann Intern Med* 96:221–232, 1982.
   Analyzes all diagnostic techniques singly and in combination.
9. Gharib H, Goellner JR, Zinsmeister AR, et al: Fine needle aspiration biopsy of the thyroid. *Ann Intern Med* 101:25–28, 1984.
   This paper tackles the knotty problem of "suspicious cytologic findings."

Case 10
Glycosuria

CARLOS A. MORENO M.D.

DATA Two-plus glycosuria is detected in an 18-year-old girl. Since her father died of diabetes and heart disease at age 42, her mother has taken her to a physician for a checkup at least once a year. These checkups have all been negative, including one 6 months ago. The urine test was done at home by the Clinitest method, since the patient's mother does interim testing too.

LOGIC Concern for the daughter is understandable. You get the impression that testing may be excessive. At any rate, further tests must now be done. While only one-third of random positive urine sugar measurements turn out to be caused by diabetes mellitus, the odds are greater with this background. You prefer urine testing by the glucose oxidase method (Clinistix or Tes-Tape), since it tests only glucose, but the mother has continued to test for any reducing substance because this was the test her husband used.

DATA Further history reveals that the patient has been very nervous and has lost weight over the past few months. Contrary to advice, she has been drinking lots of soft drinks because she likes them, though she says she has not really been thirsty. She gets up twice a night to urinate because she has a "Coke and coffee" before going to bed. She has no dysuria. In spite of weight loss, her appetite has been as good as ever. While her mother is out of the room, the patient confides that she has a boyfriend and takes birth control pills. Sometimes during the day she gets very nervous and weak and finds that a soft drink makes her feel better.

Before going further, you get another urine sample, voided in a clean container in your office, and tested by your technician using a glucose-oxidase method. It is negative. You draw blood for glucose determination and, while waiting for the results, continue with your thoughts. The time is 3 PM, 2 hours after the patient's substantial lunch.

LOGIC   On the surface, this case seems simple. But the more data you gather, the more complicated the problem becomes. Diabetes is foremost in everybody's mind because of the family history and one positive glycosuria. Was the test done accurately? Probably so, but you will never know. You have found nothing so far.

The nervousness is puzzling, although she may have enough to be nervous about. Having a boyfriend and taking birth control pills, failure to follow carbohydrate restriction, an overly concerned mother, and the stresses of adolescence—all can foster severe anxiety. The weight loss is worrisome; diabetes could be the cause, but she does not seem to have the degree of glycosuria, polyuria, and polydipsia that would be expected if diabetes were causing the weight loss. She drinks sweetened beverages and urinates twice a night, but this is difficult to evaluate. It is not a straightforward history of extreme thirst and excessive urination.

Other factors test your logic. Hyperthyroidism can cause nervousness, weight loss, and even glycosuria in the presence of a good appetite. It must be considered. Birth control pills diminish glucose tolerance and can cause glycosuria too. Nervousness and weak spells relieved by soft drinks suggest hypoglycemia. In early diabetes this can occur several hours after eating, but she cannot pinpoint the times of day; hypoglycemia would not occur if symptomatic diabetes were already present. Symptoms of this sort may be used as excuses by patients who wish to partake of sweets. Your thoughts are interrupted by the arrival of the result of the blood glucose test.

DATA   It is 100 mg/dl.

LOGIC   You press on for more data, remembering that the patient's mother had an overeractive thyroid gland removed 20 years ago and that there is an increased coincidence of diabetes and hyperthyroidism.

DATA   There has been no excessive sweating, tremor, or heat intolerance. The pulse is 80, BP 106/80, T 36.6 C, R 16. A quick branched physical examination shows no exophthalmos, lid lag, stare, or loss of convergence; the thyroid gland is not enlarged; the breasts are turgid and enlarged. This reminds you to ask if she has missed any menses. The answer is no. Since she is sexually active and takes oral contraceptives, you perform a pelvic examination; it reveals a nulliparous cervix with normal adnexae.

LOGIC   There is no evidence of hyperthyroidism, hypoglycemia, diabetes mellitus, or pregnancy. Birth control pills could cause the breast changes and the glycosuria (if it were indeed present). The weight loss is still unexplainable, though according to your own scale she has lost only 6 lb in 6 months. All the other symptoms could be explained on nonorganic bases. A normal fasting glucose does not rule out diabetes. Not wishing to miss anything, such as tuberculosis, you order additional studies.

DATA   A chest x-ray shows no evidence of tuberculosis. The T_3 resin uptake and T_4 are also in the normal range. After 3 days' preparation with a high carbohydrate intake, a standard 3-hour oral glucose tolerance test is done. The results are 96, 160, 190, 130, and 100 mg/dl at fasting, and at ½, 1, 2, and 3 hours. A trace of glucose is noted in the third urine sample. Blood count and routine urinalysis are normal.

LOGIC   This is a slightly abnormal glucose tolerance test and indicates impaired glucose tolerance. The 1- and 2-hour values are above normal, as is the trace of glycosuria. You bear in mind the fact that oral contraceptives can diminish glucose tolerance, but the family history weights your judgment. You also recall that oral contraceptives, pregnancy, and estrogen administration can elevate the T_4 (by increasing the thyroid-binding globulin) and decrease the T_3 resin uptake—thus altering your thyroid function studies. While this may have occurred in this case, the results are still within the normal range. Hyperthyroidism can be ruled out.

DATA You explain to the mother and daughter that early diabetes may exist, prescribe a sensible 1800-calorie diet, advise restriction of extra carbohydrate, and ask the patient to return in 3 months. Privately, you tell the patient to stop birth control pills and explain why. You also give her some fatherly advice about boyfriends, soft drinks, and contraception.

One year later, the patient returns. She has not been living at home and has not watched her diet, although she did stop taking oral contraceptives. Her symptoms include nausea, weight gain, frequent urination, and intense thirst.

LOGIC It sounds like severe insulin-deficient juvenile diabetes is now upon us. The nausea and weight gain do not fit the picture.

DATA Further questions elicit amenorrhea for 3 months, considerable morning nausea, bloated feeling, and swollen ankles in the evening. A rapid pregnancy test is positive and the uterus is enlarged to the size of a 3½-months' pregnancy. The blood glucose is 228 mg/dl and the urine shows 4+ glycosuria. She is pregnant and has florid diabetes (class B gestational diabetes).

LOGIC The nausea and weight gain go with her pregnancy. She manages to eat well after the nausea wears off, and much of the weight gain is salt and water retention. Hospitalization is indicated, since her diabetes will need considerable attention. This will allow control of her diabetes and permit a baseline evaluation of her vascular, renal,

and obstetric status. It is also an ideal time to educate the patient about her diabetes and nutritional needs.

DATA After 1 week in the hospital, the patient leaves much improved. Except for some persistent nausea, her symptoms are gone. She is on an 1800-calorie, 2 g sodium chloride, diabetic diet that allows for three meals daily and a bedtime snack. A split insulin regimen of 40 units of NPH insulin and 20 units of regular insulin before breakfast, and 20 units of NPH insulin and 10 units of regular insulin before dinner is required to keep her daily fasting blood glucose in the 100 to 120 mg/dl range and the urine free of glucose and acetone.

LOGIC Maternal and fetal welfare improve with tight diabetic control. Motivated patients can be taught to monitor their blood glucose at home, and good control is thus usually achievable.

DATA She is followed closely through her pregnancy with only minor adjustments in insulin dose, goes into labor, and spontaneously delivers a healthy child at 38 weeks. After promising to adhere to a strict regimen, she moves back with her mother who takes care of the baby while the patient works during the day. Now she takes 25 units of NPH insulin in the morning and 5 units of regular insulin before lunch and dinner, and she is instructed to continue her home glucose self-monitoring.

Several weeks later, her employer informs her mother, who in turn informs you, that the patient is acting strangely from time to time. Her actions seem incoordinate and she does not respond properly to questions. This is especially noticeable before quitting work for the day. A 4 PM blood glucose taken during an episode of strange behavior is 30 mg/dl. There is no evidence of perspiration, trembling, rapid pulse, or dilated pupils, which you might expect in insulin-induced hypoglycemia. Oral sweets alleviate the disorder in several minutes. Insulin dosage is reduced to 20 units daily, and the patient is advised to have a 200-calorie carbohydrate snack daily at 3 PM. The behavior disorder does not return.

LOGIC Insulin requirements generally decrease postpartum and need adjustment. The hypoglycemia might have been anticipated.

DATA You next see this lady 23 years later. She is 45 years old, has been living in another city, and has just returned. There have been several hospitalizations in the past 23 years, two for regulation of her diabetes. Several years ago she had pneumonia and was admitted to the hospital in a comatose state. While meningitis and brain abscess were suspected, it turned out to be simply ketoacidotic coma. This information is obtained by telephoning the hospital record room.

Recently her diabetes has been under "good control"; she takes insulin daily but does not monitor her glucose at home. An occasional fasting glucose is between 140 and 180 mg/dl, and the morning urine specimen is usually negative for glucose. She complains of blurred vision in both eyes.

LOGIC Visual difficulty in a 45-year-old juvenile diabetic may represent diabetic retinopathy, cataracts, or ordinary presbyopia. An examination should give the answer. You also wonder how good her diabetic control really is, since she is testing only in the morning. Whether good control delays the onset of diabetic complications or bad control hastens them is still a matter of debate. Most authorities feel that good diabetic control will delay microvascular complications.

DATA The fundi show numerous microaneurysms, small and large hemorrhages, neovascularization, and waxy exudates. No cataracts are seen. An ophthalmologist finds that she needs glasses, but these only partially correct her visual problem. Fluorescein angiography confirms the presence of diabetic retinopathy, and panretinal laser photocoagulation is recommended to prevent further deterioration.

Blood glucoses taken at different times of the day are 150 at 7 AM, 260 at 11 AM, 340 at 4 PM, and 382 at 9 PM; urine glucoses are all 4+ except for 1 + in the morning. A urinalysis shows 3+ proteinuria and occasional fine granular casts in addition to the glucose. The hemoglobin A_{1c} is 15%. The rest of the examination and laboratory tests are normal except for weak pulsations in the arteries of both legs and a creatinine of 2.1 mg/dl.

LOGIC The diabetes is poorly controlled. She now has proliferative diabetic retinopathy with early renal failure. These two microvascular complications are usually seen together. It has been demonstrated that laser photocoagulation reduces the rate of visual loss. Also the elevation of glycosylated hemoglobin corroborates poor diabetic control for at least the previous 4 to 6 weeks.

DATA The insulin dose is modified. She is to take 40 units of NPH insulin each morning and 20 units before supper. Diet and activities are again discussed, and the nature of her problems is explained.

Only 2 months later, the patient revisits you. She has had recurrent bouts of high epigastric discomfort which are unrelated to meals and unrelieved by alkali. The first episode was prolonged and occurred 5 weeks ago. Antacids did not give relief. She feels better now, but comes to see you because she still fatigues easily.

LOGIC While you consider peptic ulcer, peptic esophagitis, and cholelithiasis, your prime concern in a female patient with long-standing diabetes is myocardial infarction.

DATA An ECG shows an inferior wall myocardial infarction of undetermined age. ST segments are isoelectric so you conclude it is not acute. The ECG taken only 2 months ago was normal. You advise a month of restricted activity plus the same diabetic regimen. Just as she is about to leave your office, she mentions that her legs have been hurting over the past month. At first she says they hurt all the time, but closer questioning tells you her calves ache and get tired when she walks one or two blocks.

LOGIC   Leg pains in a diabetic person can be caused by neuropathy or vascular disease, and by arthritis or varicose veins as in anybody. If caused by arterial occlusion, the pains come with walking and go away with rest (intermittent claudication). If neuropathy is the cause, the pain is more or less constant and is associated with other sensory changes and hyporeflexia. Arthritic pain is limited to the joints and is accompanied by stiffness. In severe varicose veins, the entire leg may become achy and tired when the patient is on her feet for a long time.

DATA   Quick examination shows no joint swelling or deformity, no varicose veins, normal reflexes, and normal sensory perception. No arterial pulses are felt in either leg from the femoral arteries down, and the legs are pale and cool.

LOGIC   In addition to her other problems, she has another diabetic complication—arteriosclerosis obliterans of the lower extremities. The thought occurs to you that she may have had a saddle embolus from a mural thrombus. But remembering that her peripheral pulses were weak 2 months ago, you favor progressive sclerosis as the cause. At any rate, the result is the same. The thought of aortofemoral bypass occurs to you, but in view of all her other problems you decide to wait and see what happens. You wonder which of her many diabetic complications will eventually end her life.

DATA   As she leaves your office, she makes an appointment—for herself and her young unmarried daughter . . . .

COMMENT   The family history and subsequent development of diabetes mellitus influence our logic throughout this case study. First, we are confronted by the significance of newly discovered glycosuria and the errors that can be induced during testing. Altered glucose tolerance has three possible explanations here; pertinent negative and false positive clues are considered as we think of diabetes, hyperthyroidism, and oral contraceptives. Distracters are present in the form of nervousness, weight loss, possible polyuria, and polydipsia.

When true diabetes eventually comes, it is associated with pregnancy, so we have an overlap of symptoms that need sorting. As each diabetic complication develops, a new list of possible diagnoses appears, but odds are that they all relate to diabetes—which they do. Each new problem presents with a key clue and is easily solved with a few bits of information. The value of personally contacting a formerly used hospital for information is cited. Sequence of events and cause-and-effect are frequently used (poor control and complications, claudication following infarct, oral contraceptive and enlarged breasts).

Branching techniques are used for data gathering, sometimes to a fault. Interest in the infarct almost caused the peripheral vascular disease to be overlooked. Venn and Boole mold our thoughts as we consider the overlap of causes for glycosuria, weight loss, leg pains, epigastric pains, diminished vision in diabetics, and the presence or absence of various diabetic complications in this patient or any diabetic patient.   (*P. C.*)

Suggested Readings

1. Williams RH (ed): *Textbook of Endocrinology*, ed 6. Philadelphia, Saunders, 1981, pp 715–837.
   A comprehensive review of pancreatic endocrine function which includes all aspects of diabetes mellitus.
2. Bennett PH: The diagnosis of diabetes: new international classification and diagnostic criteria. *Annu Rev Med* 34:295–309, 1983.
3. Smith CK: Current concepts in diabetes mellitus. *J Fam Pract* 16:585–587, 591–592, 595–597, 1983.
   Excellent—covers all the newer concepts.
4. Adams DD, Knight JG, White P, et al.: A solution to the genetic and environmental puzzles of insulin-dependent diabetes mellitus. *Lancet* 1:420–424, 1984.
5. Albin J, Rifkin R: Etiologies of diabetes mellitus. *Med Clin North Am* 66:1209–1226, 1982.
6. Defronzo RA, Ferrannini E, Koivisto V: New concepts in the pathogenesis and treatment of noninsulin-dependent diabetes mellitus. *Am J Med* 74:52–81, 1983.
7. Ostman J: Can adequate control of diabetes control the vascular complications? *Acta Med Scand*, suppl 671:5–10, 1983.
8. Bell PM, Walshe K: Home blood glucose monitoring. Impact on lifestyle and diabetes control. *Practitioner* 228:197–202, 1984.
9. Rayman G, Dorrington-Ward P, Russell M, et al: Simple economical and effective home blood glucose monitoring. *Practitioner* 228:191–194, 1984.
10. Constable IJ, Knuiman MW, Welborn TA, et al: Assessing the risk of diabetic retinopathy. *Am J Ophthalmol* 1:53–61, 1984.
11. Gerich JE: Role of growth hormone in diabetes mellitus. *N Engl J Med* 310:848–850, 1984.
12. Boden G, Master RW, Gordon SS, et al: Monitoring metabolic control in diabetic outpatients with glycosylated hemoglobin. *Ann Intern Med* 82:357–360, 1980.

13. Nathan DM, Singer DE, Hurxthal K, et al: The clinical information value of hemoglobin assay. *N Engl J Med* 310:341–346, 1984.

A sobering view on the use of glycosylated hemoglobin assays.

Case 11
Weakness, Anxiety, Sweating

DAVID J. KUDZMA, M.D.

DATA   Ever more frequent spells of generalized weakness, anxiety, sweating, tremulousness, and palpitations bring a 38-year-old woman to your office. She is unmarried, an executive in an advertising agency, and has always felt well until 3 months ago when these spells began. They occur mainly in the late afternoon and while watching the late show.

LOGIC   Symptom clusters like these are common reasons for seeing a physician. Some of the features mentioned may be absent, additional ones may be present, or one or two symptoms may dominate the picture. Age, sex, and race notwithstanding, this general group of complaints would immediately suggest the following possibilities: (*a*) anxiety, (*b*) menopause, (*c*) hypoglycemia, (*d*) paroxysmal cardiac arrhythmia, (*e*) hyperthyroidism, (*f*) pheochromocytoma, or (*g*) serotonin-producing tumor. The first few conditions listed are common; the last two are rare. Some can be easily eliminated by a single question or observation.

DATA   Between episodes she is well. She has never had surgery, knows of no heart disease or murmur, and never had acute rheumatic fever. Menses are still normal and she has no flushes. There are no gastrointestinal symptoms. Appetite is normal and weight is stable. While she feels palpitations during the spells, they do not seem persistent and have no clear-cut onset or finish. During a spell, she experiences no breathlessness, dry mouth, or numbness about the mouth and fingertips. She denies being nervous or

tense but does relate that she has had to work especially hard to attain an executive position in such a "high-pressure, all male" profession.

LOGIC   These few questions immediately eliminate many possibilities. Anxiety with hyperventilation seems unlikely. The symptoms of hyperthyroidism are not episodic; furthermore her appetite is normal and she has not lost weight. Menopause can be excluded by her age and normal menses. Paroxysmal arrhythmias are unlikely in view of the description of palpitations and the absence of known heart disease. A serotonin-producing carcinoid, especially of the bronchus, produces such spells, but gastrointestinal symptoms are usually present too; in addition, this disease is rare. Four possibilities have been reasonably well eliminated. We are left with anxiety, hypoglycemia, and pheochromocytoma.

Examination of the patient during a spell would be infinitely helpful. Is the blood glucose low? Is the blood pressure high? While we may have to await an attack for final diagnosis, more information may provide an answer now.

DATA   There are no other symptoms in the history or review of systems. Her mother and older sister have hypertension, and her father is an insulin-dependent diabetic. She has remained unmarried because she chose to do so; there were several marriage offers which she declined because they would have meant giving up her career. She smokes half a pack of cigarettes a day and drinks two cups of coffee. On social occasions she has one alcoholic drink.

Physical examination is completely normal except for the blood pressure which is 160/96 in both arms and does not decline when she stands up. In particular, there are no abnormal eye signs, thyromegaly, heart murmurs, tachycardia, or tremor. Pelvic, rectal, and neurologic examinations are normal. Forty-five seconds of hyperventilation makes her dizzy but fails to produce a typical spell. ECG, chest x-ray, complete blood count, urinalysis, and 18-test chemistry profile are normal too.

LOGIC A little has been added. Hyperthyroidism is clearly excluded. So is organic heart disease. Rheumatic heart disease, a common cause of arrhythmias, is virtually ruled out by the absence of murmurs. Hypertension is often familial, though the possibility of pheochromocytoma still exists. Roughly one-third of those with the latter disease have normotension between attacks, one-third have hypertension with paroxysms superimposed, and one-third have persistent hypertension without paroxysms. So this is still possible, even though orthostatic changes are not present. The psychosocial status concerns us, though it may be of no consequence.

Three possibilities persist. Pheochromocytoma may be diagnosed by examination during an attack and by urine studies for epinephrine derivatives. Anxiety with hyperventilation remains a diagnosis to be made by exclusion and psychiatric evaluation, though this condition now seems most unlikely. But if hypoglycemia is present, we are in a different universe and a host of other considerations enter the picture. Since both pheochromocytoma and hypoglycemia have symptoms of hyperepinephrinemia, their distinction may be difficult. The former is rare; the latter is more common. Beware the frequent error of using hypoglycemia as a wastebasket diagnosis in individuals who are chronically fatigued, depressed, lethargic, "have no pep," and whose blood glucoses are borderline low. You decide that she will need careful controlled study, especially dur-

ing a symptomatic episode, so she is hospitalized.

DATA At 3 PM on her second hospital day, your patient develops another of her episodes. The blood pressure remains at its usual level. The palpitations are noted to be premature ventricular contractions. An immediate blood glucose is 40 mg/dl. Symptoms are relieved by orange juice. Urinary vanillylmandelic acid and 5 hydroxyindolacetic acid determinations are normal.

LOGIC Hypoglycemia is clearly diagnosed; pheochromocytoma and carcinoid are ruled out. Now a search for the cause of the hypoglycemia must begin. In general, there are three groups of hypoglycemias: reactive, fasting, and factitious.

Reactive hypoglycemia occurs as a reaction to a meal—often a high-carbohydrate meal. As such, it appears 2 to 4 hours after eating. If no meal is eaten, no attack occurs. Therefore, episodes of hypoglycemia resulting from a missed meal or in the early morning hours after an overnight fast must have some other cause. From the initial history, it is clear that this patient's episodes are postcibal or reactive since they only occur several hours after a meal.

There are three types of reactive hypoglycemia—functional, mild diabetic, and alimentary. The first is the most common cause of hypoglycemic attacks in adults. It is often seen in tense, striving individuals with emotional disorders or maladjustments. The fasting blood glucose is normal and remains so even after a 24- or 72-hour fast. It was thought that excessive insulin response to a normal glucose load was the cause, but insulin assays have proven this is not the case; the mechanism remains unclear. Attacks are usually short and mild, last 15 to 30 minutes, are not accompanied by central nervous system changes, and clear spontaneously. A 5-hour oral glucose tolerance test (GTT) should precipitate an attack from 3 to 4 hours after the glucose load; the blood glucose at that time should be below 40 to 50 mg/dl. Blood glucoses taken a few hours after meals often reveal similar levels.

In some instances, patients have what appear to be typical hypoglycemic episodes 1 to 2 hours after eating, yet clear-cut hypoglycemia cannot be synchronized with the attacks; here a rapidly falling blood glucose may be a factor. Complex psychosomatic elements may be operative too. Remember that some normal people may show low glucose levels during a GTT, but they do not have clinical hypoglycemic episodes.

The second most common cause of hypoglycemia is early mild diabetes mellitus. Here large amounts of insulin are released, albeit late, and the glucose falls to low levels several hours after eating. The family history of diabetes suggests this possibility.

A third type of postcibal hypoglycemia is called alimentary hypoglycemia. This is caused by an excessive insulin response to rapid glucose absorption. It is most commonly seen in patients who have had gastroenterostomies or gastric resections whereby glucose enters the small intestine rapidly. Occasionally it is seen in the absence of surgery.

DATA   A 5-hour oral GTT is done. The results are 90, 140, 150, 94, 68, 36, and 68 mg/dl at zero, ½, 1, 2, 3, 4, and 5 hours after glucose ingestion. Between 3 and 4 hours after glucose ingestion she develops the cluster of symptoms that characterized each previous attack.

A detailed nutrition history is now taken. It should have been done earlier. Breakfast consists only of coffee. But for lunch she has a sandwich, a soft drink, and ice cream. Dinner includes meat and potatoes, bread, and a sweet dessert.

LOGIC   The GTT result is characteristic of functional hypoglycemia. Early diabetes is ruled out. The initial hyperglycemia that would be seen in alimentary hypoglycemia is not present. Her diet is a bit high in carbohydrate, especially in the meals preceeding her attacks. No further studies need to be done, and treatment can be initiated. Her intake of sweets must be reduced and more frequent feedings given. Antihypertensive therapy is also begun.

On the other hand, if the patient had had attacks at 4 or 5 AM or after a missed meal, especially in the presence of vigorous exercise, organic hyperinsulinism would have been a prime consideration. A β cell insulin-secreting adenoma is both serious and curable.

Also to consider, if the attacks occurred on fasting, are severe liver disease (where the liver is depleted of glycogen), glycogen storage disease (where the liver exhibits glucose greed), pituitary or adrenal insufficiency (where hormones which counteract the falling glucose induced by insulin are lacking), severe inanition and wasting, and massive fibromas, sarcomas, or fibrosarcomas found in the chest, retroperitoneal space, or pelvis. The latter tumors cause hypoglycemia in an unclear manner. Insulin levels are normal, but these tumor cells may synthesize a polypeptide which is similar in action to insulin but not recognized immunologically as such.

An alcoholic debauch, especially in the presence of poor food intake, has become a common cause of hypoglycemia and even coma. It results from alcohol-induced impairment of hepatic gluconeogenesis.

Most of these disorders are easy to diagnose. Severe liver disease is quickly apparent on physical examination, alcoholic excess with malnutrition is solved with a question, and glycogen storage disease in children is suspected by hepatosplenomegaly and proven by biopsy. Pituitary and adrenal diseases have numerous other clues, and large connective tissue tumors are usually palpable or noted on pelvic examination or chest x-ray.

Factitious factors cause another subset of hypoglycemias. Insulin overdose and oral hypoglycemics are obvious causes in diabetics, especially if a meal is missed or late. But nondiabetics, especially relatives of diabetics whose hypoglycemic drugs are available, have been known to self-inflict mysterious attacks for secondary gain. The history gives the key clue. But if suspicion and mystery persist, the presence of insulin autoantibodies and a plasma sulfonylurea determination may give proof in spite of denial.

QUESTIONS

1. Insulin-secreting adenomas must always be considered in patients with fasting hypoglycemic episodes. A 56-year-old otherwise healthy man has convulsive seizures associated with bizarre behavior on six different mornings during the past month. Each episode occurs at 4 or 5 AM while he is still asleep, and is vividly described by his wife. Physical examination is normal. Fasting blood glucose is 60 mg/dl. You suspect an insulinoma and wish to prove it. The following reflections are all correct except one.
   (a) This disease is surgically curable, 90% of the tumors are benign, and some are associated with multiple endocrine adenomatosis (MEA type I) where adenomas occur in the pituitary and parathyroid glands as well as in the pancreatic islets.
   (b) The pattern of symptoms is repetitive in the same person, and central nervous system symptoms usually follow the less serious manifestations also seen in reactive hypoglycemias. Attacks are severe and persistent, usually requiring glucose for relief.
   (c) The fasting blood glucose is often well below 60 mg/dl. If not, a 24-hour or even a 72-hour fast may be required to elicit severe hypoglycemia (below 50 mg/dl). Since abnormal insulin-glucose homeostasis exists, the inappropriate elevation of plasma insulin concentration in the presence of hypoglycemia after an overnight or more prolonged fast remains the cornerstone of diagnosis (abnormal immunoreactive insulin:glucose ratio).
   (d) Whipple's triad is diagnostic. It consists of the clinical picture of episodic hypoglycemia, proof of hypoglycemia by blood tests during an episode, and relief of symptoms by the administration of intravenous glucose.

2. If the patient described in the logic session had not conveniently had an episode while in the hospital, you could have proven the diagnosis of functional hypoglycemia by which one of the following:
   (a) a 24-hour fast
   (b) an insulin assay
   (c) postprandial blood glucose
   (d) a stat blood glucose taken during a future episode.

3. Nonpancreatic large tumors have in recent years been identified as causes of fasting hypoglycemia. Which one of the following statements is incorrect?
   (a) Tumors are usually of mesodermal origin, grow slowly, and attain huge size before causing symptoms.
   (b) Occasionally, carcinomas with metastases will also cause hypoglycemia; hepatomas are notable in this respect.
   (c) The immunoreactive insulin:glucose ratio will be abnormally high.
   (d) A total body scan, computed axial tomography, chest x-ray, pelvic examination, and liver scan should be able to detect almost all big tumors associated with hypoglycemia.

ANSWERS

1. **(d) is correct,** since it is the only incorrect thought. Whipple's triad is present in all cases of hypoglycemia, regardless of the cause. All other statements are correct. If multiple endocrine adenomatosis is suspected, skull x-ray, serum calcium, and phosphorus must also be done. Sometimes it is difficult to be certain an insulinoma exists; insulin assays are not always conclusive. A triad of provocative tests—intravenous tolbutamide, leucine sensitivity, and glucagon administration—may be helpful.

2. **(d) is absolutely correct.** It is best to have the blood glucose measured during an attack. Postprandial blood glucose might be reasonably diagnostic too, provided the results were well below 60 mg/dl, but severe hypoglycemia at the time of symptoms would be more reliable. A prolonged fast is not helpful; the glucose would remain normal. Insulin assays too are normal here and would not help.

3. **(c) is incorrect.** The precise mechanism for hypoglycemia in these instances has not yet been resolved. It is not caused by high insulin production, and thus the immunoreactive insulin is not elevated; in fact, it is often low. Excessive utilization of glucose by the tumor is one theory. Others place blame on the tumor's secretion of insulin-like substances which lower glucose but do not immunoreact like insulin. Bear in mind that endodermal malignancies sometimes cause hypoglycemia too. The diagnostic measures listed in (d) may all be useful in locating tumors which are not externally palpable.

Suggested Readings

1. Sherwin RS, Felig P: Hypoglycemia. In Felig P, Baxter JD, Broadus AE, et al (eds): *Endocrinology and Metabolism.* New York, McGraw-Hill, 1981, pp 869–889.
   A comprehensive discussion of all the hypoglycemias.
2. Foster DW, Rubenstein AH: Hypoglycemia, insulinoma, and other hormone secreting tumors of the pancreas. In Petersdorf RG, Adams RD, Braunwald E, et al (eds): *Harrison's Principles of Internal Medicine,* ed. 10, New York, McGraw-Hill, 1983, pp 682–689.

These eight pages are packed with much valuable information covering all the causes and clinical pictures of hypoglycemia.

3. Permutt MA, Kelly J, Bernstein R, et al: Alimentary hypoglycemia in absence of gastrointestinal surgery. *N Engl J Med* 288:1206–1210, 1973.

The mechanisms of alimentary hypoglycemia in people with whole gastrointestinal tracts were carefully investigated.

4. Case records of the Massachusetts General Hospital. Weekly clinicopathologic exercises. Case 9—1984. A 64-year-old man with hypoglycemia and a thoracic mass. *N Engl J Med* 310:580–587, 1984.

An excellent case study that takes you through all the logic of solving the problem of hypoglycemia—includes exogenous, pituitary, hepatic, adrenal, pancreatic, immune-mediated, and neoplastic causes.

5. Gastineau CF: Is reactive hypoglycemia a clinical entity? *Mayo Clin Proc* 58:545–549, 1983.

6. Kwentus JA, Achilles JT, Goyer PF: Hypoglycemia; etiologic and psychosomatic aspects of diagnosis. *Postgrad Med* 71:99–104, 1982.

All causes are included with special accent on psychosomatic aspects.

7. Johnson DD, Dorr KE, Swenson WM, et al: Reactive hypoglycemia. *JAMA* 243:1151–1155, 1980.

Results given on studies of 192 patients at The Mayo Clinic; attempts to correlate blood glucose, symptoms, and Minnesota Multiphasic Personality Index scores.

8. Powers RD, Robb JF: Hypoglycemia due to insulinoma. *Minn Med* 66:13–15, 1983.

9. Kennedy T: The management of the hypoglycemic patient. *World J Surg* 6:718–724, 1982.

10. Apostolopoulos A, Lins WS: Hypoglycemia associated with large histiocytic lymphoma: case presentation and literature review. *Mt Sinai J Med* 49:318–322, 1982.

Covers hypoglycemia associated with other tumors too.

11. Williams HE: Alcoholic hypoglycemia and ketoacidosis. *Med Clin North Am* 68:33–38, 1984.

Relates alcohol ingestion to hypoglycemia in some cases.

Case 12
Obesity and Hirsutism

SAMUEL J. FRIEDBERG, M.D.

DATA In an attempt to make herself more attractive, a 38-year-old recently divorced woman seeks your advice because she is overweight and has excessive hair all over her body.

She has been in good health all her life. Although always slightly overweight (height 64 inches; weight 148 lb), in the past 3 years her weight gradually increased to 192 lb in spite of the fact that she eats "practically nothing." She is convinced there is something wrong with her glands and that her metabolism and hormones must be "out of balance." As further evidence for her opinion, she says she has been hairy ever since she can remember and would like to have this treated too.

LOGIC This lady has two chief complaints. Your first thoughts revolve around whether these are part of one endocrine disease, or are they unrelated, and are we simply dealing with a "fat hairy woman"?

Although nutrition and "nutritional value" of the diet may have become an issue of unwarranted popular concern, the greatest dietary problem in the United States remains the excessive consumption of food. In well over 95% of cases, obesity is simply the result of eating too much. This usually stems from familial and cultural eating habits, psychologic factors, lack of exercise, or combinations of these three. Only the rare fat person has an endocrine disease. Of these, we must consider hypothyroidism, Cushing's syndrome, polycystic ovaries, hypothalamic disorders and tumors, and various causes of hypoglycemia, especially insulinoma. Furthermore, diabetes mellitus and obesity often coexist. So much for the causes of obesity!

Next you quickly run through the causes of hirsutism to see if there are conditions common to both lists: familial, idiopathic, ovarian (polycystic ovaries, stromal hyperthecosis, or virilizing tumors), adrenal (virilizing tumor, congenital hyperplasia, adenoma, carcinoma, or Cushing's syndrome), porphyria cutanea tarda, and medications (steroids, androgens, diphenylhydantoin, minoxidil, danazol, diazoxide, and oral contraceptives).

A number of endocrine overlaps are noted.

You recall that *ethnic hirsutism* in Mediterranean peoples appears at puberty, worsens into the twenties, and is not associated with endocrine abnormalities. Furthermore, *idiopathic hirsutism*, the most common type, probably has some basis in androgen abnormality. In fact, 70 to 85% of women with idiopathic hirsutism have mild elevation of plasma testosterone (.8 to 2.0 ng/ml) if sophisticated measuring techniques are used. Those patients who have idiopathic hirsutism without frank virilization have abnormal secretion of various androgens from the adrenal gland or ovary; there are no detectable structural abnormalities.

If hirsutism of sudden onset is associated with menstrual disturbances and is accompanied by *virilism* (acne, frontal balding, enlarged clitoris, low-pitched voice, and increased muscle mass), then an endocrine disease caused by increased androgens must be strongly suspected and is usually clearly manifested. Virilization is most commonly secondary to an androgen-secreting adrenal or ovarian tumor. In these cases the testosterone level is over 2 ng/ml.

Harvey Cushing first described the clinical picture of bilateral adrenal hyperplasia caused by excess adrenocorticotropic hormone (ACTH) secretion from a pituitary basophil adenoma. The abundant ACTH secretion resulted in adrenal cortisol hypersecretion. This specific set of circumstances is known as "Cushing's disease."

All other clinical disorders which present the same clinical picture and which are due to the presence of excess cortisol, but in which a pituitary adenoma is *not* present are known as "Cushing's syndrome." Hypercortisolism caused by a primary adrenal tumor or adrenal carcinoma is an example of Cushing's syndrome. Recent studies reveal that the "disease" may be caused by basophilic *or* chromophobic pituitary adenomas, in addition to disorders of the hypothalamo-pituitary axis.

Notwithstanding the foregoing, by far the most common cause of Cushing's syndrome is the exogenous administration of steroids for the treatment of asthma, rheumatoid arthritis, ulcerative colitis, renal transplants, some malignancies, etc. Also, be aware of "ectopic ACTH" syndromes in which ACTH-like substances are produced by bronchogenic carcinomas and thymomas, less often by malignancies of the breast, colon, ovaries, and elsewhere.

The common substrate in all cases of Cushing's syndrome and Cushing's disease is the excessive secretion of cortisol by the adrenal cortex. If we exclude iatrogenic and ectopic causes, the pituitary gland is responsible for two-thirds of cases and autonomous adrenal disease for the remaining third.

Various textbook souces do not clearly distinguish between the disease and the syndrome. Semantics aside, from the diagnosis and treatment standpoint, it is important to know only whether the primary pathologic process results from disease in the pituitary area, disease of the adrenal cortex, tumors elsewhere, or the exogenous administration of steroids.

DATA This patient's menarche was at age 13 and sexual development was normal. However, her menses have been irregular at times, dysmenorrhea has been a problem, and she has no children. Recently her menses had become more irregular and she has not had a menstrual period for 4 months.

Excessive body hair has been present since age 15. She tells of several black hairs on the upper lip and chin which require shaving, long black hairs on the forearms, and a few hairs around her nipples and abdomen. The amount of hair present seems to have increased steadily over the years, and she shaves her legs frequently.

She also complains of frequent headaches and occasional episodes of depression. Six years ago she almost fainted on several occasions and had to eat to keep from passing out. These episodes were accompanied by weakness and sweating. A physician obtained a blood glucose and glucose tolerance test at that time; these were normal, and the episodes never recurred. A review of her current eating habits reveals that her "eating nothing" is grossly understated.

Both parents are of Mediterranean origin, and her father and one sister have diabetes mellitus. Her mother died of hypertension and a stroke. Except for easy fatigability, nocturia, and drinking three to six glasses of water daily, the rest of the history is negative. She takes no medication.

LOGIC So far we have an obese, somewhat hirsute woman with nocturia, polydipsia, menstrual irregularities, possible infertility, and past episodes suggestive of hypoglycemia. This is a complex constellation and requires much more information for its solution. The possibilities range from trivial to serious and from rare to common.

However, on the basis of the data so far obtained, you may begin to ruminate over possibilities and likelihoods. Even though myxedema and Cushing's disease are associated with obesity in the minds of many, few patients with these diseases are grossly overweight. They may even be thin. In myxedema, the facial appearance, skin color, voice, and affect are critical features. In Cushing's disease, truncal obesity with thin extremities, plethora, purple striae, and other features are the crucial determinants.

The patient's hirsutism is only mild, she is Mediterranean, and she does not so far appear to be virilized, so it is likely that what she considers excess hair is not pathologic but only cosmetically unacceptable to her. Her headaches, weakness, and fatigue are of little discriminatory value, but the family history of diabetes may be significant in view of her polyuria and polydipsia. The weak spells years ago could represent the hypoglycemia of early diabetes, though episodes of this type could be psychosomatic, insignificant, and nondiscriminatory; and it is important to realize that amenorrhea is sometimes seen in patients who gain or lose much weight rapidly.

DATA Physical examination reveals a grossly and diffusely obese woman in no acute distress. There is no moon facies, buffalo hump, centripetal obesity, or violaceous striae. The blood pressure is 185/100 in both arms lying and standing, the weight 192 lb, and the height 64 inches. She has no stigmata of hypothyroidism, is not plethoric, and her facial and body hair are as described in the history. There are no signs of virilization, and the visual fields are grossly intact. A few pale pink striae measuring 2 to 3 cm wide are noted on the breasts and abdomen. The reflexes are brisk and have a normal rate of return. Pelvic examination reveals normal-sized ovaries and uterus. There are no other positive or pertinent negative findings.

LOGIC Hypertension is now added to the pattern. The striae are simple stretch marks caused by obesity. Cushing's disease is unlikely in view of the absence of other usual findings. Polycystic ovaries (Stein-Leventhal syndrome) as a cause of hirsutism, obesity, and irregular menses cannot be ruled out even in the presence of normal-sized ovaries, since the ovaries are normal in 25% of cases. Had the ovaries been enlarged, that diagnosis would have been much more likely. Hyperthecosis of the ovaries, a variant of this syndrome, is often accompanied by hypertension and diabetes, so it is still possible. A masculinizing ovarian tumor (arrhenoblastoma) is unlikely since it was not palpated and the patient is not masculinized.

Normal visual fields and absence of other evidences of hypopituitarism with multiglandular hypofunction are against a space-occupying lesion of the pituitary, third ventricle, or hypothalamus.

Adrenal virilizing tumors which combine the features of virilization and Cushing's syndrome are now most unlikely. Numerous diagnostic possibilities seem to be eliminated, but laboratory studies are needed for confirmation.

DATA The complete blood count and electrolytes are normal. Urinalysis shows 4+ glycosuria and the fasting blood glucose is 220 mg/dl. The serum is grossly lipemic; after standing overnight in the refrigerator, the lipemia does not clear, and a creamy layer is noted on top of the serum. T_4 and T_3 resin uptake are normal. The urine vanillylmandelic acid, catecholamines, metanephrin, 17-hydroxysteroids and 17-ketosteroids, and plasma total and free testosterone are normal too. The chest x-ray and skull x-ray are normal.

LOGIC The studies are conclusive. Diabetes mellitus is present. There is no evidence for adenoma in and around the pituitary. Tumors of the adrenal cortex and medulla are excluded, and Cushing's syndrome is ruled out. Further search for an aldosteronoma is not warranted because of the normal potassium. Ovarian diseases (thecosis, tumor, or polycystic disease) causing some or all of the cluster of clues are further ruled out by the normal testosterone level. The lipemic nature of the serum probably indicates type V hyperlipoproteinemia, a common accompaniment of uncontrolled diabetes mellitus.

Instead of having one uncommon disease that causes all her problems, this woman has a concurrence of several common diseases. She is simply an obese, slightly hirsute woman with diabetes and hypertension. While most women with idiopathic hirsutism have slight elevation of plasma testosterone levels, remember that roughly one-fourth do not. The spells several years ago may well have been related to the hypoglycemia of early diabetes. Her failure to become pregnant needs further investigation, including a study of a mate's gonadal function. The recent severe weight gain may be related to her marital problems, and the amenorrhea is probably secondary to the rapidly acquired obesity.

DATA Problem list:

1. Exogenous obesity
2. Idiopathic hirsutism
3. Essential hypertension
4. Diabetes mellitus
5. Amenorrhea
6. Depression
7. Divorce.

Appropriate treatment and superficial psychotherapy were given. The patient lost weight, diabetes was controlled, hypertension was adequately lowered, and electrodesiccation successfully removed hair from her face. The menses returned. Perhaps her husband will too.

LOGIC Consider the diagnostic pathway if one or more of the above tests had turned out differently. Had the 24-hour urinary 17-hydroxysteroids been above 20 mg, you would suspect a tumor, a carcinoma, or bilateral hyperplasia of the adrenal cortex—or a micro- or macroadenoma of the pituitary gland. In that event, additional studies might have included computed tomographic scans of the sella turcica and adrenal areas and a dexamethasone test for the suppression of cortisol secretion. These would be used to distinguish the various members of the Cushing family.

If the ovaries were a suspected source for excessive androgens or 17-ketosteroids, ultrasound studies of the pelvis might detect more than the bimanual pelvic examination.

COMMENT The author started with two key clues—obesity and hirsutism—each of which had its own list of possible causes. Overlap in the two lists was immediately noted. Gradually the two clues were built into a larger pattern which could be explained by either a rare disease or a concurrence of several common ones. The latter situation turned out to be correct in this case.

Proof was obtained mainly by exclusion of all other possibilities. Some bits of irrelevant or possibly misleading information, such as headaches, "eating nothing," weak spells, and depression, had to be suppressed in order to narrow the clues to a more wieldy cluster.

Psychosocial factors were strongly related to the clinical picture, and it was often necessary to separate the functional from the organic. These factors included obesity, eating habits, sterility, divorce, and depression. Family history and racial traits helped to decide the significance and causes of hirsutism, diabetes, and hypertension. (*P. C.*)

Suggested Readings

1. Felig P, Baxter JD, Broadus A, et al: *Endocrinology and Metabolism.* New York, McGraw-Hill, 1981.
   pp 435–447: adrenal function—laboratory evaluations
   pp 465–489: adrenal hyperfunction
   pp 699–705: anovulation and hirsutism.
2. Moroulis GB, Manlimos FS, Abraham GE: Comparison between urinary 17-ketosteroids and plasma androgens in hirsute patients. *Obstet Gynecol* 49:454–458, 1977.
3. Vermeulen A, Rubens R: Adrenal virilism. In James VHT (ed): *The Adrenal Gland.* New York, Raven Press, 1979, pp 259–282.
4. Hatch R, Rosenfield RL, Kim MH, et al: Hirsutism: implications, etiology, and management. *Am J Obstet Gynecol* 140:815–830, 1981.
   Subtle hyperandrogenic states are detected in a variety of endocrine disorders.
5. Hirsutism progressing to virilization in an older woman (clinical conference). *Am J Med* 70:1255–1266, 1981.
   This clinicopathologic conference explains the entire logic tree in such a problem.
6. Braithwaite SS, Jabamoni R: Hirsutism. *Arch Dermatol* 119:279–284, 1983.
   Covers the entire subject, including endocrine aspects, in only 6 pages—excellent.
7. Margulis GB: Evaluation of hirsutism and hyperandrogenemia. *Fertil Steril* 36:273–305, 1981.
   Relates hirsutism to excessive androgen from ovary or adrenal in all cases.
8. Meikle AW, Worley RJ, West CD: Adrenal corticoid unresponsiveness in hirsute women. *Fertil Steril* 41:575–579, 1984.
   Demonstrates increased cortisol levels as a common substrate in Cushing's disease and some other causes of hirsutism.
9. Bierman EL, Hirsch J: Obesity. In Williams RH (ed): *Textbook of Endocrinology,* ed 6. Philadelphia, Saunders, 1981, pp 906–921.
10. Reyniak JV: The polycystic ovary syndrome. *J Reprod Med* 28:245–250, 1983.
    A combination of defeminization, infertility, obesity, and hirsutism.
11. Ross EJ, Linch DC: Cushing's syndrome—killing disease: discriminatory value of signs and symptoms aiding in early diagnosis. *Lancet* 2:646–649, 1982.
12. Chetkowski RJ, DeFazio J, Shamonki I, et al: The incidence of late onset congenital adrenal hyperplasia due to 21-hydroxylase deficiency among hirsute women. *J Clin Endocrinol Metab* 58:595–598, 1984.
    This enzyme deficiency may be a much more common cause of late onset hirsutism than is recognized (in adolescents too).
13. Dewis P, Anderson DC: A practical approach to the hirsute patient. *Practitioner* 226:223–244, 1982.
    An excellent British assessment of all causes on a biochemical basis.
14. Elias AN, Gwinup G: *Hirsutism.* New York, Prager, 1983.
    139 pages for those obsessed with hair.

Case 13
Nervousness and Weight Loss
PAUL CUTLER, M.D.

DATA A 36-year-old woman visits her physician because of severe nervousness and weight loss for the past 3 months. She has always considered herself to be a nervous person, but since the death of her mother she has been more so, cries easily, is jumpy and fidgety, and her hands tremble.

LOGIC This combination is not specific. You consider severe anxiety, menopause, and hyperthyroidism. Furthermore, the nervousness and weight loss may not be part of the same process; in fact, she may be losing weight because she is nervous, or she may be nervous because she is losing weight.

Either symptom, separately, has its own list of causes.

DATA Further questioning reveals that she feels warm all the time, dresses lightly even though it is winter, and argues frequently with her husband who wants the windows shut. Her appetite has remained good; she consumes more than her usual fare, yet claims to have lost 15 lb in 3 months according to her bathroom scale. She notes frequent palpitations and her legs and thighs fatigue easily, especially on walking up steps. Her menses had become scant and stopped completely 2 months ago.

LOGIC The picture is taking on a different complexion. It transcends simple nervousness and anxiety. Menopause can include almost all the symptoms, though she is quite young for that event. Cessation of menses speaks for menopause, though these may stop in severe emotional disturbances and in hyperthyroidism too. Heat intolerance is a key point favoring an overactive thyroid gland. The combination of good appetite and weight loss points to the latter diagnosis too. This duet is seen mainly in three conditions: severe diabetes, hyperthyroidism, and malabsorption. On the other hand, weight loss and anorexia indicate a totally different and usually more serious spectrum of chronic infection, malignancy, or depression.

DATA There is no cough, dyspnea, orthopnea, nocturia, frequent urination, or unusual thirst. She had had two to three formed bowel movements daily over the past few months, but the stools are not foul or greasy and do not float. She does not drink alcohol, consumes five cups of coffee, and smokes five to ten cigarettes each day. Her clothes have become too large and she needs another wardrobe; this depresses her and gives her more anxiety. Though her mother died of a heart condition, she had had some kind of thyroid disease for many years.

LOGIC Not much is added. Malabsorption and diabetes mellitus are now most unlikely. Her bowel pattern is compatible with excessive thyroid activity. Hyperthyroidism has a familial tendency and is far more common in women; these are significant facts in this case.

DATA Examination discloses a lean nervous woman in no distress. Her skin is thin, velvety, warm, and moist; this is especially noticeable on handshake. A fine rapid tremor is noted on the outstretched hands. The vital signs are: T 37.5 C, P 120 and irregular, R 20, BP 160/70. Her eyeballs are prominent and sclera is noted between the upper lid and cornea. Lid lag is present when she lowers her eyes, and she has infrequent blinking and inability to converge her eyes on a near object. Her hair is fine, silky, and scant. The thyroid gland is diffusely though only moderately enlarged, and no nodules are palpated. A systolic bruit is heard over each lower pole of the thyroid gland and a venous hum is heard in both supraclavicular areas. The heart rate is 138 and is grossly irregular, and a third heart sound is discernible at the apex. The apex beat is forceful, the left ventricular impulse is strong, and the lower portion of the neck is felt to pulsate with each heartbeat.

LOGIC The diagnosis is now beyond question. She has hyperthyroidism. Tremor, tachycardia, thyromegaly, and eye signs make an incontrovertible tetrad. But, in addition, there is also the characteristic nature of the hair and skin, evidence of high cardiac output, and high blood flow to and from the thyroid gland. The atrial fibrillation (with pulse deficit) is a common signpost. Warm sweaty hands mean hyperthyroidism, while cold sweaty hands mean anxiety. All the physical findings point in one direction.

DATA The T_4 is 16.4 μg/dl; T_3 resin uptake is 48%; serum cholesterol is 98 mg/dl; postprandial glucose is 180 mg/dl; complete blood count, urinalysis, chest x-ray, and ECG are normal except for atrial fibrillation with a ventricular rate of 132. The 18-test chemistry profile is normal except as noted above.

LOGIC Laboratory studies confirm the clinical diagnosis. The elevated glucose may be seen in hyperthyroidism, but it should be rechecked later.

DATA The primary care physician, the surgeon, the patient, and the family discuss the alternative forms of treatment and, for a variety of debatable reasons, the following course is chosen. After an appropriate 8-week period of propylthiouracil, propranolol, and preoperative potassium iodide, a subtotal thyroidectomy is performed. The patient did well in the immediate postoperative period except for transient hoarseness which cleared in a few days.

LOGIC Antithyroid drugs plus surgery were chosen over drugs alone or radioactive iodine even though there was some controversy. The hoarseness resulted from minor temporary damage to a recurrent laryngeal nerve.

DATA Three days postoperatively, the patient began to complain of twitching feelings in the face and tingling of the hands. A tranquilizer did not help, and on the sixth day she had generalized tonic contractions in the arms and legs followed by convulsions. She had positive Chvostek and Trousseau signs; the ECG showed a broad ST segment and a prolonged QT interval. The serum calcium was 6.0 mg/dl, there was no calcium in the urine, serum phosphorus was 6.0 mg/dl, and studies were otherwise normal. Intravenous calcium gluconate had already been given and the patient was begun on vitamin D even before the test results were obtained.

LOGIC Hypoparathyroidism may result from thyroidectomy since several parathyroid glands are often buried in the thyroid and the blood supply to the others may be damaged. Usually the disorder is minimal and transient, since the remaining glands take over full function. Such a clinical picture following thyroid surgery usually has this explanation. In certain cases of Graves' disease with increased alkaline phosphatase, "bone hunger" can occur after surgery, resulting in low calcium but a low phosphorus too.

DATA At discharge, she felt well and was clearly euthyroid by laboratory tests and becoming so by appearance. She was given a prescription for vitamin D and told to return in 2 weeks.

She next sees her physician 3 years later, having moved to another state in the interim. She had long ago stopped taking vitamin D and the twitchy feelings never returned. Again she complains of fatigue and weakness, but this time she has not lost weight and is not nervous. In fact, her symptoms seem diametrically opposed to the original ones. She complains of dry skin and constipation and feels cold all the time. Her husband and she still argue about the room temperature; however, now he wants the air conditioner on when she wants it off.

Her face is puffy and pale, the skin is dry and thickened, the hair is coarse, dry, and sparse, and the reflexes demonstrate a slow return to the normal position. She is definitely anemic, she appears to have gained weight, her speech is slow, and her wit is dimmed. The vital signs are T 36.6 C, P 60, R 12, BP 100/70.

LOGIC The clues are typical for hypothyroidism. Cold intolerance is a highly specific symptom except in the elderly; delayed relaxation of the deep tendon reflexes is a highly specific sign. After subtotal thyroidectomy, a small but respectable number of patients will develop insufficient thyroid function and need permanent replacement therapy.

DATA Laboratory tests confirm the obvious impression. The T_4 is 1.6 μg/dl, T_3 resin uptake is 22%, and serum cholesterol is 348 mg/dl. She is started on small doses of levothyroxine, and her dose will be titrated under careful supervision until she is again euthyroid.

LOGIC Recently the measurement of the thyroid-stimulating hormone (TSH) has come into popular usage. TSH elevation is a sine qua non for the diagnosis of primary hypothyroidism; if the TSH level is normal or subnormal, suspect that the hypothyroidism is secondary to a hypothalamo-pituitary disorder. In the patient just discussed, this determination was not necessary since by history alone the hypothyroid disorder resulted from surgery, and the TSH would have inevitably been high. But to exclude the remote possibility that pituitary gland failure is now at fault, a TSH test may be ordered.

If the clinical picture is still not clear and the tests are equivocal, an injection of thyrotropin-releasing hormone (TRH) causes a marked elevation of TSH provided the pituitary gland is intact and the thyroid hypofunction is therefore the result of disease, destruction, or ablation of the thyroid gland. On the other hand, if the TSH does not rise sharply, the thyroid hypofunction is secondary to a diseased pituitary gland.

QUESTIONS

1. You see a 28-year-old woman who has numerous signs and symptoms suggesting hyperthyroidism. Her older sister takes medication for a thyroid condition. The patient is nervous, has a tremor, rapid pulse, perspires freely, and has lost weight in spite of a good appetite. But her thyroid gland is not palpable. The T_4 and T_3 resin uptake are twice normal, but the radioiodine uptake is low. You consider:
   (a) another disease
   (b) ectopic toxic thyroid tissue
   (c) laboratory errors
   (d) thyrotoxicosis factitia.
2. Thyrotoxicosis in the aged is often overlooked because congestive heart failure tends to dominate the picture. You should be alert to this possibility if the patient has:
   (a) an enlarged nodular thyroid gland
   (b) weakness of the shoulder and hip muscles
   (c) atrial fibrillation with a rapid ventricular rate
   (d) nervousness, exophthalmos, heightened activity.
3. Most cases of hypoparathyroidism are the result of surgery as in this patient. Idiopathic hypoparathyroidism is far less common but does occur. It is characterized by all the following except:
   (a) episodes of tetany, increased bone density
   (b) high calcium, low phosphorus
   (c) calcification of basal ganglia, cataracts
   (d) evidences of autoimmune disease.
4. Though hypothyroidism in this patient clearly resulted from surgery, there are other causes. Which of the following clinical pictures can be associated with hypothyroidism?
   (a) 38-year-old woman who has had no menses since her last child was born 4 years ago
   (b) 64-year-old woman who had radioactive iodine for the treatment of a "goiter" 20 years ago
   (c) puffy, pale, comatose old woman with a temperature of 33 C
   (d) short stature, retarded bone age, and mental retardation in a 6-year-old child.

ANSWERS

1. **(d) is correct.** It is likely that the patient is taking thyroid extract or one of its analogues;

the drug is available at home and the entire clinical picture fits, though you do not yet know the psychodynamics involved. While laboratory errors are always possible, and it is necessary to consider another disease, self-induced hyperthyroidism is most likely. (b) could be correct, since ectopic thyroid tissue in the chest or ovary could become toxic, but this is most unusual and would require scanning elsewhere for detection.
2. **(a), (b), and (c) are correct.** Such patients do have large thyroids, proximal myopathy, and atrial fibrillation with frequently uncontrolled congestive heart failure. But the features of (d) are not usually present. In fact, these patients generally are apathetic and calm; eye signs are minimal. They are often mistaken for senile patients with end-stage congestive heart failure. Recognition and proper treatment effect profound improvement.
3. **(b) is correct because it is wrong.** The basic defect, lack of parathyroid hormone, results in low serum calcium and elevated serum phosphorus. Tetany and calcium deposition in bone also occur. Calcification of ganglia and cataracts result too. This disease may be seen together with other allegedly autoimmune diseases, such as pernicious anemia, thyroiditis, and Addison's disease. In addition, many cases have autoantibodies to parathyroid, lending further credence to the autoimmune etiology for the idiopathic form.
4. **All are correct.** (a) suggests a woman with Sheehan's syndrome who infarcted her pituitary gland at childbirth, then developed hypogonadism and hypothyroidism. The incidence of hypothyroidism after radioiodine treatment increases annually and approaches 100% with advancing age. The patient in (c) probably has myxedema coma, an advanced stage of hypothyroidism. And the child in (d) has juvenile myxedema.

COMMENT Problem solving was simple here. The diagnoses were fairly evident as the information unfolded. A sequence of hyperthyroidism, hypoparathyroidism, and hypothyroidism was unquestionable—the cause and effect relationship being so very obvious. Each diagnosis was proven by characteristic clusters of clues derived from all portions of the data base. (*P. C.*)

Suggested Readings

1. Spaulding SW, Utiger RD: The thyroid. In Felig P, Baxter JD, Broadus AE, et al (eds): *Endocrinology and Metabolism.* New York, McGraw-Hill, 1981, pp 301–326.
   An in-depth presentation of types, causes, pathophysiology, and clinical features of hyperthyroidism.
2. Ingbar SH, Woeber KA: The thyroid gland. In

Williams RH (ed): *Textbook of Endocrinology*, ed 6. Philadelphia, Saunders, 1981.
pp 175–208: hyperthyroidism
pp 208–226: hypothyroidism
The clinical pictures and diagnosis are presented.

3. Aurbach GD, Marx SJ, Spiegel AM: Parathyroid hormone, calcitonin, and calciferols. In Williams RH (ed): *Textbook of Endocrinology*, ed 6. Philadelphia, Saunders, 1981.
pp 936–949: parathyroid hormone, effects and assay
pp 990–996: hypoparathyroidism and pseudohypoparathyroidism.

4. Chopra IJ, Solomon DH: Pathogenesis of hyperthyroidism. *Annu Rev Med* 34:267–281, 1983.

5. Strakosch CR, Wenzel BE, Row VV, et al: Immunology of autoimmune thyroid diseases. *N Engl J Med* 307:1499–1507, 1982.

6. Volpé R: Autoimmune thyroid disease. *Hosp Pract* 19:141–151, 155–158, 1984.

7. Gooch BR, Isley WL, Utiger RD: Abnormalities in thyroid function tests in patients admitted to a medical service. *Arch Intern Med* 142:1801–1805, 1982.

8. Spaulding SW: Hypothyroidism. *Primary Care* 4:79–88, 1977.
Emphasis is placed on the early recognition of this disease and the differentiation between primary and secondary hypothyroidism.

9. Rosenthal FD: Difficulties in the clinical diagnosis of thyrotoxicosis. *Practitioner* 218:521–525, 1977.
This brief article deals with some of the less recognized presentations of hyperthyroidism.

10. Cole-Beuglet C, Goldberg BB: New high-resolution ultrasound evaluation of diseases of the thyroid gland. *JAMA* 249:2941–2944, 1983.

11. Kaplan EL, Bartlett S, Sugimoto J, et al: Relation of postoperative hypocalcemia to operative techniques. *Surgery* 92:827–834, 1982.

Case 14
Polyuria and Polydipsia

DAVID J. KUDZMA, M.D.

DATA   The patient is a 33-year-old professional lepidopterist whose relentless quest for the winged rare and beautiful has, over the past 3 months, been hampered by a too frequent need to urinate. This need exists throughout the waking day (every 2 hours) and awakens him three times nightly. Each time, the voided volume seems to be a "bladderful." There is no pain, burning, or difficulty with urination, but he is finding the problem wearisome. He has noted increasing thirst, and is aware that his fluid intake is generous; after most nocturnal trips to the bathroom he drinks a glass of water.

LOGIC   The distinctive problem here is polyuria, and its causes are multiple. It is apparent that his urinary frequency is caused by the formation of a large volume of urine rather than by the need to void small amounts frequently. Therefore he does not have common simple frequency resulting from infection or obstruction. He is too young for prostatic hypertrophy, the most common cause of obstruction in men, nor does he have the usual symptoms that go with obstruction or infection. The nocturia of congestive heart failure can easily be eliminated, since he has daytime frequency too and since patients with congestive heart failure would present with symptoms of dyspnea and fatigue rather than nocturia. Furthermore, none of these situations (obstruction, infection, congestive heart failure) causes thirst since there is no increase in total urine volume. Renal disease with waning renal function causes a compensatory increase in urine volume, but not usually to this degree.

We are left with the various *polyuric-polydipsic syndromes*: (*a*) diabetes mellitus (DM), (*b*) central diabetes insipidus (DI), (*c*) nephrogenic DI, (*d*) psychogenic polydipsia, (*e*) hypokalemia, (*f*) hypercalcemia, and (*g*) use of a diuretic.

DM causes an osmotic diuresis. Central DI is caused by a lesion of the hypothalamus or posterior lobe of the pituitary gland so that there is insufficient antidiuretic hormone. Psychogenic polydipsia is nothing more than compulsive water drinking and may be accompanied by other psychoneurotic manifestations. Nephrogenic DI results from renal unresponsiveness to antidiuretic hormone.

Even at this point, the surreptitious use of a diuretic is unlikely for a number of reasons: the effect of mild diuretics is limited to a number of days, and while potent diuretics are effective for longer periods, these patients would present with critical volume depletion, syncope, and shock rather than with polyuria. Low potassium and high calcium do not cause such severe water turnover. More historical data are needed.

DATA There is no family history of DM or polyuric syndrome. He takes no medication, drinks ethanol infrequently, and does not smoke. There is no past history of renal, stones, gastrointestinal symptoms, or conjunctival irritation. His health has remained good, he feels well, has lost no strength, and his appetite and weight have remained normal. There is no headache or visual symptoms.

LOGIC The hypercalcemia of hyperparathyroidism is not suggested because there have been no stones, gastrointestinal symptoms, or symptoms of conjunctival irritation due to deposition of calcium salts. DM is unlikely in the absence of weight loss, weakness, polyphagia, and family history. The absence of weakness is against kaliopenic nephropathy with resultant polyuria, and there is no apparent cause for low potassium. The possibility of DI due to a pituitary or hypothalamic tumor is less likely in the absence of headache and visual disturbances. But special studies are needed to explore this diagnosis more fully. Several possibilities are already reasonably well excluded and only a few remain.

DATA Physical examination discloses a healthy-looking young man. The vital signs are normal and there are no significant orthostatic changes in pulse and blood pressure. He weighs 163 lb and is 70 inches tall. With the exception of a left varicocele,

everything is normal. Specifically, visual fields, tissue turgor, and mucous membranes are normal. Band keratopathy is not present.

LOGIC Note the absence of evidence of weight loss, blood volume contraction, or dehydration. We would expect severe DM or potent diuretic abuse to cause these. The juxtacorneal calcium salt deposits resulting from prolonged or severe hypercalcemia are not present. Normal strength, normal deep tendon reflexes, normal blood pressure, absence of gastrointestinal symptoms, and the nonuse of medications are all points against hypokalemia and some of its principal causes. The varicocele is not significant. Though laboratory tests are now needed, we have already reasonably excluded most of the causes listed for the presenting cluster.

DATA Studies: urinalysis is completely normal, but specific gravity is 1.002; blood count, urine culture, ECG, and chest x-ray are normal; serum sodium, potassium, bicarbonate, chloride, glucose, creatinine, calcium, and phosphorus are all normal; serum cholesterol is 298 mg/dl.

LOGIC So much for DM, hypokalemia, and hypercalcemia! Also, renal disease in general is virtually eliminated. While hypercholesterolemia may be an important problem, it is of no consequence in this diagnostic deliberation. The often ignored urine specific gravity is significantly very low, and in the context of this patient, a dilute urine leans us toward central DI, psychogenic polydipsia (PP), or nephrogenic DI. The controlled environment of a hospital is required to explore these possibilities.

DATA The patient is hospitalized. A first-voided morning urine specimen has a specific gravity of 1.001. The 24-hour fluid intake is 7600 ml, and the concomitant 24-hour urine output is 6800 ml. Skull x-rays with specific attention to the sella turcica and suprasellar area are normal.

LOGIC Polyuria, polydipsia, and hyposthenuria are confirmed. There is no evidence of a tumor in the sellar area. Further discriminatory tests are needed.

DATA Water is rigorously withheld from 10 PM to 6 AM. At 10 PM the body weight is 160 lb and the urine osmolality is 85 mOsm/kg; at 6 AM the body weight is 156 lb and the urine osmolality is 470 mOsm/kg. After 24 hours of unrestricted access to fluids, 5 units of Pitressin* are given intramuscularly; urine osmolality rises from 80 to 310 mOsm/kg. (Some clinicians prefer to give Pitressin immediately after water restriction; others do the tests separately.)

LOGIC These results indicate that the patient is able to concentrate his urine, though imperfectly. That is, his kidneys are responsive to antidiuretic hormone and nephrogenic DI can be ruled out. Furthermore, it is typical for patients with PP to concentrate their urine more with dehydration than with Pitressin. The opposite is true of patients with central DI.

Remember that the patient with central DI drinks a lot because he urinates too much, whereas the patient with PP urinates a lot because he drinks too much. The fact that compulsive water drinkers have partially defective concentrating mechanisms because of chronic excessive water ingestion confuses the issue a bit. You can see why the patient with central DI concentrates his urine very well after Pitressin (antidiuretic hormone) but responds only partially to water deprivation. Also, it is reasonable that the PP patient concentrates well in response to water deprivation but only moderately well to Pitressin.

Though most cases of central DI are idiopathic, some result from pituitary tumors, parasellar tumors, metastatic tumors (often breast), and generalized diseases, such as the histiocytoses, sarcoidosis, and other granulomatous diseases. None of the specific causes is evident here. The abrupt onset of

---

* Antidiuretic hormone (ADH), vasopressin, and Pitressin (the commercial preparation) are all different expressions and names for the same substance. The reader should know all these terms.

symptoms and craving for ice water are characteristic of central DI; these clinical clues are not present here either.

Thus the presenting polyuria and polydipsia are most likely explained by psychogenic factors, the reasons for which should be explored with the assistance of psychiatric consultation.

The patient is asked to restrict his fluid intake to eight glasses/day, including all types of liquids, and he will need careful watching. PP and DI are often mistaken for each other—even after studies. Should symptoms continue, more detailed investigation may be needed.

While the incorporation of vasopressin radioimmunoassay into the diagnostic protocol may increase our accuracy in differentiating the causes of the polyuric-polydipsic syndromes, the role and operating characteristics of this test are not firmly established. This assay will probably be more useful in evaluating the syndrome of inappropriate antidiuretic hormone secretion (SIADH). See Case 47 for a detailed exposition of this syndrome.

QUESTIONS

1. Which of the following diagnostic procedures would give the most valuable information in evaluating a patient with a 4-week history of polydipsia and polyuria?
   (a) oral glucose tolerance test
   (b) urinalysis
   (c) fasting blood glucose
   (d) 24-hour urine collection for volume and osmolality.
2. Which of the following clues most strongly suggests DM as the cause for a 4-week history of polydipsia and polyuria?
   (a) weight loss
   (b) absence of nocturia
   (c) anorexia
   (d) bradycardia.
3. Suppose your patient with severe polyuria and polydipsia is lethargic and irritable and has no signs of dehydration. Immediate hospitalization reveals the serum sodium to be 119 mEq/liter. Otherwise, everything, including the urinalysis, is unchanged. He has a low serum sodium causing mental abnormalities and is critically ill because of:
   (a) inappropriate antidiuretic hormone secretion
   (b) diabetes mellitus

(c) diabetes insipidus
(d) compulsive water drinking.

4. Assume that our patient had responded to the test dose of Pitressin with a rise in urine osmolality to 900 mOsm/kg. Which of the following is/are correct?
   (a) Plasma level of antidiuretic hormone would be high.
   (b) Though the response is consistent with central DI, this diagnosis is unlikely because of his age.
   (c) You would expect to find DI in other members of the family.
   (d) Mild cases can exist where the urine volume is only 2000 to 3000 ml/24 hours.

ANSWERS

1. **(b) is correct.** If there is no glucose in the urine, DM can be excluded as a cause of the symptoms. The specific gravity provides other useful information regarding the concentrating ability of the kidneys. Other urine abnormalities may suggest primary renal disease. The glucose tolerance test is not of much value since, even if abnormal, heavy glycosuria is required to cause the clinical picture; this is detected by the urinalysis. For the same reason, the blood glucose is of limited value. Answer (d) fails to consider DM, the most common cause of the presenting symptom complex.

2. **(a) is correct.** Involuntary weight loss associated with the two prominent symptoms indicates DM, unless proven otherwise by an immediate urinalysis. Since polyuric patients with DM have nocturia and increased appetite, (b) and (c) are incorrect. The pulse rate is probably of little help, though under these circumstances it is more apt to be rapid than slow.

3. **(d) is correct.** Compulsive drinking can cause a dilutional hypoosmolar syndrome with low sodium, resulting mental changes, and even convulsions. Such patients who drink themselves into water intoxication are unusual. DM is excluded by the other normal laboratory tests. In DI, the stimulus to drink results from the polyuria; this is the reverse of water intoxication; the serum sodium is either normal or high. Inappropriate antidiuretic hormone secretion causes low sodium, but it is not associated with polyuria and polydipsia. Such patients have normal or low output.

4. **(d) is correct.** The dramatic response to Pitressin (exceeding the response to overnight water restriction) confirms the diagnosis of central DI. This is not an "*all or none*" disease; the deficiency of antidiuretic hormone may be mild and symptoms similarly so. The plasma antidiuretic hormone level is high in nephrogenic DI, but this diagnostic possibility is disproven by the response to Pitressin. Furthermore, central DI can occur at any age and it is not familial.

COMMENT The skilled busy physician would solve the polyuria-polydipsia cluster with alacrity. He knows the statistical likelihoods, the clues associated with these likelihoods, and how to reach his target quickly. The absence of urinary obstructive symptoms and the patient's age are against prostatic disease; further, since the total urine output does not change, thirst does not result. Good health and stable weight and appetite disqualify DM. We are now left only with the unusual.

A quick urinalysis, serum glucose, and electrolytes rule out hypercalcemia, hypokalemia, florid kidney disease, and DM. The low urine specific gravity and osmolality are helpful. You know he has dilute urine and the field is narrowed to three possibilities. The response of urine osmolality and urine output to water deprivation and Pitressin injection makes the distinction between nephrogenic DI, central DI, and compulsive water drinking.

All you've done is ask five or ten questions, examine the urine, get three blood chemical tests, and do two simple noninvasive procedures. *Et voilà!* You have the answer and you haven't even touched the patient.   (*P. C.*)

Suggested Readings

1. Barlow ED, De Wardener HE: Compulsive water drinking. *Q J Med* 28:235–258, 1959.
   An excellent, thorough, classic review.
2. Coggins CH, Leaf A: Diabetes insipidus. *Am J Med* 42:807–813, 1967.
   Diabetes insipidus clinically characterized in meticulous detail.
3. Schrier RW, Leaf A: Effect of hormones on water, sodium, chloride, and potassium metabolism. In Williams RH (ed): *Textbook of Endocrinology*, ed 6. Philadelphia, Saunders, 1981, pp 1032–1036.
   Thirst, polydipsia, and polyuria.
4. Milles JJ, Spruce B, Bayliss PH: A comparison of diagnostic methods to differentiate diabetes insipidus from polyuria: a review of 21 patients. *Acta Endocrinol* 104:410–416, 1983.
   How to differentiate three principal causes of polyuria-polydipsia by plasma arginine vasopressin levels and response to other tests.
5. Zerbe RL, Robertson GL: A comparison of plasma vasopressin measurements with a standard indirect test in the differential diagnosis of polyuria. *N Engl J Med* 305:1539–1543, 1981.
6. Singer I: Differential diagnosis of polyuria and diabetes insipidus. *Med Clin North Am* 65:303–320, 1981.
   Covers all causes with a diagnostic decision tree.

7. Scherbaum WA, Bottazzo GF: Autoantibodies to vasopressin cells in idiopathic diabetes insipidus: evidence for an autoimmune variant. *Lancet* 1:897–901, 1983.

   Autoimmunity is blamed for yet another endocrine disorder.

8. Moses AM, Notman DD: Diabetes insipidus and syndrome of inappropriate antidiuretic hormone secretion. *Adv Intern Med* 27:73–100, 1982.

   Central and renal DI and the SIADH are detailed.

9. Kern KB, Meislin HW: Diabetes insipidus: occurrence after minor head trauma. *J Trauma* 24:69–72, 1984.

10. Kimmel DW, O'Neill BP: Systemic cancer presenting as diabetes insipidus. *Cancer* 52:2355–2358, 1983.

   Metastases from lung and leukemia/lymphoma are detected in sella by computed tomographic scans.

Chapter 16

Cardiovascular Problems

Heart diseases number in the hundreds and it takes a 2000-page textbook to describe them all. Yet the ways in which patients with cardiac diseases present to the physician comprise a short list:

1. Incidental finding
2. Early chamber failure
3. Florid congestive heart failure
4. Embolus
5. Arrhythmia
6. Chest pain
7. Syncope
8. Infection
9. Combinations of the above

In recent years, more and more patients without cardiac symptoms are coming to the doctor because of abnormalities detected elsewhere on routine examination or in the course of other illnesses. These abnormal findings include murmurs, cardiac enlargement or contour abnormality seen on the chest x-ray, or any of dozens of ECG abnormalities. Many of these findings may never cause symptoms.

Beginning chamber decompensation or early congestive heart failure (CHF) brings many patients to the physician. Often the patient never knows he has a cardiac problem until the left ventricle or right ventricle begins to fail and causes symptoms. Sometimes he knows of hypertension or a heart murmur which has existed for years. While the causes of failure are many, the symptoms are generally the same. The history, physical examination, and studies will differ somewhat depending on the underlying cause for the failure and on the chamber which fails. Left ventricular failure (LVF) is by far most common, and it results in dyspnea and fatigue on exertion, orthopnea, and night cough. Mitral stenosis results in "left atrial failure," which gives the same symptoms as LVF, though palpitations may be more prominent because of atrial irritability. Right ventricular failure (RVF) causes right upper quadrant discomfort, indigestion, and swollen legs.

Florid CHF with all the signs and symptoms of bilateral chamber failure is seen in the unusual patient who does not heed the earlier warnings, in the patient who is inadequately treated, or in the patient at the end of his illness. LVF usually precedes and is the most common cause of RVF. However, florid textbook CHF is not so common as formerly since patients are treated better and the full picture is often suppressed until death occurs from a complication. But, on the other hand, as arrhythmia therapy improves, we are beginning to encounter more patients who survive despite the presence of severe myocardial dysfunction. So if the patient lives long enough, and avoids thromboemboli, pneumonia, arrhythmias, and infarctions, severe CHF is the common end point of most forms of heart disease.

An embolus may be the first indication that a cardiac problem exists. The sudden onset of a stroke, flank pain and hematuria, or a cold, painful, pulseless limb may on further study reveal mitral stenosis, atrial fibrillation, infective endocarditis, or recent unnoticed myocardial infarction—all sources of arterial emboli.

Any sort of arrhythmia may augur heart disease. The patient may come to the physician complaining of palpitations, skipped beats, or fluttering in the chest. These may be momentary, continuous, or repetitive. Correct identification can be achieved by an ECG, superimposed exercise, or even long-term monitoring. But further examination of the heart may disclose the cause (early CHF, mitral stenosis, Wolff-Parkinson-White syndrome, Barlow syndrome, coronary artery disease, hyperthyroidism) or may reveal no evidence of heart disease at all.

A common presentation is chest pain caused by angina pectoris or myocardial infarction. Bear in mind that subclinical coronary disease may often become symptomatic because of anything that might suddenly or subtly further worsen anoxia to an area of already ischemic heart muscle. This includes a paroxysm of tachycardia, gastrointestinal hemorrhage, gradually developing severe anemia for any reason, worsening of chronic obstructive lung disease, or pneumonia. The same holds true for patients with heart disease who are bordering on CHF. They can suddenly go into failure with the advent of a paroxysmal tachycardia, a small myocardial infarct, a gastrointestinal hemorrhage, pneumonia, rapid transfusions or saline infusions, or sudden severe physical or emotional strain.

One or more syncopal attacks may unveil the presence of paroxysmal tachyarrhythmia, paroxysmal bradyarrhythmia, complete heart block, sinus node disease, aortic stenosis, coronary disease, or even an atrial thrombus or myxoma.

Infection as a presenting problem refers principally to infective endocarditis, viral myocarditis, or pericarditis. Here the clinical picture varies. In endocarditis, the patient may seek help because of fever, lassitude, and embolic manifestations. Viral myocarditis usually results in arrhythmias and heart failure with dyspnea, orthopnea, and edema.

Pericarditis, with or without effusion, usually presents with chest pain, at times dyspnea, and fever, depending on the underlying cause.

Combinations of any of the common presentations may occur at the same time. A patient can present with chest pain, LVF, and arrhythmia simultaneously. In instances of this sort, you always have to determine which came first, since any one could precipitate the other two. If aortic stenosis is present, syncope, LFV, and angina can and often do coexist.

Remember that many healthy patients are seen because they only think they have heart disease. A vague chest pain, a "skipped heartbeat," a sighing deep breath, or the sudden death of a friend or relative may prompt a visit to the doctor's office.

Recent advances in diagnostic technology include: (*a*) biplane and *cineangiography* using radiopaque dyes to outline congenital and acquired anomalies, to delineate precise coronary artery anatomy, to detect valvular insufficiency, intracardiac tumors and clots, and to assess left ventricular function; (*b*) *radioisotope* scanning using technetium or thallium to measure left ventricular ejection fraction, to detect regional myocardial ischemia, to visualize, delineate, and measure infarction, and to assess regional wall motion and myocardial perfusion; (*c*) *ultrasound* to detect pericardial effusions, myocardial thickness and regional motility, valvular defects and malfunctions, vegetations, intraluminal thrombi and tumors, and septal defects; (*d*) *programmed electrical stimulation* which consists of complex electrophysiologic studies that render serious arrhythmias more diagnosable and more treatable.

The usefulness of these procedures continues to broaden, and the accuracy increases as various techniques for their application improve. The exact role for each in the theater of cardiologic diagnosis has not yet been assigned. Gated *nuclear magnetic resonance* scans (NMR) may soon offer the same diagnostic advantages in the rapidly moving heart that computed tomographic scans provide for immobile organs. By simultaneously recording the phonocardiogram, ECG, and carotid pulse tracing, the preinjection period (PEP) and left ventricular ejection time (LVET) can be measured, thus giving an indication of underlying pathophysiologic defects of ventricular function and ejection. And last, the comprehension, proof, and acceptance of the concept of coronary artery vasospasm have enabled us to understand many false negative results in the presence of coronary disease and have provided better management for some patients with atypical angina pectoris.

Especially today, when virtually 100% certainty is required before performing coronary artery bypass grafts, intracoronary thrombolysis, percutaneous transluminal coronary angioplasty (PTCA), valve replacements, and subendocardial resections, the diagnostic procedures just mentioned must be accurate and dependable. (*P. C.*)

Case 15
Abnormal ECG

PAUL CUTLER, M.D.

DATA After a routine insurance examination, a 56-year-old man was told that there was something wrong with his ECG and he should consult his private physician. A repeat ECG shows a left ventricular hypertrophy (LVH) pattern. Thereupon you proceed to ask questions and examine simultaneously.

LOGIC To solve this problem, you could easily depart from the trunk of the diagnostic tree, follow a branching pattern, and quickly arrive at a cause for the ECG abnormality. First, note the wisdom of repeating the ECG to make sure the abnormality and the patient match. True, there are negative T waves in leads 1, AVL, and V_4 to V_6, high voltage, and left axis deviation; a left atrial abnormality is also noted. You can deduce that the left ventricle is strained and hypertrophied and that the left atrium is secondarily so.

As you study the ECG, you think of the common disorders that can strain the left ventricle, especially in a man this age: hypertension, coronary heart disease, aortic stenosis, aortic regurgitation, mitral regurgitation, and cardiomyopathy. These should be easily discernible by history and examination.

If hypertension is the cause, there may be a history of it and it will be apparent in the fundi and blood pressure measurement. While essential hypertension is the usual variety, secondary causes of hypertension, like chronic bilateral renal disease, unilateral renal ischemia, primary aldosteronism, and pheochromocytoma, must also be considered if the blood pressure (BP) is found to be high. Remember that it takes moderate to severe sustained and prolonged hypertension to strain the heart. Also bear in mind that hypertension is so common that it may exist, yet not be the only cause of the patient's LVH; further examination is needed even if the BP is high.

DATA The BP is 136/58 in the right arm and 132/60 in the left arm. Ophthalmoscopy shows no evidence of present or past hypertension. Furthermore, the patient tells you he has never had high BP on previous examinations and nobody in his family has ever had it.

LOGIC So much for that! Wisely, the BP was checked in both arms since atherosclerotic occlusion or musculoskeletal deformity can make it falsely low in one arm. Next you consider another common cause for LVH: coronary heart disease. For this to be the cause, there must be a history of having had a coronary occlusion or ECG evidence thereof or angina pectoris. Diffuse ischemic cardiomyopathy may exist without any of these three being present, but it is rare.

DATA The patient has never had any chest pains, never had a heart attack that he knows of, does not have diabetes, and his ECG shows no evidence of infarction.

LOGIC The two most common causes of LVH have been eliminated. You are about to go to the next diagnostic decision point, when you realize you have not determined whether his heart is enlarged (in keeping with his ECG), nor have you decided if he is compensated or in beginning congestive heart failure.

DATA The apex beat is diffusely felt between the left midclavicular line and the anterior axillary line in the fifth and sixth intercostal spaces. A slight left ventricular heave is also noted. But there are no basal rales, neck veins are not distended at 45°, and the patient has no dyspnea on exertion, sleeps flat, and has no night cough. A quick examination of the heart reveals no murmurs, gallops, thrills, or abnormalities of S_1 and S_2.

LOGIC The heart is indeed enlarged, but there is no evidence of even beginning congestive heart failure since P_2 is not loud and there are no gallops, pulmonary congestion, or symptoms. You are becoming a bit concerned since the absence of murmurs is against rheumatic heart disease, another common cause of LVH.

Knowing that some rheumatic valvular murmurs are often overlooked, you decide to reexamine the heart more carefully. However, you have a bad cold, your nose is clogged, and you are not hearing too well that day. So first you think awhile; more examinations and questions will come later.

Aortic stenosis can be congenital or rheumatic in origin and supravalvular, valvular, or infravalvular in location. If stenosis is present, there is usually at least a grade 3/6 systolic ejection murmur heard at the base of the heart radiating into the carotid arteries, an S_4, a palpable thrill, and a slow carotid upstroke. Often, S_2 is paradoxically split and an ejection sound is heard.

Aortic regurgitation (AR) is caused chiefly by rheumatic heart disease, but infective endocarditis, syphilis, chest trauma, rheumatoid arthritis and its variants, and aortic dissection can cause it too. Uncommon hereditary diseases (Marfan's, Ehlers-Danlos, and Hurler's syndromes) would be seen in a much younger age group but could also be associated with AR. Signs of regurgitation include a wide pulse pressure and a high-pitched diastolic decrescendo murmur starting with S_2 and radiating from the aortic valve auscultatory area down to Erb's point and along the left sternal border. Confirmatory signs—such as water-hammer pulse, Corrigan's and Quincke's pulses, and Duroziez's sign—may be present.

Mitral regurgitation results from rheumatic heart disease, old myocardial infarction with papillary muscle dysfunction, and the rare hereditary diseases which also cause AR. Its hallmark is a high-pitched pansystolic murmur at the apex radiating to the left axilla or base of the heart. An S_3 or short middiastolic flow murmur is often present, and S_2 may be widely split since aortic closure is early.

DATA You reexamine the heart and again hear no murmurs, gallops, or abnormal splits, There is no history of alcoholism, and the patient does not know how long his heart has been enlarged. The tongue is not enlarged, lymph nodes are nowhere palpable, and the liver and spleen are not enlarged.

LOGIC The last common consideration—cardiomyopathy—seems unlikely. Even though this large group of diverse diseases can be caused by hereditary obstructive and restrictive muscle hypertrophy, alcohol, systemic disorders, such as sarcoidosis, amyloidosis, vasculitis, and viral infections, so far there is no evidence for any of these. Since it is often difficult to identify and verify a specific cause precisely, and since you realize cardiomyopathy is a catchall diagnosis, you may have to accept this etiology and observe the patient.

On a final review of the data, you note the pulse pressure is slightly widened. So you instill nosedrops in your nose, blow it, and inflate your middle ear with a Valsalva maneuver. Then you change stethoscopes, because you note a crack in the diaphragm you have been using. Now you can hear better.

DATA On applying the diaphragm of the new stethoscope firmly to the chest in the area of Erb's point—with the patient sitting up, learning forward, and in expiration—you hear a grade 2/4 soft, high-pitched, decrescendo murmur starting with S_2. On rechecking the BP, you find it to be 130/30 in both arms. Earlier, when your hearing was not so good, you entered the fifth Korotkoff phase too soon.

LOGIC Aortic regurgitation is clearly present. Do not berate yourself, because this murmur is easily missed if not carefully auscultated. What is the cause of the AR?

DATA　　There is no history of acute rheumatic fever or symptoms thereof (prolonged fever, chorea, joint pains, nosebleeds, lengthy bed rest as a child). The Venereal Disease Research Laboratory test is negative and the patient was never treated for syphilis. Hereditary defects are manifested at an early age. A chest x-ray merely shows moderate cardiac enlargement (cardiothoracic ratio = 18:30) but no pulmonary congestion or widening of the ascending aorta.

LOGIC　　No cause was found for the valvular lesion. Since rheumatic heart disease is the most common cause and since many cases of chronic rheumatic valvular disease give no history of a previous acute episode, the presumptive cause is rheumatic heart disease. No urgent treatment is indicated at the moment, though you might consider studies to quantitate the regurgitation in anticipation of valve replacement.

QUESTIONS

1. Assume the same patient has a grade 3/6 mitral regurgitant murmur, a grade 3/6 systolic ejection murmur and thrill over the aortic valve, a slow carotid upstroke, and a BP of 160/100 in both arms. The fundi are normal. His electrocardiographic LVH pattern is most likely caused by:
   (a) essential hypertension
   (b) aortic stenosis
   (c) mitral regurgitation
   (d) two of the above.
2. In doing a catheterization study to determine the degree of AR, before injecting the dye you would position the catheter tip in the:
   (a) left atrium
   (b) left ventricle
   (c) aortic root
   (d) right ventricle.
3. If the ECG abnormality had been right ventricular hypertrophy (RVH) each of the following would be possible except one:
   (a) mitral stenosis
   (b) tricuspid stenosis
   (c) pulmonic stenosis
   (d) multiple pulmonary emboli.
4. Change the patient's data a bit. The fundi show exudates, hemorrhages, and arteriovenous nicking, and the BP is 220/110 in both

arms. Leg pulses are strong. Two distinct murmurs are heard: a grade 2/6 systolic ejection murmur in the right second intercostal space next to the sternum, and a grade 2/6 pansystolic high-pitched murmur at the apex radiating to the left axilla. A distinct S_4 is present, and the apex beat is strong, diffuse, and displaced to the left. The cause of the patient's LVH pattern is probably:
   (a) essential hypertension
   (b) coarctation of the aorta
   (c) aortic stenosis
   (d) mitral regurgitation.

ANSWERS

1. **(d) is correct,** though the answer could be "all of the above." The hypertension is mild, probably not of long duration, and at most is contributing little to the LVH. The patient clearly has aortic stenosis as indicated by the findings. Mitral regurgitation may be present as a separate valvular lesion, but it could also result from functional insufficiency secondary to altered left ventricle geometry. Aortic stenosis would tend to make the mitral regurgitation worse. Each of (a), (b), or (c) could cause LVH. It is probable that at least two of the lesions are operative here.
2. **(c) is correct.** The dye will be seen to reflux into the left ventricle. Injection into the other chambers will not allow you to observe a regurgitant stream clearly.
3. **(b) is correct** since it is the only lesion not associated with RVH. The obstruction is proximal to the right ventricle, and only the right atrium hypertrophies. Mitral stenosis causes RVH after many years of left atrial hypertrophy, and eventually pulmonary congestion and pulmonary hypertension affect the right ventricle. (c) and (d) are obvious causes of RVH. Note that mitral stenosis does not cause LVH for the same reason that tricuspid stenosis does not cause RVH.
4. **(a) is correct.** Severe long-standing hypertension is present. Secondary forms of hypertension are statistically unlikely. Coarctation is ruled out by strong leg pulses. The aortic murmur is more characteristic of hypertension than aortic stenosis. The mitral murmur is mild and probably results from inability of the valve leaflets to coapt properly. Hypertrophied enlarged hearts often have mild mitral regurgitant murmurs regardless of the cause of the hypertrophy. S_4 is heard in any condition where the left ventricle is stiff, thick, and noncompliant.

COMMENT　　A large number of problem-solving techniques were used here. The author departed from the traditional data-gathering process and used a branching technique and decision path. First he established a list of likely common possibilities according to statistical incidence and probability theory. Positive and pertinent negative clues gave continual guidance. With a few questions and a very limited portion of the physical examination, each possibility was eliminated one by one. At each of these decision points he could have veered in one of two directions—the correct diagnosis or further information. Sequence of events was considered since long-standing hypertension with fundus changes must precede LVH if hypertension is its cause. The presence of rheumatic heart disease in the absence of a history of acute rheumatic fever invoked a negative syllogism. Overlap was under constant consideration (Venn and Boole) as we related hypertension with LVH and LVH with aortic stenosis, mitral regurgitation, and aortic regurgitation. One clue—the slightly wide pulse pressure—led the author to zero in on the diagnosis in true Holmesian fashion.

A flow chart could easily be constructed for the solution of this problem. Furthermore, a much quicker approach could have solved it: repeat the ECG, corroborate LVH by physical examination and x-ray, rule out congestive heart failure, take the BP, listen for murmurs, and rule out angina and infarct; consider cardiomyopathy if all is negative. If any step is positive (severe hypertension, characteristic murmur, etc), the search may end. In fact, proper auscultation of the heart could have solved the problem in one step. (*P. C.*).

PROBLEM-BASED LEARNING The simple problem just discussed requires that you master a wealth of material that will subsequently be of great value in solving many cardiac problems. For example, to get the most from this case study, you should know about:

1. the electrocardiographic criteria for LVH (while learning this, also learn the P, Q, R, S, and T's for *right* ventricular hypertrophy)
2. the pathophysiologic causes of LVH
3. hypertension, its criteria and physical signs, the primary and secondary causes thereof, and the symptoms, signs, and other confirmatory evidence for each possible cause
4. aortic stenosis, its various anatomic types and causes, the symptoms and signs of each cause, and how to prove each type conclusively
5. mitral regurgitation, its causes, physical signs, means of confirmation, and consequences
6. aortic regurgitation, its various causes and associated diseases, their physical signs, and their confirmation

7. coronary heart disease as it may relate to LVH
8. cardiomyopathy, its classification and causes, and how it may selectively affect the left ventricle
9. heart murmurs, gallops, and thrills and their understanding based on mastery of Wigger's diagram and the complete cardiac cycle
10. the relationship of congenital and acquired defects to the causation of valve dysfunction, to restrictive and obstructive cardiomyopathies, and to their resultant LVH
11. the vanishing but still present specter of syphilis in causing aortic regurgitation
12. chest x-ray evidence of LVH and the measurement of the cardiothoracic ratio.

Learn all this and cardiology becomes much simpler.

Suggested Readings

1. Marriott HJL: *Practical Electrocardiography,* ed 7. Baltimore, Williams & Wilkins, 1983, pp 51–55.
   Describes the features and criteria (Estes and Scott) for scoring LVH.
2. Braunwald E: Valvular heart disease. In Braunwald E (ed): *Heart Disease,* ed 2. Philadelphia, Saunders, 1984, pp 1063–1135.
   pp 1064–1074: mitral stenosis
   pp 1074–1089: mitral regurgitation
   pp 1089–1095: mitral valve prolapse syndrome
   pp 1095–1105: aortic stenosis
   pp 1105–1115: aortic regurgitation
3. Waller BF, Morrow AG, Maron BF: Etiology of clinically isolated, severe, chronic, pure mitral regurgitation. *Am Heart J* 104:276–288, 1982.
   The causes and detailed anatomic abnormalities in 97 patients are analyzed.
4. Wynne J, Braunwald E: The cardiomyopathies and myocarditides. In Braunwald E (ed): *Heart Disease,* ed 2. Philadelphia, Saunders, 1984, pp 1399–1455.
5. Devereux RB, Casale PN, Eisenberg RR, et al: Electrocardiographic detection of left ventricular hypertrophy using echocardiographic determination of left ventricular mass as the reference standard: comparison of standard criteria, computer diagnosis, and physician interpretation. *J Am Coll Cardiol* 3:82–87, 1984.
   The title tells the story—an excellent report.
6. Tsutomu I, Yasuhiko O, Yasushi K, et al: Utility of two-dimensional echocardiography in the differential diagnosis of the etiology of aortic regurgitation. *Am Heart J* 103:887–896, 1982.
   Describes the causes of aortic regurgitation as well as their diagnosis; expect to find Takayasu's disease here.
7. De Pace NL, Nestico PF, Kotler MN, et al: Comparison of echocardiography and angiography in determining the cause of severe aortic regurgitation. *Br Heart J* 51:36–45, 1984.
   Assesses the dependability of procedures to determine the four common causes of AR.

Case 16
Dyspnea on Exertion
PAUL CUTLER, M.D.

DATA A 58-year-old overweight married homemaker was rushed to the emergency room at 2 AM because of the sudden onset of severe shortness of breath. She was markedly dyspneic, orthopneic, and cyanotic, so immediate treatment with oxygen and morphine sulfate was given before further history could be obtained.

LOGIC While waiting for her to improve, a quick examination revealed BP 240/120, R 26, P 120, T 37 C, cyanosis, neck vein distention 5 cm vertically above the sternal angle, fine and coarse inspiratory rales at the lung bases, loud inspiratory and expiratory wheezes, and a large heart with a diffuse forceful apex beat. No further heart detail was obtainable because of noisy breathing.

Sudden dyspnea in the presence of severe pulmonary congestion, hypertension, and a large heart suggests a cardiac emergency such as acute left ventricular failure (LVF) with pulmonary edema, or a myocardial infarction. Were it not for the quickly obtained physical findings, sudden dyspnea might also have made you think of bronchial asthma, pneumothorax, pulmonary embolus, pleural effusion, atelectasis, or acute hyperventilation.

DATA The patient felt better in 10 minutes. Additional history revealed dyspnea and fatigue on exertion for several months. However, for the past few weeks she found it necessary to go to sleep on several pillows in order to breathe more easily, and on several occasions she awoke breathless and coughing and had to sit on the side of the bed or go to the window for relief. On the night of admission to the hospital, the dyspnea did not subside rapidly as usual but got steadily worse.

She attributes her recent difficulties to cigarette smoking since she gives a 45 pack-year history. In fact, for years she has had a morning cough productive of small amounts of grayish-white sputum. Hypertension had been present for more than 10 years, during which time she received intermittent treatment. She had difficulty adhering to a careful therapeutic regimen and, in addition, was unable to lose weight.

Both her mother and sister were hypertensive, and her mother died of a stroke. There is no history of acute rheumatic fever, joint pains, or murmur; no contact with tuberculosis or history of hemoptysis; no childhood asthma or other allergies; no chest pain or palpitations; no episodes of severe pounding headache and tremulousness; and no deep sighing breaths associated with numb sensations and lightheadedness. She takes no medication and is on no particular diet.

LOGIC It now appears that the patient has a chronic problem which seems to have culminated in an acute episode. While hypertension and LVF seem to be responsible for the picture, other concomitant or alternate possibilities must still be considered.

As for the heart, hypertension may not be the only problem; she might easily have coronary disease, valvular disease, or cardiomyopathy in addition. Her clinical course is typical of gradually worsening LVF. But the history can also be explained by a chronic progressive lung disease with a superimposed acute complication, such as pleural effusion, pneumothorax, or atelectasis. While severe anemia can cause dyspnea on exertion, it cannot account for orthopnea and the sudden acute episode.

You are left mainly with the possibilities of LVF and chronic lung disease with an acute complication. The presence of a large heart favors a cardiac etiology. But it is possible that both diseases coexist, and you must decide which is contributing principally or totally to the picture. While severe hyperventilation based on anxiety can present with what seems to be acute dyspnea, its recognition is simple, and there would not ordinarily be any evidence of heart or lung disease. The absence of certain symptoms in the history is against tuberculosis, asthma, coronary disease, pheochromocytoma, and hyperventilation—in that order.

DATA Physical examination done after marked improvement showed obesity and normal vital signs except for the BP which was 210/110 in both arms with no orthostatic changes. Cyanosis was no longer present and her color was good. The fundi showed arteriolar tortuosity, arteriovenous nicking, a few exudates, and a rare round hemorrhage. Neck veins were no longer distended at 45°. Faint bilateral expiratory wheezes and a few fine basilar rales were still present, but there was no dullness or flatness, the trachea was in the midline, and fremitus was normal. The diaphragm moved 2 to 3 cm on deep inspiration. The apex beat was forceful and diffuse in the fifth and sixth intercostal spaces at the left anterior axillary line. There was a left ventricular heave, a grade 2/6 systolic ejection murmur at the base, and a barely audible S_3. Two components of S_2 were clearly discernible, and the first component (aortic closure) was loud. The rest of the examination was normal.

Chest x-rays (posteroanterior and lateral views) showed normal lungs except for mild basilar congestion; the left ventricle was markedly enlarged. The abdominal x-ray revealed normal-sized kidney shadows. The ECG demonstrated left ventricular hypertrophy and "strain" plus a left atrial abnormality. Complete blood count, urinalysis, and 18-test blood chemistry profile were normal. Serum creatine kinase (MB isomer) was normal.

LOGIC The patient clearly has LFV, as evidenced by the x-ray, rales, enlarged heart, and S_3. The failure is caused by prolonged severe hypertension. There are no valve defects; the murmur is mild and probably relates to hypertension, not to aortic stenosis,

as there is no ejection click and the aortic component of S_2 is well preserved. There is no evidence by history, ECG, or enzyme changes for acute coronary disease. Cardiomyopathy could exist in addition to hypertension, but there are no clinical features of the hypertrophic, restrictive, or congestive forms of this entity, nor are there any etiologic factors evident.

The positive family history of hypertension, normal leg pulses, normal renal size, normal urinalysis, and normal serum potassium, and the absence of symptoms to suggest pheochromocytoma, are all indications of essential hypertension rather than hypertension secondary to another disorder.

No doubt the patient also has mild to moderate chronic obstructive pulmonary disease as denoted by the history of cough and expectoration, excessive smoking, faint expiratory wheezes, and insufficient diaphragmatic motion. The loud wheezes on admission may have been due to interstitial fluid compressing the bronchioles; the faint ones heard later may have resulted from her chronic obstructive pulmonary disease. At any rate, lung disease is probably contributing little, if at all, to her present acute problem. Pulmonary function tests will be done later.

DATA Cardiac enzymes and ECG did not change over the next 2 days. In the meantime, the patient was treated with digitalis, diuretics, antihypertensive medication, and a salt-restricted diet; improvement was marked and rapid. At discharge, the seriousness of her situation was carefully explained, and she was impressed with the need to give up smoking and adhere strictly to a drug and diet regimen.

She visited her physician at regular intervals and seemed to be doing quite well. After having missed two scheduled visits, she returned feeling weak and anorexic. Further she complained of fainting spells, leg cramps, and not feeling "clear" in her mind at times, though she insisted she was religiously observing her prescribed treatment plan. Her examination was the same as on previous visits, except that the 150/90 BP dropped to 80/60 when she stood up.

Immediate studies showed: blood urea nitrogen 42 mg/dl, serum sodium 118 mEq/liter, serum potassium 2.6 mEq/liter. The ECG was the same except for widening of the Q-T interval, prominent U waves, and multiple ventricular premature depolarizations.

LOGIC Indeed the patient had adhered quite well to her physician's treatment plan—even too well! Salt had been completely eliminated from her diet and she was taking a potent diuretic (furosemide). As a result, she had become volume, sodium, and potassium depleted. Volume depletion caused the hypotension and prerenal azotemia; sodium and potassium depletion caused the cramps, mental changes, weakness, and ECG changes. Premature beats resulted because hypokalemia made the heart more susceptible to the toxic effects of digitalis.

DATA She was given a milder diuretic, supplemental potassium salts, and a diet less restricted in sodium; she returned in several days feeling much better. This was documented by improved blood chemistry determinations, loss of symptoms, and absence of orthostatic BP changes. Pulmonary function tests at that time showed evidence of mild to moderate obstructive disease.

Two years later, the patient returned with severe dyspnea and peripheral edema. She was being treated by her husband's physician. He was not so "strict" with treatment, and her family had convinced her to change physicians. At this time she was in severe biventricular failure, was dyspneic, orthopneic, and had generalized anasarca. The BP was 220/120 and, in addition to the signs of LVF which she originally had, she also exhibited neck veins distended 12 cm vertically above the sternal angle when sitting, a large tender liver, and 4+ edema up to the mid-abdomen.

LOGIC When severe persistent LVF occurs, secondary aldosteronism resulting from decreased renal blood flow causes sodium and water retention, but peripheral edema does not ordinarily occur until right ventricular failure eventually supervenes. Then the increased capillovenous pressure works in tandem with the sodium and water retention to cause edema. This patient is now in florid congestive heart failure (CHF) because of inadequate treatment, the natural course of her disease, or complicating factors such as anemia, pulmonary emboli, etc.

DATA The ECG was unchanged; chest x-ray disclosed marked cardiomegaly, severe pulmonary congestion, and bilateral pleural effusions (right greater than left). Chemical studies showed blood urea nitrogen 45 mg/dl, sodium 122 mEq/liter, potassium 3.5 mEq/liter, chloride 84 mEq/liter, and bicarbonate 30 mEq/liter.

LOGIC Hyponatremia is again present, but this time for another reason. With severe edema and advanced CHF, the low sodium represents dilutional hyponatremia and not depletion of body sodium. Though the total body sodium is excessive, disproportionately more water is present since the kidneys somehow lose their ability to excrete water; so the sodium concentration is far below normal. This too needs treatment.

DATA She is placed at rest, severe fluid restriction is imposed, and the other components of therapy remain unchanged. Marked generalized improvement occurs as diuresis ensues, edema diminishes, and the weight comes down by 2 lb daily. After 2 weeks the patient is much better according to both symptoms and signs.

Suddenly she becomes dyspneic and cyanotic. Her legs are still slightly swollen though not tender. Chest x-ray shows cardiomegaly, absence of the previously noted effusions, and no infiltrates. A pulmonary ventilation-perfusion scan discloses a large area with absent perfusion and normal ventilation in each lung. Intravenous heparin is begun, but the patient suddenly dies the next day.

LOGIC Even though her CHF was improving, she developed clinical findings compatible with multiple pulmonary emboli and no doubt died from the last one. Emboli notoriously occur in patients who are incapacitated with severe CHF. The clinical picture and ventilation-perfusion scan are incontestable.

QUESTIONS

1. As mentioned in the case study, there are many reasons why patients with CHF get worse. Which of the following are possible causes?
   (a) excessive physical or emotional strain
   (b) superimposition of another disease causing anoxemia
   (c) excessive sodium in the diet
   (d) inappropriate medication.
2. The diagnosis of pulmonary emboli was not difficult to make in this case discussion. But it is often overlooked because it may manifest itself differently. All of the following statements regarding pulmonary emboli are true except one:
   (a) Pleuritic pain, cough, and hemoptysis may be the presenting symptoms.
   (b) Think of emboli in a bedridden patient who has unexplained low-grade fever and tachycardia.
   (c) Consider emboli if the patient is persistently dyspneic, yet is otherwise improved from his CHF.
   (d) A perfusion lung scan is highly specific for emboli.
3. You suspect a pulmonary embolus, but you are not sure. The perfusion lung scan is suggestive. You are considering the use of anticoagulants since the patient is seriously ill and might not tolerate a second embolus. But the patient also has a relative contraindication to the use of heparin. In order to make sure of the diagnosis, your most specific and sensitive test would be:
   (a) ventilation-perfusion scan
   (b) serial enzyme studies (lactate dehydrogenase, serum glutamic-oxaloacetic transaminase)
   (c) pulmonary arteriography
   (d) physical examination.
4. A 64-year-old man with both severe chronic obstructive lung disease and severe biventricular failure presents with a wide array of symptoms and signs. Which of the following clues is/are specific for one condition or the other?
   (a) markedly distended cervical veins
   (b) orthopnea and paroxysmal nocturnal dyspnea

   (c) leg edema and liver 5 cm below costal margin
   (d) S_3 at the apex and pulsus alternans.

ANSWERS

1. **All are correct.** In (a), the heart is forced to work harder. The patient who develops worsening obstructive lung disease or anemia for any reason (ulcer, cancer) will decrease his heart's work capacity by virtue of progressive anoxemia. Excessive sodium intake may occur if the patient does not care or does not understand. He may not know which foods and household remedies contain large quantities of sodium (bacon, canned soups, baking soda, etc). As for medication, errors abound regarding too much or too little digitalis, diuretics, and potassium supplementation. Other causes for apparent worsening include unidentified multiple pulmonary emboli, masked hyperthyroidism, unnoticed myocardial infarction, and an arrhythmia.
2. **(d) is untrue.** A perfusion scan is not specific since pneumonia, infiltrates, or effusions may also show decreased perfusion; it is, however, sensitive because emboli with infarcts usually show perfusion defects. In doubtful cases, a ventilation-perfusion scan will differentiate between infarct and other causes for infiltrates where both perfusion and ventilation may be impaired. (a), (b), and (c) are all different presentations for pulmonary emboli. This many-faced disease can also present as pulmonary hypertension with right ventricular failure, or sudden severe coronary-like chest pain, or pleural effusion. The source for the emboli (the leg veins) may become apparent before, during, or after the embolus—more frequently never at all.
3. **(c) is correct.** The delineation of an arterial obstruction is both highly specific and sensitive, though invasive. In this case, it may well be the procedure of choice. (a) is much more informative than a simple perfusion scan though probably not so informative as arteriography. Admittedly, some clinicians might prefer (a) in this situation. Enzyme studies are not specific and take several days. Examination is not apt to be of much definitive help even should a friction rub develop.
4. **(d) is correct.** A third heart sound and pulsus alternans are specific for CHF. They result from a high left ventricular end-diastolic pressure, decreased ventricular compliance, and alternating end-diastolic fiber length. On the other hand, (a), (b), and (c) can be seen in either condition. The patient with severe chronic obstructive pulmonary disease must often sit up to move his chest more easily, or secretions may clog his airways at night, caus-

ing him to get up. His liver is pushed down by a low diaphragm, and his legs are often swollen because his dyspnea makes him sit most of the time.

COMMENT   The presence of heart disease and lung disease in the same patient needed careful sorting to decide which disease was causing the acute problem and which clues belonged to each of the two diseases. Considerable overlap existed since the symptoms and signs for both are similar. With the sudden onset of dyspnea as the key clue, the author rapidly built an unmistakable pattern for hypertensive cardiovascular disease with LVF. Note that urgent treatment was given even before a diagnosis was made.

"Cause and effect" was extensively utilized as the two causes for hyponatremia were encountered and as the causes for worsening CHF were detailed. Also, the reader had the opportunity to follow a patient with CHF from its inception to its termination, observing the cause-and-effect relationships through a series of intermediate complications.

In detailing the many presentations of pulmonary embolism, the author had to consider the specificity and sensitivity of various diagnostic clues.   (*P. C.*)

Suggested Readings

1. Schlant RC, Sonnenblick EH: Pathophysiology of

heart failure. In Hurst JW (ed): *The Heart*, ed 5. New York, McGraw-Hill, 1982, pp 382–407.
2. Spann JF, Hurst JW: The recognition and management of heart failure. In Hurst JW (ed): *The Heart*, ed 5. New York, McGraw-Hill, 1982, pp 407–451.
   Covers all the causes, diagnosis, clinical features, complications, and treatment.
3. Braunwald E: Clinical manifestations of heart failure. In Braunwald E (ed): *Heart Disease*, ed 2. Philadelphia, Saunders, 1984, pp 488–502.
4. Weber KT, Likoff MJ, Janicki JS, et al: Advances in the evaluation and management of chronic cardiac failure. *Chest* 85:253–259, 1984.
   Shows how an understanding of the pathophysiology determines treatment.
5. Dexter L, Alpert JS, Dalen JE: Pulmonary embolism, infarction, and acute cor pulmonale. In Hurst JW (ed): *The Heart*, ed 5. New York, McGraw-Hill, 1982 pp 1227–1242.
6. Goodwin JF, Roberts WC, Wenger NK: Cardiomyopathy. In Hurst JW (ed): *The Heart*, ed 5. New York, McGraw-Hill, 1982, pp 1250–1277.
   Numerous diseases of heart muscle caused by drugs, infections, alcohol, metabolic disorders, congenital myopathies, etc are included in this catchall disease set.
7. Viamonte M Jr, Koolpe H, Janowitz W, et al: Pulmonary thromboembolism. *JAMA* 243:2229–2234, 1980.
   The radiologic diagnosis is highlighted.
8. Sasahara AA, Sharma GVRK, Barsamian EM, et al: Pulmonary thromboembolism: diagnosis and treatment. *JAMA* 249:2945–2950, 1983.
   Depicts the variable symptoms, signs, diagnostic procedures, and treatment in few pages.

Case 17
Severe Substernal Tightness
MICHAEL H. CRAWFORD, M.D.

DATA   After 1 hour of continuous tight substernal pain, a 53-year-old white male accountant is brought to the emergency room. He had been treated for hypertension for 10 years but did not adhere to his regimen nor did he see his physician regularly. Three years ago he was found to have adult-onset diabetes mellitus. He was treated with some success by diet alone but had difficulty losing weight. For the past year he has had recurrent episodes of tight substernal discomfort occurring two or three times/week. These were provoked by emotional stress or severe exertion and relieved in about 1 to 2 minutes by a sublingual nitroglycerin tablet or rest. He limited his activities to avoid these episodes.

This pattern remained stable until a month ago when he observed his chest pain becoming more severe, more prolonged, and more easily provoked. He needed two or three nitroglycerin tablets for relief. One week prior to admission he was experiencing chest pain four to five times daily. The pain during the present attack was worse than usual, radiated to the neck and down the left arm, and was unrelieved by three nitroglycerin tablets. He felt ill and was nauseated and in a cold sweat, so he came to the hospital.

LOGIC Chest pain may originate from any one of various structures in the chest. However, the information gotten about the nature of the pain, and what causes and relieves it, points directly to coronary artery disease. He has a new pattern of crescendo angina pectoris which seems to have resulted in a myocardial infarction (MI). There are two well-established risk factors here for this disease: hypertension and diabetes. Other important risk factors yet to be determined in this patient are tobacco abuse, hereditary background, and serum cholesterol. There is as yet no concrete evidence that sedentary occupation, obesity, dietary fat intake, and personality type are definite risk factors.

Angina pectoris results from an imbalance between myocardial oxygen supply and demand. When severe coronary artery disease is present, the supply of oxygenated blood to the heart muscle is limited. During exercise or emotional tension, demand increases but supply cannot match it. This imbalance results in myocardial ischemia and chest pain.

Worsening angina may be caused by increasing demand: more emotional stress, more physical exertion, or rising blood pressure. It may also worsen if oxygen availability is decreased either by the progression of coronary artery lesions, coronary artery spasm, decreased oxygen supply (chronic lung disease), or decreased oxygen-carrying capacity of the blood (anemia).

DATA Further questions reveal that the patient had decreased his activity and exposure to emotional tension over the past month. He has never smoked and has no other significant symptoms. The family history, however, is notable for a high frequency of coronary disease, hypertension, and diabetes.

The physical examination was completely normal except for the vital signs and heart:

BP 160/95, P 85 with frequent premature beats, T 37.1 C, R 18. The lungs, jugular venous pressure, and carotid pulses were normal. The apical impulse was in the fourth and fifth left intercostal spaces just lateral to the midclavicular line and was about 5 cm in diameter. A prominent presystolic wave and a sustained outward systolic thrust were palpated. On auscultation, S_1 was soft, S_2 was normal, and there was a soft S_3 and a loud S_4. No murmurs were heard.

LOGIC The family history adds another potent risk factor. The lateral displacement and enlargement of the apical impulse may be due to left ventricular hypertrophy from his long-standing hypertension and systolic expansion of a noncontractile segment resulting from the new MI. The presystolic pulsation and loud S_4 are common in both these conditions and are synchronous with the atrial infusion of blood into a noncompliant ventricle. The soft S_1 and the S_3 signify early myocardial decompensation.

DATA On admission to the hospital, the ECG showed an acute anterolateral MI and frequent ventricular premature depolarizations (VPDs). The heart was slightly enlarged, but the lungs were clear on chest x-ray. Blood was drawn for cardiac enzymes, routine chemistries, and complete blood count. Sedation, pain relief, and intravenous lidocaine were administered.

LOGIC It is now certain that our patient has an acute MI and that his worsening angina was probably related to progression of his coronary artery disease, since no cause for increased myocardial oxygen demand was found. In addition, he has the most common complication of MI—an arrhythmia. The multiple VPDs result from abnormal electrical currents in the ischemic tissue. However, other causes for VPDs which may be operant are hypoxia, electrolyte imbalance, anxiety, acidosis, alkalosis, and certain drugs (e.g. "diet pills").

DATA Pain subsided rapidly and the patient appeared much improved. The temperature rose to 37.7 C, the pulse stayed at 90, and the S_3 and S_4 persisted. Serum electrolytes, blood gases, blood pH, complete blood count, urinalysis, and other chemistries were all normal, except for the blood glucose which was 160 mg/dl. He was taking no drugs. The VPDs were undoubtedly related to the MI. After 48 hours, the lidocaine was stopped and the VPDs did not recur. Serum creatine kinase rose to 2096 mIU/liter (normal is 25 to 120), 16% of which was the MB isomer (specific for myocardium). By day 4 he looked and felt well.

Suddenly he became severely dyspneic, he could not lie flat, the BP fell to 90/65, the pulse rose to 120, and moist bibasilar rales to the midscapula could be heard. His neck veins were distended and a new loud grade 4/6 pansystolic murmur was heard at the lower left sternal border. It radiated to the apex and base of the heart. No thrill was palpable.

LOGIC   The dramatic appearance of severe biventricular failure and a new loud holosystolic murmur are consistent with either papillary muscle tear or ventricular septal rupture. Each has the same murmur and each will lead to severe heart failure. The latter has a palpable thrill 50% of the time, but the former usually has no thrill. However, the distinction is often difficult to make without right heart catheterization.

Myocardial rupture usually occurs during the first 2 weeks after infarction when the affected tissues are least strong. After 2 weeks there is enough fibrosis to strengthen the infarcted areas. Rupture of the free wall is uncommon, is rarely diagnosed premortem, and almost always results in immediate death from cardiac tamponade. Rupture of the interventricular septum leads to a sudden left-to-right shunt during systole which overloads the pulmonary circulation, decreases forward flow to the body, and causes dyspnea. When a part of the papillary muscle ruptures, the mitral valve apparatus is disrupted, and acute mitral regurgitation and severe congestive heart failure result.

DATA   Despite treatment with intravenous dopamine, nitroprusside, diuretics, and oxygen, the patient did poorly. Right heart catheterization at the bedside supported the diagnosis of severe mitral regurgitation (very high pulmonary capillary wedge pressure with a prominent "v" wave). Emergency surgery was considered, but the patient became hypotensive and died before anything further could be done. Postmortem examination showed complete rupture of the anterior papillary muscle which was involved in a large anterior MI.

LOGIC   It is important to note that this patient presented with a typical MI from the standpoint of both history and physical findings. Many infarctions are atypical. They can present with syncope, weakness, acute pulmonary edema, or an arrhythmia. Often there are no symptoms whatsoever and the infarct is discovered later on a routine ECG. The physical examination may vary from no abnormal physical findings to pulmonary edema and shock, depending on the size of the infarct.

QUESTIONS

1. You have a 65-year-old man with a moderately large MI. It is now day 3 and he is doing reasonably well. Match each of the following sudden events (letters) with its cause (numbers):
   (a)   pulse drops to 30
   (b)   tender suprapubic mass
   (c)   both legs numb, painful, and cold
   (d)   right leg painful, warm, and tender
   (e)   left hemiplegia
   (f)   left flank pain and hematuria
   (g)   obstipation for 3 days and rectal discomfort
   (h)   pulse rises to 150, chest pain returns
   (i)   pulse rises to 120, cannon waves occasionally seen in neck veins
   (j)   right pleuritic chest pain and hemoptysis.

   (1)   saddle embolus to aortic bifurcation
   (2)   ventricular tachycardia
   (3)   thrombophlebitis
   (4)   fecal impaction
   (5)   atrial flutter with 2:1 block
   (6)   complete heart block
   (7)   pulmonary embolus and infarct
   (8)   cerebral embolus and infarct

(9)   urinary retention
(10) renal embolus and infarct.
2. Which of the following factors are apt to make existing angina pectoris worse?
(a)   cold weather
(b)   hot weather
(c)   tachycardia
(d)   bradycardia
(e)   hyperglycemia
(f)   hypoglycemia
(g)   isometric exercise
(h)   obesity
(i)   severe hypertension
(j)   sudden hypotension
(k)   hyperthyroidism
(l)   hypothyroidism
(m)   lowered pO_2.
3. Which of the following chemical derangements is the most important risk factor for the development of coronary artery disease?
(a)   elevated serum calcium
(b)   elevated serum free fatty acids
(c)   elevated serum triglyceride
(d)   elevated serum cholesterol.

ANSWERS

1. **(a)-(6).** Infarction has involved the atrioventricular node and/or both bundles, and the patient has an idioventricular rhythm. There should be varying intensity of S_1 because of inconstant augmentation of ventricular filling by atrial contraction.
(b)-(9). A man of 65 with probable prostatic hypertrophy, who is put to bed and sedated, commonly develops urinary retention.
(c)-(1). Absence of pulses from the femoral arteries down would confirm this event.
(d)-(3). Thrombophlebitis or phlebothrombosis is not so common today. Anticoagulants, stockingets, early ambulation, and exercises have reduced their incidence in MIs.
(e)-(8). An embolus has traveled from a mural thrombus to the right middle cerebral artery or one of its branches.
(f)-(10). This embolus too has originated in a mural thrombus.
(g)-(4). Impactions are common unless careful attention is given to the bowels.
(h)-(5). A ventricular rate of 150/minute suggests atrial flutter, since the atrial rate is usually 300/minute with 2:1 block. However, it could be any other tachyarrhythmia. The pain returns because the fast rate increases myocardial oxygen demand.
(i)-(2). A tachyarrhythmia has occurred. The cannon "a" waves suggest there is atrioventricular dissociation with the atria sometimes contracting when the atrioventricular valves are

closed. Therefore ventricular tachycardia is likely, especially at this rate.
(j)-(7). A pulmonary embolus may originate from a mural thrombus overlying a right ventricular infarction. More commonly, it comes from the leg veins.
2. **(a) (b) (c) (f) (g) (h) (i) (j) (k) (m).** Cold weather causes peripheral vasoconstriction and increases cardiac work. Hot weather increases cardiac work by vasodilatation and then tachycardia. Rapid heart rate increases cardiac work, but slow rate decreases it. Hyperglycemia has no effect, but hypoglycemia can precipitate angina by stimulating catecholamine secretion. Isometric exercise not only increases cardiac work directly, but elevates blood pressure too. Obesity requires that the heart pump blood to a larger vascular bed. Hypertension increases cardiac work, and a sudden drop in blood pressure decreases coronary perfusion. Hyperthyroidism worsens angina by increasing the heart rate and the oxygen needs of all tissue, including the myocardium. It probably does not in itself cause angina, but only worsens it when coronary atherosclerosis already exists. Hypothyroidism would improve angina by decreasing heart work and oxygen needs. However, in the long run it will accelerate development of coronary artery disease because of associated hypercholesterolemia. Hypoxia decreases oxygen supply to the myocardium. All the above correct answers have either further decreased oxygen supply to the heart or increased the oxygen needs of the heart.
3. **(d) is the most reliable predictor.** While calcium is found in the arterial plaques, it is secondarily there and is not related to the disease process. Free fatty acids are fuel for the myocardium and are not implicated in causing coronary disease. Both (c) and (d) are associated with lipoprotein disorders, but lipoprotein disorders resulting in high cholesterol alone are almost invariably associated with early atherosclerosis. Thus (d) is the most important metabolic risk factor.

COMMENT   Here the diagnosis is easily recognized by a pattern of worsening angina in a patient with diabetes and hypertension, culminating in an acute MI. With the given risk factors, coronary disease and MI are to be expected. The sequence of events is unmistakable. The ECG is specific though not sensitive; elevation of the creatine kinase and its MB isomer is both very specific and very sensitive. The principles of cause and effect are thoroughly utilized in determining the causes for VPDs and worsening angina. With the terminal complication of myocardial tear, two possible diagnoses appear; there is considerable overlap of signs and symptoms, even though a thrill is common in one and rare in the other. An invasive diagnostic procedure is needed to make a definite distinction. *(P. C.)*

Suggested Readings

1. Hurst JW, King SB III, Walter PF, et al: Atherosclerotic heart disease, angina pectoris, myocardial infarction and other manifestations of myocardial ischemia. In Hurst JW (ed): *The Heart*, ed 5. New York, McGraw-Hill, 1982, chap 45, pp 1009–1149.
   pp 1009–1028: pathophysiology
   pp 1039–1058: diagnosis—tests and procedures
   pp 1059–1068: clinical picture
   pp 1102–1112: various anginal syndromes
   pp 1117–1133: complications of myocardial infarction
2. Cohn PF, Braunwald E: Chronic ischemic heart disease. In Braunwald E (ed): *Heart Disease*, ed 2. Philadelphia, Saunders, 1984, 1334–1362.
   Includes all forms of angina pectoris.
3. Kent KM, Rosing DR, Ewels CJ, et al: Prognosis of asymptomatic or mildly symptomatic patients with coronary artery disease. *Am J Cardiol* 49:1823–1830, 1982.
   Demonstrates the relation between symptoms, underlying coronary anatomy, and mortality rate.
4. Maseri A, Chierchia S: Coronary artery spasm: demonstration, definition, diagnosis, and consequences. *Prog Cardiovasc Dis* 25:169–192, 1982.
   All about variant angina from A to Z (195 references).
5. Patterson RE, Eng C, Horowitz SF: Practical diagnosis of coronary artery disease: a Bayes theorem nomogram to correlate clinical data with non-invasive exercise tests. *Am J Cardiol* 53:252–256, 1984.
   Shows how the physician can precisely alter disease probability with a test.
6. Detrano R, Yiannikas J, Salcedo EE, et al: Bayesian probability analysis: a prospective demonstration of its clinical utility in diagnosing coronary disease. *Circulation* 69:541–547, 1984.
   Compares pretest and posttest probabilities of having coronary disease and demonstrates the utility of Bayes' theorems in diagnosis.
7. Alpert JS, Braunwald E: Acute myocardial infarction: pathologic, pathophysiologic and clinical manifestations. In Braunwald E (ed): *Heart Disease*, ed 2. Philadelphia, Saunders, 1984, pp 1262–1300.
8. Crawford MH, O'Rourke RA: The bedside diagnosis of the complications of myocardial infarction. In Eliot RS (ed): *Cardiac Emergencies*. Mt Kisco, NY, Futura, 1977, pp 83–93.
9. Castelli WP: Epidemiology of coronary heart disease: the Framingham study. *Am J Med* 76:4–12, 1984.
   Risk factors are concisely and clearly shown.
10. ten Kate LP, Boman H, Daiger SP, et al: Familial aggregation of coronary heart disease and its relation to known genetic risk factors. *Am J Cardiol* 50:945–953, 1982.
    Indicates factors that must exist outside the well-known risks.
11. Levy RI, Feinleib M: Risk factors for coronary heart disease and their management. In Braunwald E (ed): *Heart Disease*, ed 2. Philadelphia, Saunders, 1984.
    An authoritative review by foremost experts in the area of hyperlipoproteinemias.
12. Silverman KJ, Grossman W: Current concepts. Angina pectoris. Natural history and strategies for evaluation and management. *N Engl J Med* 310:1712–1716, 1984.
    A superb, concise, very current review that includes diagnostic protocols and flow charts.

Case 18
Systolic Murmur

LAWRENCE D. HORWITZ, M.D.

DATA　During an examination for a life insurance policy, a healthy 28-year-old man was found to have a heart murmur. He consulted his private physician who confirmed the presence of a grade 2/6 midsystolic ejection murmur in the aortic and pulmonic areas but noted no other abnormalities. Symptoms of cardiac disease had not been present. Chest x-ray and ECG were normal.

LOGIC　When a murmur is unexpectedly found in a presumably healthy person, you must decide whether it is functional and without significance, or a manifestation of subtle underlying cardiac disease which can give trouble in the future.

It is important to know how long the murmur has been present. If heard at or shortly after birth, congenital lesions are suspected. But if first heard at age 28, as in this patient, it may be an acquired lesion—unless the patient had never been carefully examined in the past.

Care should be taken to establish the presence or absence of cardiac symptoms, such as chest pain, syncope, dyspnea, orthopnea, paroxysmal nocturnal dyspnea, edema, or palpitations. A history of rheumatic fever must be sought by name or by its common manifestations. Inquiries should also be made about any family history of cardiac disease.

The physical examination is of paramount importance. If a murmur is functional, the vital signs, jugular venous pulse, arterial pulse, and apical impulse should be normal, and the lungs should be clear. Abnormal precordial lifts, cyanosis, edema, and clubbing should be absent. Chest deformities must be noted; either pectus excavatum or straight-back syndrome can cause murmurs because of narrowing of the anteroposterior diameter of the chest. A third heart sound is normal only if the patient is under 20 years of age. A fourth heart sound often reflects decreased ventricular compliance, but it can be normal in those past age 55 or those who exercise vigorously. S_2 should be physiologically split and the pulmonic component audible only in the pulmonic area.

DATA In this case the history was entirely negative, the murmur was the only physical finding of note, and since the chest x-ray and ECG were normal, no further tests were deemed necessary. Based on these data the physician informed the patient that the murmur appeared to be functional but recommended a yearly examination to see if any new findings might appear.

LOGIC In reference to murmurs it should be noted that diastolic murmurs are almost always pathologic. Only systolic murmurs may be innocent or functional. If the murmur is holosystolic, high-pitched, and plateau-shaped, it is more apt to be organic, and mitral regurgitation, tricuspid regurgitation, or ventricular septal defect should be considered. These conditions are unlikely in this patient since the murmur was of the ejection type and was heard at the base.

Ejection murmurs are shorter, usually diamond-shaped, and of medium pitch. They can be functional or organic. Basal ejection murmurs may be associated with many disease states, such as aortic or pulmonic stenosis, systemic or pulmonary hypertension, high flow through the pulmonary artery as in atrial septal defect, and high flow through both sides of the heart (high output states) as in chronic anemia, beriberi, hyperthyroidism, and Paget's disease. The systolic murmur of the click-murmur syndrome is best heard at the apex in late systole and is preceded by a click. Each of these disease states has its accompanying characteristic physical findings. Since none was present here, the murmur was considered to be innocent or functional. But the physician wisely recognized that evidence of disease might appear later and recommended rechecks.

DATA The patient elected not to return and he continued to be asymptomatic until 20 years later. At age 48, while chasing an intruder on his property, he suddenly passed out for approximately 1 minute. He ignored this incident, but on two subsequent occasions over the next year and a half he had similar episodes of syncope during strenuous exertion. He began to deliberately avoid vigorous activity, but over the next 6 months he experienced numerous episodes of substernal pressure lasting 1 to 3 minutes. These came on with mild exertion, especially after meals. For the past few days he has had difficulty in getting a deep breath when sitting and watching television. Disturbed by these symptoms, he consulted a physician.

On examination he was found to have a blood pressure of 105/90 with a resting pulse rate of 90 beats/minute. The carotid and brachial artery pulses were noted to have a prolonged upstroke. The apical impulse was normally positioned but was diffuse and had a powerful, prolonged, heaving quality. A thrill was palpable in the aortic area. The first sound was normal, the second was paradoxically split, and a prominent fourth sound was present. A harsh grade 3/6 systolic ejection murmur was heard; it was loudest in the aortic area and radiated to both carotid arteries. There were no rales. On the chest x-rays, a dense calcification was noted in the vicinity of the aortic valve, the lungs were clear, the aorta was prominent, and the left ventricle appeared to be either normal or slightly enlarged. The ECG showed left ventricular hypertrophy and "strain." An echocardiogram demonstrated thickening and diminished movement of the aortic valve leaflets.

LOGIC   The findings are classical for aortic stenosis (AS). Reduced pulse pressure, prolonged or slow ejection noted at the apex and carotid artery, a heaving left ventricle, the murmur, thrill, and fourth heart sound are all the result of a hypertrophied left ventricle laboring to eject blood through a stenotic valve orifice.

Syncope, angina, and left ventricular failure, either singly or in combination, are the usual presenting symptoms in AS. Only the first two are present here. Commonly, dyspnea and fatigue on exertion appear first. This patient's "dyspnea" makes you wonder. It sounds more like hyperventilation than organic dyspnea since it occurs at rest, it is characterized by deep single breaths, and there are no signs of failure. He is probably anxious about his newly acquired symptoms.

In general, the cluster of a typical murmur and thrill is enough to diagnose AS. But thrills are not so common as once thought, since the disease is now discovered earlier and there may be concomitant chronic obstructive lung disease obscuring the abnormal vibrations. Furthermore, the murmur may be best heard at the apex, and both thrill and murmur may be difficult to detect if severe congestive heart failure supervenes. Perhaps a more reliable cluster would be a typical murmur plus a slow carotid upstroke.

Abnormality of S_2 is almost always present in advanced AS. Paradoxical splitting occurs because of a prolonged left ventricular ejection time, so that aortic closure is delayed beyond pulmonic closure; with inspiration, P_2 catches up with A_2. Sometimes A_2 is inaudible because the valve is calcific

and immobile. The S_4 results from decreased ventricular compliance due to the left ventricular hypertrophy. An ejection sound may precede the murmur.

Calcification in the aortic valve is common. Left ventricular hypertrophy is almost always present in the ECG. The causes of AS are congenital (bicuspid valve commonly) and rheumatic. Calcific AS in the elderly is probably the end result of a congenital bicuspid valve. Bicuspid valves usually develop stenosis, regurgitation, or both, although some never do. Concomitant coronary disease may also be present. However, angina often occurs in aortic stenosis with normal coronary arteries because a Venturi effect just beyond the narrowed valve tends to reduce coronary flow, and ventricular hypertrophy increases the amount of oxygen needed by the heart.

The genesis of symptoms is easy to understand. They occur on exertion since the heart is unable to increase its stroke volume when called upon to do so.

You begin to wonder about the cause of AS in this patient. As far as you can determine by history, no murmur was noted before age 28. This does not mean it was not present, since he rarely saw a physician and it may have been missed when he did. Even if no murmur had been present in childhood, stenosis of a bicuspid valve may take years to develop. The absence of a history of rheumatic fever does not in the least exclude it as a diagnostic possibility. If the mitral valve were also diseased, you would lean toward rheumatic infection, but this is not the case here.

DATA   The physician recognized that aortic stenosis was present. He advised cardiac catheterization and explained that if, as he suspected, very advanced AS were present, surgical replacement of the aortic valve with a prosthesis would be recommended. The patient refused all procedures.

He had no difficulties except occasional angina-like pain until 1 year later, when he began to notice that he would awaken from his sleep sweating profusely. He had chilly sensations or feelings of warmth during the day and had a general feeling of malaise. After 4 weeks with these symptoms, he awoke one evening with severe shortness of breath and was taken to a hospital.

At the hospital, the pulse was 120, respirations 40, blood pressure 100/40, and temperature 38.8 C. Rales were diffusely present in both lung fields. The neck veins were markedly distended. The carotid and brachial pulses were full and bounding with a rapid upstroke. The apical impulse was diffuse and located in the sixth intercostal space 10 cm from the midsternal line. S_1 was barely audible, S_2 was narrowly split, an S_3 was heard at the apex, and S_4 was not audible. The systolic murmur was present as before. A grade 3/4 high-pitched, blowing, diastolic murmur was present in early and mid-diastole along the left sternal border. A grade 2/4 short, low-pitched, mid-diastolic rumble was noted at the apex. Blood cultures drawn soon after admission grew *Streptococcus viridans* 2 days later.

LOGIC The picture was drastically changed. He had developed classic findings of aortic regurgitation in addition to the AS. This was shown by the wide pulse pressure, water-hammer pulses, and new murmurs. A high-pitched, decrescendo, early diastolic murmur along the left sternal border in association with a wide pulse pressure is virtually diagnostic of aortic regurgitation.

Pulmonary regurgitation would have no effect on the peripheral pulse and blood pressure. The mid-diastolic murmur at the apex (Austin Flint murmur) is caused by the regurgitant stream striking the mitral valve leaflet, resulting in relative mitral stenosis. The S_3 indicates either failure or rapid early diastolic filling.

However, the heart has now enlarged and both left and beginning right ventricular failure are present. In view of the sudden onset of aortic regurgitation, left and beginning right ventricular failure, fever, sweats, and malaise, you must think first in terms of valve destruction by bacterial endocarditis. This was confirmed by blood culture, and

appropriate treatment against *S. viridans* was begun. A surgeon was consulted.

You have no idea what caused the endocarditis, since there was no history of dental procedures or oral surgery—the usual causes when a mouth organism is involved. Perhaps vigorous toothbrushing can be implicated.

He had none of the other common findings of infective endocarditis, such as embolic phenomena, petechiae, enlarged spleen, and clubbing. These are often absent although they should be sought.

QUESTIONS

1. You find a grade 2/6 systolic murmur in the aortic area of a 42-year-old asymptomatic man. The murmur is audible in the neck. No lifts or thrills are present. The carotid pulses and the first and second heart sounds are normal. There is no third or fourth heart sound. You suspect AS. Which of the following is correct?
   (a) A functional murmur is likely.
   (b) AS or pulmonic stenosis is present.
   (c) Rheumatic heart disease is probably present.
   (d) If no murmur were present in childhood, a bicuspid aortic valve could not be present.

2. Assume a 16-year-old asymptomatic high school student is sent to you because his school physician noted a murmur. You suspect an atrial septal defect (ASD) because he has a grade 2/6 ejection murmur at the base, a wide fixed split S_2, and a right ventricular lift. If your suspicion is correct, which of the following is least likely to be present?
   (a) a soft diastolic murmur at the left lower sternal border
   (b) a normal chest x-ray
   (c) anomalous pulmonary veins
   (d) rSr' in V_1 of the ECG.

3. An asymptomatic 33-year-old man is found to have a grade 4/6 blowing murmur, loudest at the apex and well heard in the left axilla. The murmur begins immediately after S_1 and continues through A_2 without varying in pitch or amplitude (plateau type). It does not vary with respiration. Jugular venous and carotid pulses are normal. Aside from a 3-month illness at age 9, during which he was kept out of school because of pain and discomfort in his upper and lower extremities, he has been well. The most likely diagnosis is:
   (a) idiopathic hypertrophic subaortic stenosis
   (b) functional murmur

(c) aortic stenosis

(d) mitral regurgitation.

4. The patient described in this logic session had aortic stenosis (AS), aortic regurgitation (AR), left ventricular failure (LVF), and bacterial endocarditis (BE). They occurred in the following pathophysiologic time sequence:

(a) AS—AR—LVF—BE

(b) AS—BE—LVF—AR

(c) AS—BE—AR—LVF

(d) AS—LVF—BE—AR.

ANSWERS

1. **(a) is correct.** The absence of a slow upstroke in the carotid pulse and the absence of abnormalities of S_2 rule out significant AS. Pulmonic stenosis is unlikely in view of the location and radiation of the murmur and the lack of a wide splitting of S_2. There is no history of rheumatic fever or evidence of mitral involvement to support a diagnosis of rheumatic disease. A congenital bicuspid valve can result in AS or aortic regurgitation, and if these lesions develop, the murmur may first appear during adult life. However, since all the findings noted can be normal, a functional murmur is the most likely diagnosis. But, as in the case discussed in the protocol, what is thought to be functional today may prove to be organic years later.

2. **(b) is correct.** The chest x-ray in ASD has prominent hilar shadows and prominent distal vasculature in most cases because of the high pulmonary blood flow. The systolic murmur is caused by high flow across the pulmonic valve, and not by blood traversing the septal defect. The diastolic murmur is due to high flow across the tricuspid valve and occurs when the shunt is large. Anomalous pulmonary veins are present in approximately 25% of cases of secundum type ASD. In most centers, more than 90% of postpuberty patients with ASD have the secundum type lesion in which an incomplete right bundle branch block is common.

3. **(d) is correct.** The murmur is holosystolic and is heard best at the apex; it radiates to the axilla and does not vary with respiration. This is the usual finding in mitral regurgitation. The childhood illness was most likely rheumatic fever which is the most common cause of severe mitral valve disease. Holosystolic murmurs are not functional. The clinical features of aortic valve stenosis were discussed in the case study. Idiopathic hypertrophic subaortic stenosis is a disease which involves a functional obstruction of the aortic outflow tract below the aortic valve due to muscular hypertrophy and a supernormal contraction of the ventricular muscle. Its murmur is crescendo or crescendo-decrescendo in type, tends to be long although not holosystolic, and is often heard best at the apex; radiation to the axilla is uncommon. The carotid upstroke is often rapid and the carotid pulse bifid; S_2 is paradoxically split, though A_2 remains well heard. The echocardiogram is distinctive; it shows a markedly hypertrophied interventricular septum and an abnormal movement of the mitral valve during systole.

4. **(c) is correct.** The sequence was clearly AS, eventually BE, which in turn caused destruction of a valve leaflet and acute AR; the regurgitation brought on the LVF. Not uncommonly, LVF will be the first manifestation of AS—but not so in this case.

COMMENT The patient presented with an asymptomatic (lanthanic) finding detected on routine examination. A heart murmur became the key clue. The various causes of plateau and ejection murmurs were listed, and each was eliminated by the absence of associated findings. But after a number of years a reliable cluster formed to make the diagnosis of AS. This cluster included symptoms and physical signs, each of which exhibited varying specificity and sensitivity; but when grouped together, the weight of evidence made the diagnosis unmistakable. The thrill is specific but not sensitive; the slow carotid upstroke is both specific and sensitive; the S_4 and paradoxically split S_2 are sensitive but not specific.

Considerable overlap of three clinical presentations (LVF, angina, syncope) can occur with AS. Venn diagrams (Fig. 5.3) nicely display the various subsets whereby a patient can present with one, two, or three of these manifestations. This patient had only two. The third, LVF, was not present; dyspnea was caused by hyperventilation and could have been misleading.

Bacterial endocarditis then developed, and it was diagnosed in the absence of many signs which are often present. Sequence of events and a series of causes and effects portrayed the pathophysiologic development of AS—BE—AR—LVF (Fig. 4.6). Note too how the clinical picture changed when a new disease was superimposed (BE upon AS) and that BE and AS combined to cause one effect (Fig. 4.4), which in turn caused another. (*P. C.*)

Suggested Readings

1. Rackley CE, Edwards JE, Karp RB, et al: Aortic valve disease. In Hurst JW (ed): *The Heart*, ed 5. New York, McGraw-Hill, 1982, pp 863–892.
   Stenosis and regurgitation from all causes are included.

2. Wagner S, Selzer A: Patterns of progression of aortic stenosis. *Circlation* 65:709–712, 1982.

Progression of disease is documented by hemo-dynamic studies in the three principal subtypes of stenosis—congenital, rheumatic, and calcific.

3. Braunwald E, Lambrew CT, Rockhoff SD, et al: Idiopathic hypertrophic subaortic stenosis. A description of the disease based upon an analysis of 64 patients. *Circulation* 30 (suppl 4):3–213, 1964.
This is the original classic description of IHSS.
4. (a) Berger M, Berdoff RL, Gallerstein PE, et al: Evaluation of aortic stenosis by continuous wave Doppler ultrasound. *J Am Coll Cardiol* 3:150–156, 1984.
(b) Kligfield P, Okin P, Devereux RB et al: Duration of ejection in aortic stenosis: effect of stroke volume and pressure gradient. *J Am Coll Cardiol* 3:157–163, 1984.
These two articles correlate the pathophysiology with the anatomy and diagnosis.
5. Wood P: Aortic stenosis. *Am J Cardiol* 1:553–571, 1958.
The classic study of aortic stenosis—still of great value.
6. Durack DT: Endocarditis. In Hurst JW ed: *The Heart* ed 5. New York, McGraw-Hill, 1982, pp 1250–1277.
Covers all types, clinical picture, complications, and treatment.
7. Weinstein L: Infective endocarditis. In Braunwald E (ed): *Heart Disease*, ed 2. Philadelphia, Saunders, 1984, pp 1136–1182.
8. Brandenberg RO, Giuliani ER, Wilson WR, et al: Infective endocarditis—a 25 year overview of diagnosis and therapy. *J Am Coll Cardiol* 1:280–291, 1983.
A very practical complete coverage of the subject with emphasis on the role of echocardiography.
9. Wigle ED, Labrosse CJ: Sudden severe aortic insufficiency. *Circulation* 32:708–720, 1965.
The clinical and hemodynamic effects of sudden perforation of the aortic valve due to bacterial endocarditis.
10. Bayliss R, Clarke C, Oakley CM, et al: The bowel, the genitourinary tract, and infective endocarditis. *Br Heart J* 51:339–345, 1984.
Discusses the second most common portal of entry.

Case 19
Palpitations

PAUL CUTLER, M.D.

DATA A 38-year-old obese salesman consults his physician because he has had recurrent brief episodes of "fluttering of the heart." These have been present for several years, used to occur infrequently, but more recently have been coming almost weekly and last from 1 to 10 minutes. You, the doctor, elicit more information.

Doctor: Tell me more about these episodes.

Patient: They seem to come for no particular reason and at no special time. My heart starts to pound, I get a sinking feeling in my chest and feel a little lightheaded, but I never faint. Nothing I do seems to help. Whether I walk, sit, lie down, drink something, or eat—they just go away when they want to.

Doctor: Do the attacks seem to start and stop suddenly? (You are thinking of paroxysmal atrial tachycardia which begins and ends with a sudden "click.")

Patient: I'm not sure. I suddenly become aware of them, and when they stop I feel better, but my pulse stays fast for a while.

Doctor: Can you tell whether the pounding is regular like a clock or irregular in timing if you feel your chest or take your pulse? (The doctor taps first regularly and then irregularly on his desk.) And how fast are they?

Patient: I've never noticed the timing, and I couldn't count them.

Doctor: Do you get short of breath or do you have chest pain with these attacks?

Patient: No! It's as I told you—I get lightheaded and a little anxious, but I don't even faint. Once they're over, I feel just fine.

Doctor: Tell me about some of your habits. Do you drink Cokes and coffee? Are you taking any medications? And how are your nerves?

Patient: Well, I guess I'm an easy-going guy. Nothing seems to really bother me, and I don't have any financial or family troubles.

But I drink a couple of Cokes every day and average about two or three coffees. I don't take any medication at all now. Once a doctor gave me something to lose weight but it didn't help, so I quit. By the way, you didn't ask, but I never drink any alcohol, and I haven't smoked in years.

Doctor: What about your general health? Do you or any members of your immediate family have any illnesses?

Patient: Aside from being a little fat (chuckle), I guess I'm in pretty good shape. A few years ago I had some indigestion and a doctor told me he thought I had a hiatal hernia, but I doubt it. It doesn't ever bother me, anyway. Maybe I've got gallstones like my mother. Dad has diabetes, but nobody else in the family does. Both my parents are still doing well though, and they're pushing 80.

Doctor: Have you seen a doctor for this rhythm problem before?

Patient: Yes, I did, about a year ago. He told me I was OK as far as he could tell. He took an electrocardiogram and said it was probably my nerves. But I didn't really believe him. I've got nerves like steel.

LOGIC   This 3-minute exchange has elicited much useful information. The physician knows he is dealing with a paroxysmal arrhythmia. It is not simple sporadic ventricular or atrial premature beats since it lasts too long. In order of commonness, the patient is most apt to have (*a*) paroxysmal atrial tachycardia (PAT), (*b*) paroxysmal atrial fibrillation (PAF), (*c*) paroxysmal ventricular tachycardia (PVT), or (*d*) paroxysmal atrial flutter (PAFl). Sinus tachycardia cannot be ruled out.

PAT is the most common; PAF is a close second; PVT is a distant third; and PAFl is only one-tenth as frequent as PAF. If the patient is truly healthy you are most likely dealing with PAT, and if he has heart disease, you could be dealing with any. But even in heart disease, PAT and PAF are most common.

You know that he does not have heart disease serious enough to give him coronary

insufficiency or left ventricular failure when the rapid rate comes on. The lightheadedness could result from mild cerebral ischemia due to decreased cardiac output. Furthermore, there are no precipitating events like fright, excitement, or trauma, and he takes no possibly causative agents like excessive caffeine, nicotine, alcohol, amphetamine, or digitalis. There is no evidence for anxiety factors, either. The likelihood of sinus tachycardia is diminished.

Since PAT often starts and stops with the suddenness of a click, this negative information was of no help. Moreover, the patient was unable to tell you whether the heart is regular, slightly irregular, or very irregular. Some patients can do so, and it helps distinguish PAT, PVT, and PAF.

DATA   Complete physical examination is essentially normal except for moderate obesity (height 68 inches, weight 184 lb). In particular, the vital signs are normal; there are no heart murmurs, clicks, snaps, or gallops (except for a possible grade 1/6 short midsystolic ejection murmur over the pulmonic valve). The heart rhythm is normal and the rate is 80/minute. There is no abdominal tenderness.

While performing the physical examination, the physician fills in the rest of the history as he examines each system. No additional positive or helpful information is obtained.

A blood count, urinalysis, 6-test chemistry profile, chest x-ray, oral cholecystogram, upper gastrointestinal series, and ECG are obtained. They are all normal; in particular, the PR interval is not short, and the QRS is not prolonged.

LOGIC   On the basis of all the evidence, the patient can be reassured with reasonable certainty that he has no heart disease. The very faint murmur appears to be benign, especially since there are no concomitant findings of heart disease. There is no evidence of mitral stenosis, hyperthyroidism, or click-murmur syndrome, each of which is notorious for causing paroxysmal arrhythmias.

While the ECG is normal and gives no positive clues, at least it rules out the Wolff-Parkinson-White and Lown-Ganong-Levine syndromes. These two disorders of anomalous conduction are most often associated with PAT. Both are characterized by a short PR interval, and there is a wide QRS in the first and a normal QRS in the second. A reentrant tachycardia cannot be totally eliminated, but its likelihood is reduced.

The gastrointestinal and gallbladder x-rays were obtained to verify the situation regarding the patient's statements, though this might be considered unnecessary by some. But there are those who think diseases in these two systems may be reflexly associated with arrhythmias.

DATA Your patient is informed that there is no evidence for any significant heart disease and that his arrhythmias are almost certainly benign paroxysms of atrial tachycardia. He is further told that it would be helpful to have documentation of this fact by an ECG recording taken during an attack, before proper therapy can begin. The matter of hospitalization is raised. You both decide it would be poor hospital utilization since his attacks come only once a week, and even if he were monitored for 24 hours by Holter monitor, or for 3 days in an intensive care unit, the chance of obtaining the needed information is not great. He is therefore advised to lose weight and come to see you or visit the nearest emergency room at the next attack.

LOGIC After he leaves, you reexamine the possibilities. PAT comes and goes abruptly, is usually benign, has a ventricular rate of 150 to 250/minute, and is often stopped by carotid sinus pressure or induced vomiting.

PAF has an irregularly irregular ventricular rate ranging from 90 to 150, is usually associated with heart disease, and is only uncommonly benign. Carotid sinus pressure may slow the ventricular rate somewhat but doesn't change the rhythm.

PVT and PAFl may be slightly irregular and are almost always associated with heart disease. Carotid sinus pressure doesn't affect PVT, but it briefly stops ventricular contraction in PAFl.

DATA Ten days later, the patient returns. He has had two attacks during this time, but each one stopped before he could get to you or to a hospital. While he thinks the heart rhythm was regular and the rate about 180/minute, he is not sure. In the meantime, he has heard of a person with similar symptoms who "dropped dead," and he is now much more concerned about heart disease.

LOGIC Since you have not completely ruled out coronary heart disease with PVTs, and since the patient is now becoming very worried, you decide to do noninvasive procedures which should further strengthen your opinion—an exercise tolerance test to evaluate him for possible coronary disease and an echocardiogram to detect mitral valve prolapse (Barlow syndrome). Both are associated with paroxysmal arrhythmias.

DATA After 15 minutes of increasing exercise, the pulse rate having reached maximal levels for some time, the test is discontinued. There were no symptoms except for mild shortness of breath, no arrhythmias, and no ECG abnormalities to suggest coronary disease. An echocardiogram done with adjunctive amyl nitrite fails to detect evidence of mitral valve prolapse.

The significance of both tests and the small incidence of false negatives is explained to the patient. He feels reassured. So do you.

Three days later, you receive a telephone call from the emergency room of a hospital on the other side of town. (Your own pulse quickens.) The intern tells you, "Doctor, your patient is having an ECG-documented attack of paroxysmal atrial tachycardia. What would you like me to do?"

After a sigh of relief, you say—"Don't do anything. It will go away in a few minutes. If it doesn't, call me back. If it does, have him see me in the morning with a copy of his ECG. I'll put him on prophylactic medication. Thank you very much!"

COMMENT   Several things are worth noting in the solving of this problem. The interview started with open-ended questions which got more closed as the dialogue proceeded. Furthermore, the history pursued only one subset; the rest of the history was obtained while doing the physical examination. The remainder of the data base was obtained in a somewhat branched manner too, since pursuit of the arrhythmia was the principal issue.

Note that the physician first listed each possibility, then searched for clues of each. The weight of evidence grew for the presence of PAT and the absence of organic heart disease. Nonpertinent information, such as possible gallbladder disease, possible hiatal hernia, and slight heart murmur, had to be suppressed.

And last, Bayesian probabilities were considered. PAT is the most frequent tachyarrhythmia in the universe of people, and it is percentage-wise even more common in the set of people who do not have demonstrable heart disease. So for the most part it is benign arrhythmia. In this case, the decisive clue was the ECG taken during an attack.   *(P. C.)*

Suggested Readings

1. Zipes DP: Specific arrhythmias: diagnosis and treatment. In Braunwald E (ed): *Heart Disease*, ed 2. Philadelphia, Saunders, 1984, pp 683–743.
2. Arcebal AG, Lemberg L: Mechanisms of supraventricular tachycardia. *Heart Lung* 13:205–209, 1984.
   Reviews the mechanisms, causes, and treatment of atrial tachycardia.
3. Buxton AE, Josephson ME: Ventricular tachycardia. *PACE* 7:96–108, 1984.
   A "state of the art" review of ventricular tachycardia—diagnosis, mechanisms, electrophysiology, and treatment.
4. Coumel P, Attuel P, Flammang D: The role of the conduction system in supraventricular tachycardias. In Wellens HJJ, Lie KI, Janse MJ (eds): *The Conduction System of the Heart; Structure, Function and Clinical Implications.* Philadelphia, Lea & Febiger, 1976, pp 424–452.
   Definitive work on the complexity of evaluating supraventricular arrhythmias.
5. Marriott HJL, Myerberg RJ: Recognition of arrhythmias and conduction abnormalities. In Hurst JW (ed): *The Heart*, ed 5. New York, McGraw-Hill, 1982, pp 519–556.
   All the atrial and ventricular arrhythmias are covered in depth.
6. Cheitlin MD, Byrd RC: Prolapsed mitral valve: the commonest valve disease? *Curr Probl Cardiol* 8:10, 1984.
   A short monograph on a fascinating subject that relates to arrhythmias.

Case 20
Swollen Legs
MICHAEL H. CRAWFORD, M.D.

DATA   A 47-year-old Mexican woman was brought to the hospital by her family because of progressive weakness and swollen legs. The patient was visiting from Mexico and the family knew very little about her medical history. Not realizing the further need for an interpreter, the family left. Therefore the physical examination was done first since there were no bilingual persons immediately available.

The vital signs were: pulse 90 and regular, blood pressure 107/65, respirations 26 and labored, temperature 37.1 C. Severe pitting edema was present up to the midabdomen. The jugular veins were distended to the angle

of the jaw at 45° and there was a prominent "a" wave. Carotid pulses were weak. Chest expansion was decreased and there was poor diaphragmatic movement. Diffuse rales and wheezes were auscultated over the lung fields. There was a sustained lower left sternal border systolic impulse and a systolic pulsation in the second left intercostal space. No left ventricular apex could be felt. The first heart sound was easily heard and the second component of the second heart sound was loud. Further clarification of the cardiac examination was impossible due to the excessive pulmonary noises. Examination of the abdomen was difficult because of pitting edema of the lower abdominal wall; but liver dullness extended 15 cm from top to bottom in the right midclavicular line and the right upper quadrant was tender. There was anterior abdominal and flank distention, but no definite fluid wave or shifting dullness was noted. Peripheral pulses were weak but equal. Otherwise, the physical examination was normal.

LOGIC Two pathophysiologic events are immediately apparent: severe pulmonary hypertension (sustained right ventricular lift, palpable pulmonary artery segment, and loud pulmonary component of S_2) and right ventricular failure (neck vein distention, hepatic engorgement, edema, and probable ascites). Hypertension in any vascular bed is due to an imbalance between flow and resistance. Excessive blood flow through a normal-caliber vascular channel can cause a mild increase in pressure, but more marked hypertension can be caused only by an increase in resistance to flow. Therefore our patient must have increased resistance to blood flow somewhere downstream from the main pulmonary artery.

Some of the possibilities, in anatomic order, include: (*a*) pulmonary artery branch stenosis; (*b*) pulmonary arterial constriction (e.g. hypoxia from any cause); (*c*) pulmonary arterial obstruction (e.g. multiple pulmonary emboli); (*d*) chronic pulmonary diseases that obstruct or destroy the arteriolar-capillary bed (e.g. chronic obstructive pulmonary disease or pulmonary fibrosis); (*e*) mitral valve stenosis; and (*f*) left ventricular failure from any cause. The last item is the most common cause of pulmonary hypertension and right ventricular failure in the adult.

Pulmonic valve stenosis is not a viable consideration because of the patient's age and the presence of physical evidence of pulmonary artery hypertension. Pulmonary artery branch stenosis is not likely, since no systolic murmur was heard. The low blood pressure, weak pulses, and tachycardia suggest that the patient may have low cardiac output. In such a situation the murmur of

mitral stenosis may be markedly diminished to the point that excessive respiratory noises might obscure it. However, the lung findings suggest that the pulmonary hypertension may be due to primary pulmonary disease.

DATA To further clarify the patient's problem, an ECG and chest x-ray were done. The ECG exhibited normal sinus rhythm with right ventricular hypertrophy and left atrial abnormality. The chest x-ray was of poor quality due to an inadequate inspiration but showed generally hazy lung fields. Cardiac size or specific chamber enlargement could not be reliably evaluated.

LOGIC This information is very important in narrowing the possibilities. Absence of both hyperaeration and a flat diaphragm is against the presence of chronic obstructive lung disease, a common cause of pulmonary hypertension in adults. The presence of left atrial abnormality and the absence of left ventricular hypertrophy or myocardial infarction on the ECG places the obstruction at the mitral valve and not downstream from the left ventricle. Therefore mitral valve stenosis is the most likely diagnosis.

DATA After treatment with oxygen, aminophylline, and diuretics, the patient's respiratory rate decreased and pulmonary wheezes and rales were no longer audible. Cardiac auscultation at this time revealed a normal first heart sound and a physiologically split second heart sound with a loud pulmonary component (P_2). No opening snap was audible, but at the apex there was a grade 2/4 rumbling decrescendo diastolic murmur which started just after a P_2 that was loud enough to be heard at the apex. This murmur was best heard in the left lateral decubitus position with the bell of the stethoscope.

At the base of the heart there was a high-pitched decrescendo diastolic murmur which started with the second heart sound and was audible only during the first one-third of diastole. This murmur was best heard along the left sternal border but could also be faintly heard at the right second interspace (aortic area).

After the congestion cleared, a repeat chest x-ray showed no evidence of chronic pulmonary disease; the heart did not appear to be enlarged, but straightening of the left cardiac border and prominence of the pulmonary vasculature were noted.

More history was obtained through an interpreter. The patient denied any knowledge of acute rheumatic fever or previous heart disease. She had two children in her early twenties without complications. She has not seen a doctor since then and felt well until the last year, when she began noting progressive fatigue, dyspnea on exertion, and, more recently, swelling of her lower extremities and abdomen.

LOGIC   The low-pitched diastolic murmur at the apex is characteristic of mitral valve obstruction and confirms the suspected diagnosis. However, the clinical evaluation does not clarify the etiology of this obstruction. Only 50% of patients with rheumatic heart disease give a history of a prior illness compatible with acute rheumatic fever. Although the murmur of mitral regurgitation may appear during the acute attack, mitral stenosis does not develop until many years later. Ordinarily there is a latent period of about 10 years before the auscultatory findings of mitral stenosis can be appreciated. At this time the patient is usually asymptomatic but may become symptomatic during periods of cardiovascular stress, such as pregnancy. The asymptomatic period lasts another 10 years and then the symptoms begin in the third decade of the disease. Symptoms progress until death ensues during the fourth decade from pulmonary congestion and low cardiac output.

Our patient does not fit this classical description of rheumatic mitral stenosis. There is no history of prior acute rheumatic fever and her symptomatology has begun only recently. Also, the lack of an opening snap on physical examination raises the possibility that she has some other form of mitral valve obstruction. Another cause of such

obstruction is left atrial myxoma. This pedunculated tumor attaches to the interatrial septum and obstructs the mitral valve during diastole and then moves back into the left atrium during systole. About 25% of patients with left atrial myxoma suffer from a systemic illness with fever and arthralgias. The short duration of our patient's symptoms and the severity of the pulmonary hypertension would favor this diagnosis.

The high-pitched basal diastolic murmur is characteristic of regurgitation through a semilunar valve. In this particular case, the murmur could represent the Graham Steell murmur of pulmonary regurgitation associated with pulmonary hypertension; this murmur is commonly heard in severe mitral stenosis. However, the Graham Steell murmur is usually confined to the left sternal border and is rarely heard in the aortic area. Our patient's murmur was heard in the aortic area, which suggests that it is of aortic valvular origin. Rheumatic valvular disease often strikes more than one valve, the mitral and aortic valves being the most common. Thus, the presence of an aortic diastolic murmur would favor a rheumatic etiology for the mitral valve disease.

DATA   The patient responded well to therapy in the hospital and diuresed 30 lb in 1 week. However, one morning she complained of numbness of the left leg. It was cold and blue from the midthigh to the toes. The left femoral pulse was no longer palpable and the patient's pulse was irregularly irregular at a rate of 130. Atrial fibrillation without other changes was documented by ECG.

LOGIC   An embolic occlusion of the femoral artery has occurred. The most likely source for this embolic material would be the heart, presumably the left atrium since the occlusion was accompanied or preceded by the development of atrial fibrillation. It is common for patients with mitral stenosis, especially those in atrial fibrillation, to develop thrombi in the left atrium or its appendage; these can dislodge and embolize to the peripheral circulation. Such emboli are usually small and resolve without any difficulties, but occasionally they occlude large vessels and cause severe organ damage.

The diagnosis of rheumatic mitral stenosis has yet to be firmly established. Large vessel peripheral emboli are frequent in left atrial myxoma too. Emboli often occur from the valvular vegetations of bacterial endocarditis, and, finally, acute myocardial infarction can lead to mural thrombi which may also embolize. There is no clinical evidence to support the latter two possibilities in our patient and the choice remains between rheumatic heart disease and left atrial myxoma.

DATA Femoral embolectomy was rapidly performed under local anesthesia. Pathologic examination of the removed specimen was consistent with thrombic material without evidence of myxomatous tissue. An echocardiogram showed a thickened, poorly mobile mitral valve and an enlarged left atrium which supported the diagnosis of rheumatic mitral stenosis; there was no evidence for a myxoma.

Cardiac catheterization revealed: pulmonary artery pressure 70/26 mm Hg, mean pulmonary capillary wedge pressure 35 mm Hg, and left ventricular end-diastolic pressure 10 mm Hg. The mean diastolic mitral valve gradient was 21 mm Hg and cardiac output was 2.0 liters/minute, resulting in a calculated mitral valve orifice of 0.5 cm². At surgery the mitral valve was found to be thickened, calcified, and immobile; this probably explains the lack of an opening snap and the lack of a loud first heart sound. Mitral valve replacement was accomplished without difficulty and the patient has done well since then.

QUESTIONS

1. A 26-year-old woman complains of fatigue. Physical signs of pulmonary hypertension and right ventricular hypertrophy are present. Chest x-ray exhibits enlargement of the right atrium, right ventricle, and central pulmonary arteries. Systemic arterial blood gases are nor-

mal. At right heart catheterization the following pressures are found: mean right atrium 12; right ventricle 80/15; pulmonary artery 80/30; and mean pulmonary capillary wedge 7 mm Hg. Which of the following diagnoses is/are most likely?
   (a) multiple pulmonary emboli
   (b) primary pulmonary hypertension
   (c) restrictive pulmonary parenchymal disease
   (d) "silent" mitral stenosis.
2. In the natural course of mitral stenosis, a variety of situations can occur. Which one of the following is least likely?
   (a) dysphagia and hoarseness
   (b) sudden episodes of collapse
   (c) sustained left ventricular lift at the anterior axillary line
   (d) acute pulmonary edema.
3. Which one of the following physical findings is least likely in a patient with chronic mitral stenosis?
   (a) an early systolic decrescendo murmur at the apex
   (b) Carey Coombs murmur
   (c) an isolated presystolic murmur at the apex
   (d) Graham Steell murmur.
4. Which of the following clinical situations can be associated with right ventricular hypertrophy and failure (RVF), with resultant leg edema?
   (a) a 350-lb man with a normal chest x-ray
   (b) a 26-year-old woman with a systolic basal murmur since birth, wide fixed splitting of S₂, and marked prominence of the pulmonary arteries on x-ray
   (c) a 48-year-old beauty parlor operator with 6 months of progressively more severe dyspnea on exertion and diffuse reticular markings of the lungs on chest x-ray
   (d) a 60-year-old heavy smoker with chronic cough, expectoration, and worsening dyspnea.

ANSWERS

1. **(b) is correct.** Multiple small pulmonary emboli and primary pulmonary hypertension are very difficult to separate clinically, but multiple emboli usually cause a decreased pO₂. Both occur more frequently in young women; birth control pills increase the incidence of emboli. Both exhibit enlarged central pulmonary arteries with smaller peripheral vessel "cutoffs" seen on chest x-ray or pulmonary angiography. Most restrictive lung diseases result in pulmonary fibrosis which is detectable on chest x-ray and impairs oxygen transport, leading to decreased arterial oxygen saturation. The normal pulmonary capillary wedge pressure excludes mitral valve obstruction.

2. **(c) is correct and least likely to occur.** The obstruction at the mitral valve limits left ventricular filling, and thus this chamber is usually smaller than normal. Dysphagia and hoarseness can occur because of esophageal and recurrent larnygeal nerve compression by an enlarged left atrium. A large left atrial thrombus may act as a ball valve and intermittently obstruct the stenotic mitral valve, leading to sudden cessation of cardiac output and collapse. The change in body position moves the clot away from the orifice and circulation resumes. Excessive pulmonary venous pressure may cause fluid transudation into the pulmonary alveoli. This often occurs during pregnancy in otherwise asymptomatic women with mitral stenosis because of an obligate increase in vascular volume during this condition. It also occurs when left atrial pressure rises rapidly, as in tachycardias with decreased diastolic ventricular filling time.

3. **(b) is least likely.** The Carey Coombs murmur is a short mid-diastolic low-frequency murmur that occurs during acute rheumatic fever with carditis and is difficult to distinguish from an S_3. It is probably due to edematous mitral valve leaflets and disappears after the acute attack. Chronic mitral stenosis is often associated with a small amount of mitral regurgitation early in systole, before the stiffened valve is finally closed; this results in an early systolic decrescendo murmur. In mild mitral stenosis a diastolic gradient may occur only during atrial systole, just prior to ventricular systole; hence a presystolic murmur is heard at the apex. Secondary pulmonary hypertension may lead to pulmonary regurgitation and a Graham Steell murmur.

4. **(a), (b), (c), and (d) are all correct.** Tremendous obesity can cause hypoxia and hypercarbia because of mechanical difficulty with breathing (Pickwickian syndrome). Chronic hypoxia results in pulmonary hypertension and RVF. (b) describes a patient with atrial septal defect whose right ventricle is under chronic strain from circulatory overload. The beauty parlor operator probably has pulmonary fibrosis (hair spray related?), causing obstruction of pulmonary capillaries and pulmonary hypertension. (d) is the classical presentation of a patient with chronic obstructive lung disease. Numerous other clinical situations can cause RVF too.

COMMENT   The traditional order of data gathering was necessarily reversed and the physical examination was done first. RVF was evident and all the causes for RVF were listed. Almost all were eliminated by an absence of confirmatory clues. Only mitral stenosis and atrial myxoma remained. There was considerable overlap of signs, though some of the features (absence of opening snap, short duration of illness, severe pulmonary hypertension) favored the much less common disease—atrial myxoma. But two highly specific and highly sensitive clues (the absence of myxomatous tissue in the embolus and the echocardiogram) proved the far more common diagnosis (mitral stenosis) to be the correct one.

Not having a history, the diagnostician was at a disadvantage. Ordinarily, this case would be solved simultaneously with treatment in 24 to 48 hours. Pulmonary hypertension and right ventricular failure in the absence of previous pulmonary symptoms quickly narrow the choices. At this point, an ECG, chest x-ray, and ultrasound study would deliver the diagnosis with the same speed as rapid diuresis and the detection of typical murmurs—perhaps sooner. A more aggressive problem solver might request immediate pulmonary arteriography, Swan-Ganz catheter placement with pressure studies, and a ventilation-perfusion isotope scan. But most physicians would consider the latter studies unnecessary, wasteful, or ill-timed.   (*P. C.*)

Suggested Readings

1. Selzer A, Cohn K: Natural history of mitral stenosis. *Circulation* 45:878–890, 1972.
   A classic description of the course of this lesion produced by rheumatic fever.
2. Rackley CE, Edwards JE, Karp RB, et al: Mitral valve disease. In Hurst JW (ed): *The Heart*, ed 5. New York, McGraw-Hill, 1982, pp 892–927.
   Excellent description of this entity by a pathologist, a cardiologist, and a surgeon; diagnostic procedures are accented.
3. Colucci WS, Braunwald E: Primary tumors of the heart. In Braunwald E (ed): *Heart Disease*, ed 2. Philadelphia, Saunders, 1984, pp 1457–1467.
   An up-to-date review including sonograms of left atrial myxomas visualized by echocardiography.
4. Ross JC: Chronic cor pulmonale. In Hurst JW (ed): *The Heart*, ed 5. New York, McGraw-Hill, 1982, pp 1243–1249.
5. Grossman W, Alpert JS, Braunwald E: Pulmonary hypertension. In Braunwald E (ed): *Heart Disease*, ed 2. Philadelphia, Saunders, 1984, pp 823–848.
6. Kuida H: Primary pulmonary hypertension. In Hurst JW (ed): *The Heart*, ed 5. New York, McGraw-Hill, 1982, pp 1221–1227.
7. McFadden ER Jr, Braunwald E: Cor pulmonale and pulmonary thromboembolism. In Braunwald E (ed): *Heart Disease*, ed 2. Philadelphia, Saunders, 1984, pp 1572–1605.
   pp 1575–1589: pulmonary thromboembolism
   pp 1589–1600: cor pulmonale

Case 21
Sharp Chest Pains
LAWRENCE D. HORWITZ, M.D.

DATA After successfully concluding a malpractice suit, a 39-year-old attorney had an episode of sharp stabbing left chest pain lasting several minutes. He sat down on the steps of the courthouse until it subsided and then directly visited his physician. Within the past month he had noted six similar though milder episodes, each lasting 30 to 40 seconds. Several occurred while he was sitting at his desk, and some while walking home from work.

LOGIC A problem of recurrent left-sided chest pain is always a challenge. The principal task is to separate coronary heart disease from a multitude of benign conditions. Careful inquiry must be made into all the characteristics of the pain: when it comes, what it feels like, where it is, where it radiates, what causes it, and what relieves it. Today, when so many people are heart conscious, they usually come to the physician with sundry types of chest pains; the majority do not have serious organic disease.

Chest pain can consist of one severe episode or multiple smaller ones. In the former instance, you think of myocardial infarction, pulmonary embolus, dissecting aneurysm, ruptured esophagus, acute pericarditis, acute pleuritis, pneumothorax, and even subdiaphragmatic events like acute pancreatitis, perforated ulcer, and acute cholecystitis. By the nature of the history so far, none of these is likely since each tends to be a single event. Pericarditis and pleuritis can last for a while, but the pain is usually worse on breathing, coughing, or positioning, and the underlying cause and clues are evident.

Causes for recurrent chest pains include angina, musculoskeletal disturbances, intercostal neuralgia, postherpetic neuralgia, bone involvement by hematologic and other malignancies, hiatal hernia, peptic esophagitis, psychosomatic disorders, and breast conditions.

Musculoskeletal pain is probably the largest group and includes cervical discs, cervical and thoracic osteoarthritis, exercise of untrained muscles, fibromyositis, inflammation of the costochondral or chondrosternal articulations (Tietze's syndrome), cervical ribs, and thoracic deformities.

Remember the very important relationships of musculoskeletal pain to motion, esophageal pain to swallowing, pleuritic pain to breathing, and coronary pain to exertion.

DATA Further history reveals that the episodes of pain are sharp, involve the left upper and lower parts of the chest, do not radiate, and are not related to strenuous physical activity, swallowing, eating, mealtimes, breathing, or changes in position. He continues to play two sets of singles tennis a few times weekly and gets no pain at those times. The pain is not accompanied by dyspnea, palpitations, or a cold sweat. He has no chronic indigestion, heartburn, or any other symptoms.

LOGIC Much has been learned. Coronary pain unrelated to exertion is unlikely, unless the disease is so bad that the patient gets it even at rest; but then he would get it on exertion too, and certainly could not play tennis. Lack of relationship to the other activities mentioned is against a variety of other conditions mentioned.

It is incorrect to assume that only coronary pain radiates to the left arm. Although coronary disease is the most common cause, this type of radiation occurs occasionally with esophageal, pleuropericardial, diaphragmatic, and musculoskeletal diseases. The complexities of nerve supply and neurotomes determine the site of pain. Another important point to remember is that both coronary disease and musculoskeletal disease are very common and frequently coexist in the same individual. On careful questioning it may become apparent that the patient has two types of pain. And next, don't necessarily associate chest pain with an incidental hiatal hernia, a nonspecific ECG abnormality, or some spurs seen on the cervical or thoracic spine x-ray.

DATA   The patient has never had previous chest pain and has had a yearly physical examination and ECG which were normal. He is the youngest of three brothers and there is no heart disease in his siblings or his parents, who are still living. Neither is there a family history of hypertension, diabetes mellitus, strokes, or blood lipid abnormalities. The patient is generally under tension and smokes one to two packs of cigarettes/day, but he stays lean and does not have a high intake of dairy products or meat.

Recently, he has been working under great stress on an important case. This has involved long hours of work, irregular meals, and a reduced amount of sleep. A reason for his immediate concern is that a senior law partner died of a heart attack not long ago after suffering from angina for several years.

LOGIC   There are no risk factors for coronary disease except for the cigarette smoking. The negative family history is significant too. His high degree of tension influences you. Although some believe that environmental or emotional stress increases the risk of coronary disease, it is more likely that unusual stresses may cause a morbid preoccupation with mild discomforts which would otherwise be ignored. And the nature, location, and timing of his pain make it unlikely that he has coronary disease. But what does he have?

DATA   Complete physical examination is normal. The blood pressure is 120/80, the fundi are normal, the thyroid is not enlarged, the lungs are clear, and the heart is not enlarged and has no murmurs, ectopic lifts, S_3, or S_4. Movements of the neck and shoulders do not elicit pain. There are no areas of tenderness anywhere in the chest, including the rib cartilages and their articulations. The

abdomen and the rest of the examination are normal.

LOGIC   The normal blood pressure rules out an additional coronary risk factor, the absence of murmurs is against valvular stenoses which can cause angina-like pain, and the absence of an S_4 is somewhat against coronary disease. Tietze's syndrome is unlikely since there is no chondral tenderness; though the pain of this disease is often misleading in that it can be sharp and darting or a dull precordial ache, the affected areas should be tender. Failure of neck motions to cause pain is against cervical radiculitis or disk.

DATA   Chest x-ray is normal; a cervical rib is not present. X-rays of the cervical and thoracic spine are normal. The resting ECG is normal and unchanged from previous tracings. Blood count, urinalysis, erythrocyte sedimentation rate, and blood chemistries are all normal.

LOGIC   Normal complete blood count and erythrocyte sedimentation rate are reassuring when a patient has undiagnosed pain and you are considering a possible malignancy. X-rays rule out spondylogenic causes, and the normal ECG is comforting too. The normal serum glucose, cholesterol, and triglycerides eliminate other coronary risk factors.

Though you are reasonably assured that the patient has no serious disease, you still cannot explain the pain. However, it seems safe to conclude that the pains are related to his state of tension, to an undiagnosed but nonserious musculoskeletal condition, or to "gas under the diaphragm" associated with a splenic flexure syndrome or spastic colon.

DATA   You inform the patient of the findings and your conclusions, reassure him that he has no serious problem, and advise him to reduce his working hours, slow his pace of living, reduce or preferably discontinue cigarette smoking, and return in 6 weeks.

LOGIC In view of the almost complete absence of risk factors, the unimpressive nature of the pain, the negative family history, and the normal examination, you are comfortable in reaching this conclusion. Further tests are not indicated.

DATA He unexpectedly returns 2 weeks later. He has followed your advice but has had three more episodes of pain. They are similar to but not exactly the same as the other attacks. One came during an argument and the other while walking up steps; each lasted about 30 seconds.

Examination remains the same. A graded exercise treadmill test is done and a thallium scan is performed at the conclusion of exercise and several hours later. (Present evidence is that more than 90% of cases of serious coronary atherosclerosis are detected by thallium exercise tests.) All results are normal and there is no evidence of coronary disease or myocardial ischemia. You reassure the patient again and reschedule his visit.

He does not return at the scheduled time and you therefore assume he is well. Two months later you read his obituary notice in the newspaper, and learn that he suddenly dropped dead in court during a heated argument.

LOGIC This is a shocking bit of news. On reviewing his records, you feel completely justified in your conclusions. Was there a relation between the chest pains and his demise? There was not a single bit of evidence for coronary disease. All tests were negative, yet false negatives do occur. Should another patient with the same picture present, you would do the same thing. Here is a situation where all the evidence pointed in one direction—yet the opposite turned out to be the case.

QUESTIONS

1. Had there been indication of the existence of coronary disease in this patient and had it been urgent to establish the diagnosis, the specific thing to do would have been:
   (a) trial of nitroglycerine for pain
   (b) long-acting nitrate for prevention of pain
   (c) coronary arteriography
   (d) echocardiography.
2. A 49-year-old man complains of chest pains which frequently waken him from his sleep and occasionally occur during the day. It is a deep, burning type of pain and is relieved by antacids. At times, swallowed food seems to get stuck in his lower chest and he has considerable heartburn. To prove what you suspect, do:
   (a) upper gastrointestinal x-ray
   (b) Bernstein test
   (c) esophagoscopy
   (d) gastric analysis.
3. As for the various types and causes of chest pain, which one of the following statements is incorrect?
   (a) Pericardial pain is usually caused by inflammation of surrounding structures. The pain of pericarditis may be worse with breathing, motion, cough, or swallowing; it may be crushing in type, or synchronous with each heartbeat; or combinations of these types may exist.
   (b) Chest pains related to emotional disorders can occur anywhere, can last any length of time, are associated with fatigue, and bear no relation to activity or exercise.
   (c) Persistent though intermittent long-standing pain girdling the left chest can be the result of a previous known or unnoticed herpes zoster infection.
   (d) The chest pain of pulmonary embolus is of two types. Immediately there may be severe substernal coronary-like pain. Twelve to 24 hours later, as an infarct forms, pleuritic pain on breathing may occur.
   (e) Chest pain following a severe emotional disturbance is psychosomatic in origin.

ANSWERS

1. **(c) is correct.** Nothing is more specific than the invasive procedure of coronary arteriography. Nitroglycerine relieves many things, and prophylactic nitrates are either not helpful or inconclusive. An echocardiogram might show a poorly contractile area, so (d) might be done too, but the positive yield for (c) should be greater.
2. **(a), (b), and (c) are correct.** The Bernstein test is specific for what you expect to be present: peptic esophagitis. Acid reflux is common in the reclining position. A drip of hydrochloric acid into the lower esophagus will reproduce the pain. X-rays may be helpful in delineating a stricture or an often accompanying hiatal hernia. A fiberoptic look may also be of help to rule out another obstructing lesion. The gastric analysis will add nothing of great value.

3. **(e) is incorrect.** It is the only wrong statement. Chest pain following an emotional disturbance may very well be coronary in origin, since the release of catecholamines may elevate the blood pressure and also make the heart work harder. Thus the myocardial need for oxygen rises, and if sclerosis exists, the oxygen supply may not be increasable. The other statements are all correct and serve to characterize a variety of chest pains.

COMMENT Solving the problem of chest pain can be very simple for typical pictures but difficult for atypical ones. Generally the clinician can establish a reasonably precise disease probability—P(D)—on the basis of the history. The presence or absence of risk factors helps. The ECG is only about 50% sensitive.

Patient or doctor anxiety, or the need for more precision, may warrant additional studies, such as a treadmill test, thallium scan, and, in some cases, coronary arteriography. Digital subtraction angiography and nuclear magnetic resonance offer promise of lending greater assistance at less risk in the near future.

But always remember that all tests may be negative, yet the patient may have a variant or atypical form of angina—Prinzmetal's angina. In that case, coronary artery *spasm* occurs either at the site of a fixed atherosclerotic lesion or in a normal coronary artery. The cause for spasm remains obscure and the angina usually occurs at rest. But the results of spasm—angina, infarction, or death—are well known. Such may have been the case in the patient just discussed.   (*P. C.*)

Suggested Readings

1. Braunwald E: Chest pain. In Petersdorf RG, Adams RD, Braunwald E, et al (eds): *Harrison's Principles of Internal Medicine*, ed 9. New York, McGraw-Hill, 1983, pp 25–29.
   A succinct discussion of the causes of chest pain and how to distinguish them.
2. Bauwens DB, Paine, R: Thoracic pain. In Blacklow RS (ed): *MacBryde's Signs and Symptoms*, ed 6. Philadelphia, Lippincott, 1983, pp 139–161.
   A more detailed discussion of all cases for chest pain with special emphasis on nerve pain pathways.
3. Hurst JW, King SB III: The problem of chest pain. *JAMA* 236:2100–2103, 1976.
   The algorithmic workup of a patient with chest pain is presented.
4. Bernstein LM, Fruin RC, Pacini R: Differentiation of esophageal pain from angina pectoris: role of the esophageal perfusion test. *Medicine* 41:143–162, 1962.
5. Horwitz LD: The diagnostic significance of anginal symptoms. *JAMA* 229:1196–1199, 1974.
   A careful clinical study of the symptom complex of angina pectoris in 49 patients with proven coronary artery disease and 23 patients with recurrent chest pain but normal coronary angiograms.
6. Selzer A, Langston M, Ruggeroli C, et al: Clinical syndrome of variant angina with normal coronary arteriogram. *N. Engl J Med* 295:1343–1347, 1976.
   A brief article comparing clinical findings in patients with variant or Prinzmetal's angina who have normal coronary arteries on angiograms with those who have the syndrome with coronary atherosclerosis present.
7. Hurst JW, King SB III, Walter PF, et al: Conditions producing chest pain that must be differentiated from myocardial ischemia due to atherosclerotic heart disease. In Hurst JW (ed): *The Heart*, ed 5. New York, McGraw-Hill, 1982, pp 1029–1038.
8. Froelicher VF: Techniques of exercise testing. In Hurst JW (ed): *The Heart*, ed 5. New York, McGraw-Hill, 1982, pp 1726–1734.
9. Sheffield LT: Exercise stress testing. In Braunwald E (ed): *Heart Disease*, ed 2. Philadelphia, Saunders, 1984, pp 258–278.

Chapter 17

Pulmonary Problems

The symptoms of lung diseases are few: cough, expectoration, hemoptysis, wheeze, dyspnea, pleurisy, and fever. Scores of pulmonary diseases share one or more of these symptoms so that overlap and nonspecificity exist. A patient with cough and expectoration may have any of many diseases.

Dyspnea on exertion (one symptom) can result from the decreased partial pressure of oxygen in inspired air, from decreased oxygen-carrying capacity of the blood, or from disease and malfunction of any intervening structure. This includes: obstruction anywhere from the nasopharynx to the bronchioles; loss of functioning alveoli from edema, disease, or destruction; diffusion defects between the alveoli and capillaries because of infiltrative diseases; and perfusion defects resulting from disease in the pulmonary arterial-capillary system. Therefore high altitudes, obstruction, destruction, ventilation-diffusion-perfusion defects and mismatches, and severe anemias can all cause the same symptom. The disease processes which can do these are myriad.

Physical findings are equally nonspecific. Rales, wheezes, consolidation, atelectasis, and effusion give you some conception of the underlying anatomic-physiologic derangement. But many diseases can share a single physical finding. A portion of solid lung can be caused by pneumonia, fibrosis, collapse, cancer, or tuberculosis. Pulmonary function tests tell only the physiologic derangement, not the cause of the disease. Blood gases assess alveolar ventilation, and radionuclide scans assess ventilation and

perfusion, but these studies offer no specific diagnoses either. An exception is the almost certain diagnosis of pulmonary embolus if a well-ventilated area is poorly perfused.

Diagnosis must often be made by more specific indicators, such as chest x-ray, special x-ray techniques, comparison with former x-rays, computed tomographic scan, fiberoptic bronchoscopy, cell or bacterial identification, and biopsy.

While symptoms and physical signs may not offer many specific clues, the family history, occupational history, geographic history, and exposure history are often of great help. A diagnosis may hinge on a very small bit of evidence hidden in the patient profile.

A family history of asthma may suggest that the patient's chronic cough is the beginning of asthma. Tuberculosis in another member of the immediate family is always worrisome. A history of lung disease during childhood in other family members leads you to consider Kartagener's syndrome, congenital bronchiectasis, mucoviscidosis, or agammaglobulinemia.

The occupational history is extremely important since so many lung diseases are caused by inhalation of microparticulate irritating substances. Such job hazards include exposure to silica, asbestos, beryllium, sugar cane, nitrogen dioxide, and numerous other chemicals and molds. It is not enough to ask the occupation. You must know the patient's entire job history: how long he worked at each job, exactly what he did, and whether the ventilation was adequate. The occupation this year may be harmless, but for the previous 10 years the patient's inhalation hazard may have been great. The job may seem hazardous yet not be, and vice versa. Heavy exposure for a short time is as bad as moderate exposure for a long time.

Talc, hair spray, polluted air, and, above all, cigarette smoke are dangerous inhalants. The latter noxious agent is the worst offender insofar as lung disease is concerned. An exact smoking history must be obtained—not just what the patient is or is not smoking this month since his cough developed. Remember the suspected but still unproven hazard of inhaling somebody else's smoke.

The geographic history is important if you suspect a fungal disease. Coccidioidomycosis is endemic in central California and the southwest; histoplasmosis is seen in the Ohio and Mississippi basins and the middle Atlantic states; and blastomycosis has considerable overlap with the latter. Histoplasmosis may be caused by exposure to the excreta of birds, bats, turkeys, and chickens—on roofs, in caves, and on poultry farms. Newly acquired domestic or tropical psittacine birds can cause a bacterial pneumonia; the villain may be spotted in a cage in the living room.

The great majority of patients with lung disease come to the physician for one of the following reasons: (*a*) abnormal chest x-ray, (*b*) sudden dyspnea, (*c*) gradual progressive dyspnea, (*d*) pleuritic chest pain, (*e*) chronic cough and expectoration, (*f*) hemoptysis, (*g*) cough and fever, (*h*) wheeze and dyspnea, (*i*) cough, expectoration, and dyspnea, (*j*) weakness, weight loss, and anorexia, or (*k*) combinations of the foregoing.

While there are large numbers of lung diseases in the textbooks, for practical purposes only common ones need be considered first. These include chronic bronchitis, acute respiratory infections (tracheobronchitis and pneumonia), asthma, chronic obstructive pulmonary disease, tuberculosis, and cancer.

Remember too that certain diseases like tuberculosis, cancer of the lung, and sarcoidosis may have a broad spectrum of presentations and can affect organs all over the body as well as manifest themselves differently in the lung. Hemiplegia may be the first omen of lung cancer. Pulmonary tuberculosis can be asymptomatic or overwhelming; it may cause partial bronchial obstruction, atelectasis, fibrosis, bronchiectasis, abscess or cavity, pneumonia, effusion, pneumothorax, or an infiltrate with low-grade fever and anorexia—each with a different clinical picture, different physical findings, or different x-ray. (*P. C.*)

Case 22
X-ray Abnormality

PAUL CUTLER, M.D.

DATA   During a routine employment examination, a 52-year-old male roofer was found to have an abnormal chest x-ray and he comes to you for advice. He had always been in good health, had the "usual childhood diseases," pneumonia at 24, and an appendectomy at 44.

You decide to solve this problem quickly by a decision path or dendrogram approach with a series of stepwise questions.

DATA   1. What is the abnormality? The chest x-rays (posteroanterior (PA) and lateral views) are repeated and you see a single round 2-cm nodule in the left midlung field partially obscured by the cardiac silhouette. It has smooth borders and is surrounded by normal parenchyma. No calcium or cavitation can be seen within it. You are sure it is in the lung because it is there in both views and because you cannot feel any soft tissue lumps on the chest wall that might mislead you.

LOGIC   The description is that of a solitary pulmonary nodule (formerly called a "coin lesion"). These are most commonly caused by cancer (one-third), granulomas (one-third), and congenital hamartomas (less than one-third); miscellaneous causes, such as an arteriovenous fistula, make up the rest. The respective incidences of these categories vary with the population subset under consideration. Sixty-year-old male smokers skew the percentages toward cancer; 30-year-old male nonsmokers with nodules have a very low incidence of cancer. Granulomas include mainly tuberculosis, histoplasmosis, coccidioidomycosis, and nocardiosis.

Careful inspection of the simple chest x-ray may solve the riddle. If the nodule is round, smooth, sharp, and has calcification patterns well known to the radiologist, it is a hamartoma or granuloma. But if the nodule is irregular and fuzzy-edged, has small irregular radiating projections, and has no calcification, it is likely to be malignant. The nodule size is a variable to be considered. The larger the lesion the more likely is cancer, but smallness does not justify complacency.

Further decision nodes and branching will establish which disease exists in this case. However, your principal concern is not to establish a precise diagnosis, but to decide if this is cancer and if it is resectable. Little else matters.

DATA   2. Has a previous chest x-ray been taken, and what did it show? The patient says an x-ray taken 2 years ago was negative. He cannot recall the doctor's name so the film is unobtainable for personal review and comparison.

LOGIC   This is important though insufficient information. It would be better to have an official report rather than hearsay evidence—better yet to have the x-ray itself, since you could compare sizes and spot small lesions which are easily overlooked.

When comparing two such x-ray films, any one of four situations can exist: (*a*) the nodule was not present before, (*b*) the nodule is now smaller, (*c*) the nodule is the same size, or (*d*) the nodule is larger. If the nodule is now smaller or the same size, concern for malignancy is minimal. But if the nodule was not present before, concern is high. Difficulty arises when the lesion has enlarged and you must now concern yourself with *doubling time.* Cancers of the lung double their *volume* in 1 to 15 months (mean: 4 months); such comparative measurements are made by cubing the diameters. Thus a nodule that increases its width from 1.0 to 1.3 cm has more than doubled its volume. The assumption is made that growth is equal in all three dimensions.

If it is determined that the doubling time

is less than 1 month (very rapid growth), the lesion is apt to be inflammatory. But if it takes more than 15 months to double its size (very slow growth), the lesion is likely to be a granuloma or hamartoma. On the other hand, if the doubling time is 4 to 6 months, cancer is likely. Rare exceptions occur, especially with some metastatic tumors.

DATA   3. Are there any symptoms of cancer or tuberculosis? This includes questions about weakness, weight loss, anorexia, cough, expectoration, hemoptysis, night sweats, and fever. But tuberculomas, histoplasmomas, and hamartomas rarely become large enough to cause symptoms. Since cancer can be metastatic, a review of other symptoms (genitourinary, gastrointestinal, etc) for evidence of a primary lesion is in order too. All the answers are negative.

LOGIC   Absence of symptoms rules out nothing. Any of the above diseases can and does exist without symptoms in the early stages. Primary cancer elsewhere might be asymptomatic too.

DATA   4. How many cigarettes does the patient smoke? The answer is 2 packs/day for the past 30 years.

LOGIC   This constitutes a heavy smoking history (60 pack-years) and weights our judgment toward cancer. It is unusual to see carcinoma of the lung in nonsmokers, and a high percentage of patients with lung cancer have a strongly positive smoking history. Obviously, not everyone who smokes heavily gets lung cancer.

DATA   5. Where does the patient live, where has he lived, and where has he visited? The patient lives in South Dakota and has never been in any other part of the country except when he once visited Des Moines.

LOGIC   We are interested in establishing contact with *Histoplasma capsulatum* or *Coccidioides immitis* which are endemic in the Ohio-Mississippi basin and the southwest, respectively. Both can cause chronic

granulomas. Although he has never been in these two geographic belts, strict geographic boundaries are not completely applicable and spillovers occur.

DATA   6. Are the patient's occupation and habits such that he might have contracted one of the two aforementioned fungus diseases? He is a roofer and works where bird droppings are abundant.

LOGIC   Bird and bat droppings contain the spores of these fungi. So being a roofer, pet store owner, or spelunker might be helpful clues. But the patient does not inhabit an area where these diseases prevail, so these possibilities become less likely. Were he in South Texas where both of these disease belts cross, the question would be more relevant.

Occupation is also important in that some occupational contacts increase the incidence of lung cancer—asbestos, uranium, chromium, cobalt, nickel, arsenic, and any type of radioactivity.

DATA   7. Has the patient had prolonged contact with family members, acquaintances, or co-workers who cough a lot or who are known to have or have had tuberculosis? The answer is no.

LOGIC   This is only somewhat dependable. Had the answer been yes, your concern for tuberculosis would heighten. Hospital personnel working on open wards are subject to contact of this sort without being aware of it. Many persons have annual purified protein derivative (PPD) skin tests done, and it would be helpful to know when and if conversion had already taken place.

DATA   8. Are there physical signs of any of the suspected diseases? A lesion as small as the one under discussion would not be likely to give physical signs of itself. However, you would look for evidence of metastasis (large liver, hard supraclavicular lymph node), and signs and symptoms of a primary lesion elsewhere (breast, thyroid, lymph nodes, testicles, prostate, abdominal mass). Fever might indicate an active tuberculous process. Clubbing and periostitis might suggest cancer of the lung.

LOGIC You now have a 52-year-old man who smokes heavily; he has an asymptomatic nodule in his lung, which he says was not present 2 years ago. The probability is that he has cancer and will need surgery. However, further studies may be done first.

DATA (*a*) Intermediate strength PPD skin test is 15 mm wide; (*b*) coccidioidin skin test is negative; (*c*) complete blood count, urinalysis, and sedimentation rate are normal; (*d*) laminograms of the nodular lesion show no calcification and no cavitation; (*e*) there is no sputum, but morning gastric washings do not show any acid-fast bacilli; and (*f*) fiberoptic bronchoscopy is performed. No abnormalities are noted. Washings in the suspected area are sent to the laboratory for tumor cell, tubercle bacilli, and fungus studies. All studies are negative; you must wait 6 weeks for the results of the tuberculosis cultures.

LOGIC Laminograms may detect calcification not noted on the conventional chest x-ray, and they may also spot hilar lymphadenopathy. The computed tomographic scan may be more valuable in these two regards, but its role is not yet clearly defined.

The positive PPD is not helpful since it is common in the absence of a tuberculoma. A negative test would have more meaning in this case. Fungal skin tests are basically not helpful. Histoplasmin skin tests are contraindicated since they increase blood antibody titers and invalidate subsequent serologic tests for this disease; this skin test is useful only in epidemiologic studies. Coccidioidin skin tests are positive in exposed persons but may become negative with active dissemination, so they are of limited help. Positive blood titers (complement fixation) indicate either past or active infection and, unless very high, do not assist in determining the nature of a lesion. When negative, they are of diagnostic aid.

The study of gastric washings in patients without sputum is probably not reliable. Many saprophytic mycobacteria are present. It would have been better to try to induce sputum formation with ultrasonic saline nebulization. But even when sputum is present, the true positive yield is low.

The normal sedimentation rate merely tells us there is no active inflammation in process. Had laminograms shown calcification or cavitation, we would have leaned toward a granuloma, but these findings can occur in cancer also, though rarely. So this too is nonspecific. Bronchoscopy was not helpful. Surgery seems imminent.

DATA Liver and brain computed tomographic scans are normal. Isotopic skeletal survey is also negative for metastases. Liver function tests are normal. Blood count is normal and stools are negative for occult blood. The electrocardiogram is normal.

LOGIC Three data sets were just explored. The results of either set may stay the surgeon's hand, and they concern themselves with:

1. If the lung lesion is cancer, are there metastases present?
2. Is the lung lesion metastatic from another source?
3. Is the patient operable?

First, there is no evidence for metastases to liver, bone, or brain—common sites for spread from lung cancer. Second, there is no evidence for a primary carcinoma elsewhere resulting in a solitary lung metastasis. This was reasonably well proven by the previous normal physical examination and the absence of blood in the urine and stools. Third, the normal ECG, negative history, and normal physical examination establish that the patient is a good risk for surgical intervention.

Many do not consider such extensive preoperative screening necessary and would do only liver function tests. Bone, brain, and liver scans are done only if there are bone pains and tenderness, neurologic symptoms or signs, and an elevated alkaline phosphatase and/or an enlarged liver.

The various studies provided little help with the crucial question: Cancer? Yes or no? In certain instances, when you wish to be *more certain before proceeding with surgery*, aim for histologic identification first. Oat cells account for the 3 to 5% of solitary malignant nodules; if biopsy can establish the presence of this cell type, surgery should not be performed since this disease is invariably generalized. Then too, if the patient has other diseases that substantially *increase his surgical risk* to 5% or 10%, greater diagnostic certainty is desirable before thoracotomy is done.

Under these circumstances, choose between flexible *fiberoptic transbronchial biopsy* and *percutaneous transthoracic thin-needle biopsy*. The former method is most effective for central larger lesions. The latter is preferable when the lesion is peripheral, but it has a higher complication rate. Neither method is highly sensitive, false negatives are common if the lesion is missed, specific diagnoses are not made with great regularity, and frequent reports of "chronic inflammation" do not instill confidence. Since negative biopsies are not dependable, when surgery seems likely the physician often goes directly to thoracotomy, open biopsy, frozen section, and excision. This approach is as close to 100% specific and 100% sensitive as is possible—a gold standard test.

On occasion, mediastinoscopy is performed first when enlarged hilar nodes are suspected by previous radiographic procedures. Its risk is low, metastases may be confirmed, and a high-risk patient may be spared an operation whose mortality is much higher than the possible harm of this diagnostic procedure. Affected nodes are unlikely, however, if the lesion is small and peripheral, and mediastinoscopy is not indicated if tomography shows no enlarged mediastinal nodes.

DATA   On the basis of the entire clinical picture, surgery is deemed advisable. The nodule and a segment of adjacent lung are removed. The pathologic diagnosis is tuberculoma. No evidence of tuberculous activity is noted, though a Ziehl-Neelsen stain shows some tubercle bacilli at the center of the nodule.

LOGIC   The decision for surgery was wise, even though cancer was not found. Evidence for malignancy was strong—age, heavy smoking, an allegedly normal x-ray 2 years before, plus no indication that the lesion might be infectious. You do not know if the nodule is recent or was simply obscured on the previous x-ray. The latter situation is more likely.

COMMENT   In spite of newer technologies, the diagnostic approach to this sort of problem is much the same in the '80s as in the '60s. Better out then doubt!

The road we have just traversed is simply an academic exercise, because we want to know only if this is a primary cancer and if it is operable. For, given a lung nodule in an otherwise healthy man, unless *obviously* long present or *clearly* caused by a granulomatous disease, intermediate procedures may be omitted, and open biopsy with possible additional surgery *must be done*. It's fast, it's relatively safe, it often cures, and it eliminates doubt and observation.

But in our double aim to avoid unnecessary surgery and avoid missing a curable lesion, we are like Ulysses riding the straits between Scylla and Charybdis. It is easy to veer too much in one direction. The approach to each case must therefore be individualized.

It should not be necessary to remove 20 benign lesions to find one that is malignant. But in *this* case, a benign lesion was justifiably removed. Solving the problem here lent itself handily to using many techniques. First, bits of information were gathered via a decision path invading only the pulmonary subset of the data base. This patient had a lanthanic presentation for which such a technique can be readily used. Clues of all types were present—negatives (absence of certain expected features) and false positives (heavy cigarette smoking, yet no cancer). Some clues were misleading (occupation, "negative x-ray" 2 years ago). Geography, occupation, and contact history were considered but were of limited help.

Tuberculosis was present in spite of no history of contact, no symptoms, and no specific x-ray evidence.

The specificity and sensitivity of clues were an integral part of logic as we considered various points in the history and modes of testing. According to probability theory, this patient was likely to have cancer. But probabilities did not provide a correct solution in this case. Both Venn and Boole were resurrected many times in considering the overlap of smokers, nonsmokers, and cancer; the reliability of fungal tests; the significance of positive and negative PPDs with tuberculosis; the existence of diseases with and without symptoms or signs; and the presence of nodules with or without calcification.

The operating characteristics of various procedures and the concept of imperfect information were explored as each diagnostic modality was considered and its value placed into proper perspective. And in this era of cost containment, the rationale of using so many procedures was bared for debate.

Hanging like an invisible shroud over the entire diagnostic process in this case were the Bayesian theorems of probability and probability revision plus newer notions of medical decision making. (*P. C.*)

Test Your Judgment by devising a clinical strategy for each of the following patients. The strategy should consider and include one or more of the stated options in proper sequence. The author's choices and explanations follow. Do not be disturbed if you disagree. Oncologists sometimes do too. And strategies may be revised as more data are obtained about various diagnostic procedures.

Options

1. Do nothing
2. Recheck in 1 to 2 months
3. Do laminography
4. Do transbronchial biopsy
5. Do percutaneous biopsy
6. Do mediastinoscopy
7. Do metastatic screen
8. Do open biopsy
9. Do lobectomy if 8 is positive for cancer.

Patient 1. A 26-year-old male is seen for a 2-cm nodule in the right upper lung field. He has lived in Sacramento, California, all his life and smokes one pack of cigarettes daily. The lesion has a ring of calcium. There are no symptoms or signs, and routine tests, smears, and cultures are normal or negative. All skin tests are positive. No previous x-rays are available.

Patient 2. Consider the same patient. The lesion is in the right midlung field near the hilum and it is not calcified. An x-ray taken 2 years ago shows the same lesion, but its diameter was 1.5 cm. All else is the same.

Patient 3. This is a 56-year-old man who smokes two packs daily. He has a 2-cm nodule in the right midlung field. It shows no calcifica-

tion by conventional radiography and laminography. However, the right upper hilar nodes are questionably enlarged. No previous x-rays are available. PPD skin test shows 15-mm erythema after 48 hours, and he lives in New Mexico. Bronchoscopic examination, brush cytology, and stains for acid-fast bacilli and fungal spores are all negative. He is otherwise quite well.

Patient 4. A 75-year-old man with moderately severe coronary artery disease and mild congestive heart failure has a 2-cm nodule in the right midlung field equidistant between the hilum and the pleura. Previous x-rays are unavailable. He has never smoked. Laminography shows no calcification and no enlarged hilar nodes. Skin tests are negative except for mumps and *Candida* antigens.

Answers to "Test Your Judgment"

1. Do nothing. This is an obvious granuloma, probably a histoplasmoma.
2. This case is more difficult. The lesion has grown but probably too slowly to be considered malignant; its doubling time is slightly less than 2 years. Yet it is not calcified. It may be asking too much to expect a 28-year-old to live with even a 3% specter of cancer. As always, the patient must enter the decision-making process. I would do laminography hoping to find calcification. If not found, and no mediastinal nodes were noted. I would bypass options 4, 5, and 6, do a minimal 7 (alkaline phosphatase), and go directly to 8—open biopsy. Others may disagree. What would you do?
3. The patient's age, smoking, and noncalcified nodule far outweigh the distractions of his habitat and positive PPD skin test. In addition, hilar adenopathy is worrisome but does not necessarily preclude surgical cure. Do 6, 7, 8, and 9, each step depending on the results of the previous one. If mediastinoscopy and node biopsy are negative for cancer, do a metastatic screen; if the screen shows no metastases, proceed with open biopsy and surgery if biopsy is positive. There is no unanimity of opinion if mediastinal biopsy is positive. Most would stop at this point and begin radiation and/or chemotherapy. A few would not consider hilar node involvement a contraindication to extensive surgery and would continue with steps 7, 8, and 9.
4. This patient has a high risk for thoracotomy (approximately 10%). Therefore be sure he has cancer without metastases before performing surgery. Option 4 or 5 or both are in order. While these procedures have risk, the risk is small compared to option 8. A tissue diagnosis assumes first priority. If 4 or 5 is positive for

cancer, proceed with 7, 8, and 9 unless metastases are found. Lung cancers are seen in nonsmokers too. But if 4 and 5 are fruitless, consider 2 or 8. When all studies are equivocal in a high-risk patient and some clinical features suggest this may not be cancer (e.g. no smoking, positive PPD skin test, spelunking history, etc), you may justifiably wait and recheck the patient in 2 months. Even if it were cancer, considering the doubling time, the disease has already existed for a few years and a short wait would have no great impact on the outcome. Others would disagree and see nothing to gain by waiting. Most would proceed with steps 7, 8, and 9 as indicated. Decision analysis and the construction of a decision tree using the patient's values and your researched data might be helpful here. Doubt may be preferable to surgery.

The last word! Admittedly there are gray zones between each of the four categorized patients just described, where diagnostic management decisions are closer calls or tossups.

And just one more question!

1. A 2-cm diameter pulmonary nodule is noted in retrospect to have had a 1-cm diameter 1 year ago. What is its doubling time? Is it probably malignant?

Answer. Doubling time equals 4 months. The volume has increased 8-fold ($2 \times 2 \times 2$) in 1 year ($1 \to 2 \to 4 \to 8$). The lesion is probably malignant.

PROBLEM-BASED LEARNING To learn all about this patient and this type of presentation, the student should read referable to the following subjects:

1. how to interpret a chest x-ray
2. other chest film abnormalities that may be asymptomatic
3. the causes and prevalence of each cause of pulmonary nodules and their associated clinical manifestations; this includes a large array of uncommon diseases (e.g. Osler-Weber-Rendu's disease with a pulmonary arteriovenous fistula) in addition to the common ones described in the text
4. lung cancer, its cell types, relationship to cigarettes, and the broad spectrum of its clinical presentations
5. the very special paraneoplastic syndromes associated with specific types of lung cancer
6. pulmonary tuberculosis, its clinical manifestations, PPD skin test interpretation, and the varied modes of presentation
7. pulmonary mycoses, their clinical features and laboratory diagnosis

8. hamartomas
9. simpler tests such as sputum smears, cultures, and cytology
10. the indications for and limitations of bronchoscopy (rigid and flexible); bronchography; mediastinoscopy; transbronchial, percutaneous, and open biopsy; and computed tomographic scan
11. when, if, and how to confirm extrapulmonary metastases.

All this information will add another 5% of medicine to your rapidly expanding knowledge base.

Suggested Readings

1. Godwin JD: The solitary pulmonary nodule. *Radiol Clin North Am* 21:709–721, 1983.
   A radiologist presents an excellent review of the causes, clinical features, and diagnostic modalities.
2. Lillington GA: The solitary pulmonary nodule. *Am Rev Respir Dis* 110:698–707, 1974.
   An excellent discussion of the facts behind the decision-making process in the patient with a pulmonary nodule.
3. Gracey DR, Byrd RB, Cugell DB: The dilemma of the asymptomatic pulmonary nodule in the young and not-so-young adult. *Chest* 60:479–483, 1971.
   A round-table discussion which dwells mainly on the relationship between age and cause of lung nodules.
4. Nathan MH: Management of solitary pulmonary nodules. *JAMA* 227:1141–1144, 1974.
   An organized approach based on growth rate and statistics.
5. MacMahon H, Courtney JV, Little AG: Diagnostic methods in lung cancer. *Semin Oncol* 10:20–33, 1983.
   Includes all procedures from innocuous to highly invasive.
6. Westcott JL: Direct percutaneous needle aspiration of localized pulmonary lesions: results in 422 patients. *Radiology* 137:31–35, 1980.
7. Contesse DA: Solitary pulmonary nodule; observe, operate, or what? *Chest* 81:662–663, 1982.
8. Lillington GA, Stevens GM: The solitary nodule; the other side of the coin (editorial). *Chest* 70:322, 1976.
   Discusses the doubling time.
9. Libshitz HI, McKenna RJ, Haynie TP, et al: Mediastinal evaluation in lung cancer. *Radiology* 151:295–299, 1984.
   Compares the sensitivity of various imaging techniques using node sampling as the gold standard.
10. Stevens GM, Jackman RJ: Outpatient needle biopsy of the lung: its safety and utility. *Radiology* 151:301–304, 1984.
   Utility and cost effectiveness are demonstrated; so are the complications.
11. Elliott JA: Pre-operative mediastinal evaluation in primary bronchial carcinoma—a review of staging investigations. *Postgrad Med J* 60:83–91, 1984.
   Imaging, mediastinoscopy, and surgical means are compared.

Case 23
Wheeze and Dyspnea

GARY D. HARRIS, M.D.
W. G. JOHANSON, JR., M.D.

DATA A 28-year-old man became acutely dyspneic while vacationing in the mountains with his family. The dyspnea was associated with cough and wheezing which was readily apparent to the patient and his family. A local physician was consulted.

LOGIC Wheezing indicates airway obstruction. It is important that the physician differentiate the site of obstruction and the nature of the obstructing process. The location of the obstruction may be in the *upper, central,* or *peripheral* airways.

Upper airway obstruction in the region of the epiglottis and larynx may produce wheezing. Such lesions usually cause inspiratory as well as expiratory obstruction and result in stridor, a crowing noise during inspiration. Stridor is typically caused by inflammatory processes in infants or carcinoma of the larynx in adults.

Central obstruction involving the trachea or major airway may be due to foreign bodies or tumors, either benign or malignant. Foreign body aspiration in adults is usually associated with a known or suspected episode of aspiration; such episodes are frequently less obvious in children or in obtunded alcoholics. Central airway obstruction due to foreign body or tumor may mimic the physical findings of peripheral airway disease and must be carefully considered in all patients with the new onset of wheezing. The obstruction is usually relentless, leading to persistent symptoms unless relieved by therapy.

Obstruction of peripheral airways is a much more common cause of dyspnea with wheezing and is usually due to asthma, chronic obstructive pulmonary disease, or left ventricular failure. Rarely, the acute onset of dyspnea with wheezing is caused by viral bronchiolitis, toxic fume exposure, or pulmonary embolism.

DATA Additional history revealed that the patient had enjoyed excellent health previously. None of his family members had experienced fever or other symptoms of respiratory infections. He recalled noticing nasal congestion and sneezing since arriving in the mountains but had attributed these symptoms to the low relative humidity in the area. He had asthma each autumn as a child while living in the midwest but had no such episodes after age 12 when he and his family moved to the southwest.

On physical examination, the patient was in moderate respiratory distress. Yet the vital signs were normal. The nasal mucosa was boggy and bluish in hue, and a thin watery exudate was present. Examination of the chest revealed bilateral expiratory wheezes. The cardiac examination, including auscultation in the left lateral decubitus position, was entirely normal. A chest radiograph was also within normal limits. A smear of the nasal mucosa showed numerous eosinophils. The peripheral blood leukocyte count was 7500/mm^3 with 12% eosinophils.

LOGIC Absence of chronic cough or absence of impairment in exercise capacity is strong evidence against chronic obstructive pulmonary disease (COPD). The normal blood pressure, cardiac examination, and chest radiograph rule out the presence of any cardiac disease which might present in this fashion. Mitral stenosis may be difficult to detect by auscultation alone, but other features of this patient's disease do not support that diagnosis. Rather, the patient demonstrates typical findings of acute bronchial asthma.

Bronchial asthma is a condition of widespread airway narrowing which changes rapidly in severity either spontaneously or as the result of treatment. Reversibility of obstruction is the key feature of asthma. Patients with asthma have *reactive airways* which serve to separate them from normal individuals and, to a large extent, from patients with COPD.

Immediate hypersensitivity, mediated by immunoglobulin E (IgE) and the release of substances from mast cells, is the most common mechanism triggering asthma attacks. In these hypersensitive individuals, a genetic predisposition to atopic disorders (rhinitis, asthma, or eczema) is usually present in other family members. Other allergic disorders may be present in this patient, although many have only asthma. Episodes of asthma occur predictably upon exposure of a patient to the agent or agents to which he is sensitive, i.e. to which he has formed specific IgE antibody. Such episodes may be explosive in nature, as with anaphylaxis, or more gradual in onset, as was the case in this patient. Partial symptomatic improvement occurs promptly with appropriate therapy, although factors not well understood may perpetuate bronchial obstruction of varying severity for prolonged periods in some patients.

DATA The physician prescribed oral and inhaled bronchodilator drugs and the patient improved. The next day he and his family left the mountains and returned home where he consulted his own physician. Physical examination at that time revealed a few scattered expiratory wheezes although the patient felt he had returned to normal.

Spirometry was obtained (Table 17.1).

LOGIC These results were interpreted as showing moderately severe airway obstruction with significant ($> 15\%$) improvement following the administration of a bronchodilator.

Airway obstruction in asthma is due to: (*a*) bronchospasm from contraction of bronchial smooth muscle, (*b*) edema and inflammation of airway walls which encroach on the bronchial lumen, and (*c*) retention of tenacious secretions within the airways. Both the relative importance of these various mechanisms and the site of major obstruction within the bronchial tree vary among patients as well as among different attacks in the same patient.

The markedly reduced FEF_{25-75} (forced midexpiratory flow) in this patient indicates obstruction principally in small, peripheral airways which may require days or weeks of therapy before returning to normal. This divergence of symptoms and measured lung function is common in asthma. The patient's subsequent therapy will depend in part on the physician's assessment of the cause of his asthma attack.

Based on the presence of previous allergic disorders, the absence of virus infection, and the lack of exposure to known nonspecific irritants, it was reasonably presumed that the attack was due to exposure to an allergen to which the patient was sensitive, and he was referred to an allergist for further evaluation.

DATA Skin testing was performed with a number of likely antigens, and flare and wheal reactions occurred to many. A brisk reaction developed to an extract of mountain cedar pollen which had been in season at the time the patient had visited the area. In light of the prompt response of the patient to avoidance of this antigen and to sympto-

Table 17.1.
Spirometry Results

Measurement	Units	Predicted Normal	Before Bronchodilator	After Bronchodilator
Forced vital capacity (FVC)	liters	5.72	4.50 (79%)	5.50 (96%)
Forced expiratory volume ($FEV_{1.0}$)	liters	4.47	2.50 (56%)	4.20 (94%)
$FEV_{1.0}$: FVC		0.78	0.56	0.76
Forced midexpiratory flow (FEF_{25-75})	liters/second	4.64	1.00 (22%)	1.80 (39%)

matic therapy, it was decided not to undertake hyposensitization injections.

LOGIC Avoidance of the offending antigens is without doubt the ideal management of allergic disorders. When the patient's symptoms are due to well-defined agents, such avoidance may be readily accomplished. Unfortunately, in many patients, symptoms are produced by a number of antigens, exposure to which can be reduced but frequently not altogether eliminated. Immunotherapy, or "allergy shots," is of proven benefit for some patients with allergic rhinitis, although it is less well documented in the case of asthma. However, if avoidance is successful, such therapy is unnecessary.

DATA Therapy with an oral theophylline preparation was continued for several weeks and the patient remained asymptomatic. Spirometry performed 1 month after the attack was entirely normal. It was concluded that the patient's asthma was due to hypersensitivity to mountain cedar. With continued avoidance of this antigen he remained well and therapy was discontinued.

Two years later the patient became ill with an upper respiratory infection followed by the development of cough, dyspnea, and wheezing. During an episode of severe coughing at home he experienced a marked sudden increase in dyspnea associated with sharp pain in the right chest. Alarmed by his extreme air hunger, his wife called for an ambulance which arrived shortly and transported the patient to a nearby hospital.

LOGIC Sudden marked dyspnea is an uncommon symptom which indicates a catastrophic derangement in cardiopulmonary function. It may occur in asthmatic patients as a result of widespread bronchospasm triggered by exogenous agents. In any patient with excessive airway secretions, acute worsening may be a manifestation of plugs of material moving centrally from the periphery of the lung, thus obstructing a greater fraction of the total airway. Such movement of secretions occurs commonly during re-

cumbency in patients with COPD, resulting in episodes of nocturnal dyspnea which may be difficult to differentiate from those due to left ventricular failure. Cardiovascular events, including myocardial infarction, rupture of a papillary muscle, or pulmonary embolism may produce sudden severe dyspnea. Last, a pneumothorax may produce symptoms which vary from only mild chest discomfort to severe dyspnea and death. The occurrence of chest pain suggests that diagnosis but does not rule out other possibilities.

DATA On arrival at the hospital, the patient's vital signs were: pulse 140/minute, BP 60/40, respirations 40. He was cyanotic and in obvious severe respiratory distress. A rapid examination revealed distended neck veins, tracheal shift to the left, tympany, absent breath sounds, and absent respiratory movements of the right hemithorax. Heart sounds were inaudible due to wheezing and rhonchi over the left lung. A clinical diagnosis of tension pneumothorax on the right was made, and a 15-gauge needle was inserted through an intercostal space. Gas under pressure quickly escaped and the patient's blood pressure improved. A portable radiograph was obtained, and a chest tube was inserted with prompt improvement in the patient's dyspnea, cyanosis, and heart rate. The radiograph showed approximately 30% collapse of the right lung at the time of chest tube insertion, with a shift of the mediastinum to the left.

LOGIC Spontaneous pneumothorax results when the visceral pleura ruptures, exposing the pleural space to air within the lung. Pneumothoraces occur most commonly in young healthy men with tall asthenic physiques or in patients with emphysema. In the former case, pneumothorax is usually due to a small rupture of a thin-walled bleb at the lung apex. In emphysema, pneumothorax is due to the rupture of bullae formed as part of the disease process. While bullae are typically associated with emphysema, smaller (occasionally only microscopic) cysts also develop in fibrosing disease of the lung such as eosinophilic granuloma. In asthma, a valve type obstruction of a small bronchiole may lead to progressive hyperinflation of a region of lung and its ultimate rupture. Spontaneous pneumothorax most commonly occurs in association with exercise or cough but may occur at rest or even during sleep.

A special category of pneumothorax is that associated with a rise in pleural pressure above atmospheric pressure—a tension pneumothorax. The increased pleural pressure impairs venous return, leading to circulatory collapse as well as collapse of the lung. A tension pneumothorax develops when the communication between the intrapulmonary air spaces and the pleura contains a valve-like mechanism preventing reentry of air from the pleural space into the lung, but allowing further accumulation in the pleural space during inspiration.

DATA   Examination of the patient's sputum revealed numerous polymorphonuclear neutrophilic leukocytes, a few eosinophils, and small pleomorphic gram-negative organisms. *Haemophilus influenzae* was isolated in the sputum culture. Treatment with intravenous aminophylline, oral ampicillin, and terbutaline was initiated and the asthma rapidly improved.

LOGIC   Whereas the previous attack had been precipitated by a specific allergen, this attack followed an infection. Such infection may trigger attacks in all asthmatic patients and may be the sole precipitating cause in some patients. Differentiation of attacks due to infections or other irritant exposure may be difficult but can usually be made on the basis of the history and examination of the patient's sputum.

DATA   Following an uneventful course in the hospital the patient was discharged, the chest tube having been removed on the third hospital day. He was maintained on symptomatic therapy for his airway disease.

QUESTIONS

1. Shortness of breath, wheezing, and production of purulent sputum in a 14-year-old girl with asthma:
   (a) usually indicates acute bronchitis due to a viral infection
   (b) occurs episodically and will disappear without treatment
   (c) requires a chest radiograph for proper evaluation
   (d) may be due to either allergy or infection.
2. A 50-year-old businessman has noted persistent cough and wheezing since he choked on a mouthful of popcorn at a ballgame 1 week ago. His symptoms can be attributed to bronchial irritation alone when:
   (a) his chest radiograph is shown to be free of infiltrates
   (b) physical examination is found to reveal diffuse and not localized wheezing
   (c) his chest examination is found to be normal
   (d) bronchoscopy fails to reveal a foreign body and the chest radiograph is normal.
3. Arterial blood gases during asthmatic attacks:
   (a) usually show mild hypoxemia and hypocarbia during mild to moderate attacks
   (b) show hypercarbia early in the attack
   (c) may show decreases in PaO_2 following bronchodilator therapy
   (d) show hypoxemia refractory to oxygen therapy.
4. Which of the following findings is helpful in distinguishing severe dyspnea due to obstructive lung disease from that due to left ventricular failure and pulmonary edema?
   (a) wheezes on physical examination
   (b) tachycardia
   (c) elevated jugular venous pressure
   (d) a chest radiograph showing cardiomegaly and vascular congestion.

ANSWERS

1. **(d) is correct.** It is important to know that increases in the number of either eosinophils or polymorphonuclear neutrophilic leukocytes in sputum will cause purulence due to the enzymes contained in these cells. Thus, either infection or allergy could be responsible for the patient's symptoms. A smear of the sputum will be more informative than the chest radiograph, especially in the absence of fever.
2. **(d) is correct.** Foreign bodies may not be radiopaque and may not completely obstruct bronchi. Their presence may be heralded by only cough, occasionally by wheezing. With

the history provided, it would be mandatory to examine the patient's tracheobronchial tree endoscopically to be certain that a foreign body is not present.

3. **(a) and (c) are correct.** Blood gases in asthma display rather characteristic changes—alveolar hyperventilation (low $PaCO_2$) and mild hypoxemia early, with CO_2 retention and severe hypoxemia occurring only when airway obstruction is extremely severe. In a significant percentage of patients, bronchodilator therapy causes worsening hypoxemia, apparently due to the release of pulmonary arterial vasoconstriction caused by regional hypoxia. Hypoxemia in asthma is usually due to ventilation-perfusion mismatching and responds readily to oxygen therapy.

4. **(d) is correct.** Wheezes and rhonchi occur commonly in acute pulmonary edema and may mask the characteristic alveolar rales. Tachycardia occurs in most dyspneic patients and is not a useful differential sign. Jugular venous pressure may be elevated or normal in either condition. The chest radiograph is usually diagnostic if physical findings are inconclusive.

COMMENT Numerous distinctions and decisions must be made in the patient who wheezes. Simple inspection tells you if there is difficulty in "getting air in" or "getting air out." The former results from high tracheal or laryngeal obstruction, the latter from airway obstruction lower down. Wheezes are high-pitched sounds of appreciable duration, most pronounced during expiration when the airways become naturally more narrow. They are caused by constriction or partial obstruction from within or compression from outside the airway.

Left ventricular failure may cause "cardiac asthma" because of bronchiolar constriction resulting from congestion and edema. But the physical signs of heart disease should be readily observed.

You are then left with the two lung diseases that most commonly cause wheezes—asthma and COPD. Patients with asthma demonstrate complete remissions and are usually well between attacks; their pulmonary function tests are normal then too. In COPD, the illness is chronic and progressive, with episodes of acute worsening but no complete remissions. Function tests show reduced air flow and reduced FEV_1 (forced expiratory volume) at all times, and the ECG and chest x-ray are often abnormal. Differentiation in this case was easy.

Wheezes localized to one lobe suggest an area of partial obstruction by a foreign body or tumor. Both can lead to infection and abscess. Bronchoscopy is mandatory. A chest x-ray during expiration may show an area of hyperaeration due to trapping even when the routine film taken on inspiration is normal.

Asthma is a recurrent lifelong disease, treatment is only partially successful, and emergency rooms generally harbor several asthmatic patients at any one time. Either they get well in a few hours, spend the night in a holding area, or are admitted to the hospital if treatment doesn't help, if the pCO_2 rises, or if they become exhausted.

To solve the problem of the patient who wheezes, decisions are based on age, diffuseness or localization of wheezing, elimination of left ventricular failure, and the distinction between COPD and bronchial asthma by history and examination. The chest x-ray, ECG, and pulmonary function tests solidify your impression. (*P. C.*)

Suggested Readings

1. (a) Schwartz HJ, Tuthill TM: Bronchial asthma. In Baum GL, Wolinsky E (eds): *Textbook of Pulmonary Diseases*, ed 3. Boston, Little, Brown, 1983, pp 635–650.
   (b) Johnston RG, Green RA: Pneumothorax. In Baum GL, Wolinsky E (eds): *Textbook of Pulmonary Diseases*, ed 3. Boston, Little, Brown, 1983, pp 1327–1341.
   Detailed textbook descriptions.
2. Boushey HA, Holtzman MJ, Sheller JR, et al: State of the art: bronchial hyperreactivity. *Am Rev Respir Dis* 121:389–413, 1980.
   A detailed review of the mechanisms of hyperreactivity and its relationship to airways disease.
3. Middleton E Jr, Atkins FM, Fanning M, et al: Cellular mechanisms in the pathogenesis and pathophysiology of asthma. *Med Clin North Am* 65:1013–1031, 1981.
   A general review of mechanisms of bronchoconstriction and their applications in planning therapy for asthma.
4. Hiller FC, Wilson FJ Jr: Evaluation and management of acute asthma. *Med Clin North Am* 67:669–683, 1983.
   Discusses the inciting factors, physical findings, gradation of severity, and care.
5. Fletcher CM, Pride NB: Definitions of emphysema, chronic bronchitis, asthma, and airflow obstruction: 25 years on from the Ciba symposium (editorial). *Thorax* 39:81–85, 1984.
   Adds clarity to a difficult distinction.
6. Stempel DA, Boucher RC: Respiratory infection and airway reactivity. *Med Clin North Am* 65:1045–1053, 1981.
   A review of the mechanisms by which infection may enhance airway reactivity.
7. Frick OL: Role of viral infections in asthma and allergy. *Clin Rev Allergy* 1:5–17, 1983.
8. Fischl MA, Pitchenik A, Gardner LB: An index predicting relapse and need for hospitalization in patients with acute bronchial asthma. *N Engl J Med* 305:783–789, 1981.

Provides a basis for objective assessment of severity of asthma and response to treatment.

9. Eliakim R, Halperin Y, Menczel J: A predictor index for hospitalization for patients with acute asthmatic attack. *Isr J Med Sci* 20:202–206, 1984.

10. Butcher BT, Hendrick DJ: Occupational asthma. *Clin Chest Dis* 4:43–53, 1983.
    A most important consideration for 10% of all asthmatics.

11. Marks MB: Respiratory tract allergy to household pet birds. *Ann Allergy* 52:56–57, 1984.
    Birds may be greater offenders than dogs and cats: how a cockatoo can be bad for you.

12. Brown PJ, Greville HW, Finucaine KE: Asthma and irreversible airflow obstruction. *Thorax* 39: 131–136, 1984.
    Shows how the air flow obstruction in asthma may eventually become irreversible.

Case 24
Coughing of Blood
PAUL CUTLER, M.D.

DATA   After coughing up a cupful of bright red blood, a 48-year-old female office worker is brought to the emergency room. For the previous 3 months she has had a chronic cough productive of whitish-gray mucoid sputum which had become slightly blood-streaked for the past few weeks. She had also noticed increasing fatigability, dyspnea on exertion, and difficulty in sleeping for a few months.

LOGIC   Hemoptysis is usually a serious presenting symptom and invariably brings the patient to the physician. You wonder why this patient did not come in sooner, considering the variety of symptoms. Initially you think of the common causes of hemoptysis:

1. carcinoma
2. tuberculosis
3. bronchiectasis
4. bronchitis
5. heart failure
6. pulmonary infarct
7. mitral stenosis.

Less common causes include pneumonia, abscess, parasites, fungi, anticoagulants. Goodpasture's syndrome, Wegener's granulomatosis, and periarteritis nodosa.

We are no doubt dealing with hemoptysis rather than hematemesis or nasopharyngeal bleeding because of the associated pulmonary symptoms.

The distinction between hemoptysis and hematemesis is sometimes not simple. If the amount of blood is large, the patient himself may not know if it was coughed or vomited. In hemoptysis the blood is frothy, red, and alkaline. Vomited blood is usually darker red, acid, and may contain food particles. If in doubt, gastric intubation helps you decide.

In view of chronic cough and expectoration, diagnoses 1, 2, 3, and 4 are all serious considerations. Congestive heart failure is also suggested by the additional symptoms of fatigue, dyspnea on exertion, and difficulty in sleeping. Cancer or tuberculosis could cause the additional symptoms too if there were destruction of much tissue or an associated pleural effusion. At this point it is not known if the sleeping problem is from orthopnea, severe cough, or ordinary insomnia.

DATA   The patient has smoked two packs of cigarettes daily for the past 30 years and drinks eight to ten cups of coffee a day, but she has had no known medical illnesses. She has had a hysterectomy for fibroids, cholecystectomy for stones, and a subsequent laparotomy for adhesions. The last operation was 5 years ago. Her appetite has been excessive. She has gained 60 lb in the past 5 years and now weighs 230 lb. She attributed her many symptoms to obesity and smoking and did not seek medical care until she coughed a large quantity of blood. There has been no chest pain, night sweats, or fever.

LOGIC Such a cigarette history always raises the specter of cancer. The coffee intake is not significant here. No relation can be established between the three surgical procedures and her present problems. Too much time has elapsed for emboli and there has been no pleuritic pain. Weight gain plus hearty appetite tend to negate cancer and tuberculosis. Heavy smoking might relate to chronic bronchitis or chronic obstructive lung disease. This, plus the additional burden of severe obesity and its resulting alveolar hypoventilation, might explain the fatigue and dyspnea. Do not infer that all obese patients have alveolar hypoventilation. Occasionally, in extreme obesity, massive accumulations of fat prevent adequate mechanical ventilation, and hypoxemia and hypercarbia may result.

DATA Further history reveals that her father died of tuberculosis at 56 when she was 20, and that one of her close co-workers developed a "chest condition" 6 months ago for which she was hospitalized and is still under treatment. Pulmonary tuberculosis is still a common cause of hemoptysis and must always be seriously considered, especially in those living in inner cities and in recent immigrants from Haiti and southeast Asia. There has been no history of leg injury or a recent long automobile trip, and she takes no birth control pills.

LOGIC You now know that she has had close contact with tubercle bacilli and that there is no obvious reason why she should have leg vein thrombosis with emboli. But remember that visceral carcinoma can increase the propensity toward venous thromboemboli. So can wheelchair or bed confinement, congestive heart failure, postsurgical status, leg trauma, and a history of thrombophlebitis—none of which is present in this patient.

DATA A review of systems reveals nervousness, headaches, insomnia, occasional ringing in the ears, rare double vision, bad taste and dryness in the mouth, nocturia 3×, occasional burning on urination, painful menses, slight vaginal discharge, constipation, progressively worsening dyspnea on exertion, worsening of her cough at night, and the need to sleep on three pillows for comfort. Her mother died in an auto accident many years ago, she has no siblings, and she has three well children: ages 25, 21, and 18.

LOGIC The multiplicity of symptoms needs weeding out. She gives many positives, most of which are unrelated to her main problem. In fact, some are clearly psychosomatic and others are what anybody might have from time to time. They should, however, be closely checked since additional problems may exist. The dyspnea and orthopnea do seem genuine and suggest left ventricular failure.

DATA Physical examination discloses a markedly obese woman in no acute distress, though appearing quite apprehensive. The vital signs are T 37 C, P 106 with slight irregularity, R 18, and BP 106/80. General inspection shows no remarkable abnormalities. In particular, there is no malar flush, no clubbing, and no hypertrophic pulmonary osteoarthropathy.

LOGIC A rich amount of material may often be harvested from the physical examination in patients with hemoptysis. Considering the common possibilities, you may find rales at the apex, rales at the bases, metastatic nodes, Horner's syndrome, pleural friction rub, tracheal deviation, pleural effusion, enlarged nodular liver, tender calf, or positive Homans' sign. Basal rales or rhonchi may represent aspirated blood and not pinpoint the bleeding site. The significance of each of these findings should be apparent. In this case the apprehension and rapid pulse are understandable, though the irregularities in the pulse need clarification. A malar flush might suggest rheumatic mitral valve disease. Absence of clubbing and hypertrophic pulmonary osteoarthropathy are against lung cancer and bronchiectasis, though certainly do not rule them out, since only a minority of patients with these diseases exhibit such features. Absence of fever is against pneumonia or abscess, as is the long history of symptoms.

DATA Further examination shows no lung abnormalities except for a few coarse wet rales at both bases; there are no friction rubs or wheezes. An occasional premature beat without a compensatory pause is noted. The second heart sound is loud; its second component (P_2) is not only heard all over the precordium but felt over the pulmonic valve area. At the apex of the heart, an opening snap (OS) is heard shortly after S_2 (S_2-OS time = 0.05 second). This is followed by a low-pitched, rumbling, decrescendo-crescendo murmur terminating in a loud S_1. The apex beat is normally situated, and no thrill is felt. The remainder of the examination is normal. In particular, there is no neck vein distention, hepatomegaly, or leg edema. The calves are not tender and Homans' sign is negative.

LOGIC Mitral stenosis is well established. Premature atrial contractions denote atrial irritability, a loud P_2 suggests pulmonary hypertension, and tight severe mitral stenosis is indicated by the short S_2-OS interval, opening snap, typical murmur, and loud S_1. Obesity obscures the thrill and a malar flush is not always present. The murmur was probably present at the times of surgery, though one can only guess why it was not noted. There is as yet no evidence for right ventricular strain or failure.

The basal rales represent either pulmonary congestion from the stenotic valve, blood still present in the lower airways, or concomitant lower airway bronchial disease. Bronchiectasis, chronic bronchitis, or chronic obstructive lung disease could be present too and may warrant later investigation. The absence of general or local wheezes lessens the likelihood of chronic obstructive lung disease and partial airway

obstruction from a neoplasm. For the moment, one diagnosis can easily explain the entire picture.

DATA The 18-test chemistry profile, blood count, and urinalysis are normal. Intermediate strength purified protein derivative skin test is negative. The sputum is negative for acid-fast bacilli and tumor cells on three occasions. Platelet count, prothrombin time, and partial thromboplastin time are done to rule out a bleeding diathesis; they are normal. The ECG shows evidence of left atrial abnormality and occasional premature atrial contractions but is otherwise normal. Chest x-ray demonstrates no pulmonary parenchymal lesions, a normal-sized heart, straightening of the left cardiac border with a prominent convexity at its midportion, mild pulmonary edema, and distended upper lobe veins. Barium swallow radiography shows a very large left atrium in the right anterior oblique position.

LOGIC The normal serum calcium, alkaline phosphatase, and transaminases are against lung cancer, especially with liver metastases. The diagnosis is now certain. The x-ray and ECG are characteristic; negative tests help rule out other possibilities. Without doubt, the mitral orifice is small, the valve gradient is high, left atrial and pulmonary capillovenous pressure is high, pulmonary congestion exists, and a pulmonary varix has ruptured. Prior to valve replacement, the patient will be encouraged to lose weight, stop smoking, and restrict activity. Cardiac catheterization and an echocardiogram will be performed to round out the picture. Fiberoptic bronchoscopy might be considered only if the patient were still bleeding and there were a need to locate the bleeding site should massive hemoptysis occur prior to valve surgery.

In fact, flexible fiberoptic bronchoscopy is extremely useful in cases of this type. With it one may discover a small intrabronchial adenoma or carcinoma still too small to be visible by chest x-ray, and bronchial washings for smear, culture, and cytologic study often solve the problem when the diagnosis is not otherwise apparent. In this case it was not reasonable to search further.

With the advent of fiberoptics, bronchograms are becoming of less value but are still useful in localizing bronchiectasis amenable to resection. If repeated emboli were under consideration a ventilation-perfusion scan and pulmonary arteriography might be performed.

QUESTIONS

1. Consider the same patient with the following variations: she has signs and x-ray evidence of a large right pleural effusion. The chest film is otherwise normal and there is no evidence of mitral stenosis. The ECG is normal. Furthermore, she has lost weight and has anorexia. Your diagnostic spectrum shifts considerably. You should:
   (a) remove 10 ml of fluid for study
   (b) remove all fluid and do a bronchogram
   (c) study sputum for tumor cells and tubercle bacilli
   (d) remove all fluid and repeat the chest x-ray.
2. As a matter of Bayesian statistical likelihood, a 46-year-old woman who smokes heavily and has hemoptysis most commonly has:
   (a) no disease
   (b) carcinoma of the lung
   (c) chronic bronchitis
   (d) tuberculosis.
3. If the data in this patient were rearranged so that you suspected multiple pulmonary emboli, which procedure might give you the highest yield at the lowest risk?
   (a) venogram of lower extremities
   (b) ventilation-perfusion lung scan
   (c) pulmonary arteriogram
   (d) blood gases.
4. Assume that your 48-year-old patient presented with chronic cough and expectoration, hemoptysis, weakness, weight loss, and anorexia. She is a heavy smoker and has had exposure to tuberculosis. Chest x-ray showed an infiltrate in the right upper lobe, though the physical examination was negative. The diagnosis would be most reliably established by:
   (a) purified protein derivative skin test
   (b) bronchogram
   (c) fiberoptic bronchoscopy
   (d) isotope lung scan.

ANSWERS

1. **(c) and (d) are correct.** The likelihood rests between cancer and tuberculosis. The long history, weight loss, and anorexia point away from repeated pulmonary emboli, though this is still a consideration. Heart failure is ruled out by the normal heart. Bronchitis and bronchiectasis do not give pleural effusions. Both (c) and (d) should be done. A simple sputum examination might provide the answer. But the fluid would have to be removed for therapeutic purposes as well as to study it and x-ray the underlying lung. To remove only 10 ml might give the answer, but it is almost as easy to remove it all and then x-ray again. Bronchogram would probably be worthless, since bronchiectasis is unlikely in view of the effusion.
2. **(c) is correct,** since it is by far the most common cause of hemoptysis. (a) is most unlikely in view of the clinical picture. (b) and (d) are possibly correct, though less common.
3. **(b) is correct.** The positive yield is high and risk is almost nil. Venograms are formidable, time consuming, and may show nothing since the clots may be coming from sites other than the legs. Blood gases would show anoxemia, which is nonspecific. An arteriogram is invasive and not without risk, though the yield of positive information would be high. It might be done if the scan were inconclusive or if the insertion of a vena cava filter is being considered.
4. **(c) is correct.** The most likely diagnoses in these circumstances are carcinoma of the lung and tuberculosis. With fiberoptic bronchoscopy, biopsy of a visible lesion or bronchial washings for tumor cell study and acid-fast bacilli could both be obtained. Simple sputum examination might be most helpful but it was not mentioned in the list of possibilities. A positive purified protein derivative skin test would be of no value, though a negative one would be helpful. A bronchogram, no longer commonly done, would be of value if bronchiectasis were suspected; this is not the case here since an apical lesion was noted. A lung scan would help diagnose pulmonary embolus, not suggested by the clinical picture.

COMMENT First, we invoked the law of probabilities in dealing mainly with common diseases. Second, a large amount of information was gathered in the history, much of which was irrelevant. Then extraneous material was filtered out by suppression of information in a patient who seemed prone to answer yes to most inquiries. Pertinent negatives were an important part of the data base—e.g. absence of weight loss, night sweats, and fever; lack of clubbing; lack of pulmonary infiltrate; and negative sputum examination. The absence of a rheumatic fever history represented a false negative clue. False positive clues like the contact with tuberculosis had to be dealt with. Venn diagrams, and sets and subsets were subconsciously employed in considering the overlap of pulmonary findings, cardiac findings, and hemoptysis.

Bayes' theorems were an integral part of the reasoning. In considering the causes of hemoptysis, we began by considering the incidence of diseases in the general population. The seven diseases first listed have a relatively high incidence in this country. However, in certain areas of the Orient, paragonimiasis would have been the prime consideration. In addition, we weighed the likelihood of hemoptysis given a certain disease and the likelihood of a disease given the symptom of hemoptysis.

This problem could probably have been very quickly solved by an experienced clinician. Presented with a patient who coughed blood, he would have gotten a stat chest x-ray, asked five or ten pertinent questions while examining the heart and lungs, and out would have come the diagnosis of mitral stenosis. He would have then completed his data base at leisure, ruling out the other already unlikely possibilities, establishing concomitant diseases, and confirming his first impression. (*P. C.*)

Suggested Readings

1. Pierce JA: Cough and hemoptysis. In Blacklow RS (ed): *MacBryde's Signs and Symptoms*, ed 6. Philadelphia, Lippincott, 1983, pp 317–334.
   A careful analysis of each symptom, its causes, and how to distinguish between the causes.

2. Gong H Jr, Salvatierra C: Clinical efficacy of early and delayed fiberoptic bronchoscopy in patients with hemoptysis. *Am Rev Respir Dis* 124:221–225, 1981.
   One hundred twenty-three cases are reported and the role of bronchoscopy in diagnosis and clinical decision making is reviewed.

3. Carroll D: Obscure causes of hemoptysis. *Md State Med J* 24:87–90, 1975.
   Unusual causes are well presented and illustrated by case studies.

4. Jokinen K, Palva T, Nuutinen J: Haemoptysis. A bronchological evaluation. *Ann Clin Res* 9:8–11, 1977.
   This is a study of 342 patients with hemoptysis and a determination of the causes.

5. Colman RW, Rubin RN: Update on pulmonary embolism—modern management. *DM* 29:1–41, 1982.
   Forty tiny pages cover the subject from leg to lung; emphasis is on diagnosis, anticoagulants, and thrombolytics.

6. Detels R, Sayre JW, Tashkin DP, et al: The UCLA population studies of chronic obstructive respiratory disease. VI. Relationship of physiologic factors to rate of changes in forced expiratory volume in one second and forced vital capacity. *Annu Rev Respir Dis* 129:533–537, 1984.
   Documents the year-to-year changes in patients with a disease that has high prevalence in the Los Angeles area.

7. Stevens RS, Moolgavkar SH: A cohort analysis of lung cancer and smoking in British males. *Am J Epidemiol* 119:624–641, 1984.
   A good study in a country where tobacco isn't grown.

Case 25
Cough, Fever, Chill

GARY D. HARRIS, M.D.
W. G. JOHANSON, JR., M.D.

DATA A 53-year-old insurance agent calls his physician after having a single shaking chill. One week ago the patient, along with several members of his family, had experienced an upper respiratory illness consisting of fever, cough, headache, and myalgias. Recovery had taken 3 to 4 days and he had felt reasonably well except for a lingering cough. This morning the patient awoke with fever, pain in the left chest aggravated by deep breathing, and increased sputum production. While eating breakfast he had a shaking chill which lasted for 5 minutes.

LOGIC This is a characteristic history for bacterial pneumonia. The physician knows that influenza had reached epidemic proportions in his community several weeks ago and reasonably assumed that the febrile illness experienced by the patient and his family was influenza. The association of other viral infections with bacterial pneumonia has been less well documented. However, many patients with bacterial pneumonia give a history of antecedent upper respiratory symptoms for 24 to 72 hours prior to the development of symptoms of lower respiratory tract disease.

During influenza epidemics, or even during outbreaks of other viral respiratory diseases, enormous numbers of people may become acutely ill. In the great majority, this illness will be mild, self-limited, and require only self-administered symptomatic therapy. However, in this patient, the recrudescent nature of the symptoms clearly indicates that he has either developed a complication of influenza or a new unrelated problem and further investigation is required. The physician agrees to meet the patient in the hospital emergency room because of the necessity for studies.

DATA Physical examination reveals an acutely ill patient with flushed face, slight cyanosis of the nail beds and lips, and frequent episodes of cough which elicit severe left chest pains. Vital signs are: temperature 39.4 C, pulse 110/minute, BP 120/85, respirations 24/minute.

The left hemithorax shows diminished expansion with dullness and increased tactile fremitus posteriorly. Breath sounds in this area are increased in intensity and distinctly bronchial in quality; whispered pectoriloquy is present. Numerous fine inspiratory rales are heard over the lower third of the left chest posteriorly. No pleural friction rub is heard. The rest of the physical examination is normal.

LOGIC The chest findings are those of consolidation with a patent bronchus. Diminished expansion is due to the combined effects of consolidation plus severe pleural pain with splinting, although physical signs of pleuritis are not present. Obstruction of a lobar bronchus with distal atelectasis leads to dullness and absent breath sounds.

Pneumonia is the most reasonable diagnosis. Examination failed to reveal signs of infection at other sites which might have been the cause of the pneumonia or have

resulted from it. Now the physician's problem is to determine the etiology of this pneumonia so that appropriate therapy can be given.

DATA Chest radiographs including posteroanterior, lateral, and left lateral decubitus views disclose extensive consolidation of the left lower lobe but no pleural effusion. The right lung and left upper lobe are normal. The leukocyte count is 23,500/mm^3 with 90% polymorphonuclear leukocytes (PMNs). Arterial blood gases reveal: (FIO$_2$ = 0.21) pH 7.46, pCO$_2$ 30 mm Hg, pO$_2$ 52 mm Hg, 84% saturation. A Gram stain of expectorated sputum shows sheets of PMNs and numerous gram-positive, encapsulated diplococci. A sputum culture and three blood cultures are obtained.

LOGIC The markedly elevated leukocyte count strongly supports bacterial infection since normal or low values are usually found in patients with viral or other nonbacterial pneumonias. Alveolar hyperventilation is present, as indicated by the low arterial pCO$_2$. Hypoxemia in pneumonia is due to ventilation-perfusion mismatching and to the development of shunts in regions of alveolar consolidation which maintain some perfusion without ventilation.

A presumptive diagnosis of postinfluenza pneumococcal pneumonia has been made. A predisposing factor such as viral infection or underlying chronic disease is present in at least 70% of people with bacterial pneumonia. The usual organisms associated with bacterial pneumonia are *Streptococcus pneumoniae* (pneumococcus), *Streptococcus hemolyticus*, *Staphylococcus aureus*, *Haemophilus influenzae*, and various gram-negative bacilli, especially *Klebsiella pneumoniae*. *Legionella* species must also be considered.

Influenza markedly increases the likelihood of staphylococcal pneumonia and this agent must therefore be sought with great care. Staphylococcal pneumonia typically involves multiple lung segments, is usually bilateral, and is associated with early lung necrosis, abscess formation, and empyema. The absence of cavitation and pleural effusion, the localized nature of the process, and the apparent absence of the organism in sputum argue against a staphylococcal etiology.

Pneumonia due to *S. hemolyticus* occurs principally in young persons and typically produces an early exuberant empyema. Community-acquired pneumonias due to *H. influenzae* or enteric bacilli such as *K. pneumoniae* are uncommon among previously healthy adults, occurring principally in individuals with chronic diseases like obstructure lung disease, alcoholism, and perhaps diabetes.

DATA   The patient is admitted to the hospital and given procaine penicillin 600,000 units intramuscularly every 12 hours, oxygen at 4 liters/minute, and codeine for pleuritic pain.

LOGIC   Blood cultures are positive in one-third of such patients and, if positive, provide by far the best means of establishing the bacterial agent responsible for pneumonia. Pleural fluid is the second best source and a sample should be obtained if fluid is present. This was the reason for the lateral decubitus film in this patient. Sputum cultures are difficult to evaluate because the rates of both false positivity and false negativity approach 25%. Cultures are important in this patient to detect staphylococci not seen microscopically.

Transtracheal aspiration avoids the resident flora of the upper respiratory tract and tends to reduce the number of potentially pathogenic bacteria isolated. This procedure is usually indicated in attempting to establish that anaerobic bacteria are present in the lower respiratory tract and is occasionally indicated in the evaluation of complicated cases of pneumonia. Because of the morbidity of the procedure, it is not indicated in the usual case of uncomplicated pneumonia.

Similarly, transthoracic lung aspiration may be used to obtain material directly from the lung parenchyma for stain and culture; the rate of complications with this procedure

is too high to permit its use in the routine evaluation of pneumonia, at least in adults. Fiberoptic bronchoscopy is a safer means of obtaining specimens from the distal lung. A sterile brush protected by an outer catheter is used to sample secretions in the area of pneumonia.

Nonbacterial pneumonia may present similarly to this patient. Pneumonias due to viruses or mycoplasma are generally more diffuse, lack shaking rigors, and are not associated with numerous bacteria in respiratory secretions.

DATA   The patient partially improved with treatment. However, on the fourth day he still had an oral temperature of 38.3 C and complained of persistent discomfort in the left chest. Physical examination revealed flatness to percussion, absent tactile and vocal fremitus, and markedly diminished breath sounds over the left lower lobe. Radiographs confirmed the presence of a moderately large pleural effusion. Thoracentesis was performed with the removal of 1000 ml of slightly cloudy fluid containing 6000 leukocytes/mm^3, 85% of which were PMNs. Gram stains of the fluid did not reveal organisms and both anaerobic and aerobic cultures were subsequently negative. Following aspiration of the pleural fluid, the patient's recovery was uneventful.

LOGIC   This effusion represents a parapneumonic effusion. These are common with pneumococcal pneumonia, although, as with this patient, they usually develop after several days of treatment and are sterile. The important differential diagnosis of this effusion concerns other bacterial agents which may have been present from the onset or which have been acquired during therapy with penicillin. Empyema is particularly common with pneumonia due to staphylococci, gram-negative bacilli, or anaerobic bacteria. The patient's original sputum culture yielded only pneumococci and his blood cultures were sterile. Empyema due to inadequately treated lung infection produces grossly cloudly pleural fluid with leukocyte counts exceeding 25,000/mm^3, and usually reveals organisms by stain and culture. Pleural fluid pH is helpful in deciding which exudative effusions will require tube drainage. If the pH in a parapneumonic effusion is less than 7.2, a tube thoracostomy will be necessary.

After 3 to 4 days of antibiotic treatment, continuing fever in a patient with pneumonia requires investigation. Most commonly, an incorrect choice of antibiotics is responsible, such as penicillin treatment of mycoplasma pneumonia. However, other problems including lung abscess, pericarditis, meningitis, or other remote foci of infection need to be considered and ruled out by physical examination or special procedures. Last, "drug fever" may be responsible, although this diagnosis should not be entertained until other causes of fever have been eliminated.

QUESTIONS

1. Agents which commonly cause early pleural effusions in pneumonia include:
   (a) *S. aureus*
   (b) anaerobic streptococci
   (c) *K. pneumoniae*
   (d) *Mycoplasma pneumoniae.*
2. Isolation of *S. pneumoniae* from which of the following specimens would prove the etiology of a pneumonia beyond any reasonable doubt?
   (a) expectorated sputum
   (b) pleural fluid
   (c) transtracheal aspirate
   (d) blood.
3. Necrotizing pneumonia with abscess formation is a common complication of pneumonias due to:
   (a) *S. pneumoniae*
   (b) *K. pneumoniae*
   (c) adenovirus, type 4
   (d) *S. aureus.*
4. Pneumonia due to *K. pneumoniae* would be a likely event in which of the following patients?
   (a) a 64-year-old malnourished alcoholic
   (b) an intubated patient with emphysema who requires continuous ventilatory support
   (c) a patient with leukemia receiving chemotherapy
   (d) a 19-year-old army recruit in basic training.

ANSWERS

1. **(a), (b), and (c) are correct.** Pleural effusions may occur in the course of pneumococcal

pneumonia; most such effusions occur after several days of illness and are not present on admission of the patient to the hospital. However, the presence of an early pleural effusion should alert the physician to the likelihood of another etiologic agent, since such effusions are commonly associated with pneumonia due to *S. aureus*, anaerobic organisms, gram-negative bacilli, and *S. hemolyticus*. Mycoplasma pneumonia may produce effusions in up to 20% of patients, but these are almost always small and frequently undetected.

2. **(b) and (d) are correct.** The finding of pneumococci in sputum is difficult to interpret since the rate of false positives is about 25%. In a similar percentage of patients with pneumococcal pneumonia, the organism cannot be recovered in cultures of sputum (false negatives); in such patients a Gram stain of sputum may be more rewarding than the culture. Transtracheal aspiration improves the yield somewhat, but there remain yet a significant number of both false negative and false positive specimens. However, isolation of *S. pneumoniae* from either pleural fluid or blood is incontrovertible evidence of infection due to the organism. Pleural fluid should always be examined and blood cultures drawn before initiating therapy.

3. **(b) and (d) are correct.** Necrotizing pneumonia and abscess formation are much more common with pneumonia due to organisms other than the pneumococcus. Gram-negative bacilli, *S. aureus*, and anaerobes are the most common causes of this serious complication. Pneumococcal infection rarely, if ever, causes cavitation of the lung, except perhaps in infection due to the heavily encapsulated type III strain. Viral pneumonias do not produce cavitation unless complicated by a superimposed bacterial infection, most commonly *S. aureus*.

4. **(a), (b), and (c) are correct.** Pneumonias due to gram-negative bacilli occur almost exclusively among patients with underlying diseases. Hospital-acquired pneumonias are usually due to gram-negative bacilli, and patients who are seriously ill or immunosuppressed are particularly susceptible. Pneumonias among military recruits, or among other groups of healthy young people, are generally viral or mycoplasmal in etiology and are rarely due to gram-negative bacilli.

COMMENT Problem solving was simple in this case where the symptoms, physical signs, and chest x-ray were typical for lobar pneumonia; the sputum examination clearly identified the causative organism as the pneumococcus (*S. pneumoniae*). The presenting pictures for all types of pneumonia are not so characteristic. This is especially true for viral pneumonias, Legionnaires' disease, psittacosis, mycoplasma pneumonia, and those due to more virulent bacterial organisms.

It is important to quickly identify pneumonia when it exists and to try to determine its microbiological cause since treatment may differ. Distinctions are made by the clinical picture, the nature of the radiologic changes, and special laboratory procedures. Some features suggest one organism rather than another. If herpes labialis is present, suspect the pneumococcus. If bullous myringitis is present, suspect *Mycoplasma*. In an outbreak among middle-aged male smokers who attended a convention 1 month ago, suspect *Legionella pneumophila*. Think of Q fever (*Coxiella burnetii*) if there was recent contact with infected livestock. And consider aspiration pneumonia (mouth organisms) if there was a preceding episode of altered consciousness caused by alcohol, epilepsy, stroke, or drug overdose.

Cough and *fever* are generally present in all pneumonias. Other than direct identification by smear and culture (tests which have varied sensitivity and specificity depending on the source of tested material), rising titers of cold agglutinins (IgM antibodies) in mycoplasma infection and the detection of direct fluorescent antibody in *Legionella* infection may help make the diagnosis.

Always to be considered is pneumonia in the *immune-compromised host*. If the patient is a promiscuous male homosexual, has hemophilia, takes steroids for any disease, has a renal transplant with suppressed immunity, or has leukemia or lymphoma, he is highly eligible for developing infection. This often takes the form of pneumonia and may be caused by ordinary bacteria; but notable in these patients is the development of infection with gram-negative bacilli, *Candida, Aspergillus fumigatus*, cytomegalovirus, mycobacteria, and *Pneumocystis carinii*.

Since so many antibiotics are available for treating pneumonias, you should choose the antibiotic on the basis of a clinical assumption, better yet on the basis of direct or indirect organism identification. Use the drug that kills the bug! (*P. C.*)

Suggested Readings

1. Harris GD, Johanson WG Jr: Acute respiratory tract infections. In Guenter CA, Welch MH (eds): *Pulmonary Medicine*, ed 2. Philadelphia, Lippincott, 1982, pp 294–388.
   A comprehensive discussion of clinical features of various pneumonias.
2. Muder RR, Yu VL, Zuravleff JJ: Pneumonia due to Pittsburgh pneumonia agent; new clinical perspective with a review of the literature. *Medicine* 62:120–128, 1983.
   A review of newer agents associated with pneumonia.
3. Louria DB, Blumenfeld HL, Ellis JT, et al: Studies on influenza in the epidemic of 1957–1958: pulmonary complications of influenza. *J Clin Invest* 38:213–256, 1959.
   A classic study of the effect of influenza infection on pulmonary function.
4. Anderson LJ, Patriarca PA, Hierholzer JC, et al: Viral respiratory illness. *Med Clin North Am* 67:1009–1030, 1983.
   Review of clinical syndromes produced by specific viruses.
5. Pierce AK, Sanford JP: Aerobic gram-negative bacillary pneumonias. *Am Rev Respir Dis* 110:647–658, 1974.
   A classic paper on pathophysiology and treatment of these pneumonias.
6. Verghese A, Berk SL: Bacterial pneumonias in the elderly. *Medicine* 62:271–285, 1983.
   A reminder of the special features of host defenses and bacterial pneumonias in the geriatric patient.
7. Louria DB: Bacterial pneumonias. In Baum GL, Wolinsky E (eds): *Textbook of Pulmonary Diseases*, ed 3. Boston, Little, Brown, 1983, pp 407–430.
   A textbook description of all bacterial pneumonias and their complications.
8. Reimann HA: Landmark article: Dec. 24, 1938. An acute infection of the respiratory tract with atypical pneumonia: a disease entity probably caused by a filtrable virus. *JAMA* 251:936–944, 1984.
   A Philadelphia landmark.
9. Levin S: Landmark perspective. The atypical pneumonia syndrome. *JAMA* 251:945–948, 1984.
   "Atypical pneumonia" is viewed 46 years later.
10. Esposito AL: Community acquired bacteremic pneumococcal pneumonia. Effect of age on manifestations and outcome. *Arch Intern Med* 144:945–948, 1984.
    The classic features no longer prevail; they differ with age.
11. MacFarlane JT, Miller AC, Smith WHR, et al: Comparative radiographic features of community acquired Legionnaires' disease, pneumococcal pneumonia, mycoplasma pneumonia, and psittacosis. *Thorax* 39:28–33, 1984.

Case 26
Sudden Shortness of Breath

GARY D. HARRIS, M.D.
W. G. JOHANSON, JR., M.D.

DATA A 48-year-old woman noticed shortness of breath one morning while climbing a flight of stairs to her office. She had been aware of discomfort in her right chest for several days but related this symptom to chronic cigarette smoking. On further questioning the patient reported that she had enjoyed excellent health except for a fracture of the left femur sustained in an automobile accident 3 years earlier. Since that time she had experienced recurrent swelling and mild pain in the left lower extremity, aggravated by prolonged standing or walking, and relieved by rest and elevation of the leg.

LOGIC Dyspnea of sudden onset is usually due to a major cardiopulmonary event. Acute myocardial infarction with pulmonary congestion is probably the most common cause, although the patient's age, sex, and lack of angina type pain make the diagnosis unlikely in this case. Acute cardiac failure can occur from other causes, but it is usually preceded by a long history of heart disease. Tachyarrhythmias may produce dyspnea and are usually abrupt in onset; many are accompanied by "palpitations," a sensation not experienced by our patient.

Pulmonary embolism is frequently followed by dyspnea and chest pain. Most patients with pulmonary embolism have a predisposing cause such as congestive heart failure, prolonged immobility, or abnormalities in the veins of the pelvis or lower extremities. The history of venous disease manifested by unilateral orthostatic edema must raise the physician's index of suspicion.

Pneumonia may certainly present with the sudden onset of dyspnea, although associated symptoms of fever, cough, and sputum production usually dominate the clinical picture.

Spontaneous pneumothorax may produce symptoms which vary from mild to severe depending on the extent of lung collapse, the pressure within the pleural space, and the presence or absence of underlying lung disease.

The symptoms of pleural effusion may be acute or chronic and vary widely depending on the cause of the effusion, the rapidity of its development, and the presence of underlying cardiopulmonary disease.

DATA The patient's vital signs were normal except for a respiratory rate of 24 breaths/minute. Examination of the head and neck was unremarkable; the neck veins were flat with the patient elevated to 45°, and the trachea was not deviated. The heart was normal in size, and auscultation was entirely normal. Examination of the chest revealed diminished expansion of the right hemithorax, flatness to percussion on the right to the level of the midscapula posteriorly, and markedly diminished breath sounds over the right lower chest. Tactile and vocal fremitus were diminished in the same area. There was a firm, nontender, 2-cm nodule in the upper outer quadrant of the right breast; several enlarged axillary lymph nodes were also palpable. The left lower extremity was mildly edematous and the left calf circumference was 3 cm greater than the right. Neither lower extremity was tender to palpation, venous cords were not found, and Homans' sign was negative.

LOGIC The physical findings indicate the presence of a large right pleural effusion which is the probable cause of the patient's symptoms. The physician must now determine the cause of the effusion in order to plan effective therapy. The most common causes of pleural effusion include:

1. congestive heart failure
2. cirrhosis of the liver

3. nephrotic syndrome
4. pneumonia
5. pulmonary embolism
6. tuberculosis
7. cancer
8. connective tissue diseases.

The first three produce transudation fluid; the rest cause exudates. On the basis of history and physical examination, we can rule out all but the last four. Connective tissue disease would be unlikely in the absence of other symptoms. The physical findings provide clues which support malignancy or pulmonary embolus. At this point, radiographic studies and analysis of the pleural fluid are indispensable.

DATA   Radiographs of the chest were taken in posteroanterior, lateral, right lateral decubitus, and left lateral decubitus positions. The posteroanterior film showed a large right pleural effusion; the cardiac and mediastinal structures appeared normal. With decubitus positions, the fluid layered out along the chest wall, indicating that the fluid was not loculated. The left lateral decubitus film was taken to better evaluate the right lower lobe of the lung. No lesions were identified in the right lung. An intermediate purified protein derivative (PPD) skin test was applied.

Thoracentesis was performed in the ninth intercostal space in the posterior axillary line. Several hundred milliliters of serous fluid were easily obtained. Multiple pleural biopsies were performed in the same needle tract with an Abrams needle. These specimens were submitted for the following tests: total protein, lactate dehydrogenase (LDH), glucose, cell count and differential, specific gravity, Gram stain, fluorochrome stain, and cultures for aerobic and anaerobic bacteria, mycobacteria, and fungi. Cytologic preparations were made from the unspun fluid and a cell block was prepared from the sediment following centrifugation.

One piece of pleural tissue was homogenized and cultured for mycobacteria; the other pieces were fixed in formalin. A simultaneous blood specimen was submitted for measurement of total protein, LDH, and glucose. The resultant data were:

	Pleural Fluid	Serum
Total protein	4.5 g/dl	7.0 g/dl
LDH	240 IU/liter	80 IU/liter
WBC	800/mm^3 (84% lymphocytes)	
Glucose	88 mg/dl	100 mg/dl
Specific gravity	1.021	

LOGIC   Transudates usually have low cell counts and a specific gravity less than 1.015. Exudates and transudates can be distinguished more reliably on the basis of the ratio of pleural fluid:serum protein and LDH concentrations, and the absolute pleural fluid LDH concentration. If the pleural fluid:serum ratio exceeds 0.6 for protein and 0.5 for LDH, and the pleural fluid LDH exceeds 200 IU, the fluid is an exudate. If these criteria are not met, the fluid is a transudate. Total cell and differential counts show large variations and are of less help, except when great numbers of polymorphonuclear leukocytes are present, indicating pyogenic infection. Thus, our patient has an exudative pleural effusion without underlying lung infiltration.

It is of interest to know that as little as 200 ml of pleural fluid can be detected in a simple upright chest x-ray film and that a lateral decubitus film may detect even less. Sometimes the film is not so typical, and effusions may be subpulmonic, loculated, or interlobar.

Thoracentesis is almost always necessary for a diagnosis. Except for cases of obvious congestive heart failure, the fluid must be removed and studied. The diagnostic yield is very high. Appearance alone may guide you. A milky chylothorax usually suggests lymphoma or cancer obstructing the thoracic duct. Turbidity is caused by lipid or leukocytes. Blood-tinged fluid results from 10^3 to 10^4 red blood cells/mm^3 and may be seen with pulmonary infarction, congestive heart failure, cancer, etc. Grossly bloody fluid indicates 10^5 or more red blood cells/ mm^3 and is seen in cancer and trauma.

The distinction between transudate and exudate is most important, and, as already noted, it is made on the basis of the fluid's protein, glucose, and LDH content, its white blood cell count, and its specific gravity. Transudates are seen in congestive heart failure, hepatic cirrhosis, and the nephrotic syndrome. Exudates are generally seen with tuberculosis, connective tissue diseases, pneumonia, and infarction. The predominance of polymorphonuclear leukocytes or lymphocytes may predict the diagnosis. And the pleural effusions seen with pancreatitis are usually exudates with high amylase content.

Remember that thoracentesis is not a completely benign procedure and may cause pneumothorax, hemorrhage, empyema, and puncture of the liver or spleen.

DATA The PPD skin test was negative, resulting in only 3-mm induration after 48 hours. Gram, fluorochrome, and acid-fast stains of the pleural fluid did not reveal organisms.

LOGIC The negative intermediate PPD skin test is helpful since at least 90% of patients with tuberculous effusions have positive (> 10 mm) skin tests. However, 15 to 50% of adults may have positive tests, and this finding would not have proved the etiology of the patient's effusion. The pleural biopsy will reveal granulomas in about 40% of patients with tuberculous effusions, and another 30% will have positive cultures from either pleural fluid or pleural tissue. Thus, a definite diagnosis of tuberculosis can be made in about 70% of cases.

Similarly, malignant cells will be recovered from pleural fluid, the sediment sectioned as a cell block, or the pleural biopsy in about 75% of patients with malignant effusions. In both circumstances, the pleural biopsy significantly increases the diagnostic yield from thoracentesis.

While awaiting the results of these studies, the physician still faces the possibility that a pulmonary embolism is the cause of the patient's symptoms and pleural effusion.

The chemical findings in the pleural fluid would be compatible with that diagnosis although blood-tinged fluid is more typical. Arterial blood gases usually reveal hypoxemia (pO_2 < 80 mm Hg) following pulmonary embolism. However, this finding is nonspecific and a large pleural effusion would be expected to produce hypoxemia, regardless of its etiology, due to impaired ventilation of the underlying lung.

A perfusion (or, better yet, a combined ventilation and perfusion) lung scan can be performed rapidly with no hazard to the patient. It must be kept in mind that the effusion alone will cause diminished perfusion and ventilation to the right lower lobe. Thus, a perfusion defect in this region will not be interpretable; pulmonary emboli can be diagnosed in this situation only when multiple defects are found, including areas of lung which appear normal in the chest radiographs. However, a delay in instituting anticoagulant therapy may place the patient in jeopardy of having further embolic events.

DATA A perfusion lung scan was performed immediately after removal of all possible fluid by thoracentesis. The perfusion scan showed only nonsegmental decreased perfusion in the right lower lobe and anticoagulants were not begun. The pleural biopsy showed nests of malignant cells compatible with metastatic carcinoma of the breast. Biopsy of the right breast mass revealed a tumor with similar histology. All cultures were subsequently negative for mycobacteria. The diagnosis is now certain—carcinoma of the breast with pleural metastases.

LOGIC In this instance, the diagnosis is clearly evident. But the perfusion scan was indeterminate, and had the pleural and breast biopsies been negative for cancer, further studies to exclude a pulmonary embolus might have been indicated. This could necessitate a repeat perfusion scan coupled with a ventilation scan and possibly more. The decision of whether to give anticoagulants sometimes requires a greater certainty of diagnosis. Establishing such a certainty might in some cases require pulmonary arteriography. The use of ultrasound and digital subtraction angiography may prove to be highly helpful in this regard in the coming few years. Should emboli become repetitive, absolute certainty of the diagnosis and knowledge of the source of emboli is needed before doing a surgical blocking procedure. And this, in turn, would mandate both pulmonary arteriography and an assessment of the deep leg veins by venography and/or impedance plethysmography. In this patient, had pulmonary emboli been found the source was already apparent in her left leg.

QUESTIONS

1. The mediastinum may shift:
   (a) toward the side of a large pleural effusion
   (b) toward the side of a pneumothorax
   (c) toward the side of pneumonia
   (d) toward the side of atelectasis.
2. A region of decreased perfusion visualized on a perfusion lung scan:
   (a) indicates decreased capillary blood flow in that region relative to other regions of the lungs
   (b) indicates pulmonary vascular obstruction, usually due to emboli
   (c) strongly suggests embolism only if no corresponding infiltrate or ventilation defect is present
   (d) is helpful in diagnosing pulmonary embolism in the presence of emphysema.
3. In evaluating patients with pleural effusions:
   (a) Therapy for the suspected disorder should be instituted promptly and thoracentesis reserved for those patients who do not respond promptly.
   (b) Pleural biopsy adds significantly to the diagnostic accuracy of thoracentesis.
   (c) It is advisable to obtain only small amounts of fluid initially since more can be readily obtained later if needed.
   (d) Serum should always be obtained simultaneously for comparison of certain values between pleural fluid and serum.
4. Pleural effusion due to malignant disease:
   (a) is always associated with the presence of malignant cells in the fluid
   (b) is frequently bloody
   (c) always indicates inoperable disease
   (d) may be due to mediastinal obstruction of lymphatic flow.

ANSWERS

1. **(d) is correct.** Shift of the mediastinum is an important sign which indicates either loss of

volume of one lung or an increase in the volume of the other. It is detected by tracheal deviation and displacement of the apex beat. Since both pleural effusions and pneumothorax increase the volume of the involved hemithorax by the addition of either air or fluid, mediastinal shift, if present, should be away from the side of involvement. Such shift may be an important clue to the presence of tension pneumothorax. In spite of the large effusion, the mediastinum did not shift in the patient just discussed. It may have been fixed. Shift of the mediastinum toward the involved lung indicates atelectasis of the underlying lung.

2. **(a) and (c) are correct.** Regionally depressed activity on a perfusion lung scan indicates decreased capillary blood flow but does not clarify the reason for such a decrease. A decreased capillary bed—as in emphysema, regional alveolar hypoxia and vasoconstriction due to airway disease, or alveolar filling as in pneumonia—may decrease capillary blood flow without causing vascular obstruction. This may mislead the clinician into a diagnosis of pulmonary embolism. Such regions will usually display impaired ventilation as well. Thus, combined ventilation and perfusion scans provide the most definitive information in suspected cases of pulmonary embolism. Segmental perfusion defects with normal ventilation are diagnostic of the latter.

3. **(b) and (d) are correct.** Failure to obtain pleural fluid before initiating therapy may delay making the proper diagnosis and complicate interpretation of the results. Pleural fluid should always be obtained if the diagnosis is in doubt. In inflammatory conditions, pleural fluid may loculate rapidly and render subsequent attempts at thoracentesis unsuccessful. Therefore, aspiration of all obtainable fluid is advised. Pleural biopsy adds only a small risk to thoracentesis in the hands of experienced operators and the diagnostic value far exceeds this added risk. The comparison of pleural fluid:serum levels of protein, LDH, and glucose may provide more valuable data than the pleural fluid levels alone since serum levels may vary widely among individuals; thus, simultaneous serum should always be obtained.

4. **(b) and (d) are correct.** Malignant disease produces pleural effusion through several mechanisms: by infiltration of the pleura directly; by producing bronchial obstruction with subsequent atelectasis and pleural effusion; and by lymphatic obstruction due to involvement of mediastinal nodes. Malignant cells are usually not found in pleural fluid in the latter two situations. Most often, pleural effusion is due to pleural involvement with tumor, resulting in blood and malignant cells in the fluid. Such tumors are not amenable to resection for cure.

Similarly, mediastinal node involvement indicates metastatic and therefore nonresectable disease. However, localized tumors which produce atelectasis and effusion may be resected. Each patient with cancer and pleural effusion must be carefully evaluated before inoperability is decided.

COMMENT The principal problem-solving technique here was the use of the key clue. First it was acute dyspnea; next it was a pleural effusion. Each was pursued by considering the major causes, eliminating most by the absence of concomitant features, and proving the existence of only one. Emboli from thrombophlebitis and metastatic cancer from a palpable breast lesion became the dominant Bayesian likelihoods as the author pondered the specificity-sensitivity of the PPD skin test, the isotope lung scan, and the studies of pleural fluid and pleura. The finding of metastatic cancer cells was the clue with the greatest three-dimensional magnitude. The presence of old thrombophlebitis and cigarette smoking were misleading positive clues. A direct approach using a chest x-ray, thoracentesis, scan, and study of the pleura and its fluid would have solved the problem quickly—no questions asked or examination done until later. (*P. C.*)

Suggested Readings

1. Pierce AK: Pleural disease. In Guenter CA, Welch MH (eds): *Pulmonary Medicine*, ed 2. Philadelphia, Lippincott, 1982, pp 555–606.
   A comprehensive review of the pathophysiology, differential diagnosis, and evaluation of pleural effusion.

2. Black LF: The pleural space and pleural fluid. *Mayo Clin Proc* 47:493–512, 1972.
   An excellent review of the basic mechanism of pleural fluid formation.

3. Johnston RJ, Green RA: Pleural inflammations and pleural effusion. In Baum GL, Wolinsky E (eds): *Textbook of Pulmonary Diseases*, ed 3. Boston, Little, Brown, 1983, pp 1299–1325.
   A textbook in-depth description of pleural diseases with a detailed discussion of effusions.

4. Good JT Jr, Taryle DA, Maulitz RM, et al: The diagnostic value of pleural fluid pH. *Chest* 78:55–59, 1980.
   Documentation of the ability to narrow the differential diagnosis of pleural effusion by use of pH.

5. Poe RH, Israel RH, Utell MJ, et al: Sensitivity, specificity, and predictive values of closed pleural biopsy. *Arch Intern Med* 144:325–328, 1984.
   Demonstrates that closed pleural biopsy and simultaneous fluid analysis are extremely valuable in the diagnosis of tuberculosis and cancer.

6. Sasahara AA, Sharma GVRK, Barsamian EM, et al: Pulmonary thromboembolism. Diagnosis and treatment. *JAMA* 249:2945–2950, 1983.
   Clinical features and diagnostic modalities are measured in the light of contemplated alternate treatments.

7. Sahn SA: The differential diagnosis of pleural effusions. *West J Med* 137:99–108, 1982.
   A good review of the causes, types, and diagnoses.

8. Pardee NE, Winterbauer RH, Allen JD: Bedside evaluation of respiratory distress. *Chest* 85:203–206, 1984.
   Predicting outcomes by clinical signs.

9. Rosa VW: Pleural effusion. How to avoid a diagnostic stalemate. *Postgrad Med* 75:253–268, 1984.
   A stepwise approach to finding the cause—much valuable information in only ten pages.

Case 27
Chronic Cough and Expectoration

GARY D. HARRIS, M.D.
W. G. JOHANSON, JR., M.D.

DATA A 64-year-old unemployed alcoholic man comes to the emergency room because of a change in his chronic cough. He has had a chronic cough productive of scant mucoid sputum for more than 10 years. At least once each year he experiences episodes of acute bronchitis, characterized by increased amounts of sputum which is yellow or slightly green in color. Antibiotic therapy results in gradual improvement. About 3 weeks ago he noted slightly increasing amounts of purulent sputum in the early morning. On two occasions, including the morning of admission, he saw streaks of blood after episodes of vigorous coughing.

LOGIC The patient has chronic bronchitis, which is defined as the presence of a productive cough on most days for at least 3 months over the past 2 years. Chronic bronchitis is a common disease, affecting as many as 25% of adults in some surveys. However, it should be recognized for what it is—a chronic inflammatory disease of the airways accompanied by mucous hypersecretion—and not dismissed as "smoker's cough."

Although smoking is the most common cause of chronic bronchitis, a variety of other conditions may give rise to similar symptoms. Persistent or repeated episodes of cough may be the only symptoms of mild asthma. Chronic inflammation of the airways may result from recurring inhalation of dusts or fumes during occupational or other exposures. Hair spray may be one such offender. A frequently overlooked cause of chronic bronchitis is gastroesophageal reflux with nocturnal aspiration. Specific pulmonary diseases such as bronchiectasis, tuberculosis, or lung cancer may be manifested only by chronic cough, and these must be excluded before a diagnosis of chronic bronchitis due to smoking is made. In most patients with chronic cough and sputum production, the history, physical examination, and chest radiograph will provide an adequate evaluation.

Hemoptysis is a serious symptom which requires investigation. While no cause other than chronic bronchitis can be identified in some patients, hemoptysis commonly heralds the presence of lung cancer, tuberculosis, lung abscess, or bronchiectasis.

It is important to note that the patient's usual pattern of chronic bronchitis with acute flare-ups has changed. The current episode differs from previous episodes in that the onset was gradual, sputum purulence was not prominent, and blood streaking of sputum had occurred. These symptoms suggest the presence of a new problem complicating his chronic bronchitis.

DATA   The patient lives in a house for derelict men. He has smoked two packs of cigarettes daily for nearly 50 years and drinks 2 quarts of wine every day. His last chest x-ray was taken 6 months ago and was normal as far as he knew. He has lost weight over the past few months but could not estimate an amount. He has not had fever, chills, or night sweats.

Physical examination revealed a thin, elderly appearing man in no acute distress. Vital signs were normal. Examination of the chest disclosed an area of tubular breath sounds and whispered pectoriloquy anteriorly beneath the right clavicle and in the right supraclavicular fossa. The trachea was shifted to the right. Scattered coarse rhonchi were heard throughout the remainder of both lung fields and expiration was prolonged. The liver was enlarged with a vertical span of 15 cm. The spleen was not palpable. Definite clubbing of the fingers was present and pressure over the distal radii elicited pain. Numerous spider angiomata were seen over the upper thorax, shoulders, neck, and face. Palmar erythema was noted.

LOGIC   The physical findings in the chest indicate volume loss and consolidation of the right upper lobe. The presence of pectoriloquy in this region must be interpreted with caution; although its presence usually indicates a patent bronchus, in the upper lobes, tracheal deviation may be sufficient to permit tracheal sounds to be transmitted to a segment which is totally obstructed and atelectatic. He has signs of cirrhosis of the liver and chronic obstructive pulmonary disease too.

DATA   Posteroanterior and lateral chest radiographs revealed a density in the right upper lobe consistent with partial atelectasis of the lobe. The trachea and mediastinum were deviated to the right and the right diaphragm was elevated. Air bronchograms were not visible in the right upper lobe. Radiographs of the distal radius revealed periosteal elevation and new bone formation. Attempts to locate the patient's previous radiographs were unsuccessful.

LOGIC   This chest x-ray is not helpful in distinguishing volume loss of the right upper lobe due to bronchial obstruction from that due to a chronic inflammatory process. Tuberculosis, fungal infection, or bacterial pneumonia could present in this fashion, although the absence of specific symptoms makes the latter unlikely. Bronchial obstruction, most commonly due to carcinoma, remains a distinct possibility.

Digital clubbing may be found in chronic liver disease, ulcerative colitis, bacterial endocarditis, atrial myxoma, and a wide variety of thoracic diseases. Occasionally, clubbing is congenital and not associated with disease. Carcinoma of the lung is a common cause. Chronic obstructive pulmonary disease alone rarely causes clubbing. The presence of long bone tenderness, usually best demonstrated in the forearm or above the ankle, suggests periostitis due to hypertrophic pulmonary osteoarthropathy (HPO). The radiographs of the arm confirm this diagnosis. Patients with this disorder usually, but not necessarily, have clubbing as well. Chronic inflammatory diseases of the lung including tuberculosis and bronchiectasis formerly were common causes of HPO; currently, the great majority of cases are due to lung cancer. It is important to recognize that extrathoracic causes of clubbing are rarely, if ever, associated with HPO. Thus, while this patient has definite signs of chronic liver disease and chronic airway obstruction, his clubbing and HPO are most likely due to the process in the right upper lobe.

DATA Skin tests were applied with intermediate strength purified protein derivative (PPD), coccidioidin, mumps, and *Candida* antigens. Serum was obtained for latex-agglutinating and complement-fixing antibody titers against *Histoplasma capsulatum* and *Coccidioides immitis.* Two early morning sputa were examined by Ziehl-Neelsen and fluorochrome stains and were negative for acid-fast bacilli. Two expectorated sputa did not contain malignant cells.

LOGIC A positive PPD skin test will indicate only past infection with *Mycobacterium tuberculosis* and will not be helpful in assessing whether the infection is active at this time. Positive skin tests for the fungal agents have the same limitation. *Candida* and mumps antigens were used as controls to determine whether this debilitated patient's delayed hypersensitivity mechanisms were intact. Since the skin test data will be nondiagnostic and sputum cultures for mycobacteria and fungi will not be available for several weeks, further workup should proceed without delay in situations in which such infections are not highly probable. Results of smears are valuable since they both establish the diagnosis and are good indicators of the infectiousness of the patients. All four skin tests were positive (had the PPD skin test been negative and others positive, tuberculosis would have been unlikely, especially with negative sputum smears).

DATA Fiberoptic bronchoscopy was performed with topical anesthesia. The orifice of the right upper lobe bronchus was completely occluded by a friable endobronchial mass. Biopsies of this lesion revealed squamous cell carcinoma.

LOGIC At this point, the diagnosis is established. The presence of extrathoracic manifestations of cancer of the lung (clubbing and HPO) does not eliminate the consideration of resection. Hypercalcemia is generally associated with squamous cell tumors. Other endocrine abnormalities such as the syndrome of inappropriate antidiuretic hormone, ectopic adrenocorticotropic hormone production, or gynecomastia are usually seen with small or oat cell tumors. All extrapulmonary manifestations of lung cancer tend to regress with effective treatment of the primary lung tumor except, of course, metastatic lesions.

In our patient, three issues must be addressed before his treatment plan can be formulated:

1. whether the lesion is resectable, a question which will require mediastinal exploration for definitive answer
2. whether the hepatic enlargement is due to cirrhosis or metastatic disease, a

question which will require a liver scan and possibly a liver biopsy for resolution

3. whether the patient's pulmonary function is such that he would be able to withstand a curative lobectomy or a possible pneumonectomy, since he has clinically evident obstructive pulmonary disease. This question will require tests of total lung function and an assessment of regional contributions to overall function by isotope scanning techniques.

DATA   The liver scan was compatible with cirrhosis rather than metastatic disease. However, pulmonary function studies revealed severe airway obstruction with an $FEV_{1.0}$ (forced expiratory volume) of only 0.7 liter. It was concluded that the patient was not a candidate for resectional surgery because of underlying lung disease, and further staging procedures, i.e. mediastinoscopy and node biopsy, were not performed. The upper lobe lesion was treated with irradiation.

The final problem list is:

1. carcinoma of the lung
2. chronic obstructive pulmonary disease
3. cirrhosis of the liver
4. chronic alcoholism
5. cigarette abuse.

The patient's two excesses—alcohol and tobacco—are at the root of all his problems.

LOGIC   Since lung cancer may have as short a doubling time as 1 month, diagnostic delays must be avoided. The physician must rapidly make the diagnosis, determine the cell type, and decide on operability. The success of surgery depends on an absence of metastases, absence of serious visceral disease that might preclude a surgical procedure, and the patient's willingness to undergo surgery. In the great majority of patients found to have lung cancer, the disease is inoperable because of already existing metastases and/or abnormal pulmonary function tests resulting from concomitant lung disease.

Assessment of pulmonary function is important. An $FEV_{1.0}$ that is less than 2 liters and a maximal breathing capacity that is less than 50% of the predicted value are bad omens. The presence of hypercapnia ($pCO_2 > 45$ mm Hg) and a poor functional history preclude surgery.

Autopsies on patients who die of lung cancer show metastases to lymph nodes in 70% and to brain, liver, and bone in 30 to 40%. Therefore, the search for metastases may begin with the biopsy of a palpable scalene node, mediastinoscopy if large nodes are suspected by x-ray studies, and thoracentesis if pleural fluid is present. The latter is highly sensitive if cancer is the cause of the effusion. Beyond this, some clinicians routinely scan the brain, liver, and bones, bearing in mind that false positives and false negatives do exist. Needle biopsy of a suspected metastatic site is chancy. Other clinicians search only if symptoms, physical signs, or chemical screens suggest possible disease at these sites. If we are dealing with oat cell cancer, bone marrow biopsy is done, surgery is precluded, and we must treat a medical disease which is unquestionably already widespread.

Depending on the cancer's location and extent in the lung, the symptoms and signs may vary greatly. They may include those of bronchial obstruction, atelectasis, a hilar mass, rib erosion, superior vena cava obstruction, hoarseness, Horner's syndrome, brachial plexus involvement, and hemidiaphragm paralysis.

It is interesting to note the many faces of lung cancer. Often patients are seen with asymptomatic pulmonary lesions detected by chest x-ray. Most often the initial presentation is with pulmonary symptoms of cough, expectoration, hemoptysis, etc. Not infrequently it is a metastasis that brings the patient to the doctor—neurologic manifestations, severe backache, jaundice, etc. Less commonly a patient is seen because of a nonmetastatic manifestation—hypercalcemic symptoms, myopathy, neuropathy, cerebellar degeneration, periostitis, etc. Frequently these various subgroups are seen in concert.

QUESTIONS

1. The development of digital clubbing in a 55-year-old heavy cigarette smoker:
   (a) is usually due to chronic bronchitis and/or emphysema
   (b) if associated with lung cancer, will regress with treatment of the tumor
   (c) is so common that extensive investigation is not indicated
   (d) is usually not associated with pulmonary osteoarthropathy.
2. Hemoptysis occurring for the first time in a 60-year-old smoker with a normal chest radiograph:
   (a) can be safely dismissed as being due to chronic bronchitis
   (b) should be evaluated with repeated chest radiographs at monthly intervals
   (c) should be evaluated with multiple examinations of sputum for mycobacteria
   (d) should be evaluated by sputum examinations for malignant cells and fiberoptic bronchoscopy.
3. Bronchiectasis should be considered in the presence of:
   (a) recurring bacterial pneumonias
   (b) persistent coarse basilar rales
   (c) persistent purulent sputum
   (d) hemoptysis.

ANSWERS

1. **(b) and (d) are correct.** Clubbing of the digits occurs commonly in association with bronchiectasis, pulmonary fibrosis, and cancer of the lung. The development of this finding in a cigarette smoker should not be attributed to "chronic obstructive pulmonary disease" until other causes have been ruled out. Effective treatment of the primary lung tumor is usually followed by regression of clubbing. HPO is much less common than clubbing.
2. **(d) is correct.** Chronic bronchitis is the most common cause of hemoptysis, but the initial occurrence of this symptom should prompt a thorough evaluation of the patient. Carcinoma of the bronchus may not be visible on radiographs of the chest until the tumor has been present for 3 to 4 years. Since such tumors begin in the bronchial mucosa, hemoptysis may occur before any abnormality can be detected by radiography. Awaiting sufficient growth of the tumor to permit detection by x-ray makes little sense. Sputum cytology may indicate the presence of a tumor, and may in fact be positive even when the tumor cannot be visualized endobronchially. Such tumors represent in situ malignancies and, if localized by bronchial brushing or biopsy, have a high cure rate following resection. (c) is reasonable too, but (d) is obligatory.

3. **All are correct.** Most patients with bronchiectasis differ from patients with bronchitis alone in that they expectorate persistently purulent sputum, have coarse basilar rales, and experience recurring episodes of pneumonia. Persistent infection leads to episodes of hemoptysis.

COMMENT Hemoptysis superimposed on chronic cough and expectoration indicated a change in the nature of a chronic cluster and warranted an investigation. The most likely and most common possibilities were considered. Solving the problem was complicated by the fact that the patient did indeed have two coexistent lung diseases—cancer and chronic obstructive pulmonary disease—wherein there was a broad overlap of clues. But HPO and clubbing lay outside the zone of overlap. Probability theory (Bayes) was used to evaluate this 64-year-old heavy smoker with a cluster of symptoms and signs that statistically could mean only cancer. The decisive clues were delivered by x-ray, bronchoscopy, and biopsy—in order of their specificity. (*P. C.*)

Suggested Readings

1. Rohwedder JJ: Neoplastic disease and mediastinal disorders. In Guenter CA, Welch MH (eds): *Pulmonary Medicine*, ed 2. Philadelphia, Lippincott, 1982, pp 795–932.
   A broad review of neoplastic disease in the thorax.
2. Anderson HA, Prakash UBS: Diagnosis of symptomatic lung cancer. *Semin Respir Med* 3:165–175, 1982.
   A general discussion of the techniques for diagnosis of thoracic malignancy.
3. Coury C: Hippocratic fingers and hypertrophic osteoarthropathy. *Br J Dis Chest* 54:202–209, 1960.
   A classic description with illustrations of the causes of clubbing and HPO.
4. Lamb D: Histologic classification of lung cancer (editorial). *Thorax* 39:161–165, 1984.
   Differentiating the undifferentiated—a knotty problem.
5. Stead WW: Tuberculosis among elderly persons: an outbreak in a nursing home. *Ann Intern Med* 94:606–610, 1981.
6. Glassroth J, Robins AG, Snides DE Jr: Tuberculosis in the 1980s. *N Engl J Med* 302:1441–1448, 1980.
   The current diagnosis, prevention, and treatment.
7. Koh HK, Prout MN: The efficient workup of suspected lung cancer. *Arch Intern Med* 142:966–968, 1982.
   Rapid triage makes the diagnosis and determines the stage and operative status.
8. Morgan WKC, Hales MR: Bronchogenic carcinomas. In Baum GL, Wolinsky E (eds): *Textbook of Pulmonary Diseases*, ed 3. Boston, Little, Brown, 1983, pp 1045–1086.
   Complete textbook coverage.
9. Morgan WKC, Andrews CE: Extrapulmonary syndromes associated with tumors of the lung. In

Baum GL, Wolinsky E (eds): *Textbook of Pulmonary Diseases*, ed 3. Boston, Little, Brown, 1983, pp 1125–1143.
   Covers the gamut of strange endocrine, neurologic, dermatologic, myopathic, electrolyte, and connective tissue disorders seen in lung cancer.

10. Spiro SG: Lung cancer—areas of progress. *Postgrad Med J* 60:218–224, 1984.
    Includes diagnosis, staging, and treatment.
11. Geddes DM: Chronic airflow obstruction. *Postgrad Med J* 60:194–200, 1984.
    Portrays the magnitude of the problem.

Case 28
Worsening Shortness of Breath

GARY D. HARRIS, M.D.
W. G. JOHANSON, JR., M.D.

DATA   This 26-year-old woman consults her physician because of shortness of breath and cough. These symptoms have been present for about 6 months. Dyspnea has increased in severity to the point that she is unable to perform her usual housekeeping tasks. The cough is not prominent.

LOGIC   This constellation of symptoms is a common mode of presentation of a variety of disease processes. The patient relates that specific activities have become increasingly difficult for her to perform, establishing the progressive nature of the process. Almost certainly this represents either chronic pulmonary or cardiac disease. One could now approach this problem in one of several ways: pursue a detailed history; go directly to a physical examination to separate the possibilities; or obtain screening tests to facilitate and guide the evaluation. Let us begin with a limited examination in this patient.

DATA   The vital signs are: P 88 and regular, BP 110/70, R 28, T 37 C. The heart is normal in size. Neither right nor left ventricular hypertrophy is apparent by palpation. S_2 splits normally with inspiration, but the pulmonic component is accentuated. No murmurs or abnormal sounds are present. The chest is normal by inspection and expansion is equal bilaterally. There is no dullness to percussion. Coarse midinspiratory rales are present at both lung bases. Expiration is not prolonged, no wheezes or rhonchi are present, and the patient can exhale her vital capacity in less then 3 seconds. The rest of the physical examination is normal.

LOGIC   Several findings of significance are present. The increased P_2 suggests an increase in pulmonary artery pressure, although the absence of a parasternal lift indicates that this increase is not so severe as to have produced clinically detectable right ventricular hypertrophy. Pulmonary hypertension may result from left ventricular failure. However, in the absence of cardiomegaly, displacement of the apex beat, an S_3, or any cause for left ventricular hypertrophy, such failure is unlikely. Pulmonary hypertension may be caused by an increase in left atrial pressure due to mitral valvular stenosis. The absence of a diastolic murmur, no opening snap, and no increase in intensity of S_1 make this unlikely. Thus, cardiac disease does not appear to account for either our findings or the patient's symptoms.

Pulmonary hypertension can be the result of narrowing of the pulmonary arteries due to intimal and/or muscular hyperplasia. In the absence of chronic pulmonary disease, alveolar hypoxia, or cardiac disease, this process is called "primary pulmonary hypertension." This unusual disorder typically affects young women, producing progressive limitation of exercise capacity and cor pulmonale. Our patient's history and physical findings are compatible with that diagnosis with two exceptions: this diagnosis would not account for the patient's rales, and it would be unusual for primary pulmonary hypertension to produce such severe symptoms without more impressive signs of right ventricular hypertrophy on physical examination.

The category of disease which fits her symptoms and findings best is interstitial lung disease; this would explain all the features of her illness—progressive dyspnea, rales, and loud P_2. Having suspected this diagnosis, the physician will obtain chest radiographs and pulmonary function studies.

DATA   The radiographs reveal a diffuse process throughout both lungs characterized by both accentuated linear interstitial markings and areas of alveolar opacification. There is bilateral hilar lymphadenopathy. Pulmonary function studies are shown in Table 17.2.

Arterial blood gases while breathing air show pH 7.44, pCO_2 30 mm Hg, pO_2 76 mm Hg, and 93% saturation. During moderate exercise the pO_2 decreases to 60 mm Hg and the saturation to 88%.

LOGIC   These studies show:

1. proportionate reductions in TLC, FVC, and $FEV_{1.0}$ indicating that the patient's lungs are abnormally small
2. the ratio of $FEV_{1.0}$:FVC is normal and expiratory flow rates are reduced only in proportion to loss of lung volume,

indicating that airway obstruction is not present
3. oxygen transport is markedly abnormal as shown by the decreased diffusing capacity and desaturation of arterial blood with exercise.

These findings are characteristic of diffuse interstitial processes in which the reduction of lung volume is due to abnormal stiffness of the lung (decreased lung compliance). The reduced diffusing capacity may result from several factors including loss of lung units (i.e. volume), thickening of the alveolocapillary membrane, and mismatching of ventilation and perfusion.

Diffuse lung disease may be caused by a wide variety of processes. Infectious etiologies may be ruled out in this case by the history, the absence of fever, and the long duration of symptoms. Major considerations in this patient would be:

1. pulmonary fibrosis associated with a systemic disease, especially those associated with altered immunity (such as connective tissue diseases, thyroiditis, or chronic active hepatitis)
2. hypersensitivity pneumonitis, an immunologically mediated response to inhaled organic antigens
3. idiopathic pulmonary fibrosis
4. sarcoidosis.

Less common causes of this presentation would include chronic drug reactions (busulfan, methysergide, nitrofurantoin), fungal infections (either histoplasmosis or coccidioidomycosis), or lymphangitic spread of malignancy in the lungs.

Table 17.2.
Pulmonary Function Studies

Measurement	Units	Predicted Normal	Observed
Total lung capacity (TLC)	liters	5.00	2.50 (50%)
Forced vital capacity (FVC)	liters	4.01	1.52 (48%)
Forced expiratory volume ($FEV_{1.0}$)	liters	3.12	1.65 (53%)
$FEV_{1.0}$: FVC		0.78	0.86
Forced midexpiratory flow (FEF_{25-75})	liters/second	3.43	2.06 (60%)
Diffusing capacity, single breath (DL_{COSB})	ml/minute/mm Hg	22.10	7.70 (35%)

DATA The patient is a housewife with no history of other employment for the past 8 years. She takes no medication regularly and has not traveled to areas in which histoplasmosis or coccidioidomycosis is endemic. She is an avid gardener, maintaining a greenhouse with a wide assortment of plants, but is unable to associate her symptoms temporally with exposure to her working materials. A review of other systems reveals intolerance of fatty foods and occasional dysmenorrhea.

Further examination shows slight hepatic enlargement; the liver edge is palpable 3 cm below the right costal margin and liver height is 13 cm by percussion. The spleen is not palpable and there is no lymphadenopathy in any region. All else is normal.

LOGIC The physician now faces a diagnostic and therapeutic dilemma. On the basis of the accumulated evidence, he is certain that the patient has a diffuse pulmonary disease and that this process is the cause of her symptoms. Its progressive nature by history dictates that therapy should be started. However, while some possible diagnoses can be excluded, he is left with a list which includes a chronic infectious process, hypersensitivity pneumonitis (presumably related to her gardening hobby), lymphangitic spread of malignancy, sarcoidosis, and idiopathic interstitial pneumonitis. Certain features of the clinical presentation may point toward one diagnosis or another; however, tissue will be required to make a definitive diagnosis.

Hilar adenopathy is a common feature of sarcoidosis, chronic infections, and malignancy but not of the other possible diagnoses. The patient's age and lack of evidence of a primary malignancy on physical examination are against lymphangitic spread of tumor. The absence of weight loss and fever is strong evidence against a chronic infectious process. Thus, sarcoidosis or hypersensitivity pneumonitis becomes most likely.

DATA A battery of serologic tests including antibody titers against common fungal agents, *Aspergillus*, and thermophilic actinomycetes is ordered. An 18-test blood chemistry profile is normal except for an alkaline phosphatase of 125 units. Skin tests with purified protein derivative, *Candida*, and mumps antigens are applied; all are negative at 48 hours.

LOGIC Although the role of circulating antibody in the pathogenesis of hypersensitivity pneumonitis (*extrinsic allergic alveolitis*) is not entirely clear, demonstration of antibody against the suspected antigen provides a valuable diagnostic aid. Thus, individuals with "farmer's lung" usually have precipitating antibody against thermophilic actinomycetes, fungi which multiply in moldy hay. This patient might have been exposed to these organisms through her gardening activity. Failure to demonstrate antibody in this patient, however, may mean only that the appropriate antigens were not tested. Some investigators have found it useful to visit a patient's home or place of work to identify potential sources of antigenic material and to test the patient's serum against the agents isolated.

Absence of delayed hypersensitivity against common agents such as *Candida* and mumps suggests anergy, which is found in 70% of patients with sarcoidosis.

At this point, tissue is needed. Possible sites of biopsy are (*a*) mediastinal lymph nodes via mediastinoscopy, (*b*) lung, (*c*) liver, and (*d*) peripheral sites including nodes, muscle, or skin. As a general rule, sites which are clinically involved provide a much higher yield of positive biopsies, and thus either mediastinoscopy, lung biopsy, or liver biopsy would be preferred in this case. Since granulomata in the liver may be nonspecific, the other sites offer the best chance of making a specific diagnosis.

DATA A transbronchial biopsy of the lung was performed via a bronchofibroscope. The lung parenchyma was extensively infiltrated with noncaseating granulomas, typical of sarcoidosis. The serologic tests were negative and all cultures, including cultures of lung tissue, were negative for fungi and mycobacteria.

LOGIC   Thus we have established that the patient's problems are due to a diffuse pulmonary process, and that histologically the process is compatible with sarcoidosis. Mild liver function abnormalities are consistent with sarcoidosis as well and it was not considered necessary to perform a liver biopsy since the remainder of her illness was typical of sarcoidosis.

DATA   The patient was treated with long-term corticosteroid therapy and improved physiologically, radiographically, and symptomatically.

LOGIC   It is significant to note that sarcoidosis is most frequently seen in the third and fourth decades and that it is twice as common in women as in men. Furthermore, blacks are ten times more affected than whites in the United States.

Recent advances in the understanding of sarcoidosis granuloma formation have provided a number of new diagnostic tests and procedures. Some are related to immunologic aspects and are reflected by elevations of the serum angiotensin-converting enzyme (ACE), of the serum lysozyme activity, and of the serum unsaturated vitamin B_{12}-binding capacity. Radioactive gallium concentrates especially well in sarcoid lung tissue. An increase in T lymphocytes is found in the fluid derived from bronchoalveolar lavage.

These tests all exhibit variable sensitivity and specificity so that false negatives and false positives must always be considered. But tests that are positive in combination have greater significance, especially if they are not interdependent. For example, a positive gallium lung scan seen together with an increased ACE is considered by some to be 99% specific.

Of course, the standby Kveim-Siltzback skin test that uses ground sarcoid lymph node antigen is still a reasonably reliable test if the reagent is available. Though this test is 98% sensitive, it is tarnished by an occasional false positive.

COMMENT   One wonders why a patient with worsening dyspnea waits 6 months before consulting a physician. Perhaps it represents denial, reluctance, procrastination, or misinterpretation. At any rate, the chief complaint—dyspnea on exertion—is the *key clue.*

A variety of alternate pathways for gathering data appeared. The physician chose to do the physical examination first, and by finding evidence of diffuse lung disease, pulmonary hypertension, and a normal heart, he pinpointed the diseased organ. A chest x-ray and pulmonary function tests narrowed the diagnostic list to *diffuse fibrosis.*

Not uncommonly, patients of this sort are given a radiologic diagnosis of "pulmonary fibrosis." But lifting the lid of the pulmonary fibrosis box releases a swarm of exotic diseases. You must now consider collagen disorders (rheumatoid arthritis, systemic lupus erythematosus, and scleroderma), drugs as previously listed, radiation exposure, hemosiderosis, histiocytosis X, alveolar proteinosis, lymphangitic carcinomatosis, idiopathic pulmonary fibrosis, Hamman-Rich syndrome, sarcoidosis, and so forth. Closely competing pictures are presented by environmental lung diseases such as those caused by asbestos, silica, beryllium, and other inhaled nuisance organic dusts.

In this situation, other aspects of the history and physical examination may offer help. For example, the presence of lymphadenopathy, polycythemia, arthritis, or clubbing may guide you. And, as always, one simple question regarding the patient's occupation may furnish the answer. You must be aware of the special roles of age, gender, race, occupation, and inhalation hazards which may serve as clues in the various diseases included under pulmonary fibrosis.

Had a chest x-ray been done first, the diagnostic possibilities would have diminished rapidly, and a specific line of data gathering could have branched from that point. Studies might have been differently sequenced and the physician might have opted for a lung biopsy before all else.

Had the initial probe been into the history, the problem solver would have found a dearth of cardiac clues—no history of rheumatic fever, heart disease, murmur, orthopnea, or palpitations. This would have led him back to the lung as the disease site. As is frequently the case, the distinction between heart and lung disease as the cause of symptoms had to be made. Here it was simple. When both organs exhibit disease, it may be difficult to decide which one, or perhaps both, contributes to the chief complaint of dyspnea.

Most often, the clinical picture is diagnostic and tissue confirmation may not be deemed necessary. Otherwise, tissue diagnosis can be made by open, transbronchial, or percutaneous lung biopsy. At times, mediastinoscopy and lymph node biopsy is the chosen route. In the patient presented here, transbronchial biopsy furnished the *decisive clue*.

Note that the most *common feature* of sarcoidosis was present in this case. Pulmonary disease exists in 90% of such patients. But generalized adenopathy, present in two-thirds of cases, was not found here. Also, there was no hypercalcemia, hyperglobulinemia, arthralgias, rash, or ocular, parotid, lacrimal, cardiac, or renal manifestations. Only the liver seemed involved.

Since sarcoidosis is a generalized disease, it has many faces and can present in numerous ways. Multiple noncaseating granulomas may exist in the lung, lymph nodes everywhere, liver, spleen, joints, heart, kidneys, phalanges, skin, uveal tract, lacrimal glands, and parotid glands. Thus the patient may be seen first by the chest specialist, the cardiologist, the dermatologist, the ophthalmologist, the rhematologist, etc. The lungs and nodes are most commonly involved.

Sarcoidosis may be asymptomatic. On the other hand, the patient may be critically ill with severe dyspnea and cyanosis. Between these extremes is the patient with hepatosplenomegaly, McKulicz' syndrome (dry eyes and dry mouth), joint pains, panhypopituitarism, etc—depending on which organ system is predominantly affected. (*P. C.*)

Suggested Readings

1. Weg JG: Chronic non-infectious parenchymal diseases. In Guenter CA, Welch MH (eds): *Pulmonary Medicine*, ed 2. Philadelphia, Lippincott, 1982, pp 607–662.
   A general review of all non-infectious causes of interstitial lung disease and the evaluation of the patient.
2. DeRemee RA: The roentgenographic staging of sarcoidosis: historic and contemporary perspectives. *Chest* 83:128–133, 1983.
   Definition of staging and its relationship to clinical parameters as a predictor of prognosis and clinical course.
3. DeRemee RA, Gracey DR: Diffuse interstitial lung disease. *DM* 29:1–56, 1983.
   A comprehensive clinical review of the diseases causing this roentgenographic presentation.
4. Crystal RG, Bitterman PB, Rennard SI, et al: Interstitial lung diseases of unknown cause. Disorders characterized by chronic inflammation of the lower respiratory tract. *N Engl J Med* 310:154–165, 235–243, 1984.
   A detailed review of the current theories of pathogenesis of this specific disease pattern. Covers the broad ill-defined field of interstitial disorders.
5. *Clin Chest Med* 3:455–653, Sept 1982.
   This entire issue is devoted to interstitial lung diseases. It includes 14 separate articles on the related radiology, pathology, and hypersensitivity; sarcoidosis; collagen-vascular diseases; idiopathic fibrosis; vasculitis; histiocytosis X; drug- and occupation-induced fibrosis, and more.
6. Merrill WW, Reynolds HY: Bronchial lavage in inflammatory lung disease. *Clin Chest Med* 4:71–84, 1983.
   Sheds light on the immunopathogenesis of this group of diseases.
7. Kerr IH: Interstitial lung disease: the role of the radiologist. *Clin Radiol* 35:1–7, 1984.
   Diagnostic pointers covering the many members of this group of diseases—from the basic plain chest radiograph.
8. Niederman MS, Mathay RA: New techniques for the assessment of interstitial lung disease. *Radiol Clin North Am* 21:667–681, 1983.
   Includes lavage, nuclear scans, and a complete clinical approach.
9. Louw SJ, Bateman ED, Benatar SR: Cryptogenic fibrosing alveolitis. Clinical spectrum and treatment. *S Afr Med J* 65:195–200, 1984.
   Forty-two patients with a serious variant of pulmonary fibrosis.
10. Fan K, D'Orsogna DE: Diffuse pulmonary interstitial fibrosis. Evidence of humoral and antibody mediated pathogenesis. *Chest* 85:150–155, 1984.
    Good electron microscopic photos seem to prove this point.
11. Sharma OP: Diagnosis of sarcoidosis. *Arch Intern Med* 143:1418–1419, 1983.
12. James DG: Sarcoidosis. *Postgrad Med J* 60:234–241, 1984.
    An excellent short review of all aspects of sarcoidosis.
13. Fajman WA, Greenwald LV, Staton G, et al: Assessing the activity of sarcoidosis: quantitative 67 Ga-citrate imaging. *AJR* 142:683–688, 1984.
    Demonstrates 84% sensitivity in detecting active disease.

Chapter 18

Gastrointestinal Problems

A consideration of gastrointestinal (GI) diseases must also include the diseases of this tract's appendages: the liver, gallbladder, and pancreas. We are therefore looking at a very large number of organs and diseases, from the mouth to the anus. The symptoms and signs are abundant, and ancillary studies are also of great value.

Principal symptoms are dysphagia, anorexia, nausea, vomiting, "indigestion," pain, bleeding, mass, trauma, diarrhea, constipation, distention, and jaundice. Each in itself may be a patient's chief complaint, though combinations are common.

In addition to the finding of a palpable mass, tenderness, distention, jaundice, hepatomegaly, or the various stigmata of cirrhosis, much help may be obtained from the physical examination.

However, various studies must often be done before the final solution is reached. These include studies of the stool and urine, blood chemistry determinations, hepatic and pancreatic function tests, contrast x-rays, radionuclide studies, ultrasound, endoscopy, biopsies, computed tomographic scans, arteriography, percutaneous transhepatic cholangiography, and endoscopic retrograde cholangiopancreatography—an armory of diagnostic weapons. The exact roles, indications, benefits, risks, and preferential order of these studies are still to be delineated.

The most frequent GI problems seen in office practice may not be serious. The 1- or 2-day episode of nausea, vomiting, and diarrhea—acute gastroenteritis—is the single most common disorder; it clears spontaneously and needs little problem solving. Also frequent are acute gastric insults, indigestion, dyspepsia, psychogenic GI symptoms, and constipation; the latter two must be regarded with caution. Needing more thought and resolution, though less common but still not uncommon, are ulcer, hepatitis, ileitis, ulcerative colitis, acute and chronic pancreatitis, acute cholecystitis, cholelithiasis, appendicitis, intestinal obstruction, and bleeding. Cirrhosis of the liver is in a class by itself since it is so very common in special subsets of the population. And at the tail end of this list are hemorrhoids—very common and easily diagnosed, yet often the scapegoat for symptoms originating in a more serious lesion higher up.

Lurking in the background, waiting to be mistaken for almost every disease just mentioned, is carcinoma occurring anywhere in the GI tract. It must not be overlooked.

Diverticulosis, gallstones, and hiatal hernia are common radiographic or autopsy findings (15 to 35% of adults have one or more of these three); therefore the patient's symptoms are not necessarily attributable to these usually asymptomatic situations. The fact that a hiatal hernia can be demonstrated does not mean the patient's symptoms are due to the hernia; the same can be said for the other two x-ray findings.

To be remembered is the fact that many GI symptoms originate from diseases other than in the GI tract. Nausea, anorexia, and vomiting are commonly seen in uremia, Addison's disease, and congestive heart failure; medications being taken for another illness may cause these symptoms too. Diarrhea or constipation may result from disease of the thyroid, parathyroid, or adrenal gland.

Perhaps nowhere in medical practice must there be closer liaison between the primary care physician, the surgeon, and the radiologist than in GI tract disease. For obvious reasons, the distinction between medically and surgically treated disease must be made; the dividing line is often not clear, overlap may occur, and continuing consultation is often needed. Medically treated diseases develop surgical complications and vice versa. A bleeding ulcer should be seen concurrently by the surgeon and primary care physician; the surgeon should not be hurriedly consulted at the last minute.

Two more points should be made. First, the reader should have an idea of the relative incidence of GI diseases. Expect to see a Zollinger-Ellison syndrome or Whipple's disease once in a lifetime, cancer of the stomach once every few years, cancer of the colon once every few months, a new peptic ulcer once a month, and a simple GI upset or psychogenic GI reaction daily.

Second, the reader must appreciate the fact that several GI diseases have many faces and can present to the physician in any one of many ways. Peptic ulcer can first be seen with classical symptoms, nondescript indigestion, perforation, hemorrhage, or obstruction. Regional enteritis can present with fever of unknown origin, right lower quadrant pain, intestinal obstruction, or an anal fistula. Cirrhosis can first be noted by asymptomatic hepatomegaly, a swollen abdomen, massive hemorrhage, acute alcoholic hepatitis with jaundice, or liver failure and impending coma. (*P. C.*)

Case 29
Difficulty in Swallowing
PAUL CUTLER, M.D.

DATA   A 60-year-old woman visits your office with an 8-month history of difficulty in swallowing. The patient first noticed the problem when she was unable to eat a steak while dining in a restaurant. Since then she has had intermittent difficulty swallowing both liquids and solids and has lost 10 lb.

LOGIC   Dysphagia must always be taken seriously. A few critical questions will determine the order of statistical likelihoods and the urgency with which tests must be done.

First—what is the location of the dysphagia? Difficulty in the neck may be functional, neurologic, obstructive, or referred from a lower lesion. While the sensation of dysphagia from lower lesions may be referred up, the reverse is not true. The classic teaching that the patient can point to the site of the obstruction is only partially correct. If the symptom is high in the chest, you cannot be sure of its origin; but if it is lower in the chest, it may indeed indicate the location of the obstructing process.

Second—what kind of dysphagia is it? If only solids are involved, a mechanical obstruction that calibrates the food passing through it is suspect. This allows liquids and small particles to pass freely, but obstructs foodstuffs that approach the diameter of the opening. On the other hand, if the patient has difficulty with both solids and liquids, then the passageway is pinhole in size (unlikely), or the problem is due to functional spasm of the lower esophageal sphincter (achalasia) or the body of the esophagus (diffuse esophageal spasm).

Third—is the dysphagia continuous or intermittent? Progressive continuous worsening, first involving solids and later liquids too, suggests organic obstruction by cancer or stricture. Intermittency makes you think of a spastic lesion which waxes and wanes, or an organic lesion like a diverticulum which empties itself, thus temporarily reliev-

ing symptoms. Achalasia can be either continuous or intermittent, though not so progressively relentless as cancer.

DATA   On asking these questions, you learn that the discomfort on swallowing is in both the xiphoid area and the base of the neck. The dysphagia involves both liquids and solids, though the severity of the obstruction varies from time to time.

LOGIC   This information makes you think mainly in terms of a disturbance of esophageal motility and/or a spastic, hypertensive lower esophageal sphincter. But since many other serious diseases of the esophagus exist, you recall the various problems that can cause dysphagia and wish to rule them out.

Cervical dysphagia (difficulty arising in the neck) can be caused by globus hystericus; this is a feeling of a lump in the throat that occurs between meals and causes no real dysphagia. It is a manifestation of anxiety. Various neurologic diseases involving the brain stem or bilateral corticobulbar tracts cause difficulty in initiating the act of swallowing. In this instance, the patient chokes, coughs, and regurgitates through the nose, especially when trying to swallow liquids. Zenker's diverticulum in the hypopharynx can fill with food and obstruct swallowing until the pouch empties itself by regurgitation; this allows a brief symptom-free interval. Myasthenia gravis creates difficulty because of weakness of voluntary muscles which initiate swallowing. The Plummer-Vinson syndrome causes upper dysphagia because of high esophageal webs.

DATA   With this foreboding list in mind, you inquire about and note no other neurologic abnormalities, no difficulty with eye movements, no drooping eyelids, no feeling of a constant "lump in the throat," no history of regurgitation of undigested identifiable food, and no regurgitation of liquids through the nose. There is no evidence of anemia, the nails are not spoon-shaped, and the tongue is not smooth. Reflexes and cranial nerves are normal. No mass is felt in the side of the neck.

LOGIC This quick subset of the history and physical examination has ruled out all the conditions associated with cervical dysphagia. A neurologic disease would not selectively affect only swallowing, nor would myasthenia gravis. There are no clues to speak in behalf of Plummer-Vinson syndrome and Zenker's diverticulum.

You now concern yourself with the rest of the esophagus, and the list of possibilities is equally formidable. Mainly you consider cancer, achalasia, and peptic esophagitis with stricture. Diffuse esophageal spasm and scleroderma are less common. Caustic stricture is easily eliminated by the lack of a history of swallowing a caustic. Diverticuli in the mid- and lower esophagus occur, but they rarely if ever cause symptoms.

DATA There is no history of heartburn, indigestion, regurgitation of undigested non-acid material, choking and coughing which awaken the patient during sleep, anorexia, or weakness. Also, there are no symptoms or signs of arthritis, Raynaud's phenomenon, or tightening of the skin.

LOGIC Absence of heartburn is against peptic esophagitis. While there is no evidence of scleroderma, dysphagia can be its first manifestation. This disease affects the smooth muscle and results in aperistalsis and secondary acid-peptic reflux due to a weakened lower esophageal sphincter. Progressive acid reflux will cause a lower esophageal stricture to form, just as in peptic esophagitis.

You suddenly remember that diseases outside the esophagus can also cause dysphagia, so a quick search is made.

DATA The thyroid gland is not enlarged or hard; there is no auscultatory hint of mitral stenosis, nor can you feel, hear, or see evidence of an aortic aneurysm or a medias-

tinal mass. A normal chest x-ray rules out the latter three possibilities. While waiting for this film, you complete the physical and neurologic examinations. All is normal there too.

LOGIC The diagnostic field has been narrowed to either cancer of the esophagus or a motility disorder. The latter seems most likely.

DATA Further discussion with the patient discloses that she has always considered herself to be "a slow eater," and over the past 10 years she has habitually "washed down" her food with liquids. The dysphagia is worse when she is out in company, but better when she can eat at her own pace at home. She tells of dysphagia which at times "hurts my heart."

LOGIC This history is becoming classic for achalasia. In this disease there is degeneration of the myenteric plexus in the esophageal submucosa. Nerve transmission is severed and the signal for peristalsis or lower esophageal sphincter relaxation cannot be transmitted. Large quantities of food and liquid create enough pressure, especially when the patient is erect, to intermittently force material into the stomach. Often, during sleep, liquid and food regurgitate from a distended esophagus, causing the patient to choke, cough, and sometimes even develop aspiration pneumonia. However, these symptoms are not present in this case.

On the basis of history, you may not be absolutely certain of the cause of dysphagia, though you can determine likelihoods and guide those who will do further diagnostic procedures. The investigation of dysphagia is stereotyped. It includes an esophagram, upper GI series, and esophagogastroduodenoscopy in all cases. A blood count for anemia, a stool examination for occult blood to detect an ulcerating gastroesophageal lesion, and a chest x-ray complete the workup. Because of similar visceral innervation, esophageal pain can sometimes mimic cardiac pain, so an ECG and exercise tolerance test may be necessary.

An esophagram is the safest of the first

three studies mentioned, but it misses a significant number of carcinomas and other esophageal abnormalities, especially in the upper third. GI x-rays may detect carcinoma of the cardia. Fiberoptic esophagogastroduodenoscopy is most reliable but has more risk. It should generally follow an esophagram so that areas of potential hazard and sites of biopsies can be identified beforehand. The esophagram allows the fluoroscopist to watch peristalsis and the movement of the barium bolus—not generally possible with endoscopy.

DATA An esophagram demonstrated a dilated esophagus with narrowing at the esophagogastric junction. Endoscopy revealed a macerated esophagus with retained food and a sharp narrowing at the lower esophageal sphincter. However, with gentle pressure the endoscopist was able to guide his 13-mm endoscope through this narrowing with a definite "pop" as the instrument was advanced. On withdrawing the scope, no evidence of a mucosal lesion was noted. A functional abnormality of the esophagus was therefore further suspected. X-rays of the stomach and duodenum were normal. An esophageal motility study was then done. It found aperistalsis in the body of the esophagus and a hypertensive lower esophageal sphincter that relaxed only 50% (from 60 mm Hg to 30 mm Hg) upon deglutition, whereas complete relaxation is normal. Complete blood count and urinalysis are normal. The stool is negative for occult blood.

LOGIC Achalasia is now established. Diffuse esophageal spasm, like achalasia, is a disease of the visceral afferent nerves of the esophagus resulting in uncoordinated spasms demonstrable by motility studies. It is less common than achalasia and its pathophysiology is poorly understood. Treatment may now begin.

QUESTIONS

1. Given a patient with solid food dysphagia and a history of severe "heartburn" for many years, the most likely cause is:
   (a) carcinoma of the distal esophageal seg-

   ment
   (b) reflux esophagitis with secondary stricture formation
   (c) Schatzki's ring
   (d) scleroderma with secondary stricture.
2. If the patient's complaint had been cervical dysphagia, which of the following diagnoses could have been excluded with absolute certainty?
   (a) globus hystericus
   (b) pseudobulbar palsy
   (c) carcinoma of the lower esophageal segment
   (d) none of the above.
3. Anginoid pain is sometimes seen in patients with achalasia, diffuse esophageal spasm, or reflux esophagitis. This pain closely simulates angina because:
   (a) food lodging in the esophagus presses on the heart and causes cardiac pain
   (b) visceral afferent fibers from the lower esophagus and from the heart enter the spinal cord at the same level
   (c) both pains are relieved by nitroglycerin
   (d) patients with thoracic pain ofter fear the worst and imagine their chest pain to be cardiac in origin.
4. In which of the following esophageal diseases would a motility study be least likely to help?
   (a) scleroderma
   (b) carcinoma of the esophagus
   (c) peptic stricture
   (d) achalasia.

ANSWERS

1. **(b) is correct.** The presence of solid dysphagia indicates a structural abnormality that blocks the passage of food. Heartburn leads one to believe that reflux esophagitis has been present and therefore the most logical diagnosis would be a peptic stricture. Carcinoma must always be excluded; biopsy of the lesion at endoscopy is a necessity. Schatzki's ring, an indentation at the squamocolumnar junction, is also possible but is not usually associated with heartburn and is almost always asymptomatic. Scleroderma with reflux and peptic stricture is rare.
2. **(d) is correct.** Cervical dysphagia generally points the clinician toward disease of the upper esophagus. However, it is a well-established clinical observation that obstruction of the lower esophageal segment can be perceived by the patient as cervical dysphagia. Therefore, the history alone cannot absolutely exclude carcinoma of the lower esophageal segment. Choices (a) and (b) give symptoms in the neck, though, strictly speaking, globus does not cause true dysphagia. Pseudobulbar palsy is caused by bilateral partially resolved strokes; phonation and deglutition are disturbed since

the lower cranial nerves on both sides are affected.

3. **(b) is correct.** The angina-like pain that sometimes accompanies dysphagia is due to stretching and stimulation of the visceral afferent fibers of the esophagus. These pain fibers enter the spinal cord at the same level as pain fibers from the heart, and they are often perceived as a squeezing chest pain that is at times virtually indistinguishable from angina. Therefore the older patient may have coexistent angina, or angina rather than esophageal disease. An ECG or exercise tolerance test may be indicated. (c) and (d) are both true; however, neither explains the similar nature of the pains. (a) has no pathophysiologic basis.

4. **(b) is correct.** A study of esophageal motility is expected to help uncover motor disturbances. Scleroderma is characterized by aperistalsis and hypotension of the lower esophageal sphincter. Peptic stricture in general demonstrates normal peristalsis but a hypotensive sphincter that allows reflux of gastric contents. Achalasia has the combination of aperistalsis and a hypertensive lower esophageal sphincter. There are usually no characteristic abnormalities in carcinoma of the esophagus.

COMMENT This case study confronts us with a single key clue that may have multiple causes. Therefore the problem solver forms initial hypotheses—in this case a long differential diagnosis. On the basis of three historical points—location, type, and discontinuity of dysphagia—the list is rapidly narrowed. Other bits of pertinent negative information exclude additional diagnostic possibilities.

Two hypotheses remain plausible—cancer and achalasia. The diagnostic protocol is routine and a diagnosis is clearly made on a preconceived diagnostic sequence of esophagram, fiberoptic endoscopy, and motility-pressure studies. The patient has achalasia.

But in recent years it has become increasingly clear that peptic esophagitis with resulting spasm and stricture is very common. Careful studies of the lower esophageal sphincter have shown a causal relationship between a patent lower esophageal sphincter and gastroesophageal reflux. This results in frequent heartburn, eventual peptic esophagitis, and even stricture with dysphagia. The link to hiatal hernia is unproven, but reflux is abetted by the delayed gastric emptying seen in unrelated disease states such as diabetes. Furthermore, the patient with frequent heartburn due to reflux knows that caffeine, nicotine, alcohol, and chocolate exacerbate the reflux and the heartburn. To prove the existence of gastroesophageal reflux, manometry is impractical, endoscopy is widely used, the Bernstein test is good, a standard acid reflux test using a pH electrode is helpful,

and barium radiography may give information in more advanced states. Radionuclide scintiscanning may be useful; the stomach is loaded with a nonabsorbable isotope, and a gamma camera records the reflux over the lower end of the esophagus.

Technology for the diagnosis of esophageal disorders is barreling rapidly into the '90s.

(P. C.)

PROBLEM-BASED LEARNING Dysphagia leads to a study of many diseases both inside and outside the esophagus. Begin with a standard textbook for general orientation. There you learn a little about all conditions associated with difficulty in swallowing. Then progress to a textbook of gastroenterology for further details about the individual diseases. A complete study requires that you read recent literature where you will find that there is much ongoing research in the area of the lower esophageal sphincter. When finished, you should know all about:

1. the causes of dysphagia
2. neuromuscular diseases such as pseudobulbar palsy, amyotrophic lateral sclerosis, multiple sclerosis, myasthenia gravis, and myotonia dystrophica—each of which may cause dysphagia
3. how collagen disorders such as scleroderma and dermatomyositis cause dysphagia
4. disorders of esophageal motility—diffuse esophageal spasm and achalasia
5. dysfunction of the lower esophageal sphincter, gastroesophageal reflux, and peptic esophagitis
6. strictures caused by acid or lye
7. the possible role of hiatal hernia
8. esophageal diverticuli (including Zenker's)
9. carcinoma of the esophagus
10. Schatzki's ring
11. globus hystericus
12. Plummer-Vinson syndrome and esophageal webs
13. extraesophageal diseases, such as thyroid cancer, lung cancer, substernal thyroid, aortic aneurysm, and mitral stenosis—each of which may cause dysphagia
14. how esophageal disease causes chest pain
15. the various diagnostic procedures needed to assess dysphagia—manometry, the Bernstein test, barium radiography, endoscopy, and scintiscanning: their uses, limitations, operating characteristics, and interpretation.

And that's a lot to swallow!

Suggested Readings

1. Pope CE II: Heartburn, dysphagia, and chest pain of esophageal origin. In Sleisenger MH, Fordtran

JS (eds): *Gastrointestinal Diseases*, ed 3. Philadelphia, Saunders, 1983, pp 145–148.
   An analysis of esophageal symptoms.
2. Sleisenger MH, Fordtran JS (eds): Gastrointestinal Diseases, ed 3. Philadelphia, Saunders, 1983.
   Chapters 26, 27, 28, 29, 30, and 31, respectively, report on motor disorders, gastroesophageal reflux diseases, rings and webs, tumors, diverticula, and systemic diseases affecting the esophagus in adequate depth for the student or house officer who wants complete textbook coverage.
3. *Ear Nose Throat J* 63, Jan 1984.
   This entire issue (eight articles) is devoted to esophageal disorders and is well worth reading. It contains an excellent survey of the anatomy, physiology, pathology, and diagnosis of esophageal diseases in very few pages.
4. Wilkins WE, Walker J, McNulty MR, et al: The organisation and evaluation of an open-access dysphagia clinic. *Ann R Coll Surg Engl* 66:115–116, 1984.
   Easy access and quick diagnosis are highlighted.
5. Richter JE, Castell DO: Gastroesophageal reflux.

Pathogenesis, diagnosis, and therapy. *Ann Intern Med* 97:93–103, 1982.
   Discusses the diagnosis and magnitude of lower esophageal sphincter problems.
6. Richter JE, Castell DO: Diffuse esophageal spasm: a reappraisal. *Ann Intern Med* 100:242–245, 1984.
   How to verify this entity as a cause of chest pain.
7. Webb WA, McDaniel L: Endoscopic evaluation of dysphagia in 293 patients with benign disease. *Surg Gynecol Obstet* 158:152–156, 1984.
   A view of all causes of dysphagia through the endoscope.
8. Blackwell JN, Castell DO: Oesophageal chest pain: a point of view. *Gut* 25:1–6, 1984.
9. *Surg Clin North Am* 63, Aug 1983.
   Numerous excellent articles in this issue cover esophageal motility, reflux, diverticuli, esophagitis, stricture, cancer, spasm, and achalasia through the eyes of surgeons.
10. Jacob H, Berkowitz D, McDonald E, et al: The esophageal motility disorders of polymyositis. *Arch Intern Med* 143:2262–2264, 1983.

Case 30
Vomiting of Blood
PAUL CUTLER, M.D.

DATA   The ambulance arrives at the emergency room with a 55-year-old man who has just vomited huge quantities of blood, is passing purplish liquid stools, and has fainted several times within the past 2 hours. This had never happened to him before. The blood pressure is 90/70, the pulse is 120, and the patient is pale.

LOGIC   The patient needs prompt treatment; diagnosis is secondary. But as you institute emergency measures, you are thinking of what might be wrong. Primary considerations are duodenal or gastric ulcer, cirrhosis with varices, and acute hemorrhagic gastritis. Other common possibilities include Mallory-Weiss syndrome, peptic esophagitis, and stomach cancer. More unusual causes are vascular malformations, leiomyoma of the stomach, aorticoduodenal fistula, and hereditary hemorrhagic telangiectasia.

DATA   A central venous line is inserted;

intravenous fluids are started and followed by blood as soon as available. A nasogastric tube is passed and the stomach is washed with iced saline. Vital signs and hematocrit are frequently checked to assess the circulatory status and rate of blood loss. Clotting studies are also rapidly assessed by requesting a platelet count, prothrombin time, and partial thromboplastin time. Inquiry into the cause of the problem is proceeding at the same time and must be done with the least number of questions and examining techniques.

Fiberoptic gastroduodenoscopy will be done as soon as hemodynamic stabilization is attained; the various causes mentioned will be sought. In the meantime, you seek selected data. Is the patient alcoholic, has he had hepatitis, and are there stigmata or cirrhosis present (large liver, spleen, ascites, distended abdominal veins, spider nevi, etc)? Is there a history of indigestion suggesting peptic ulcer or esophagitis? Has the patient been ingesting aspirin, alcohol, steroids, or other drugs that can cause ulcer or gastritis? Have there been recent indigestion, early satiety, anorexia, and weight loss? Are there evidences of metastases (Virchow node, nodular liver)? Is there an epigastric mass or abnormal epigastric pulsation? Did the patient vomit several times before any blood came up? Are there many telangiectases noted on the skin or mucous membranes?

LOGIC All this information can be obtained in a few minutes, and together with endoscopy you can be reasonably sure of the diagnosis. Remember that the presence of cirrhosis does not mean that you are necessarily dealing with bleeding from varices, nor does the absence of symptoms preclude ulcer or cancer. However, if there are no stigmata of cirrhosis, varices are a very unusual cause of bleeding.

DATA The answer to all the above questions and physical maneuvers was "no." Hematemesis stopped, tube drainage was slightly pink, and the vital signs stabilized promptly. Coagulation studies were normal. A plain film of the abdomen showed no masses, abnormal gas patterns, or calcifications suggesting aneurysm. Endoscopy revealed a 1-cm-wide bleeding duodenal ulcer.

LOGIC You are not surprised. Ulcer is a common disease in the universe of people; given a patient with ulcer, the incidence of bleeding is 10 to 25%; and given a patient with upper GI bleeding, ulcer is the most common cause (25 to 50%). The latter figure is even more true in the universe of 55-year-old men who do not have cirrhosis of the liver.

DATA The rest of the data base was obtained over the next 24 hours as the patient improved. It revealed the presence of symptomatic benign prostatic hypertrophy and asymptomatic hyperglycemia. There was no evidence of hyperparathyroidism, gastrinoma, or other diseases associated with ulcerogenic activity. Bleeding stopped, transfusions were discontinued, tubes were removed, and medical therapy, including antacids and ranitidine, was begun.

A surgical consultation was obtained while the patient was still in the emergency room. (This should be done for all upper GI hemorrhages, but especially in the setting of a middle-aged man with massive bleeding unheralded by symptoms. In the latter situation, surgery is more apt to be needed.)

LOGIC Not all cases of gastrointestinal hemorrhage are so easily diagnosed and managed as this one. Often it is difficult to establish the site and determine the cause of the bleeding. Especially here, there is need for cooperation between the primary care physician, the surgeon, and the radiologist. Most patients (80 to 90%) will stop bleeding. The surgeon may have to manage the rest. The radiologist can advise on the diagnostic sequence and may even offer treatment in selected cases.

First, decide if the bleeding is from the upper or lower GI tract; the ligament of Treitz is the dividing point. It is upper GI bleeding if there is hematemesis or if a nasogastric tube delivers a bloody aspirate. If there is no blood in the aspirate, upper GI bleeding cannot be excluded; the bleeding may already have stopped or the bleeding may originate distal to the stomach and not be brisk enough to reflux.

Next you must choose between (*a*) endoscopy, (*b*) radionuclide imaging, (*c*) selective arterial angiography, and (*d*) contrast barium radiography.

Endoscopy has its greatest value in upper GI hemorrhages and is done first in most cases. While there is a 1% risk of complications, some serious, this technique provides a high degree of accuracy. It is especially good for small tears or erosions that conventional radiography does not detect. Wait if bleeding is massive, don't do it if an ulcer was previously diagnosed, and it is not nearly so helpful for lower GI bleeding.

Radionuclide imaging is especially good for patients who are still bleeding. The use of isotopes or isotope-tagged red blood cells can locate an approximate site of bleeding if the blood pool is created by .1 to 1.0 ml of bleeding/minute. While this technique has no morbidity, it may merely locate the site but not define the lesion.

Angiography is best for lower GI lesions. The pooling of dye may demonstrate the approximate site if the bleeding rate is as slow as .5 ml/minute. This technique may also identify the bleeding lesion and it is especially good for vascular malformations. But remember that vascular malformations are not uncommon and, when found, are not necessarily the cause for the bleeding. Know too that this procedure carries a respectable morbidity.

Contrast radiography is the conventional diagnostic modality; it uses barium of varying fluidity, often with air constrast. It is best for patients whose bleeding has already stopped and is especially good for lesions of the colon and stomach. This technique provides acceptable accuracy in the stomach (70%) and colon. Endoscopy is preferred for upper GI bleeding. And don't do radiography first for a lower GI lesion if there is active bleeding because the barium coating precludes successful endoscopy.

Since each patient with GI bleeding confronts the physician with a multivariate analysis, diagnostic management must be individualized. At times, exploratory surgery is necessary to locate the bleeding site and remove the lesion.

QUESTIONS

1. If the patient had been an alcoholic and had shown all the stigmata of cirrhosis including severe portal hypertension, then the cause for the bleeding would have been:
   (a) varices
   (b) ulcer
   (c) gastritis
   (d) any of the above.
2. The syncope that occurred in this patient is caused by:
   (a) sight of blood
   (b) effect of blood loss on cardiac function
   (c) depletion of blood volume and cerebral ischemia
   (d) severe anxiety and probable hyperventilation.
3. On admission to the emergency room, you would have expected the patient's hematocrit to be:
   (a) 40%
   (b) 64%
   (c) 34%
   (d) 24%.

4. Since hyperparathyroidism and Zollinger-Ellison (Z-E) syndrome may cause duodenal ulcer disease, these two conditions are unlikely in the presence of the following laboratory results:
   (a) normal serum calcium, normal serum gastrin
   (b) low serum calcium, high serum gastrin
   (c) high serum calcium, low serum gastrin
   (d) high serum calcium, high serum gastrin.
5. Mallory-Weiss syndrome is more common than was originally thought. It occurs in a patient who is vomiting or retching violently and then starts to vomit blood. The cause is:
   (a) alcohol-induced gastritis
   (b) steroid-induced ulcer
   (c) tear of gastric mucosa near esophagogastric junction
   (d) tear of gastric mucosa near gastroduodenal junction.

ANSWERS

1. **(d) is correct.** Patients with alcoholic cirrhosis commonly bleed from any of the three. While varices are common, bleeding may occur from ulcer or gastritis even if varices are present. In fact, gastritis may be as common as varices as a cause for bleeding in the cirrhotic patient.
2. **(c) is correct.** While any of the choices could cause syncope in selected instances, depletion of blood volume is by far the principal factor here. In the presence of decreased circulatory volume, not enough blood reaches the brain with the patient in the erect position. A tilt test is superfluous under the circumstances.
3. **(a) is correct.** A low nearly normal hematocrit, 40%, would be most likely in spite of severe blood loss. Not enough time had yet elapsed for hemodilution to take place. It would certainly not be 64% unless the patient had preexisting polycythemia. Over the next 24 hours it would have dropped to a level reflecting the blood loss, were it not for transfusion therapy. A lower hematocrit could be present if there were previous occult blood loss.
4. **(a) is correct.** While these diseases are not common, they must be considered, especially in cases of recurrent and difficult-to-heal ulcers. High serum calcium is a very sensitive and reliable indicator for hyperparathyroidism, and a high serum gastrin is strongly suggestive of a Z-E syndrome (gastrin-producing tumor of pancreatic non-β islet cells).
5. **(c) is correct.** The tear occurs because a sudden increase in intragastric and intraabdominal pressure results in forceful traction through the hiatus against the fixed crux of the diaphragm. This causes a tear of the gastric mucosa at or just below the gastroesophageal junction. Bleeding can be minor or very se-

vere. This usually occurs in alcoholics or in patients with hiatal hernia.

COMMENT The brevity of this logic session is commensurate with the speed with which this emergency was handled. Shortcuts were necessary because of the urgency of the situation. An invasive procedure (endoscopy) was used because of its high instant yield. Selected information was sought via a branching technique, and only a subset of the data base was explored. Possible causes for bleeding were quickly eliminated and the real cause was proven. The absence of indigestion did not preclude the diagnosis of duodenal ulcer, since bleeding may be its initial manifestation. Patients with ulcer, gastritis, or varices who bleed can be diagrammed by Venn or formularized by Boole in order to express the overlap which exists. Bayes' theorems were invoked as we considered the likelihoods, probabilities, and statistics of patients with ulcer and bleeding, as well as the specificity and sensitivity of some of the diagnostic aids which were used. (*P. C.*)

Suggested Readings

1. Peterson WL: Gastrointestinal bleeding. In Sleisenger MH, Fordtran JS (eds): *Gastrointestinal Diseases*, ed 3. Philadelphia, Saunders, 1983 pp 177–207.
   This chapter assesses the patient with, details the causes of, and introduces the reader to the diagnosis of upper, lower, and obscure GI bleeding.
2. Sleisenger MH, Fordtran JS (eds): *Gastrointestinal Diseases*, ed 3. Philadelphia, Saunders, 1983.
   Various subheadings related to GI bleeding, under different authorships, are found as follows:
   pp 725–728: peptic ulcer bleeding
   pp 902–904: diverticular bleeding
   pp 1609–1612: fiberoptic endoscopy
   pp 1674–1677: radionuclide imaging
   pp 1765–1774: angiography
3. Luk GD, Bynum TE, Hendrix TR: Gastric aspiration in localization of gastrointestinal hemorrhage. *JAMA* 241:576–578, 1979.
   Proves the value of aspiration in triaging the bleeding site.
4. Larson DE, Farnell MB: Upper gastrointestinal hemorrhage. *Mayo Clin Proc* 58:371–387, 1983.
   Management and causes are detailed.
5. Steer ML, Silen W: Current concepts. Diagnostic procedures in gastrointestinal hemorrhage. *N Engl J Med* 309:646–649, 1983.
   Explains the roles of endoscopy, radionuclide imaging, angiography, contrast radiography, and surgery in locating the bleeding site.
6. Conn HO: To scope or not to scope. *N Engl J Med* 304:967–969, 1981.
   An editorial comment on 6 controlled investigations as well as a further study on pp 925–929. The value of early endoscopy in upper GI hemorrhage is still controversial.
7. Schoppe L, Roark GD, Patterson M: Acute upper gastrointestinal bleeding in patients with portal hypertension: a correlation of endoscopic findings with etiology. *South Med J* 76:475–476, 1983.
   Verifies the overriding importance of varices (86% of cases).
8. Reynolds TB: Hemorrhage from esophageal varices. In Schiff L, Schiff ER (eds): *Diseases of the Liver*, ed 5. Philadelphia, Lippincott, 1982, pp 410–415.
   These pages are preceded by a section on portal hypertension and its consequences (pp 393–410).
9. Wilson MA, Hellman RS: The detection of gastrointestinal bleeding using nuclear medicine techniques: a local experience and review. *Wis Med J* 83:15–19, 1984.
10. Langman MJ, Coggon D, Spiegelhalter D: Analgesic intake and the risk of acute upper gastrointestinal bleeding. *Am J Med* 74:79–82, 1983.
    Aspirin is blamed; acetaminophen is partially vindicated. Neither drug is as guilty as was thought.
11. Stewart JG, Ahlquist DA, McGill DB, et al: Gastrointestinal blood loss and anemia in runners. *Ann Intern Med* 100:843–845, 1984.
    Another reason for joggers to beware.

Case 31
Indigestion

ERNEST URBAN, M.B.B.S.

DATA Intermittent episodes of "indigestion" for 5 years bring a 45-year-old Mexican-American mother of three teenagers to your office. She describes the indigestion as an upper abdominal fullness associated with gurgling noises and gas. This discomfort comes 1 to several hours after meals, lasts for a variable number of hours, then gradually disappears. There is no pain or heartburn. Over the last few months these symptoms became more frequent, occurred several times per week, and lasted for longer periods of time.

LOGIC The symptom complex of patients with indigestion can be vague and nonspecific or it may be clear-cut and suggest a specific disorder. For example, duodenal ulcer may cause heartburn and epigastric pain several hours after eating; this is relieved by food or alkali. By contrast, the pain of gastric ulcer occurs on eating and subsides when the stomach empties. Peptic esophagitis causes symptoms like those of peptic ulcer; dysphagia may also be present. Stomach cancer causes anorexia and early satiety. Gallbladder disease was thought to cause indigestion after eating fried or fatty foods, but this is probably not so. Right upper quadrant pain is characteristic of gallstones, though stones do not cause indigestion. Gastrointestinal symptoms of anxiety states are vague, variable, and often nondescript.

Descriptions of indigestion vary. They include complaints such as gas, belching, heartburn, dyspepsia, bloating, discomfort, pain, gurgling noises, fullness, distention, and cramps. Typical syndromes are uncommon. Usually there is an overlap of symptoms from one digestive disease to another, and it is difficult to be certain of a diagnosis without studies.

DATA Further history does not elicit much additional significant information. The patient has experimented by avoiding spicy and fried foods, broiling meat, and omitting various vegetables and desserts. She has the impression that fatty and fried foods could be responsible for her symptoms. Antacids are of no help. Her appetite is good and her weight has remained constant at 170 to 175 lb for at least 10 years. Occasional headaches are relieved by salicylates; she does not smoke and rarely drinks alcohol.

Her first child was delivered by cesarean section 18 years ago because of severe toxemia of pregnancy; the other two children are twins, 2½ years younger. Menses have been normal both before and since the pregnancies. A few weeks after the birth of her last two children she had several episodes of severe colicky upper abdominal pain that woke her at night. She felt distended each time, but the pains rapidly abated and she sought no medical advice.

Otherwise, the past medical history is negative. She has three healthy younger sisters and a healthy 70-year-old mother. Her father died of a myocardial infarction at 62. The patient is a homemaker who left paid employment when she married.

LOGIC The fact that the patient is fat, female, fecund, and fortyish suggests gallstones. Several episodes of pain years ago could represent gallstone pain or the passage of stones or gravel. Incomplete intestinal obstruction from postoperative adhesions was possible. The constancy of weight and duration of symptoms are against cancer. Her dietary experimentation led nowhere. There is no pattern of periodicity, symptom relation to meals, or relief by alkali. The picture remains unclear.

DATA Physical examination disclosed a healthy-appearing but overweight woman. Everything was normal or negative, including the rectum, pelvis, stool for occult blood, and sigmoidoscopy. A low midline scar was noted. There was no epigastric tenderness, and no abdominal masses or organs were palpated.

LOGIC Again no help! A stool without occult blood and the absence of pallor preclude a bleeding gastrointestinal lesion but do not rule out intermittent bleeding. No masses or organs were palpable, but her obesity makes this negative finding unreliable. The absence of tenderness is fairly reliable and would eliminate an active ulcer, and certainly an acutely inflamed gallbladder.

We must now distinguish between *functional* and *organic* disease. This is a vital distinction. There is much information to show that "functional disorders" result from alterations in motility or dyskinesias of the gastrointestinal tract. Psychologic disturbance *may* play a role. But future clinical studies and new disease concepts may disprove the nervous or functional aspects of some subsets of this hodgepodge of gastrointestinal disorders. Organic diseases, on the other hand, have identifiable pathologic or structural lesions. Those disorders resulting from known hormonal or enzyme deficiencies are either considered to be organic or belong in a gray zone.

About 50% of patients with "indigestion" have no organic disease. Middle-aged women predominate. The onus on the physician is great. A label of "functional gastrointestinal disorder" or "nervous stomach" is difficult to erase once established. This label must often be revised if symptoms change or new symptoms develop. Remember that patients with functional disorders develop organic disease with the same frequency as the general population.

With these thoughts in mind, you list the traditional causes of indigestion for further consideration. These include:

1. peptic esophagitis
2. peptic ulcer
3. cancer of the stomach
4. chronic cholecystitis with cholelithiasis
5. aerophagia and other functional disorders
6. malabsorption
7. chronic pancreatitis
8. pancreatic pseudocyst
9. right ventricular failure with visceral congestion
10. anginal equivalent
11. abdominal epilepsy or migraine
12. lack of proper dentures.

A number of the listed entities can be rapidly screened by history and examination. The absence of diarrhea, no abdominal pain, no history of acute pancreatitis, no evidence for heart failure, no relation of symptoms to exertion, and the presence of teeth easily rule out most of diagnoses 6 to 12. The first five are the most common and merit the most consideration.

DATA　You order a series of tests: blood count, urinalysis, ECG, chest x-ray, plain film of the abdomen, 18-test blood chemistry profile (including bilirubin, transaminase, alkaline phosphatase, and proteins), erythrocyte sedimentation rate, oral cholecystogram (OCG), and upper gastrointestinal x-rays.

All tests are normal except for the OCG. The gallbladder does not visualize, but flecks of contrast material are present in the large bowel. The plain film of the abdomen shows normal renal sizes, no radiopaque calculi in the gallbladder or urinary tract, and no abnormal gas patterns. The normal erythrocyte sedimentation rate and blood chemical tests point away from organicity.

LOGIC　A diseased gallbladder seems likely. But you are not sure. There are several causes for nonvisualization of the gallbladder in an OCG. Perhaps the patient did not take the dye the night before; this is negated by the presence of dye in the colon. Abnormal liver function causes reduced excretion of contrast material into the biliary tree, but liver function tests are normal here. Third, abnormal gallbladder function may exist. A diseased gallbladder loses its ability to absorb water and concentrate the bile (or the contrast material). Hence, that organ may not visualize even if the patient has cholelithiasis and chronic cholecystitis.

DATA　You order a repeat study of the gallbladder using a double-dose technique. The x-rays now show a faintly visualized gallbladder containing several round contrasting radiolucent areas. The radiologist is confident that these are stones.

LOGIC　A dose of contrast material (six tablets of Telepaque) was given on each of 2 consecutive evenings. This allows for a prolonged period of dye concentration and an increased change of radiologic visualization of the gallbladder. About 80% of biliary tract calculi are radiolucent cholesterol stones; not surprisingly, none was seen on the plain film of the abdomen. This is in contradistinction to renal calculi where more than 80% of stones are radiopaque.

If the gallbladder does not visualize in a single-dose OCG, most physicians prefer an *ultrasound study*. This saves time; it is relatively inexpensive, safe, generally available, and highly reliable; and it is not subject to the vagaries of the OCG. In fact, its 95% sensitivity for biliary calculi makes it a first-line definitive diagnostic procedure that is consigning the OCG to obsoletion.

You are not surprised to find stones. There is an increased incidence of cholelithiasis in Mexican-Americans; it is most likely a reflection of the increased incidence of cholelithiasis seen in the American Indian. Also, approximately 10 to 20 million Americans of all ethnic backgrounds have gallstones—i.e. 5 to 10% of the population.

But are the stones related to the symptoms? You recall the episodes of pain many years ago. Now she may have fatty food intolerance in addition to her other symptoms of indigestion. But the association of symptoms (other than pain) with gallbladder disease is chancy. In fact, the relation of fatty food intolerance and gallstones is purely fortuitous. It has been nicely demonstrated that fatty food intolerance is more frequent in patients with normal than with abnormal cholecystograms. So much for a popular but mistaken concept introduced as far back as 1908 and still not expunged.

DATA   After careful consideration, consultation, and discussion with the patient, surgery was advised. Cholecystectomy was performed. The gallbladder wall was thickened and showed chronic inflammation. There were 12 stones of varying sizes within the gallbladder. The common duct was of normal caliber and felt normal. Recovery was uneventful.

LOGIC   Even though the symptoms and diagnosis could not be definitely related, surgery was indicated. An elective procedure in a healthy patient bears little risk. One-third to one-half of patients with gallstones will develop severe symptoms or serious complications. At that point, the surgical risk is much higher. Furthermore, cancer of the gallbladder can result from stones. And, since chenodeoxycholic acid for dissolution of biliary calculi is slow, only partially effective, and does not prevent stone recurrence, surgery is still the best treatment.

DATA   Six months later the patient consults you again. For a few weeks after the cholecystectomy she seemed to be relieved of her symptoms, but over the past few months her indigestion returned and now seems to be getting worse. She has noticed an increasing amount of bloating and gas, and there have also been several bouts of diarrhea. She has not been out of the country and no family members have had similar symptoms. Examination is completely normal. The cholecystectomy scar is well healed and not tender.

LOGIC   This situation is not rare. Was the diseased gallbladder unrelated to the symptoms? Was her original disease not uncovered? Does she have a new disease? Is she psychoneurotic? Diarrhea has been added to the cluster of symptoms, but it does not seem to be of infectious origin.

DATA   Further inquiries are made. Her home situation does not seem to be stressful in spite of three children. She does not seem disturbed, anxious, tense, or depressed. The stools are watery but contain formed solid material. Borborygmi frequently precede a sudden need to go to the toilet. The solid part of the stool is of normal caliber and there is no blood, mucus, or pus.

LOGIC   Again the matter of organicity arises. At least on the surface, no psychologic problems are present. You know that irritable bowel syndrome is the most common chronic gastrointestinal disorder seen in clinical practice. Mucous colitis, spastic colitis, and nervous colon are popular aliases for this condition. While it causes much distress, it has no serious consequences. It is characterized by chronic abdominal crampy pains and constipation, or chronic intermittent watery diarrhea, or a combination of both. The stools may contain much mucus and are sometimes pencil-like; or the stool may be passed frequently in small amounts, yet there be no increase in the total amount of stool. A fact that must always be considered when seeing patients with such complaints is that these symptoms mimic more serious or curable diseases.

Mistakes in this area are common. The absence of blood, pus, and mucus in the stool makes infectious or ulcerative colitis less likely but does not exclude them. And be aware that the common denominator for all forms of irritable bowel syndrome is alteration in intestinal motility for which psychologic disturbances may or may not be responsible.

DATA Sigmoidoscopy is normal. Stool culture shows only normal flora, and no ova or parasites are seen on careful microscopic examination. Barium enema is normal. You are perplexed and ready to label the symptoms functional in spite of the absence of environmental stress. The patient tells you again that she has explored dietary manipulations without success.

LOGIC Suddenly an idea flashes through your mind. Lactose intolerance of *varying degrees* occurs in 50% of adult Mexican-Americans, 70% of black Americans, and almost 100% of orientals and American Indians, but in less than 15% of whites of northern European ancestry. The symptoms are wholly consistent with lactose intolerance. Milk products containing lactose are widely present in foods, often being added as fillers or extenders. They are present in such items as cream of chicken soup, some breads, and many cookies, as well as the more obvious dairy products.

DATA You inquire in detail about the use of milk and dairy products. She drinks several cups of coffee with milk or cream each day, eats ice cream, and has milk with cereal for breakfast. She has not liked the taste of milk since her late teens but never thought much about it and never related her indigestion to milk or milk products.

An oral lactose tolerance test is done. After 50 g of oral lactose, the blood glucose levels are: 86, 89, 94, and 96 mg/dl at fasting, 30, 60, and 90 minutes after ingestion. The patient complained of considerable bloating, gas, and several loose, watery bowel movements during and for several hours after the test.

LOGIC Lactose intolerance is now proven.

The amount of lactose used is equivalent to that found in about 1 liter of milk. The blood glucose results indicate a flat curve (a rise of less than 20 mg/dl). These values plus the exacerbation of symptoms are excellent evidences that the patient is lactase deficient and therefore lactose intolerant. Recall that lactose is split by the mucosal enzyme lactase into glucose and galactose prior to absorption. Unsplit lactose remains in the intestinal lumen where it exerts an osmotic effect. When the lactose and greater amount of water reach the colon, enteric bacteria flourish and some even split lactose. Thus, gas, bloating, and diarrhea result. This is a specific malabsorption, and absorption of all other nutriments by the small intestine remains unimpaired.

DATA The patient is given detailed instructions about a low-lactose diet and calcium supplementation because elimination of a wide range of foods containing lactose may lead to osteopenia. She is informed of the need to read labels for the composition of the packaged foods she buys. Since you watch the national news and read the latest medical information, you tell her about the yogurt story and also prescribe a new commercial lactase preparation which, when added to milk, hydrolyzes the lactose and makes it drinkable.

Two months later she reports back to you—free of symptoms.

COMMENT Two problems existed in this patient. Both were organic and each could have caused some of her symptoms. Fortunately, a psychoneurotic label was avoided. It would appear that lactose intolerance probably caused her symptoms and that the gallstones were coincidental. Nevertheless, surgery was indicated. The combination of cholelithiasis and lactose intolerance is not so unusual. Chance alone dictates that two fairly common conditions will occur together in a smaller but definite number of people. (*P. C.*)

Suggested Readings

1. Gray GM: Maldigestion and malabsorption: clinical manifestations and specific diagnosis. In Sleisenger MH, Fordtran JS (eds): *Gastrointestinal Diseases*, ed 3. Philadelphia, Saunders, 1983, chap 15, pp 228–256.

   The chapter is a comprehensive physiologic approach to the wide spectrum of maldigestion and malabsorption. The many clinical and laboratory tests are discussed in depth. Disaccharidase deficiencies are specifically addressed on pp 242–243.

2. Way LW, Sleisenger MH: Cholelithiasis and chronic cholecystitis. In Sleisenger MH, Fordtran JS (eds): *Gastrointestinal Diseases*, ed 3. Philadelphia, Saunders, 1983, chap 84, pp 1383–1389.
   This short chapter discusses diseases of the gallbladder and the differential diagnosis of chronic cholecystitis.

3. Welsh JD: Carbohydrate malabsorption. In Bayless TM (ed): *Current Therapy in Gastroenterology and Liver Disease, 1984–1985*. Philadelphia, Decker, 1984, pp 135–138.
   A succinct account of the principles of treatment regarding lactose malabsorption.

4. Thistle JL: Gallstones: medical-surgical aspects. In *Current Therapy in Gastroenterology and Liver Disease, 1984–1985*. Philadelphia, Decker, 1984, pp 457–460.
   A brief discussion of elective cholecystectomy and stone dissolution therapy including who should undergo dissolution therapy.

5. Koch JP, Donaldson RM: A survey of food intolerance in hospitalized patients. *N Engl J Med* 271:657–660, 1964.
   Hospitalized patients (655) were investigated for the incidence of selected food intolerances as a cause of gastrointestinal symptoms. The results may surprise you.

6. Bayless TM, Rothfeld B, Massa C, et al: Lactose and milk intolerance; clinical implications. *N Engl J Med* 292:1156–1159, 1975.
   This excellent study reports on the clinical importance of tolerance tests to determine lactose intolerance in 166 hospitalized patients.

7. Garfield E: The worldwide problem of lactose intolerance. *Curr Contents* 23:5–8, 1980.
   A provocative editorial that focuses on the world-wide extent of lactose intolerance. It questions the American attachment to milk.

8. Ferguson A, MacDonald DM, Brydon WG: Prevalence of lactase deficiency in British adults. *Gut* 25:163–167, 1984.
   Shows how irritable bowel syndrome and lactase deficiency can be similar.

9. Newcomer AD, McGill DB: Irritable bowel syndrome: role of lactase deficiency. *Mayo Clin Proc* 58:339–341, 1983.

10. Rosado JL, Solomons NW: Sensitivity and specificity of the hydrogen breath-analysis test for detecting malabsorption of physiologic doses of lactose. *Clin Chem* 29:545–548, 1983.

11. The influence of colonic pH on the hydrogen breath-analysis test. *Nutr Rev* 40:172–175, 1982.
    Explains the chemical rationale for the test.

12. Newcomer AD, McGill DB: Clinical importance of lactase deficiency. *N Engl J Med* 310:42–43, 1984.

13. Kolars JC, Levitt MD, Aouji M, et al: Yogurt—an autodigesting source of lactose. *N Engl J Med* 310:1–3, 1984.

14. Brand JC, Gracey MS, Spargo RM, et al: Lactose malabsorption in Australian aborigines. *Am J Clin Nutr* 37:449–452, 1983.
    An investigation of the incidence of lactose intolerance in Australian aborigines who represent a surviving remnant of the world's largest and perhaps oldest hunter-gatherer society. In common with most human adults, the aborigines are lactase deficient, suggesting that this deficiency also existed in archaic *Homo sapiens*.

Case 32
Sudden Upper Abdominal Pain
CARLOS PESTANA, M.D.

DATA A 43-year-old man arrives at the emergency room at 6 AM complaining of severe abdominal pain which he has had all night. He is accompanied by his wife. As you start your evaluation of the problem, you notice that he is lying on the stretcher on his back, with his knees drawn up, and he is retching and vomiting a very small amount of greenish fluid. While you are asking your first few questions he changes position twice, lying on his side but still with the knees drawn up. It is obvious that he is in great pain.

LOGIC Your initial observation and the complaint with which he registered have already given you several clues. The problem is acute, has lasted about 12 hours, and is a problem of abdominal pain. His appearance and the fact that he sought help at a rather inconvenient hour suggest that the pain is severe. Furthermore, even though you were trained to take a history first and then do a physical examination, you cannot help but notice his position and the fact that he moves around seeking relief. The fetal position is frequently assumed with pancreatic pain.

Acute abdominal pain brings to mind perforated ulcer, acute pancreatitis, mesenteric thrombosis, biliary colic, ureteral colic, and a host of other disorders. It is unusual to thrash around seeking relief if there is an irritating fluid loose in the belly, so that perforated ulcer, bile peritonitis, free perforation of a diverticulum, or other examples of visceral perforation are less likely. Let us go on and get the details about the pain.

DATA   The patient relates that he was in his usual state of good health until last night. He began to experience epigastric pain at about 8 PM, shortly after he returned home from a party at which he ate and drank heavily. The pain began gradually, and built up to full intensity in about ½ hour. It was constant in nature, very severe, radiating straight through to the back, and was accompanied by nausea and vomiting shortly after its onset. He vomited 1 or 2 cupfuls of greenish material, but later he simply retched without bringing up much. The pain has remained constant in nature, location, and intensity. He has taken no medications for it.

LOGIC   An experienced clinician would already have a tentative diagnosis, based on pattern recognition. The description is classical for acute pancreatitis. You would not easily elicit such a concise summary from a patient or his wife, but you could achieve it only by careful questioning. We start by setting the time of onset: he says last night. You press on: does he really mean last night, or has he been sick for 2 or 3 days and things got worse last night? No, he was fine until last night. OK, how did it begin? What was he doing at the time? It makes a big difference if he got the pain right after being run over by a truck, as opposed to lying quietly in bed. It turns out that he had just returned home after an unusual meal—a heavy one, with lots of drinking.

This pattern fits pancreatitis, but also would fit acute alcoholic gastritis, a flare-up of an otherwise tame duodenal ulcer, food poisoning, or plain old upset stomach of the television commercial variety. The latter is unlikely, in view of the duration and severity of the pain. In food poisoning, we would

expect vomiting and diarrhea, and the pain would be of a colicky nature (intermittent pain with a crescendo-decrescendo pattern). An angry duodenal ulcer can give much pain, particularly one that penetrates into the pancreas or, even more so, one that perforates. The fact that he is moving around is a small clue against the latter, but does not rule it out. Acute alcoholic gastritis should have been somewhat relieved with vomiting, and would have produced bleeding—it sounds unlikely.

We press on with the details. Just how sudden was the onset? If he had been calmly reading the paper, and suddenly, on line 10 of column 2, he was struck by a bolt out of the blue, you would think of a perforation, most commonly a perforated ulcer (but it could also be a diverticulum). If it were almost as sudden, but then took on a colicky pattern, you would think of a stone suddenly moving—biliary or ureteral. On the other hand, the slow buildup suggests an inflammatory condition: pancreatitis, diverticulitis, appendicitis, etc. But he has already located his pain in the epigastrium and it has not moved from there, so lower abdominal conditions are less likely.

He next told us that the pain was constant in nature, again what you expect from inflammation of a solid organ or from irritating fluid loose in the belly. The radiation straight through to the back is typical for pancreatic pain. Nausea and vomiting may accompany many acute abdominal conditions, including pancreatitis. If vomiting had preceded the pain, one would have seriously considered a perforation of the lower esophagus, but it was the other way around.

We have been building a clinical picture that we recognize as pancreatitis. But we must rule out other possibilities. The anatomic approach is a good way to make a list. Persistent epigastric pain suggests disease of organs in that vicinity: stomach, pancreas, duodenum, biliary tree, liver, lower esophagus, and colon on the abdominal side; and heart and lungs just above the diaphragm. We quickly consider possibilities: gastritis, gastric or duodenal ulcer perforation, acute cholecystitis, biliary colic, acute hepatitis, esophageal perforation, colonic perforation, lower lobe pneumonia, pulmonary embolus, or myocardial infarct. We have already cast doubt upon some of these; the others are still possible. Further information will help.

DATA A review of systems is quickly done. There are no other symptoms referable to the gastrointestinal tract. Specifically, there is no bleeding, no diarrhea, and no dysphagia. The respiratory system offers no additional clues. There is no cough, shortness of breath, or sputum, and the epigastric pain has no relationship to respiratory movements. Cardiovascular symptoms are also absent. The pain does not radiate to the left arm, is not perceived as tightness in the chest, and is not accompanied by palpitations. The urinary system is also noncontributory. There is no dysuria and no radiation of the pain to the inner thigh or scrotum. Other systems are equally negative. He has never had an episode like this before, and "has never been sick."

LOGIC The negative information gleaned from the review of systems makes us doubt that there is pulmonary or cardiac disease. The urinary tract, never seriously in our thoughts, recedes even further into the background. The upper gastrointestinal tract and its adjacent organs (liver, biliary tree, and pancreas) are the most likely sources. Let us proceed with the physical examination.

DATA Vital signs were taken before you arrived: temperature is 37.2 C, blood pressure is 70/50, pulse rate is 140, respirations are 36/minute. You recheck them yourself, and he is indeed that hypotensive. You also note that the pulse is feeble and fast but regular. The patient is clearly dehydrated. Head, neck, and chest are not remarkable, but the abdomen is. There is generalized distention, tenderness to deep palpation in the epigastrium, muscle guarding, and rebound tenderness. The lower abdomen is somewhat tender also, but not so much as the epigastrium; there is no rebound or muscle guarding in the lower abdomen. Percussion does not help much; it does not sound like a drum, but it is not dull either. You

cannot quite decide whether there is ascites or gaseous distention. The pain on deep palpation discourages further investigation. Bowel sounds are present but very sporadic. Rectal examination is unremarkable.

LOGIC "Pattern recognition" again: shock, signs of an acute upper abdomen, and relatively subdued abdominal findings are what you expect from pancreatitis. A perforated ulcer should give you a board-like abdomen throughout, with rebound everywhere, and probably no bowel sounds at all. Shock would be expected also. Another devastating catastrophe, mesenteric occlusion, might lead to shock but would give more alarming generalized findings except in the very old. Mesenteric occlusion would be more likely in an older person or in someone with an irregular pulse or a recent myocardial infarct. Acute hepatitis or acute cholecystitis would have localized the findings to the right upper quadrant and would ordinarily not lead to shock. Lower thoracic pathology, although unlikely on the basis of the review of systems, is still a faint possibility.

DATA You start a central venous line where you read a central venous pressure of zero and then proceed to infuse Ringer's lactate rapidly until plasma arrives from the blood bank. A Foley catheter goes in to monitor hourly urinary output. You draw blood for the laboratory and order a hemoglobin, white blood cell count, serum amylase, and serum calcium. Your hospital offers an automated collection of tests for the same price, so you get all the electrolytes, as well as several liver enzymes. A nasogastric tube is placed, and various people arrive to do an ECG, a chest x-ray, and an upright film of the abdomen which you have ordered. Urine has not yet begun flowing.

Shortly thereafter, results begin to pour in: the hemoglobin is 20 g/dl, white blood cell count is 8200/mm³, serum amylase is 1250 units/dl and serum calcium is 5 mg/dl (normal is 10). The other electrolytes are unremarkable, as are the liver enzymes. Bilirubin, however, is 4 mg/dl with 2.5 mg direct. The ECG and chest x-ray are normal.

The film of the abdomen shows several distended loops of small and large bowel, no air-fluid levels, and no free air under the diaphragm. You do not quite see it, but the radiology resident points out a loop of small bowel in the midabdomen and the fact that there is no gas beyond the midtransverse colon; he calls these a "sentinel loop" and a "colon cutoff sign."

LOGIC　　Things have fallen into place. The serum amylase, along with a different clinical picture, would not diagnose pancreatitis, since other diseases can elevate the amylase; but in this instance it does. It is a severe case, as evidenced by the degree of hemoconcentration and the hypocalcemia. Hemoconcentration results from decreased intravascular fluid; lowered serum calcium is caused by binding of calcium to saponified fats in the abdominal wall and retroperitoneal tissue, although recent studies cast doubt on this mechanism. The mild hyperbilirubinemia probably results from an inflamed head of the pancreas and partial obstruction of the common bile duct. You decide not to scan the pancreas because computed tomography is not very helpful in acute pancreatitis and the diagnosis is already reasonably certain.

This brings us to a consideration of etiology. Does he have pancreatitis secondary to biliary tract disease (unusual in the male), or is it due to alcohol abuse? You will eventually visualize the gallbladder, but it is not essential that you do so right now. The initial treatment is identical for either type of pancreatitis. To rule out biliary tract disease a sonogram is the procedure of choice; it is at least 95% sensitive for stones in the gallbladder. But even before doing this simple, noninvasive, cheap, and highly reliable test, you rethink the history. As you ponder the question of when to get the sonogram, you realize that you did not ask about alcohol intake.

DATA　　The patient says that he drinks only socially and usually in moderation. You wonder if he indeed has biliary tract disease, but at that point his wife calls you aside: "Doctor," she says, "he drinks at least two fifths of whiskey every week. I wish you

would get him to stop." "Madam, I will try," you respond.

QUESTIONS

1. Several pathologic entities are listed in the numbered column. In the lettered column, descriptions of different types of pain are listed. Match the pain descriptions with the diagnoses.

(1) acute myocardial infarct

(2) pulmonary embolus to a lower lobe

(3) perforated peptic ulcer

(4) penetrated peptic ulcer

(5) acute pancreatitis

(6) mesenteric artery occlusion

(7) biliary colic

(8) acute rupture of the lower esophagus

(a) colicky pain in the right upper quadrant of the abdomen, nausea, and vomiting

(b) cyclic epigastric pain relieved by meals, that changes to constant pain radiating to the back, unrelieved by meals

(c) crushing type epigastric pain, radiating to the left arm

(d) sudden severe epigastric pain following repeated vomiting

(e) epigastric pain of sudden onset, aggravated by deep breathing, in a patient immobilized in bed for a hip fracture

(f) generalized constant abdominal pain in a 78-year-old man, 5 days after a myocardial infarct.

(g) constant epigastric pain radiating to the back in an alcoholic patient who just had a heavy meal

(h) generalized abdominal pain of sudden onset in a patient with chronic indigestion

2. Assume we have the same patient as the one discussed in this case presentation. The history and physical findings are the same, except that he has had pain for only 6 hours and his blood pressure is normal. The laboratory values are: hemoglobin 16; white blood cell count 8200; serum amylase 180 units; serum calcium 8 mg; bilirubin 1.2 mg. These values in such a

patient:
(a) rule out pancreatitis
(b) are nondiagnostic, thus suggesting the need for exploratory laparotomy
(c) are nondiagnostic, thus suggesting the need for further observation and additional tests
(d) confirm the presence of early pancreatitis.

3. Given a history and physical findings identical to those described in the case presentation, but of 48 hours' duration instead of 12 hours, what would be the significance of a serum amylase of 180?
(a) It would rule out pancreatitis.
(b) It would be nondiagnostic, indicating the need for exploratory laparotomy.
(c) It would be nondiagnostic, indicating the need for an additional test.
(d) It would confirm the diagnosis of acute pancreatitis.

4. A 43-year-old man has severe, constant, generalized abdominal pain of sudden onset and of 6 hours' duration. He lies quietly in the supine position, perspiring profusely. He is in shock and has a rigid silent abdomen. There is free air under the diaphragm in an upright film of the abdomen. What significance does a serum amylase of 1250 have in this case?
(a) It confirms a diagnosis of acute pancreatitis.
(b) It suggests that a duodenal ulcer has penetrated into the pancreas.
(c) It suggests that gas-forming organisms have produced acute suppurative pancreatitis.
(d) none of the above.

5. A 56-year-old obese woman sees you for acute severe epigastric pain and vomiting on and off for 24 hours. She does not drink alcohol, but smokes one pack daily and has diabetes mellitus. Over the past 2 years she has had similar though much milder episodes. Examination shows tenderness and mild rigidity in the epigastrium and right upper quadrant. The temperature is 38.3 C and no jaundice is visible. Which of the following is correct?
(a) The negative alcohol history rules out pancreatitis.
(b) Perforated peptic ulcer is likely and a gastrointestinal x-ray series is indicated.
(c) Acute cholecystitis is likely and a DISIDA scan is apt to clinch the diagnosis.
(d) Acute cholecystitis is unlikely because there is no jaundice.
(e) An ultrasound study that shows gallstones makes the diagnosis of acute cholecystitis certain.

ANSWERS

1. (1–c), (2–e), (3–h), (4–b), (5–g), (6–f), (7–a), (8–d).

2. **(c) is correct.** The clinical picture is very suggestive of pancreatitis, even if limited to a duration of 6 hours. A normal serum amylase early in the course of the disease does not rule out its presence; it may take several more hours for the values to go up. Because of the relatively localized and mild degree of signs of peritoneal irritation, it would be safe to initiate conservative medical management (fluid replacement, nasogastric suction) and repeat the tests several hours later. This short period of observation would also allow collection of urine for a 2-hour urinary amylase—another valuable test to diagnose or rule out pancreatitis. Only if repeated determinations continue to show normal serum amylases and the urinary values are normal, or if the clinical signs become worse, might an exploratory laparotomy be needed.

3. **(c) is correct.** Elevation of the serum amylase occurs early in the disease, although it can be missed in the first few hours. It also disappears early—in about 1 or 2 days. This patient could have had elevated values before he was seen and tested. If he had been under observation for 48 hours and multiple tests had persistently shown normal values, the diagnosis would be ruled out. But if first seen at 48 hours, your best test would be the urine amylase. It rises a bit more slowly than the serum amylase, but it stays elevated for a longer time. If that is negative, you may have to look inside the abdomen. If pancreatitis is found, the exploration per se does not add to its morbidity or mortality.

4. **(d) is correct.** The description is classical for a perforated hollow viscus, and a perforated ulcer would be the most likely possibility. An elevated serum amylase is not pathognomonic of acute pancreatitis; it can occur in other acute abdominal conditions, including a perforated duodenal ulcer. A penetrated ulcer does not produce the acute abdomen described in this question. There is no need to invoke the pancreas to explain the high serum amylase. This case is one where the clinical picture vastly outranks other findings in making a correct diagnosis.

5. **(c) is correct.** Pancreatitis can occur in teetotalers. Barium x-rays are certainly not indicated for possible perforation on an ulcer; an upright film for free subphrenic air should be obtained. Jaundice is present if the common bile duct is obstructed or if there is extensive inflammation, but its absence certainly does not exclude cholecystitis. Both (c) and (e) are correct, but (c) is more correct. The presence of gallstones does not guarantee that the acute episode is related since stones are so common in obese middle-aged diabetic women. The DISIDA isotope scan is considered most help-

ful; if no radioactivity is promptly detectable over the gallbladder, the cystic duct must be obstructed by stone, inflammation, or both. In doubtful cases, (c) and (e) might be considered equally correct. If a patient has repeated episodes of right upper quadrant pain and you are seeing her between episodes or when the picture is not acute, ultrasound imaging is the procedure of choice.

COMMENT An upper abdominal catastrophe requires a quick direct approach. You cannot spend the time required for a complete data base. Anatomically we are dealing with the upper abdomen and its contents. A cluster of pain, vomiting, and shock makes a recognizable pattern of fairly typical acute pancreatitis. The other possibilities quickly pass through your mind and you rule them out, proving pancreatitis most likely by a series of well-chosen questions and a brief localized examination. The conclusive studies are the markedly elevated serum amylase, low calcium, and absence of air under the diaphragm. Probability theory may be invoked to predict the presence of pancreatitis in an alcoholic. Sequence of events (pain preceding emesis) was considered to rule out a perforated esophagus. The reliability, specificity, and sensitivity of the serum amylase were detailed in several examination questions.

The author has taken you into the inner recesses of his mind and told you the multitude of thoughts he experienced in seconds. He would have no doubt solved this problem in the time it took you to read the first paragraph. An acute upper abdomen plus shock in a boozer would mean acute pancreatitis—"nine times out of ten"; then a few tests to confirm the hypothesis. (*P. C.*)

Suggested Readings

Author's Note: Patients do not present to a physician with a diagnosis of acute pancreatitis or any of the other acute abdominal conditions. They present with severe abdominal pain. Although our example turned out to

be pancreatitis, one cannot diagnose the latter without an understanding of the acute abdomen as a diagnostic challenge. As of the mid-1980s, we are still handling the acute abdomen in the same manner as we have for the past 50 years. It is primarily a clinical diagnosis which is helped by laboratory and x-ray studies, but in which there has not been a single spectacular diagnostic breakthrough. One is needed. In an era when hormonal assays, sonograms, and computed tomographic scans have given us great diagnostic accuracy in many conditions, we still accept with equanimity negative exploratory laparotomies for what was clinically believed to be an acute abdomen. Worse yet, because those negative explorations hound us, there is the occasional patient who is not operated on until it is too late and the signs are painfully obvious for everyone to see. Until the day arrives when nuclear magnetic resonance, positron emission tomography, or some exotic procedure tells us exactly what is happening inside the painful abdomen, we can only refer you to readings that summarize the diagnosis of the acute abdomen. (*C. P.*)

1. Beal JM: The acute abdomen. In Sabiston DC Jr (ed): *Davis-Christopher's Textbook of Surgery.* Philadelphia, Saunders. 1981, pp 875–895.
   This is the most concise yet complete description of the acute abdomen to be found in current textbooks.
2. Cope Z: *The Early Diagnosis of the Acute Abdomen.* New York, Oxford University Press, 1963.
   A standard classical monograph on the early diagnosis of the acute abdomen.
3. Gardner B: Acute abdominal pain. In Polk HC Jr, Stone HH, Gardner B (eds): *Basic Surgery,* ed 2. Norwalk, CT, Appleton-Century-Crofts, 1983, pp 319–352.
   This book approaches the problem from a patient presentation standpoint rather than from traditional organ disease discussions.
4. Nardi GL: The pancreas. In Hardy JD (ed). *Textbook of Surgery,* ed 6. Philadelphia, Lippincott, 1983, pp 679–702.
   Acute pancreatitis is very well covered here.
5. Leclerc P, Forest J-C: Variations in amylase isoenzymes and lipase during acute pancreatitis and in other disorders causing hyperamylasemia. *Clin Chem* 29:1020–1023, 1983.
6. Neff CC, Ferrucci JT Jr: Pancreatitis. *Surg Clin North Am* 64:23–36, 1984.
   Do ultrasound and CT really help?

Case 33
Diarrhea and Weight Loss
ELLIOT WESER, M.D.

DATA Watery, nonbloody, non-mucus-producing diarrhea brings a 48-year-old man to your office. Though these symptoms have been present for 12 years, they got worse especially over the past 2 years. He now has

several stools daily and gets up at night to go to the toilet. The diarrhea is accompanied by abdominal cramps, excessive flatulence, and loud noises in the abdomen. During the past 2 years he has lost 20 lb. Several physicians told him he had a "nervous colon" and one had a barium enema performed, which was normal. Otherwise he has always been well.

LOGIC You react with surprise and disbelief that such severe symptoms could possibly be considered functional, especially with weight loss. Many organic diseases characterized by chronic diarrhea come out of your memory tape: (*a*) parasitic diseases such as amebiasis, giardiasis, strongyloidiasis; (*b*) primary small or large bowel disease such as regional enteritis, ulcerative colitis, and tuberculosis; and (*c*) an endocrine-induced diarrhea caused by hyperthyroidism, gastrinoma, carcinoid, or diabetes.

The absence of gross blood in the stool makes a mucosal ulcerating disease such as ulcerative colitis unlikely, and the chronicity is against a bacterial dysentery. Cancer is unlikely in view of the 12-year illness, unless cancer of the colon was more recently superimposed on another chronic diarrheal disease. It is important to consider a malabsorption disorder since there has been recent documented weight loss. The cramping and borborygmi indicate increased peristalsis and therefore disease of the small intestine.

DATA The stools are bulky, frothy, float, and smell foul. Despite other symptoms, the patient's appetite is excellent and food intake remains normal. He drinks no coffee or alcohol and takes no laxatives.

Examination shows normal vital signs, evidence of weight loss, scattered ecchymoses of the skin, cracking at the corners of the mouth (cheilosis), a smooth red tongue, and a protuberant abdomen with increased bowel sounds. There is no tenderness or organ enlargement in the abdomen. Moderate pretibial and ankle edema are present. All else, including proctosigmoidoscopy, is normal.

LOGIC Normal sigmoidoscopy makes ulcerative colitis and amebiasis unlikely since these diseases usually involve the rectum and sigmoid. However, the rectum may be spared in Crohn's disease of the colon or

regional enteritis in the gastrointestinal tract since skip areas are common.

The character of the stools almost certainly indicates that the patient has steatorrhea and malabsorption. Fat and fermentation gas entrapped in the stool give it the observed appearance with a density less than water.

Excellent appetite in the face of weight loss and diarrhea implies that calories are either not being absorbed (malabsorption) or are being readily used (hyperthyroidism). But the latter is unlikely in the absence of common corroborative symptoms and the usual physical findings.

Ecchymoses suggest a clotting defect such as hypoprothrombinemia resulting from fat-soluble vitamin K deficiency. The cheilosis and smooth tongue indicate vitamin B complex deficiency, and the edema is compatible with hypoproteinemia.

Malabsorption seems likely. The causes include intestinal lymphoma, regional enteritis, celiac sprue, severe liver disease, bacterial overgrowth in the small intestine (blind loop syndrome), Whipple's disease, intestinal lymphangiectasia, and chronic pancreatic insufficiency. The absence of fever, abdominal mass, or specific tenderness reduces the likelihood of regional enteritis and lymphoma. There are no stigmata of liver disease. Tests are needed to corroborate malnutrition and malabsorption. As we proceed, it is important to distinguish between digestion and absorption, since an increased loss of nutrients in the stool can reflect a disorder of either process.

Digestion begins in the mouth and stomach (pepsin), but occurs mainly in the upper small intestine (SI) under the influence of the pancreas (lipase, amylase, trypsin) and small intestinal cells (disaccharidases). The sites where various nutrients are absorbed are: iron, calcium, water-soluble vitamins, and fats in the proximal SI; hexose sugars in the proximal and mid-SI; amino acids all over the SI but mainly in the mid-SI; bile salts and B_{12} mostly in the distal SI; and water and electrolytes in the proximal colon.

DATA Blood count shows a mild anemia

(hematocrit 35%, hemoglobin 10 g/dl) with a nondiagnostic blood smear. Serum potassium is low (2.8 mEq/liter); thyroid function (T_4 and T_3 resin uptake) is normal; serum calcium is low (7.8 mg/dl); total protein is low (5.1 g/dl) with a low albumin (2.2 g/dl); liver function tests are normal except for the prothrombin time (22 seconds: control 12 seconds); serum cholesterol is reduced (96 mg/dl), as are the carotene (18 μg/dl) and triglycerides (42 mg/dl). Blood glucose, 5-hydroxyindoleacetic acid in the urine, and serum gastrin are normal.

The chest x-ray is normal. Upper gastrointestinal and small bowel x-ray series show moderate diffuse dilatation of the small bowel and thickened folds, compatible with a malabsorption pattern; pancreatic calcifications and narrowing of the ileum are not present. Barium enema is normal. An intermediate strength purified protein derivative skin test is negative. The stool is negative for ova, parasites, and blood (Hemoccult test).

LOGIC These tests substantiate malnutrition and suggest but do not absolutely document malabsorption or indicate its cause. Diabetic autonomic neuropathy, carcinoid, and gastrinoma are now unlikely. Low potassium may result from chronic diarrheal loss. The other low blood chemistry values are related to depleted lipid and nitrogen stores caused by poor fat and protein absorption. Protein may also be lost by "weeping" of albumin into the intestinal lumen through a damaged mucosa. The low total serum calcium may be caused by decreased binding to reduced serum albumin and a decrease in ionized serum calcium from reduced absorption. Calcium malabsorption is the result of two factors: binding of calcium to malabsorbed fatty acids, and vitamin D deficiency caused by this vitamin's fat solubility and subsequent poor absorption. Tetany may result.

Fat-soluble vitamins (A, D, and K) are poorly absorbed and cause the low carotene and low prothrombin. B complex deficiency accounts for the tongue and cheilosis, though B_{12} malabsorption can smooth the tongue too. Anemia can result from poor

absorption of iron, B_{12}, or folic acid and its cause needs clarification with more studies.

The x-rays do not show changes characteristic of regional enteritis, ulcerative colitis, or any abnormality of the gastrointestinal tract that might indicate bowel stasis and bacterial overgrowth (multiple diverticula, fistulas, or blind loop). There are no pancreatic calcifications, epigastric pain, history of alcoholism, or episodes of acute pancreatitis to suggest chronic pancreatitis and pancreatic insufficiency. The normal chest x-ray and negative purified protein derivative skin test make intestinal tuberculosis unlikely. Intestinal parasites are excluded by the stool study.

It is important to exclude cirrhosis and chronic pancreatitis even though they are uncommon causes of maldigestion and consequent malabsorption.

If, contrary to the stated data, the patient drinks much alcohol and has epigastric pains, diabetes, severe steatorrhea, and pancreatic calcifications, marked deficiency of exocrine pancreatic function is your first diagnostic consideration. Such an obvious instance needs no further tests. But in doubtful, on-the-fence cases, you might wish confirmation. The *secretin* test measures duodenal fluid and bicarbonate after intravenous secretin. The *combined secretin-cholecystokinin* test measures intraluminal duodenal amylase, lipase, trypsin, and chymotrypsin after an intravenous infusion of the secretagogue. Or you can simply measure the *fecal chymotrypsin* content.

If the liver size and feel are normal and there are no stigmata of chronic severe liver disease, the liver may be virtually eliminated as the cause of malabsorption. When severe liver disease is clearly evident by history and physical examination, another cause for malabsorption may still be present and must be sought.

DATA A *d*-xylose absorption test (25-g oral dose) reveals a low urinary excretion of 2.3 g (9.2%). The 3-day fecal fat excretion is increased and averages 16 g/day (16% of daily fat intake). A pancreatic secretin stimulation test indicates normal pancreatic function.

Finally, a peroral jejunal biopsy is performed. It shows histologic evidence of total atrophy of the intestinal villi with a dense infiltrate of lymphocytes and plasma cells in the lamina propria. Celiac sprue is diagnosed and the patient is treated with a strict gluten-free diet. Within 2 weeks his diarrhea gradually subsides, he gains 20 lb during the next 6 months, and a repeat jejunal biopsy 1 year later is normal.

LOGIC Tests clearly demonstrate generalized malabsorption involving fat, protein, carbohydrate, vitamins, and calcium. It is important to reemphasize that malabsorption may be caused by maldigestion (pancreatic disease, inadequate bile salts, or lack of intestinal enzymes due to organic intestinal disease). But digestion may be normal yet malabsorption occur as a result of a small bowel disease where mucosal transport is affected.

The small intestinal biopsy shows specific changes in celiac sprue, Whipple's disease, intestinal lymphangiectasia, and abetalipoproteinemia (acanthocytosis). In this patient, the clinical and laboratory evidence of malabsorption, the characteristic changes on biopsy, and improvement on a gluten-free diet establish the diagnosis with certainty.

While general malabsorption exists in this case, it is possible to have a disorder in which there is malabsorption of a specific nutrient such as lactose in primary lactase deficiency, B_{12} deficiency in the blind loop syndrome where bacterial overgrowth utilizes the vitamin, and glucose or galactose malabsorption in monosaccharide transport carrier deficiency. Even some celiac sprue patients can present with isolated abnormalities which do not initially suggest sprue. For example, iron deficiency anemia, hypoprothrombinemic bleeding, or bone pain with demineralization may each be the presenting picture due to malabsorption of either iron, vitamin K, or calcium—yet no diarrhea or overt steatorrhea be present.

QUESTIONS

1. Steatorrhea may occur in all but one of the following:
   (a) isolated lactase deficiency
   (b) severe liver disease
   (c) a patient with chronic abdominal pain, alcoholism, and mild diabetes
   (d) intestinal lymphoma.
2. A 38-year old juvenile-onset diabetic man has gastric surgery for severe peptic ulcer disease. Subsequently, he develops steatorrhea and weight loss in spite of a good appetite. Which of the following statements is/are correct?
   (a) Diabetes may be causing the problem.
   (b) Macrocytic anemia might be present.
   (c) He may have a "blind loop syndrome."
   (d) Gastrointestinal x-rays must be done.
3. Increased fecal fat excretion with a normal *d*-xylose test suggests:
   (a) celiac sprue
   (b) ulcerative colitis
   (c) diffuse intestinal lymphoma
   (d) pancreatic insufficiency.
4. Intestinal biopsy is particularly helpful in the diagnosis of:
   (a) regional enteritis
   (b) pancreatic insufficiency
   (c) intestinal lymphoma
   (d) celiac sprue.
5. You see a 30-year-old woman who has had bloody diarrhea and crampy abdominal pains for 3 weeks. She feels sick, has lost weight, has a fever (38.3 C), and the abdomen is slightly distended and diffusely tender. Inflammatory bowel disease is likely and you consider ulcerative colitis (UC) and Crohn's disease (CD) in that order. Knowing that there is considerable overlap in the clinical features of both diseases, you draw tentative conclusions from each of the following bits of information. Which conclusion is *wrong*?
   (a) Severe rectal tenesmus is present. This favors UC.
   (b) This episode was preceded by several years of recurrent right lower quadrant pain and fevers; once she was thought to be obstructed. This favors UC.
   (c) Proctosigmoidoscopy reveals intense inflammation of the rectum and sigmoid; biopsy shows no granulomas. This favors UC.
   (d) She has had aching joints and "eye" inflammations several times over the past year. This favors neither UC nor CD.
   (e) Suddenly her abdomen distends, bowel movements cease, and she appears critically ill. This favors UC.

ANSWERS

1. **(a) is correct.** Isolated lactase deficiency is a specific defect that impairs only the digestion (and thus the absorption) of lactose; fat digestion (hydrolysis) and fat absorption are not

affected. Severe liver disease can cause steator-rhea. Bile salts play a minor role in the digestion and absorption of fats. This is done by effecting the proper pH in the duodenum, by emulsifying fats and permitting pancreatic lipase to split them, and by forming mixed micelles of bile salts with split fats to facilitate absorption. These salts are made in the liver, secreted in bile, and resorbed in the ileum. Severe liver disease, bile duct obstruction, and failure to recycle bile salts can each cause steatorrhea and all of its by-products. Bile salts will not be recycled if there is severe ileal disease, ileal resection, or chelation with cholestyramine. In each of these events, bile salt depletion will occur and fat absorption will be decreased.

The patient in (c) probably has chronic pancreatitis, lipase deficiency, inability to digest fats, and thus malabsorption. Lymphoma may directly impair the mucosal transport of fat and bile salts.

2. **All are correct.** Diabetes can cause steatorrhea for many reasons: decreased motility with bacterial overgrowth, neuropathy, and accompanying exocrine pancreatic insufficiency, among others. The usual backdrop is a juvenile-onset, poorly controlled, diabetic man with other complications of diabetes also present.

Bacterial overgrowth in the small intestine may result in malabsorption. Decreased intestinal motility, postsurgical blind loops, fistulae, and multiple small intestinal diverticula create stasis which permits bacterial proliferation (blind loop syndrome). Bacteria deconjugate bile salts and thereby inhibit proper micelle formation. In so doing, they cause steatorrhea; but the bacteria utilize B_{12} and prevent its absorption too. This type of malabsorption then is characterized by steatorrhea, fat-soluble vitamin deficiencies, and macrocytic anemia; d-xylose absorption remains normal. X-rays will be helpful in discovering a blind loop or other abnormalities leading to stasis. Postgastrectomy patients develop malabsorption because of improper mixing of food with enzymes, as well as bacterial proliferation.

3. **(d) is correct.** Pancreatic insufficiency results in lipase deficiency which impairs the hydrolysis of fat and thus reduces its absorption. Intestinal mucosa function is usually normal, and therefore a d-xylose absorption test should also be normal. Celiac sprue and intestinal lymphoma are likely to have impaired mucosal transport and the d-xylose absorption test should be abnormal. Ulcerative colitis is a disease of the colon and does not affect absorption of fat or d-xylose.

4. **(d) is correct.** There are specific mucosal diseases which can be diagnosed by histologic examination. Celiac sprue is the most common, and a patient with malabsorption and typical histologic changes in the jejunal mucosa most likely has this disease. Pancreatitis does not alter the intestinal mucosa. In regional enteritis and lymphoma, the biopsy is not specific enough and you are moreover apt to miss the disease area.

5. **(b) is correct.** It doesn't fit UC, but does suggest CD. The inflammatory bowel disease issue compels you to read about the pithy subjects of *CD* and *UC*. Ulcerative colitis almost invariably involves the rectum as well as a portion of the colon; tenesmus is present and granuloma formation is absent. Crohn's disease is a granulomatous process affecting various areas of the gastrointestinal tract from top to bottom, but it is noteworthy for normal areas interspersed with diseased areas; mostly it affects the terminal ileum but can also affect the colon, thus mimicking UC. However, CD often presents after several years of intermittent right lower quadrant pain, fevers, and perianal fistulae—sometimes with intestinal obstruction. Both diseases may be accompanied by joint, eye, mouth, biliary tract, and skin inflammations. Toxic megacolon (e) is a calamitous complication of UC, but is rare in CD.

COMMENT　In a more traditional approach to solving this problem, the author gathers an orderly complete data base, verbalizing his thoughts and forming hypotheses all along the way.

Lists of diagnostic possibilities are formed several times—first for diarrhea, later for malabsorption. Diagnoses are eliminated one by one as the author collects pertinent negative data. Final diagnoses are reached by positive undeniable evidence. Malabsorption is proven by fairly specific and sensitive clues such as poor d-xylose absorption, steatorrhea, and avitaminoses. The jejunal biopsy and response to treatment establish celiac sprue as the cause for malabsorption in a way which leaves no room for false positivity. Reasons for the different presentations of malabsorption in general and sprue in particular are well explained.

This session is notable for the extensive use of many of the cause and effect relationships discussed in Chapter 4 (Figs. 4.1 to 4.11). Low calcium results from three causes: malabsorption of protein, calcium, and vitamin D. This in turn causes tetany. Steatorrhea can have three or more coacting causes in diabetes mellitus. A lack of bile salts (many causes) can bring about both maldigestion and malabsorption. The latter two relate to one effect: malnutrition. Furthermore, severe liver disease can result in a lack of bile salts, which in turn causes fat malabsorption via three separate paths: the failures to create a proper duodenal pH, to emulsify fats, and to form mixed micelles. Low serum protein results from loss through the mucosa and lack of absorption through the mucosa—two causes linked to one musosal disease. The *one cause-one effect* relationship is ubiquitous.

In this case study, pancreatic function tests might well have been bypassed and the small intestinal biopsy done first. You might also question the need for a 72-hour stool collection and analysis. It is neither pleasant nor practical, though it may be of assistance in borderline cases. Qualitative microscopic examination of a random stool for muscle fibers or Sudan III-stained fat may suffice (or be superfluous) if the sample is greasy to the naked eye. The three-stage Schilling test was not done. If needed, it determines whether B_{12} malabsorption results from lack of intrinsic factor, distal ileal disease, or bacterial overgrowth.

Diagnosis related groups and the intelligent thoughtful practice of medicine may very well turn out to be good partners in eliminating unnecessary tests, shortening hospital stays, and reducing health care costs. (*P. C.*)

Suggested Readings

1. Gray GM: Maldigestion and malabsorption: clinical manifestations and specific diagnosis. In Sleisenger MH, Fordtran JS (eds): *Gastrointestinal Diseases*, ed 3. Philadelphia, Saunders, 1983, pp 238–256.
   An excellent review of symptoms, signs, and diagnostic tests for malabsorption. Detailed analyses of separate subheadings are written by different authors:
   pp 1023–1030: blind loop syndrome
   pp 1030–1039: Whipple's disease
   pp 1040–1049: tropical sprue
   pp 1050–1068: celiac sprue
2. *Clin Gastroenterol* 21 (issue 2), May 1983.
   This entire issue is devoted to *malabsorption*. Its 17 articles (including one by the author of this case) cover all aspects of the problem: physiology, malabsorption of protein, fat, carbohydrate, calcium, and vitamins; blind loop syndrome, intestinal immunity, short gut, gluten enteropathy, parasitic causes, small bowel diseases (inflammatory and neoplastic), a diagnostic approach, small intestinal biopsy, and the use of breath tests.
3. Finlay JM, Hogarth J, Wightman KJR: A clinical evaluation of the *d*-xylose tolerance test. *Ann Intern Med* 61:411–422, 1964.
   This reference documents the clinical usefulness of the commonly used *d*-xylose absorption test in cases of malabsorption.
4. Trier JS: Diagnostic usefulness of small intestinal biopsy. *Viewpoint Dig Dis* 9:1–4, 1977.
   A review of the diagnostic specificity of small bowel biopsy with emphasis on histologic changes in selected small bowel diseases causing malabsorption.
5. Trier JS, Falchuk ZM: Celiac sprue and refractory sprue. *Gastroenterology* 75:307–316, 1978.
   A detailed clinical conference on pathogenesis, pathophysiology, and treatment of celiac sprue.
6. Goldstein F: Mechanisms of malabsorption and malnutrition in the blind loop syndrome. *Gastroenterology* 61:780–784, 1971.
   Good pathophysiologic review of malabsorption caused by bacterial overgrowth in the small bowel.
7. Kirsner JB, Shorter RG: Recent developments in "nonspecific" inflammatory bowel disease (2 parts). *N Engl J Med* 306:775–785, 837–845, 1982.
8. Crohn BB, Ginzberg L, Oppenheimer GD: Regional ileitis. A pathologic and clinical entity. *JAMA* 251:73–79, 1984.
   A landmark article first printed in *JAMA* Oct 15, 1936.

Case 34
Lower Abdominal Pain
ARTHUR S. McFEE, M.D., Ph.D.

DATA Brought to the emergency room by his father, an 8-year-old boy complains of abdominal pain which has been present for several days. The pain started in the middle of his abdomen and was like a "cramp." It settled in both lower quadrants and became steady and sharp but hard to localize; his right side seemed more uncomfortable.

More history reveals anorexia and nausea but no vomiting, and he has not felt like taking any food or water for 2 or 3 days. He has not had a bowel movement for 24 hours. Several of his bothers and sisters have recently been sick with gastrointestinal "flu" which they presumably contracted at school. Each had been ill for 2 to 3 days. Their illnesses were associated with nausea, vomiting, diarrhea, and persistent cramping pain relieved by the bowel movements.

This is the patient's third visit to the emergency room in 4 days. After brief examinations he was discharged at the first two visits with a diagnosis of viral gastroenteritis.

LOGIC   With this history and in this age group, you think primarily of acute appendicitis. Other possibilities merit some consideration too. A few very simple initial thoughts pertain. The character of the pain has changed. In the first few hours it was colicky and periumbilical, indicating a source of obstruction within the nerve distribution of the appendix and small bowel. As time passed, it became sharp and constant but poorly localized. The mechanisms causing the two types of pain are different; local irritation of the peritoneum followed obstruction of an organ. Tenderness should also be demonstrable in the area of suspected inflammation since it promptly follows the development of local peritoneal irritation. Presumably no such change occurred with the siblings who were ill.

Poor localization of the pain tends to steer you away from an immediate diagnosis of classical appendicitis. In addition, the fact that considerable acute bowel disease has been present among siblings is important.

The history gives two important additional clues regarding acute inflammatory disease of the gastrointestinal tract: nausea and anorexia. Each is a nonspecific symptom and is present in many diseases. Anorexia is, however, the single most common symptom seen in acute appendicitis. Its presence does not indicate the diagnosis, but its absence casts doubt.

The patient has not had a bowel movement in 24 hours. This finding is highly significant and does not support a diagnosis of the common gastrointestinal infectious disorders which as a group cause mucosal irritation and diarrhea.

The length of the history is important. Acute appendicitis is a short-lived process. Ordinarily, if untreated, rupture occurs 18 to 24 hours after its onset. Accordingly, after some days you must seek signs consistent with complicated or ruptured appendicitis.

The fact that this patient had been discharged from the emergency room prior to this visit underlines a very important consideration. After the first 24 hours, the clinical picture of right lower quadrant inflammatory disease, especially appendicitis, is usually not clear. It very frequently is not clear in the pediatric patient. Admission to the hospital for observation *by one doctor* would have been appropriate at either visit and would have led to a much more expeditious diagnosis. Observation over a period of time by a single individual is invaluable in defining the existence and nature of inflammatory intraabdominal problems.

DATA   A physical examination is done. The young boy is lying very quietly in bed and does not move much. He appears ill and has poor skin turgor and a dry mouth. Moderate tenderness is present in both lower abdominal quadrants. Bowel sounds are present. Point tenderness cannot be elicited at the junction of the lateral and middle thirds of a line joining the right anterior superior iliac spine and the umbilicus (McBurney's point). Neither forced hyperextension (psoas sign) nor forced external rotation (obturator sign) of the right thigh causes pain. No masses can be defined in the groins or femoral canals.

A rectal examination reveals an area of exquisite tenderness at the tip of the examining finger on the right side. A mass is felt in this area and the central portion is distinctly soft. No stool is present in the rectal vault.

LOGIC   The physical examination is most significant. The patient with peritonitis tends to lie quietly in bed. Motion and occasionally breathing hurt. The demonstration of localized point tenderness within the pelvis on the right side indicates an inflammatory lesion in this area. The presence of a mass with a softened center suggests a fluctuant abscess. In a young male patient with such a history for over 24 hours, the diagnosis of a ruptured appendix must be strongly considered.

Constipation and the absence of stool in the rectum tend to confirm an acute perirectal inflammation with a segmental ileus at that point. Bowel sounds are present and indicate that the inflammatory process has been quite efficiently walled away in the pelvis and has not caused diffuse peritonitis and ileus. Dehydration accounts for the general appearance of the patient since he has neither eaten nor drunk well for 2 to 3 days.

This examination is most helpful in ruling out alternate considerations. The patient with ureteral colic ordinarily does not have peritoneal irritation; he may seek a comfortable position and thrash about in bed. Furthermore, his pain is persistently colicky, does not localize, tends to radiate downward, and is often accompanied by urinary frequency and hematuria.

A tender palpable mass in the groin would indicate an inguinal or femoral hernia with obstruction and strangulation as the source of the problem. In either case obstructive symptoms of nausea, vomiting, and cramps would precede the development of sharply localized peritoneal signs in the hernia sac.

For this patient to have "classical" appendicitis, one would expect to find well-localized right lower quadrant tenderness in keeping with the peritoneal irritation in that area. The localized point tenderness is now in the pelvis. Nevertheless, it is regarded, as in other areas, as the single most important sign confirming the presence of intraabdominal acute inflammation. In simple uncomplicated acute appendicitis in the right lower quadrant, tenderness is most often localized at McBurney's point. After rupture, it overlies the abscess which has formed. This sign may be difficult to demonstrate depending on the location of the abscess, but its importance as an indicator of intraabdominal inflammation cannot be minimized.

DATA Final studies are done and include: a normal chest film, flat and upright abdominal films which reveal a 6- to 8-cm air-filled loop of ileum in the right lower quadrant, hemoglobin 16.5 g/100 ml, hematocrit 49%, 20,000 white blood cells (WBCs) with 79% polymorphonuclear leukocytes, and a urinalysis with 15 red blood cells and 10 WBCs/high-power field. The temperature is 38.8 C.

LOGIC The additional information confirms an acute inflammatory process in the right lower quadrant (elevated WBC count, fever, and sentinel ileal loop). The term sentinel loop refers to a single area of small or large bowel distended with gas. It signifies that peristalsis is deficient or absent at this point, and gas, which normally does not collect sufficiently to cause distension, is delayed in its passage. It signals the presence of an adjacent inflammatory process.

Pyuria and hematuria suggest a urinary tract disorder but do not exclude appendicitis. These urine abnormalities may result from inflammation adjacent to the bladder or ureter and may indeed be seen as a result of appendicitis itself. The elevated hemoglobin and hematocrit indicate hemoconcentration and dehydration.

Since this patient is a young male, one need not consider sources of inflammation associated with the female pelvic genitalia. Those problems would include: ectopic pregnancy, pelvic inflammatory disease, tuboovarian abscess, and ovarian cysts with their complications of rupture or twisting.

One should not overlook other more obscure problems such as muscle strain in an active young male. A strain, while producing severe abdominal wall signs, is rarely associated with colic. A mass may even be present if an intramuscular or rectus sheath hematoma exists.

Acute appendicitis can produce a number of variations of the basic clinical signs. The appendix is a mobile, mesenteric organ and can reside in a 360° circle of rotation in several planes. Accordingly, right upper quadrant pain and tenderness (simulating cholecystitis), absence of right lower quadrant tenderness (retrocecal appendix), or the picture described here can be seen. In each, a sequence of colicky pain followed by peritoneal signs referable to the localization of the appendix is present. You must seek to demonstrate the local tenderness in the area where the appendix might lie.

Some diseases of the ileum and right colon mimic appendicitis and are often indistinguishable except at the operating table. Right colon diverticulitis, Crohn's disease of the ileum, cecal ulceration, perforating cecal carcinoma, appendiceal obstruction by cecal carcinoma, and appendiceal carcinoid tumors are examples. In the foregoing diseases, with the exception of those which cause appendiceal obstruction, the element of periumbilical cramping may not be seen, and right lower quadrant pain is predominant. Almost all are associated with varying degrees of nausea and anorexia.

In the patient who seeks medical care late in the course of the disease, both the computed tomographic scan of the abdomen and ultrasound may be helpful. The computed tomographic scan may reveal an area of significantly decreased density that displaces adjacent structures and is suggestive of an abscess. The sonographic study may indicate a right lower quadrant or pelvic cystic structure which is also consistent with an abscess. *Neither study is used in the primary diagnosis of appendicitis.* Both may produce such information in the long-standing, neglected, or complicated patient. A gallium isotope scan is another procedure that may be useful in locating an occult abscess.

At the extremes of age—in the very young and the very old—appendicitis is a very difficult diagnosis to make because it is not suspected and demonstrates few localizing signs. In the pediatric patient, fever is common early in the course of the disease and the history is that of an "upset stomach," possibly diarrhea, and poor feeding. In the older patient, fever is rarely seen without rupture. The physical examination in the pediatric patient may be very revealing, must be carefully and gently done, and may be the only means of securing a diagnosis. In the aged patient, physical signs and complaints may be few until a well-established abscess is present and sepsis has occurred. It

must therefore be a diagnosis of suspicion in everyone without clear findings who has not had an appendectomy.

A history of multiple visits to the emergency room with the innocuous diagnosis of viral gastroenteritis should raise the suspicion of some other inflammatory disease. Ordinarily, the diagnosis of gastroenteritis in these instances is supported by the presence of diarrhea along with cramping, nausea, and vomiting. More important, this type of problem is usually limited to 2 or 3 days; the more severe inflammatory diseases are not.

The value of repeated examinations *by a single individual* for the patient in whom the diagnosis is initially uncertain cannot be overemphasized. Admission to the hospital or emergency room observation ward is easily effected and a diagnosis is ordinarily clear within 8 to 12 hours. In our patient, by all odds, the best consideration is a ruptured pelvic appendicitis with abscess formation.

DATA This was confirmed at the operating table.

QUESTIONS

1. A 38-year-old woman has had severe, crampy right lower quadrant pains for several days. They are getting progressively worse. There was no preceding epigastric or periumbilical pain, significant fever, or anorexia. She has had a similar episode in the past. Each of the following is possible except one:
   (a) T 38.8 C, tender right lower quadrant, diarrhea, and anal fistula
   (b) physical examination normal, 20 red blood cells/high-power field in urine
   (c) acute appendicitis, even if there is no anorexia and the temperature is normal
   (d) a small tender mass in the right inguinal area.
2. You elicit a history of severe left lower quadrant pain for 2 days in a 48-year-old woman. The pain is constant, there is marked tenderness, the temperature is 38.3 C, and the WBC count is 18,500 with 86% polymorphonuclear leukocytes. Rectal and pelvic examinations are refused. Which of the following is possible?
   (a) acute diverticulitis
   (b) acute appendicitis
   (c) torsion of an ovarian cyst
   (d) peridiverticular abscess.

3. The most sensitive clue in the diagnosis of acute appendicitis is:
   (a) tenderness over McBurney's point
   (b) leukocytosis
   (c) right lower quadrant pain
   (d) anorexia.
4. The most specific clue in the diagnosis of acute appendicitis is:
   (a) tenderness over McBurney's point
   (b) leukocytosis
   (c) right lower quadrant pain
   (d) anorexia.
5. You see a 42-year-old woman who seems to have a classical case of acute appendicitis. She has been sick for 12 hours, leukocytosis is present, urinalysis is normal, the temperature is 37.7 C, and the rectal and pelvic examinations are normal. She has a 3-inch distorted right lower quadrant scar. An operation was performed at age 22, 2 years after her marriage. She does not know exactly what was done but thinks her appendix may have been removed. Drainage and healing took 6 weeks. Her parents and relatives are dead or unavailable. She has been in excellent health. You should:
   (a) perform prompt appendiceal exploration
   (b) observe for 24 to 48 hours
   (c) obtain old hospital records
   (d) do complete barium x-ray studies of upper and lower gastrointestinal tracts

ANSWERS

1. **(c) is correct.** Acute appendicitis is unlikely in the presence of crampy pain for several days; there was no preceding epigastric or periumbilical pain, and there is no fever or anorexia. By this time, fever would invariably be present. The others, however, are all distinct possibilities. (a) describes a patient with regional enteritis. The type of pain and hematuria (b) suggest a ureteral calculus. A tender inguinal mass with crampy pain (d) points to an incarcerated, possibly strangulating, hernia.
2. **All are correct.** Diverticulitis is most likely and presents in this manner. Appendicitis cannot be ruled out—the appendix may be on the left side (malrotation). Pelvic disease of various types can cause this picture. The inflamed diverticulum or, for that matter, the appendix may have already ruptured and resulted in an abscess.
3. **(d) is correct.** Anorexia is almost universally present, though it is nonspecific. Leukocytosis may not be present in the event of poor host response. McBurney's point is tender only if the appendix is in the classic location. Right lower quadrant pain may not be present if the appendix is ectopic, in the case of infants who

cannot give pain descriptions, or in the aged who may overlook or fail to appreciate pain.
4. **(a) is correct.** The classically located inflamed appendix gives point tenderness at McBurney's point. Leukocytosis is very nonspecific. So is anorexia. Right lower quadrant pain can be caused by a host of illnesses. Questions 3 and 4 show the difference between clue specificity and clue sensitivity.
5. **(a) is correct.** This is a judgment decision. Were it not for the old scar there would be no decision to make. But the scar could represent drainage of an appendiceal abscess or some other operation and the appendix might have been left intact (not ordinarily done today). Twenty-year-old hospital records are not usually obtainable. X-ray studies take time and offer little. Regional ileitis may be suspected by upper gastrointestinal x-rays, but if surgery must be done anyway, this can be confirmed on the table with very little added risk. Observation for 24 to 48 hours is risky and may result in perforation with abscess formation. But observation for 8 to 10 hours permits a more firm distinction between nonspecific abdominal pain and acute appendicitis, and therefore some physicians might prefer to observe the patient for several hours. Her health is good and a surgical disease, probably appendicitis, is likely. The risk of surgery is small compared to the risk of doing nothing.

COMMENT This was *not* a textbook case of acute appendicitis, for typical cases hardly exist anymore. Many clues in the data base make you think of other possibilities—"flu" in the family, pain in *both* lower quadrants, earlier "viral gastroenteritis," absence of tenderness over McBurney's point, and an abnormal urinalysis.

Consideration was given to Crohn's disease, ureteral calculus, and viral gastroenteritis. In other age and gender subsets, such a presentation might include a consideration of colon cancer with perforation, urinary tract infection, diverticulitis, pelvic inflammatory disease, etc.

The author of this case led you gently from one bit of evidence to another and rendered a clear exposition of his logic as he reached a conclusion. Further expansion of the clinical reasoning process is found in the mini-cases (questions and answers). (*P. C.*)

Suggested Readings

1. Fitz RH: Perforating inflammation of the vermiform appendix with special reference to its early diagnosis and treatment. *Trans Assoc Am Phys Phil* 1:107, 1886. Reprinted in *Medical Classics* 2:459. Baltimore, Williams & Wilkins, 1937–1938.
   Our knowledge of the pathology of appendicitis

dates from the publication of this classic study in which the concept of typhlitis was laid to rest.

2. Condon RE: Appendicitis. In Sabiston DC Jr (ed): *Davis-Christopher's Textbook of Surgery: The Biological Basis of Modern Surgical Practice*, ed 12. Philadelphia, Saunders, 1981, pp 1048–1063.

    A standard surgical textbook description of all forms of appendicitis. The controversial issue of the incidental appendectomy is included.

3. Law D, Law R, Eiseman B: The continuing challenge of acute and perforated appendicitis. *Am J Surg* 131:533–535, 1976.

    In a review of 216 patients, the authors present a logical decision tree for the management of acute appendicitis. Complications attendant on perforation are presented and analyzed.

4. Wangensteen OH, Dennis C: Experimental proof of obstructive origin of appendicitis in man. *Ann Surg* 110:629–647, 1939.

    The pathophysiology of the disease was first stated over 45 years ago—a classic experiment.

5. Beal JM: The acute abdomen: acute appendicitis. In Sabiston DC Jr (ed): *Davis-Christopher's Textbook of Surgery: The Biological Basis of Modern Surgical Practice*, ed 12. Philadelphia, Saunders, 1981, pp 887–889.

    A brief three-page description.

6. McFee AS, Hollimon PW, Dewan SR: Diagnosing appendicitis in the pediatric patient. *Infect Surg* 1:42–49, 1982.

    From the author's own institution, experience with 430 consecutive cases of pediatric appendicitis is presented.

7. Buchman TG, Zuidema GD: Reasons for the delay of the diagnosis of acute appendicitis. *Surg Gynecol Obstet* 158:260–266, 1984.

    Covers unusual presentations.

8. Edwards FH, Davies RS: Use of a Bayesian algorithm in the computer-assisted diagnosis of appendicitis. *Surg Gynecol Obstet* 158:219–222, 1984.

    Surgical diagnosis is modeled by statistical algorithms using a conditional probability matrix.

9. Teicher I, Landa B, Cohen M, et al: Scoring system to aid in diagnosis of appendicitis. *Ann Surg* 198:753–759, 1983.

    A system to avoid overdiagnosis and underdiagnosis.

10. Scott JH 3rd, Amin M, Harty JI: Abnormal urinalysis in appendicitis. *J Urol* 129:1015, 1983.

    Only 1 page, but worth reading.

Case 35
Black Stools

ERNEST URBAN, M.B.B.S.

DATA A 68-year-old retired police officer is brought to the hospital several hours after fainting while on the commode. He had passed a few, black, malodorous stools each day for the past 5 days; these were attributed to something he "must have eaten." He did feel a little lightheaded from time to time, and on the day of admission he actually passed out while again passing considerable black stool. The color was noted and verified by his son, who drove him to the emergency room several hours later.

On arrival, he felt weak and looked pale but had no other complaints. Nothing like this had ever happened before. The patient thought he was in excellent health and had no other symptoms, previous serious illnesses, or operations. He was taking no medications regularly.

LOGIC Before delving into the specific causes for such a presentation, you must concern yourself with two issues. First, how severe is the blood loss and how urgently is treatment needed? Second, is the bleeding from the upper or lower gastrointestinal (GI) tract?

DATA The vital signs are T 37 C, R 16, BP 130/80, pulse 104 and of good strength. The tilt test is negative. A nasogastric tube is gently passed into the stomach and the gastric aspirate is clear and negative for occult blood using Gastroccult. A stat hematocrit is 28%. Intravenous fluids are begun while the patient is being typed and cross-matched; blood is drawn for other studies too.

LOGIC Normal vital signs (with only a slightly rapid pulse) plus a negative tilt test suggest that the patient is not in immediate danger and that he has an adequate blood volume. This has no doubt been effected by a continual 5-day process of hemodilution whereby fluid is drawn from the extravascular tissue spaces into the vascular tree to make up for the loss of blood. Even during the few hours since the syncopal episode, the blood volume was sufficiently restored to make the tilt test negative. Treatment is moderately urgent since the hematocrit is below 30%, but the patient seems far from shock and not critical at the moment.

A tilt test is positive if the pulse rate increases more than 20 beats/minute or the systolic blood pressure drops more than 20 mm Hg when the patient is moved from the supine to a sitting position. It indicates significant acute blood volume loss, usually greater than 1000 ml in adults. The actual volume loss required for a positive tilt test will also depend on the ability of the patient's vascular system to respond with peripheral vasoconstriction.

The absence of blood from the gastric aspirate usually indicates that bleeding is not originating proximal to the ligament of Treitz. Rapid bleeding from a duodenal ulcer may reflux into the stomach, but slow bleeding may not. Tube trauma may cause blood in the gastric aspirate, so the tube must be passed gently.

Acute gastritis, a common cause of bleeding, is usually caused by drugs (notably aspirin) and alcohol. The patient takes neither, but the absence of blood in the stomach rules out bleeding from this site anyway.

DATA Further inquiry is not helpful. Apart from an appendectomy 50 years ago, there have been only minor upper respiratory infections. The patient smokes three packs of cigarettes/week, drinks a bottle of beer every few days, and has coffee once daily. About once a month he takes two aspirins for a headache and an occasional antacid for indigestion. There has been no persistent diarrhea, constipation, indigestion, nausea, anorexia, weight loss, or abdominal pain.

Physical examination is entirely normal except for pallor and black stool which is 4+ guaiac positive (dark blue-green with Hemoccult). The vital signs are now all normal,

the pulse having slowed to 90 beats/minute. There is no tenderness or masses in the abdomen and the liver is not enlarged.

LOGIC It is ordinarily important to test a black stool for blood. In this case, however, you may be sure that the black color was caused by blood because of the syncope, pallor, and odor of the stool. But in other cases, black stools may be caused by the ingestion of iron and bismuth medications and large quantities of spinach, licorice, green beets, and certain berries. It takes at least 5 to 10 ml of blood/day to make the stool positive 50% of the times with Hemoccult test, and 30 ml of blood/day results in 93% positive reactions. But it requires at least 60 ml, and more likely over 100 ml, to make the stool black.

The source of blood in the stool cannot always be determined by the color. Generally speaking, bleeding from the midtransverse colon down is red, and more proximal bleeding is black. But this varies with the amount of bleeding and the transit time of the blood. Massive upper GI bleeding can be black, purple, or red, depending on how long it takes to reach the rectum and whether there is enough time to permit bacterial action on the hemoglobin. Bright red rectal bleeding originating in the lower GI tract may come from polyps, cancer, diverticuli, angiodysplasias, or hemorrhoids. The latter three conditions are very common in older people and the presence of any one does not guarantee that it is the source of bleeding. A direct relationship must be established. The presence of only black stool does exclude blood loss from the descending colon down.

Consider too the facts that the absence of hematemesis and lack of abdominal pain do not exclude a bleeding duodenal ulcer, and that 60 to 70% of GI hemorrhages originate in the upper tract. Accordingly, the upper tract will be investigated first even though there was no blood in the stomach.

DATA Repeat hematocrit is 26%. The red blood cells (RBCs) are hypochromic and microcytic on the blood smear and by the determination of indices. Platelets are adequate and prothrombin time and partial thromboplastin time are normal. Two units of packed RBCs are given. Fiberoptic esophagogastroduodenoscopy is performed the next morning and no abnormal findings are noted. Proctosigmoidoscopy is also done to a full length of 25 cm. Nonbleeding internal hemorrhoids are seen, but the rectal mucosa is normal, and there are no polyps or other lesions visible. Black stool is present above the tip of the instrument.

LOGIC The small drop in hematocrit probably represents further hemodilution, though you must be alert for continued bleeding. Packed RBCs are given rather than whole blood because only the RBCs are needed and blood volume is adequate. Tests disclose no evidence of a bleeding disorder. Hypochromic microcytic anemia indicates that chronic blood loss has antedated the acute hemorrhage; therefore the bleeding lesion has existed for some time and blood loss had been occult.

Why was proctosigmoidoscopy done if the stools were black? The presence of only black stools without any red blood virtually excludes a distal lesion. But the rectum and sigmoid are the sites of 70% of large bowel malignancies; in about 5% of cases there is a synchronous lesion present elsewhere in the colon. That is why the patient could have a lower large bowel nonbleeding cancer in addition to some other colon lesion (malignant or benign) that is the source of the blood loss.

So far, the upper GI tract to the first or second portion of the duodenum and the terminal 25 cm of the GI tract are cleared of suspicion. The patient appears to have stopped bleeding, or he is bleeding only minimally.

DATA It is day number two. The vital signs are stable, and the hematocrit has stabilized at 32% after 2 units of packed RBCs. There have been no more bowel movements, so the material in the rectum is still black.

LOGIC What next? The choice lies between early angiography, barium studies, radioisotope scanning, or urgent colonoscopy. Angiography, if done, must be performed before barium studies; otherwise critical vascular detail may be obscured, and time must be allowed after barium studies for the GI tract to rid itself totally of barium. This can take days! Your patient is no longer bleeding rapidly, so angiographic material may not be seen pooling in the intestinal lumen after exuding from the yet undiscovered mucosal lesion. Blood loss of at least 5 ml/minute is necessary to visualize the bleeding site by angiography. A vascular malformation (including abnormal vasculature in a tumor) may, however, be seen. Angiography is a specialized procedure and is usually less readily available than barium studies. In this 68-year-old patient there is also an increased risk of dislodging an atheromatous plaque during cannulation of the aorta, the two mesenteric vessels, and celiac axis. Thus barium studies are commonly performed next.

Would you order a barium enema or an upper GI series with a small bowel follow-through as the next examination? A barium enema is the procedure of choice. The large bowel is the second most common site of blood loss after the upper GI tract and the latter site has already been eliminated. Common lesions include carcinoma, polyp, diverticular bleeding, bowel ischemia, and inflammatory bowel disease. The small bowel is an uncommon site of bleeding—vascular malformations, tumors such as leiomyomas and peptic ulceration in a Meckel's diverticulum being the most likely causes.

DATA A barium enema is performed. The bowel preparation was not good. The radiologist reports considerable stool residue; he is unable to obtain reflux of barium into the terminal ileum, but the examination in his opinion is otherwise grossly normal.

LOGIC What do you do now? It is impossible for the radiologist to distinguish a polyp from stool residue in the above study. Furthermore, the radiologist's inability to reflux barium into the terminal ileum (or fill the lumen of the appendix) indicates a degree of uncertainty that the entire cecum was filled and outlined with barium. Thus a mass lesion in the cecum could easily be missed.

Shall the study be repeated after better bowel preparation? No! An air contrast barium enema should be done. In fact, it should have been done in the first place. A small amount of thicker barium is followed by the injection of air into the colon. This distends the bowel and coats it with a thin layer of barium, giving superior mucosal detail.

DATA The bowel is properly prepared, and an air contrast barium enema produces excellent visualization of the entire colon. This time the study shows an irregular mass occupying the medial aspect of the lower cecal wall, highly suggestive of carcinoma.

LOGIC Carcinoma of the cecum is well known as a site of silent GI blood loss. Obstructive symptoms occur late, if at all, because ileal efflux is liquid. Lymphoma, ameboma, and tuberculoma are other cecal mass lesions. The last two are uncommon. Travel to an ameba-infested area might be a clue, and *Amoeba histolytica* serologic studies are indicated if this is suspected. Tuberculosis of the bowel is usually the result of swallowing infected sputum from pulmonary tuberculosis. He has no symptoms of any of these diseases.

The cecal lesion is most likely the source of this patient's blood loss. Because a malignancy is strongly suspected, bleeding is likely to worsen as the lesion grows. Surgical excision is indicated. However, before this is done, recall that in about 5% of cases of colon carcinoma there is a second synchronous lesion elsewhere in the colon. It may not have been detected on barium enema. Thus, colonoscopy with biopsy of any abnormal mucosa is desirable if the procedure is available.

DATA Colonoscopy is done; no additional lesions are found. Biopsy of the cecal mass

shows adenocarcinoma; the radiologic diagnosis is confirmed.

LOGIC An upper GI and small intestinal barium study is now considered unnecessary. Should the surgeon attempt a curative or palliative resection? The fundamental problem is the extent and spread of the lesion. The final decision will be made at surgery.

But a search must be made for metastatic spread before operation. This consists of a chest x-ray, liver function tests, and a computed tomographic liver scan. Unless disease is very extensive and far advanced, surgery will be performed for palliation of bleeding and prevention of obstruction even if a few metastases do exist. It is, however, very important to test the carcinoembryonic antigen titer; it is elevated in 70% of colon cancer cases. If positive, the success of surgery can be gauged and the patient can be subsequently observed for evidence of recurrence by repeated carcinoembryonic antigen tests.

DATA There were no indications of metastatic deposits. The patient is taken to surgery, and an ulcerating cecal carcinoma is found. A right hemicolectomy is performed with excision of a few centimeters of terminal ileum. The remaining distal ileum is anastomosed to the transverse colon. The liver appears uninvolved. Histologic examination of the resected specimen reveals adenocarcinoma; 5 of 29 lymph nodes are also positive for malignancy. After recovery from the surgery, an oncologist is asked to see the patient and advise on chemotherapy.

LOGIC The cause of bleeding was easily discovered in this case. But what if the colon x-ray were negative? Then a GI series with small intestinal follow-through might uncover a lesion missed on endoscopy or a lesion lower down such as a Meckel's diverticulum with ulceration or a benign small intestinal tumor. However, barium now beclouds the field and precludes arteriography if it is necessary.

Failing to locate the bleeding source, and

if the patient still evinces evidence of continued bleeding (positive stool, falling hematocrit), further steps are necessary. This brings to mind the entire scenario of what diagnostic sequence to follow for *any type* of GI bleeding—upper or lower, fast or slow, continuing or already stopped.

In hospital situations where all diagnostic modalities are available, it may be difficult to decide what to do first—endoscopy, contrast radiography, nuclear scintiscan, or arteriography. *The order must be tailored to the individual patient!* Consider the age, general health, rapidity of blood loss, hemodynamic status, and the likelihoods of upper vs lower GI bleeding.

Endoscopy is very good for upper GI lesions, cannot be done if bleeding is massive, and is not so helpful for colonic bleeding. Barium studies are good though less sensitive and give more information if bleeding has stopped. Scintiscan of the abdomen after the intravenous injection of ^{99m}Tc sulfur colloid, better yet ^{99m}Tc-labeled autologous RBCs, detects small pockets of radioactivity from blood loss as slow as 0.1 ml/minute. This technique locates the general area of bleeding but does not identify the lesion; it is not useful in upper GI bleeding where liver and spleen scintillation dominate the field. Selective arteriography may locate and define a lesion or at least demonstrate an intraluminal collection of dye. For example, an arteriovenous malformation or angiomatosis may be visualized; bleeding from an ulcer in a Meckel's diverticulum may be noted. However, if barium has already been given, arteriography is worthless until the field is clear—perhaps 3 or 4 days.

The present general consensus (*always subject to debate and change*) is:

1. Decide if bleeding is likely to be from the upper or lower GI tract on the basis of history, examination, and nasogastric tube aspiration.
2. If upper GI bleeding is likely, do endoscopy first, when the patient is stable. This procedure is 90% sensitive. For the rest, do arteriography if bleeding continues and barium studies if bleeding stops.
3. If lower GI bleeding is likely and the bleeding seems to have already stopped, do proctosigmoidoscopy followed by air contrast colonography, and then small bowel radiography (oral barium or enteroclysis).
4. If lower GI bleeding is likely and is continuing, do proctosigmoidoscopy followed by isotope scan if necessary. Arteriography may be helpful in conjunction with the scintiscan, especially if bleeding is severe.
5. Steps 3 and 4 localize the area of bleeding; may define the lesion; can suggest the need for interventional therapeutic radiologic procedures, colonoscopy, or repeat barium studies; or may guide the exploring surgeon.

But remember that since each case has unique features, a consensus of consultants may be needed to devise the diagnostic plan. The presence and quality of hardware and software are additional determining factors.

COMMENT   The author gives you a very clear insight into his thought processes and decision making. He aptly demonstrates the dynamics of problem solving. Note that the order of gathering data is altered by the semiurgency of the problem. First he assesses the need for urgent therapy and then performs endoscopy and gastric aspiration even before the results of routine studies are known, and before a detailed data base is obtained.

Actually, he has created his own decision tree, and followed a stepwise approach that could easily be transformed into a flow chart:

1. assess the hemodynamic status
2. begin treatment if needed
3. a few pertinent questions and a branched examination to consider or rule out possibilities
4. gastric aspiration to assess the possibility of upper GI bleeding
5. endoscopy
6. barium studies, isotope scan, or selective arteriography.

At any step in this decision tree, further pursuit may be halted if a diagnosis is reached.

The reliability of data obtained from tilting,

testing for occult blood, gastric aspiration, and color of the stool is carefully set forth. Also, the choice of further diagnostic procedures—such as endoscopy, conventional barium radiography, and angiography—vis-à-vis their sequence, sensitivity, risk, and reliability is discussed with clarity.

Probability theory is utilized. Once upper GI bleeding (especially peptic ulcer) is ruled out, carcinoma of the colon is the next most likely cause of melena in this age group. (*P. C.*)

Suggested Readings

1. Many of the suggested readings in **Case 30** are equally valuable for the study of this case too. They apply to lower as well as upper GI hemorrhage.
2. Schiff L: Hematemesis and melena. In Blacklow RS (ed): *MacBryde's Signs and Symptoms*, ed 6. Philadelphia, Lippincott, 1983, pp 393–421.
   A short chapter covering all causes and their diagnosis—very up-to-date.
3. Gupta S, Luna E, Kingsley S, et al: Detection of gastrointestinal bleeding by radionuclide scintigraphy. *Am J Gastroenterol* 79:26–31, 1984.
   The authors demonstrate high sensitivity and specificity using labeled red blood cells.
4. Winzelberg GG, Froelich JW, McKusick KA, et al: Scintigraphic detection of gastrointestinal bleeding: a review of current methods. *Am J Gastroenterol* 78:324–327, 1983.
   Especially good for bleeding from diverticuli.
5. Forde KA: Colonoscopy in the diagnosis and management of colonic bleeding. *Bull NY Acad Med* 59:301–305, 1983.
   Clarifies the roles of colonoscopy and arteriography.
6. Thoeni RF, Venbrux AC: The value of colonoscopy and double contrast barium enema examinations in the evaluation of patients with subacute and chronic lower intestinal bleeding. *Radiology* 146:603–607, 1983.
   Compares the relative merits of the two methods.
7. Eckstein MR, Athanasoulis CA: Gastrointestinal bleeding. An angiographic perspective. *Surg Clin North Am* 64:37–51, 1984.
   Ably describes the various diagnostic approaches and attempts to localize the bleeding site.
8. Winn M, Weissmann HS, Sprayregen S, et al: The radionuclide detection of lower gastrointestinal bleeding sites. *Clin Nucl Med* 8:389–395, 1983.
9. Pingleton SK: Gastrointestinal hemorrhage. *Med Clin North Am* 67:1215–1231, 1983.
10. Winawer SJ, Sherlock P: Malignant neoplasms of the small and large intestine. In Sleisenger MH, Fordtran JS (eds): *Gastrointestinal Diseases*, ed 3. Philadelphia, Saunders 1983, pp 1220–1249.
    The pathology and clinical features of colorectal cancer constitute the first 15 pages of Chapter 72.

Case 36
Jaundice and Pain
PAUL CUTLER, M.D.

DATA A 70-year-old woman who retired to Mexico 6 months ago returns to the United States because of nausea, vomiting, jaundice, and right upper quadrant pain for 1 week.

Her illness began with the gradual onset of anorexia and right upper quadrant discomfort, followed the next day by nausea and vomiting. By the third day her husband noted that her skin and eyes were slightly yellow, and she observed the urine getting dark and the stools becoming light. The pain got much worse and became a dull steady ache which seemed to wax and wane and did not radiate to the back or to anywhere else in the abdomen. On admission to the hospital she was still vomiting, could not eat, and was complaining of pain.

LOGIC The diagnostic possibilities in an elderly woman with jaundice and pain are many, but principal concern centers around whether this problem needs medical or surgical treatment.

The combination of jaundice, dark urine, and light stools tells you that obstruction to the flow of bile (*cholestasis*) exists. Your job is to determine whether the cause is *intrahepatic* (hepatocellular disease) or *extrahepatic* (stone, stricture, sclerosing cholangitis, cancer of the bile ducts, ampulla of Vater, or pancreas; or metastatic cancer to the porta hepatis from many possible primary sites). The mode of treatment depends on this important distinction; for if the patient has hepatitis or metastatic cancer to the liver, treatment is medical. If there is a removable or bypassable obstruction, the treatment is ultimately surgical.

The tenet that painless jaundice means cancer and painful jaundice means biliary tract stone is no longer reliable, because pain may be present or absent in either condition. Furthermore, hepatitis may be present with pain of variable degree and varying types. In general, though, colicky pain suggests bile duct obstruction by a stone, whereas a constant dull ache points more in the direction of hepatitis, cholecystitis, pancreatitis, or pancreatic carcinoma. In this case the pain is not clearly colicky nor is it constant, so that cancer, stone, and hepatitis all merit concern.

Even with the minimal history obtained so far, additional judgments can be made. Viral hepatitis is extremely common in Mexico and deserves strong consideration. Miliary tuberculosis and amebic abscess, while also frequent in Mexico, are less likely to cause prominent jaundice and severe pain. Gallbladder disease (acute cholecystitis with cholelithiasis) is common in this age group, regardless of the geography. Think of bile duct stricture if there has been previous surgery in the area.

Drug- or alcohol-induced hepatitis are additional considerations. Almost any drug may rarely cause hepatitis. But notorious in this regard are: anesthetics (halothane, chloroform); tranquilizers (phenothiazines, haloperidol, diazepam, chlordiazepoxide); antidepressants (iproniazid, tricyclics); anticonvulsants (phenytoin, carbamazepine); antiarthritics (gold, allopurinol, probenecid, nonsteroidal antiinflammatory drugs); all the hypoglycemics; antithyroidal drugs; some antimicrobials (clindamycin, isoniazid, rifampin, sulfonamides); cardiac drugs (methyldopa, quinidine); and most cancer chemotherapeutic agents.

Cancer always hovers in the background at this age. But a sudden onset of symptoms, the absence of weakness, weight loss, and anorexia, plus the absence of symptoms indicating a primary site would weigh against it.

DATA   Additional history reveals that the patient felt perfectly well until this episode. She ate well, slept well, and never had similar symptoms before. There were no prodromes of arthritis, arthralgia, pruritus, or urticaria (to suggest hepatitis B) nor had there been any change in bowel habit except for 2 weeks of nonbloody diarrhea shortly after arriving in Mexico. She had had no cough, sputum, hemoptysis, fever, or weight loss. The rest of the systems review was equally devoid of positive symptoms.

Past history indicated no previous surgery. She had had mild diabetes mellitus for 12 years, controlled by diet alone, and recent hypertension treated with hydrochlorothiazide; no other drugs have ever been taken. She smoked one pack of cigarettes daily until 10 years ago but gave up the habit as a result of widespread antismoking publicity, and she has been drinking one to two glasses of wine with supper nightly for the past 20 years. Otherwise she consumes no alcohol. Family history is negative for gallbladder disease, stone, or cancer, and nobody in her home or family was recently jaundiced. She eats no raw seafood and has had no injections or transfusions in the recent past. The patient is a successful artist, and her husband is an author.

LOGIC   The additional history is helpful in eliminating or discounting certain possibilities. Previous good health is against cancer. Drug hepatitis is unlikely since hydrochlorothiazide only rarely causes hepatitis. Alcohol consumption is very modest and chronic liver disease is unlikely. Viral hepatitis is rendered less likely by the absence of common prodromes and by the absence of factors such as eating raw shellfish, contact with jaundiced people, or a history of injections. The episode of severe diarrhea 6 months ago was probably infectious, though we do not know the cause, and amebiasis is always possible. There are no symptoms to suggest active pulmonary tuberculosis.

DATA Physical examination disclosed a somewhat anxious, obese, obviously jaundiced woman complaining of persistent abdominal discomfort. Vital signs were T 38.5 C, P 90, R 18, BP 160/90, and the head, neck, and chest were normal. The liver was enlarged (15 cm by percussion in the right midclavicular line, and palpated 4 cm below the rib cage) and exquisitely tender on palpation and percussion, but the spleen was not palpable, the abdomen was not distended, and there was no evidence of ascites. In addition, there were no stigmata of chronic liver disease. Pelvirectal examination was negative and the stool was light tan and negative for occult blood. There was no asterixis and Babinski signs were absent.

LOGIC The absence of stigmata of chronic liver disease is against a long-standing or decompensated liver disorder. Fever and tenderness are consistent with acute cholecystitis, hepatitis, or liver abscess. The blood pressure seems well controlled. Cholestasis is confirmed by the light stool and dark urine, though you cannot yet decide if the obstruction is intrahepatic or extrahepatic. There is no evidence of hepatic encephalopathy.

More studies are urgently needed. It is necessary to decide if and when surgery should be performed, and medical therapy may be urgent if you are dealing with an abscess or cholangitis. Surgery in the face of acute hepatitis might be disastrous (10% mortality), and biliary tract obstruction and subsequent infection together with diabetes have an even higher mortality.

DATA Except for 4+ bilirubin, the urinalysis is normal; urobilinogen is absent. The complete blood count shows no anemia and there are 10,000 white blood cells/mm^3 with 50% lymphocytes and 50% polymorphonuclear leukocytes (5% of the lymphocytes are atypical). Electrolytes, creatinine, and amylase are normal. Blood glucose is 240 mg/dl. Prothrombin time is 3 seconds longer than the control. Total bilirubin is 12.0 mg/dl (direct 7.0, indirect 5.0 mg); SGOT is 1100 and SGPT 800 IU/liter (normal is less than 100); alkaline phosphatase is 200 IU/liter. Hepatitis B surface antigen (HBsAg) test is negative, as is the serologic test for amebiasis. The hepatitis A virus antibody of the IgM type (HAVAB-M) is also negative. Twenty-four hours after intramuscular vitamin K, the prothrombin time falls to equal the control. Chest x-ray, ECG, and plain abdominal film are normal. In particular, there are no radiopaque calculi, no air in the biliary tree, and no ileus.

LOGIC The absence of polymorphonuclear leukocytosis is against abscess and cholecystitis, whereas the lymphocytosis is consistent with hepatitis. Urobilinogen is absent from the urine because no bile is entering the gut. Precluding hemolytic jaundice are the absence of anemia, the relatively low indirect bilirubin, the high total bilirubin, and the marked bilirubinuria. Diabetes is confirmed by the high glucose, but it is difficult to evaluate control in the presence of an acute process. The slight prothrombin time prolongation responded well to vitamin K, suggesting that liver function in this regard must be adequate, and that a relative lack of bile salts in the gut may have accounted for this abnormality. More important, the normal prothrombin will permit invasive procedures.

The enzymes are quite high whereas the alkaline phosphatase is only two or three times normal. This suggests acute liver disease rather than bile duct obstruction where the reverse would be true. Less than 25% of gallstones in the United States are radiopaque, and biliary tract sepsis can occur in the absence of biliary tract air, so these negative findings are of limited usefulness.

Acute liver necrosis seems likely. The negative HBsAg cannot exclude viral hepatitis. The surface antigen is positive in 90% of cases of hepatitis B, and the core antigen (HBcAg) may also be positive slightly later in the course of the disease. The antibody test for hepatitis A (HAVAB-M) is highly sensitive, but it may take 10 to 12 days to become positive. There are as yet no dependable serologic tests for non-A non-B hepatitis and it is therefore a diagnosis of exclusion. It is interesting to note that, in the recovery phase, many weeks later, other tests for A and B become positive (HAVAB-G, HBs antibody, HBc antibody). A small percentage of transfusion-related hepatitis is caused by the B virion, but most cases are caused by the non-A non-B viruses for which there are as yet no known serum markers. The latter type of hepatitis probably has numerous routes of transmission and may be caused by a variety of different viruses. A breakthrough seems imminent here.

More sophisticated diagnostic techniques are necessary. There is a wide variety of noninvasive and invasive procedures available. When the serum bilirubin exceeds 4 mg/dl, ordinary cholecystographic techniques do not visualize the gallbladder or ducts. Other available procedures include liver-spleen isotope scan, ultrasound, computed tomography (CT), thin needle percutaneous transhepatic cholangiography (PTC), liver biopsy, and endoscopic retrograde cholangiopancreatography (ERCP)—each of which has its specific indications, values, and limitations. How to decide which to do? The least invasive test with the highest yield is best. But these two criteria may not coincide. Under certain circumstances you might be forced to do the most invasive procedure first, since it has the highest yield, and time may be a cogent factor.

DATA   A liver-spleen isotopic scan demonstrated uneven uptake in an enlarged liver without discrete filling defects and without significantly increased uptake in the spleen and marrow. An abdominal sonogram was unfortunately of poor quality and dilated intrahepatic ducts could not be excluded. CT was not available.

LOGIC   The isotope scan is consistent with a diffuse liver disease; the absence of a "cold area" is against bacterial or amebic abscess,

or large metastatic nodules, and the lack of increased uptake by the spleen is against portal hypertension. Sonography in experienced hands may detect stones in the gallbladder, but even if they are present they may not necessarily explain the patient's jaundice since stones are so common in this age group. On the other hand, sonographic or CT demonstration of dilated intrahepatic ducts would strongly imply biliary tract obstruction and laparotomy might be justified. The sonogram should also detect an abscess.

So far, then, the cholestatic jaundice appears to arise from acute diffuse liver disease. A diagnosis requiring surgery seems less likely, but the persistence of severe pain is worrisome. If you were certain of hepatitis, you might wait and watch. But the picture is neither black nor white, and you decide that, since greater certainty is needed, invasive procedures that visualize the biliary tree should be done.

DATA   All the previously mentioned studies had been obtained during the first 48 hours after admission. During this time, the patient received analgesics for pain and intravenous fluids with insulin coverage. The pain abated somewhat, but persisted.

On day 3, thin needle PTC was performed and failed to visualize the biliary tree. Before terminating the procedure, a Menghini needle biopsy was done and yielded a 3-cm core of brown tissue.

LOGIC   When properly done, thin needle cholangiography successfully visualizes *dilated* bile ducts in 100% of cases and demonstrates normal ducts in 60 to 70%, so that failure to visualize the biliary tree made extrahepatic obstruction highly unlikely. Needle biopsy of the liver was therefore unlikely to enter a dilated duct and could be considered a safe procedure. Its purpose was to confirm a diagnosis of hepatocellular disease and to further justify a conservative course of close observation.

DATA   The biopsy was followed by hypotension, tachycardia, right upper quadrant rebound tenderness, and a decrease in hematocrit. She was given 2 units of packed red blood cells. On the following day the biopsy revealed acute viral hepatitis with cholestatic features but was without bridging necrosis or fatty infiltration. By this time she had recovered from her biopsy complication of probable liver tear with hemoperitoneum.

Over the next 5 days the patient improved clinically. Pain and tenderness subsided and at the time of discharge she was feeling and eating well. The bilirubin and liver enzymes gradually returned to normal in the ensuing 6 weeks. The patient refused further immunologic studies to determine the viral agent. These tests would be of prognostic significance. It was presumed that the hepatitis was type non-A non-B, source unknown.

LOGIC   One might justifiably question the wisdom of doing invasive risky procedures when the diagnosis of acute hepatitis was already reasonably certain. But the primary care physician and collaborating surgeon did not wish to overlook a surgical lesion in a patient exhibiting some atypical features. In their judgment this was the wisest course to follow.

QUESTIONS

1. Assume the patient just presented had a prothrombin time of 25 seconds which was not correctable by vitamin K. Needling the liver would have been precluded. The sonogram was of no help and the patient continued to be sick with pain, jaundice, and fever. Your next step would be:
   (a) exploratory laparotomy
   (b) give antibiotics
   (c) ERCP
   (d) wait and watch.
2. If this patient had no palpable liver, a very high alkaline phosphatase, only slightly elevated liver enzymes, normal prothrombin time, colicky pains, and leukocytosis, and no invasive procedures had yet been done, you would:
   (a) do surgery
   (b) give antibiotics
   (c) order ERCP
   (d) order "skinny" needle PTC.
3. A 60-year-old man becomes jaundiced after a 2-month period of anorexia and weight loss. Serum bilirubin is 10 mg/dl, SGPT twice nor-

mal, alkaline phosphatase ten times normal, and serum glucose 220 mg/dl. Which of the following could explain the entire picture?
   (a) carcinoma of the pancreas
   (b) carcinoma of the stomach with liver metastases
   (c) diabetes mellitus
   (d) (b) plus (c).
4. Return to the patient in the protocol. Suppose the x-ray of the abdomen had revealed radiopaque stones in the general area of the gallbladder and the CT liver scan showed a 6-cm single round posterior filling defect near the porta hepatis. Also suppose that ultrasound of the liver found that the defect was cystic. No invasive studies had yet been done, and the blood count showed a marked polymorphonuclear leukocytosis. The probabilities are that the disease causing the patient's acute problem is:
   (a) acute cholecystitis with cholelithiasis
   (b) hepatitis
   (c) cancer with metastases
   (d) amebic liver abscess.

ANSWERS

1. **(c) is correct.** Provided an expert endoscopist is available, this procedure should tell if there is common bile duct obstruction. If (c) were unavailable, (b) and (d) would be the best choices because surgery in the face of severe hepatocellular disease carries enormous risks. If there were no improvement, a therapeutic dilemma would be present, and the surgeon's hand might be forced.
2. **(c) or (d) still remain the best choices** because even typical cases of seeming extrahepatic obstruction occasionally turn out to have intrahepatic cholestasis and surgery may be dangerous under such circumstances. The techniques which distinguish *extrahepatic* (surgical) from *intrahepatic* (nonsurgical) forms of jaundice are among the most significant recent advances in hepatology. They should be utilized when available because they are reasonably safe and are far more accurate than clinical judgment alone. In their absence, you would initiate antibiotic therapy and you would probably perform surgery at a time which would be determined by the clinical course.
   Legitimate differences of opinion may exist in this instance. Some clinicians might go directly to surgery since the clinical picture seems so characteristic of common duct obstruction.
3. **(a) and (d) are correct.** Cancer of the pancreas may cause obstructive jaundice, and diabetes may develop if the neoplasm extensively re-

places the body and tail. Common genetic diabetes mellitus may also occur, but it does not account for the other symptoms. Stomach cancer with metastases may be present, but it does not explain the diabetes. (d) represents a concurrence of diseases which explains the whole picture.

4. **(d) is correct.** The "hole" in the liver, fever, leukocytosis type of pain and tenderness, and her residency in Mexico all point to amebic abscess which can cause jaundice if adjacent to the common duct. While the patient also has stones, it is less likely that this is causing her illness; it does not account for the large single filling defect, although it could cause multiple abscesses by ascending suppurative cholangitis. Hepatitis could not account for a large filling defect either. Cancer with metastases is unlikely in view of previous good health; furthermore, the filling defects are more apt to be multiple, and cancer is not so apt to cause an acute picture such as is seen here.

COMMENT Papers that propose to solve the common riddle of cholestatic jaundice still flood the journals. These attest to the fact that this issue is not yet solved, and diagnostic procedures and sequences are variable. No single strategy is optimal for all patients, for, as always, there are many individual variables, and each case must be handled differently.

Yet some facts are well established and a few protocols are strongly advocated for the patient who has cholestatic jaundice. But do we need *diagnostic road maps* or can we get to the same destination by simply following the *road signs*? Must we rely on the preconceived plans of others, or do we have sufficient gray matter to think our own way through the morass of procedurists who beckon this way or that?

The diagnostic accuracy of the combined history, physical examination, and laboratory tests should approach 90%. For example, given a 22-year-old healthy patient with the recent onset of nausea, anorexia, cholestatic jaundice, and an enlarged tender liver, the diagnosis is infectious hepatitis—almost for certain. Given a 56-year-old reasonably healthy woman with repeated episodes of right upper quadrant pain who now has colic, fever, and cholestatic jaundice, the diagnosis is stone in the common bile duct with retrograde infection—almost for certain. And given a 65-year-old man with a 3 months' downhill course, recurrent diffuse abdominal pains, an enlarged nodular liver, and cholestatic jaundice, the diagnosis is metastatic cancer to the liver—almost for certain.

But there are great numbers of patients who cannot be so neatly categorized. For them you must perform diagnostic procedures. And for those whose diagnosis is reasonably certain, some procedures may be necessary too. The question is: which procedure for whom, when, and in what order? Today's consensus may change as diagnostic techniques become more refined and their operating characteristics are firmly established.

The procedures of greatest use are (a) ultrasound, (b) CT scan, (c) PTC, (d) ERCP, and (e) liver biopsy. Ultrasound is good for detecting gallbladder stones, liver abscesses or metastases, and intrahepatic biliary duct dilatation; it has no risks and is not costly. The CT scan is of equal value but is more costly and may involve the injection of intravenous dye. PTC and ERCP are both good for visualizing the biliary tree and detecting extrahepatic obstruction with radiopaque contrast dye. The former has a respectable morbidity and is best for upper biliary obstructions. The latter has less risk but requires great skill; however, it is especially good for detecting pancreatic and ampullary lesions, and obstructions closer to the lower parts of the biliary tree. Both are costly. Liver biopsy has its risks, especially if ducts are dilated.

The disease spectrum with which we deal has already been presented in the case discussion. If you are not satisfied with the degree of probability established by the clinical picture, further procedures must be done. The sensitivity, specificity, success rate, complications, and cost of each procedure is well established in good institutions with expert procedure performers. Since the figures for the operating characteristics of each test are in the 75 to 90% range, the tests have high accuracy and reliability. But the results are not that good everywhere. This must be borne in mind when the report is "equivocal," "compatible with," "of poor quality," "suggestive of," "unobtainable," or "suboptimal reading."

If the patient almost certainly has hepatitis, do nothing. But if the clinical estimate of hepatitis likelihood is .80 or less, then the P(D) for extrahepatic cholestasis is .20 or more. In that event, do an ultrasound study.

The sonogram has a 90% sensitivity for dilated intrahepatic ducts and a 10% false negativity rate. Therefore, if the ducts are not visibly dilated, observe the patient. If the patient gets well, hepatitis is almost certain and nothing further needs to be done. But if the patient continues to exhibit unremitting cholestatic jaundice, a liver biopsy should be obtained. A biopsy showing hepatitis warrants continued observation; but if such is not the case, and especially if the biopsy shows bile duct dilatation, then opacification of the biliary system is indicated. You may have encountered one of the 10% of patients whose ultrasound study is falsely negative. Do a PTC or ERCP.

Go back to the original setting, but suppose the sonogram shows dilated intrahepatic ducts. Proceed directly to PTC or ERCP, or both if necessary, and be prepared to request arteriography, guided needle biopsy, and whatever is required on your voyage of discovery.

In this case, and especially in other cases where the probability of extrahepatic biliary obstruction is even greater, you must establish the cause of obstruction. Some form of surgery may be necessary, and surgeons generally prefer to know in advance what they will encounter. (*P. C.*)

Suggested Readings

1. Schiff L: Jaundice: a clinical approach. In Schiff L, Schiff ER (eds): *Diseases of the Liver*, ed 5. Philadelphia, Lippincott, 1982, pp 379–392.
   A common-sense discussion devoid of high-tech procedures. Chapters 37, 39, and 40 elaborate on scanning techniques, ERCP, PTC, and angiography.
2. Tan EGC, Warren KW: Diseases of the gall bladder and bile ducts. In Schiff L, Schiff ER (eds): *Diseases of the Liver*, ed 5. Philadelphia, Lippincott, 1982, pp 1513–1543.
   This portion covers stones, cholecystitis, and their complications.
3. Koff RS, Galambos J: Viral hepatitis. In Schiff L, Schiff ER (eds): *Diseases of the Liver*, ed 5. Philadelphia, Lippincott, 1982, pp 461–610.
   Hepatitis from Hippocrates to DNA; 1041 references from A to Z.
4. Combes B, Schenker S: Laboratory tests for liver disease. In Schiff L, Schiff ER (eds): *Diseases of the Liver*, ed 5. Philadelphia, Lippincott, 1982, pp 259–302.
5. Sleisenger MH, Fordtran JS (eds): *Gastrointestinal Diseases*, ed 3. Philadelphia, Saunders, 1983.
   Subjects related to the problems of Case 36 can be found in:
   chap 82, pp 1356–1369: gallstones

   chap 83, pp 1374–1381: acute cholecystitis
   chap 85, pp 1389–1400: biliary obstruction
   chap 93, pp 1514–1526: carcinoma of the pancreas
   chap 102, pp 1688–1705: ultrasound
   chap 104, pp 1727–1742: ERCP
   chap 105, pp 1745–1760: PTC
6. Richter JM, Silverstein MD, Schapiro R: Suspected obstructive jaundice: a decision analysis of diagnostic strategies. *Ann Intern Med* 99:46–51, 1983.
   Portrays the optimal strategy for varying diagnostic likelihoods—a fascinating mathematical approach.
7. Siegel JH, Yatto RY: Approach to cholestasis. An update. *Arch Intern Med* 142:1877–1879, 1982.
   Presents an algorithmic workup using a logical sequence of procedures.
8. Scharschmidt BF, Goldberg HI, Schmid R: Approach to the patient with cholestatic jaundice. *N Engl J Med* 308:1515–1519, 1983.
   Readings 6, 7, and 8 depict approaches to the same problem from Boston, New York, and San Francisco, respectively.
9. O'Connor KW, Snodgrass PG, Swonder JE, et al: A blinded prospective study comparing four current non-invasive approaches in the differential diagnosis of medical vs. surgical jaundice. *Gastroenterology* 84:1498–1504, 1983.
   Assesses the sensitivity, specificity, and accuracy of clinical evaluation, scintiscans, CT, and ultrasound: leads into the subject of invasive techniques.
10. Teplick SK, Haskin PH, Matsumoto T, et al: Interventional radiology of the biliary system and pancreas. *Surg Clin North Am* 64:87–119, 1984.
    Documents the radiologist's role in diagnosis and treatment.
11. Mueller PR, van Sonnenberg E, Simeone JF: Fine-needle transhepatic cholangiography—indications and usefulness. *Ann Intern Med* 97:567–572, 1982.
12. La Russo NF, Wiesner RH, Ludwig J, et al: Primary sclerosing cholangitis. *N Engl J Med* 310:899–903, 1984.

Case 37
Cramps and Nausea
ARTHUR S. McFEE, M.D., Ph.D.

DATA A 45-year-old woman comes to the emergency room complaining that she has had "intestinal flu" for the past 3 days. This began with cramping, periumbilical pain, anorexia, and nausea; the episodes of cramping were severe and frequent at first, but then came less often and nearly disappeared by the second day, at which time she felt she was better. She denies diarrhea and indeed notes that she has had no stool nor has she passed gas for 2 days.

Toward the end of the second day she began to feel uncomfortably full and her clothes felt tight. That night she began to vomit and continued to do so until admission on day 3. Her last vomitus was particularly foul-tasting and consisted of dark greenish-brown liquid material (feculent vomiting). Several hours before admission she noted a different type of abdominal pain which was steady, sharp, and localized in the left lower quadrant (LLQ).

LOGIC   This is a characteristic history of distal small bowel obstruction. The patient thought she had "intestinal flu" because of the cramping. If that were so, she should have had diarrhea too. Occasionally, as in this case, the patient assumes improvement as the cramping pain diminishes. Actually she is much worse.

Vomiting can be a late sign with distal obstruction. Nausea and anorexia are common symptoms which give no clues to the specificity of the diagnosis. Often the patient with a distal lesion may not seek help for several days until distention and feculent vomiting occur. Feculent vomitus originates in the small bowel. It indicates distal small or large bowel obstruction and is noted only after prolonged incessant vomiting has emptied the proximal GI tract.

The advent of a new, more steady pain indicates peritoneal irritation and a different pain mechanism. It is a very significant symptom which tells you something else is happening.

The concurrent onset of vomiting and cramps usually indicates a more proximal obstruction and causes the patient to seek aid much earlier in the course of the disease.

DATA   Past history reveals good health with no major diseases. She has three children all delivered by cesarean section; the youngest is 14. Ten years ago she underwent an abdominal hysterectomy for fibroids. The systems review, family history, and patient profile are negative or normal.

LOGIC   Fibrous adhesions within the celom are the preponderant cause (80%) of bowel obstruction in the patient who has undergone an abdominal operative proce-

dure. Although most develop this obstruction within 1 or 2 years of surgery, it can occur much later. In the patient who develops a similar picture in the absence of prior surgery, the most common cause of obstruction is an internal or external hernia. Other causes of distal bowel obstruction include colon cancer, volvulus, intussusception, foreign body, gallstone, and regional ileitis.

DATA   Physical examination discloses a very sick patient who is lying quietly in bed. The vital signs are T 38.7 C, P 105, R 24, BP 90/70. Skin turgor is poor, mucous membranes are dry, and the eyes are sunken. While the heart and lungs are normal, the diaphragm moves poorly. There is marked abdominal distention and bowel sounds are absent. Point tenderness and rigidity can be defined in the LLQ at the site of her present pain. The abdomen is tympanitic and a succussion splash is elicited, but no masses can be palpated. Pelvirectal examination reveals marked left adnexal tenderness and an empty rectal ampulla. No inguinal, femoral, or umbilical herniae are noted. There are midline and transverse lower abdominal incisions; each is well healed, firm, and without hernia.

LOGIC   The prime impression is that you have a very ill patient who exhibits many signs of dehydration and has an acute surgical abdomen. By itself, it means nothing that the patient is lying quietly in bed. But together with LLQ pain, point tenderness, and rigidity, it indicates the presence of peritoneal irritation and confirms the historical report of a different type of pain starting hours before admission. Other significant physical findings are present in the abdomen.

The first is marked distention due to dilated air- and fluid-filled loops of intestine; this is indicated by tympanites and a succussion splash and is characteristic of distal bowel obstruction. If the bowel were obstructed at the gastric outlet, duodenum, or proximal few feet of the small intestine, abdominal distention would not be noted because the upper bowel empties itself quite well by early vomiting and the process is largely concealed beneath the costal margin.

Second, lack of bowel sounds can result from several causes. In the absence of peritonitis, a distended edematous bowel gradually loses its ability to sustain effective peristalsis. Bowel sounds and cramps diminish as peristalsis decreases, and they may indeed vanish altogether. In the presence of peritonitis from any cause, a reflex paralysis or ileus of the bowel occurs; this may be localized to the area adjacent to the inflammation, or generalized if the peritonitis is widespread or severe. Extracelomic processes, such as pelvic or spinal fractures and pneumonia, can also cause reflex ileus with absent bowel sounds.

Left adnexal tenderness can result from acute tuboovarian disease causing secondary bowel obstruction or it may simply mean that inflamed tender bowel is being felt in this area. Hysterectomy does not necessarily include removal of the adnexae. The fact that no masses were palpable in the abdomen may merely reflect the difficulties of examination in the presence of tenderness and distention.

An empty rectum is compatible with obstruction.

The physical examination buttresses the history's impression of distal mechanical bowel obstruction followed by an inflammatory process. This can only mean that obstruction with strangulation or perforation has occurred. A rapid workup and treatment are mandatory.

DATA Chest and abdominal x-rays show a normal chest with an elevated diaphragm, and a marked layering "stepladder" pattern of air-filled bowel with air-fluid levels apparent in the upright position. It is impossible to define a normal colon pattern of gas, and no air is seen in the distal large bowel.

Complete blood count shows hemoglobin 16.5 g/dl, hematocrit 47%, white blood cell count 21,800, 91% polymorphonuclear leukocytes. Only 30 ml of urine are obtained; specific gravity 1.034, ketones positive, but all else is normal or negative. Serum sodium is 126, potassium 3.2, bicarbonate 15 mEq/liter; blood urea nitrogen is 46, glucose 100, and creatinine 1.6 mg/dl.

Proctosigmoidoscopy is normal to 25 cm though some difficulty is encountered due to tenderness. After some discussion on the appropriateness of radiologic contrast studies, a barium enema is performed; it is normal.

LOGIC The x-rays confirm obstruction; the site is not apparent, but it is certainly not in the colon. Blood and urine studies indicate dehydration, hemoconcentration, electrolyte depletion, ketosis, acidosis, and decreased renal blood flow with prerenal azotemia and scant concentrated urine. The marked leukocytosis suggests an acute inflammatory process.

In this setting, contrast x-rays are not generally productive of more information than can be adduced by history and examination. However, a barium enema is reasonably innocuous and rules out obstruction in the colon. Most carcinomas of the colon (60 to 70%) causing obstruction should be visible by proctosigmoidoscopy, so that colon malignancy causing obstruction can be effectively ruled out by these two studies. Furthermore, the absence of anemia and no history of rectal bleeding are also against colon or rectal cancer.

An upper gastrointestinal series is contraindicated in this patient for several reasons. It is doubtful if the contrast medium could be made to pass into the bowel at all; the admixture of the agent with large quantities of retained fluid would hinder good visualization; and if the contrast material passed all the way to the point of obstruction, the study would indicate only the point of obstruction but not its nature.

New imaging techniques are available but none will produce helpful information in this case. Ultrasound is rendered useless by the large amount of air-distended bowel. A gallium scan for infection or abscess is not warranted here. A CT scan might reveal an obstructing mass lesion. But enough clinical information is already at hand, and prompt operative intervention is necessary anyway.

DATA   Over the next 4 hours, the patient is intensively prepared for surgery with intravenous fluids, colloids, appropriate electrolytes, gastrointestinal suction, and antibiotics. The blood pressure rises, the pulse falls, and urinary output rises to 30 to 50 ml/hour. Ketosis, acidosis, and electrolyte disorders are rapidly ameliorated.

Exploratory laporatomy reveals an area of extensive fibrous adhesions surrounding a left cystic ovary. Approximately 1½ feet of proximal ileum are entrapped within this cystic mass and are strangulated. The adhesions are lysed, the ovary and tube are removed, gangrenous small bowel is resected, and an anastomosis is performed. The patient makes an uneventful recovery and is discharged well in 2 weeks.

LOGIC   Several important lessons are to be learned. The exact cause for obstruction must not necessarily be known, but surgery is mandatory to relieve both the effects of the obstruction and the obstructing mechanism.

In most cases of simple mechanical intestinal obstruction, preoperative treatment can proceed on a planned basis at a leisurely pace—unless the obstruction is high. Proximal high obstruction rapidly depletes body fluid and electrolytes and poses the danger of aspirated vomitus, pneumonia, or asphyxiation. If an obstruction results in intestinal strangulation, signs of peritoneal irritation are additionally present (fever, tenderness, rigidity). Therefore, in case of high obstruction or peritoneal irritation, treatment prior to surgery must proceed rapidly. A dead or perforated viscus cannot be long tolerated, for systemic sepsis and shock cause the patient's death.

QUESTIONS

1. Assume the same clinical presentation: cramping pain followed by increasing distention and vomiting. The patient is 62 and has had no previous surgery. While the bowels had always been normal, large amounts of laxatives were taken over the previous 3 months for increasingly more severe constipation. Physical examination is normal. The most likely diagnosis is:
    (a) cancer of the sigmoid colon
    (b) acute diverticulitis
    (c) obstruction in a femoral hernia
    (d) Crohn's disease of the colon.

2. A 23-year-old woman has the acute onset of cramping abdominal pain, distention, and vomiting. She had an appendectomy at age 8. Distention and very active borborygmi are present. Bilateral inguinal adenopathy is felt to be the result of fungal infection of the feet. A tender mass, 1 cm in diameter, is noted near one lymph node just inferior to Poupart's ligament on the left. The most likely diagnosis is:
    (a) acute inguinal lymphadenitis
    (b) Richter's femoral hernia
    (c) inguinal hernia
    (d) fibrous adhesions in the abdomen.

3. A 14-year-old boy is hit by an automobile and sustains a severely fractured pelvis and a pulmonary contusion. No intraabdominal bleeding is demonstrated on peritoneal lavage. Four days later he develops pneumococcal pneumonia. Six days after the accident, abdominal distention is still present, bowel sounds are absent, and he has passed no stool or gas. He has never complained of colicky pain. The abdomen is soft and not tender. He has:
    (a) fibrous adhesions as a result of lavage
    (b) obstruction from an internal hernia
    (c) reflex paralytic ileus without obstruction
    (d) need for urgent surgery.

4. A 58-year-old man with a clear-cut picture of intestinal obstruction had an operation for the repair of two inguinal hernias 1 year ago and an appendectomy for a ruptured appendix 2 years ago. For the past 6 months he has had bright red rectal bleeding with most bowel movements, but no change in bowel habit. Examination shows distention but no tenderness, a large, easily reducible, right recurrent inguinal hernia, and internal hemorrhoids which are not bleeding at that moment. After reduction of the hernia, evidence of obstruction continues. The obstruction is most likely caused by:
    (a) carcinoma of the left hemicolon
    (b) recurrent right inguinal hernia
    (c) adhesions from previous surgery
    (d) carcinoma of the cecum.

ANSWERS

1. **(a) is correct.** Diverticulitis is associated with tenderness and guarding. A femoral hernia is

not present. (d) does not present in this manner. A distal bowel obstruction in this age group, under these circumstances, is most likely caused by cancer. The left colon is narrow and cancers there are usually of the "napkin-ring" constricting type, so obstruction occurs early.

2. **(b) is correct.** A small tender mass in the femoral canal, associated with the picture of intestinal obstruction, indicates an obstructed femoral hernia. Since this canal is small, it is common for the obstruction to be caused by only a knuckle of bowel rather than an entire loop; this is called a Richter's hernia. While (a) could account for a tender mass, it could not cause obstruction. Postappendectomy adhesions could cause obstruction but would not cause a tender femoral mass. The location of the mass is against an inguinal hernia; besides, femoral hernias are more common than inguinal hernias in women.

3. **(c) is correct.** Both a retroperitoneal hematoma resulting from fractured pelvis and pneumonia can cause reflex paralytic ileus. The clinical picture of obstruction (colic and borborygmi) is not present, and there are no findings of peritoneal irritation (tenderness and guarding). Adhesions from lavage are rare. Surgery is not indicated and bowel activity will return with appropriate nonsurgical measures.

4. **(c) is correct.** Admittedly, there is an overlap of findings and possibilities here. With rectal bleeding, cancer of the left colon is a distinct possibility at this age, even though hemorrhoids are present; the absence of change of bowel habit is against this impression. The larger recurrent hernia is probably not the cause of obstruction because of its size, easy reducibility, and lack of improvement after it was reduced. Cancer of the right colon rarely causes obstruction unless it is at the site of the ileocecal valve; this is because the right colon is wide and lesions there tend to be fungating rather than constricting. Thus they present with anemia, occult bleeding, and unexplained fatigue. This leaves us with adhesions, the most common cause of obstruction in a patient with previous surgery. Of course, proctosigmoidoscopy and barium enema prior to surgery are especially indicated in this patient.

COMMENT A complete data base was gathered via a traditional approach. But quite early a pattern of intestinal obstruction was established; most symptoms and signs were by themselves nonspecific, but the combination was incontestable. Likelihoods and probabilities were frequent considerations as the patient's age, operative history, and presence or absence of certain clues entered the picture.

As the author mulled over each new finding, he verbalized his logic with numerous intricate cause and effect relationships. This was especially notable in his selection of tests and x-rays and the order of their performance. The need for speed and the timing of treatment received careful attention. And overlapping sets were an obviously important issue in solving question 4.   (*P. C.*)

Suggested Readings

1. Jones RS: Intestinal obstruction. In Sabiston DC Jr (ed): *Davis-Christopher Textbook of Surgery: The Biologic Basis of Modern Surgical Practice*, ed 12. Philadelphia, Saunders, 1981, pp 995–1004.
   A brief, extremely informative analysis of the subject in an excellent standard textbook.
2. Stewardson RH, Bombeck CT, Nyhus LM: Critical operative management of small bowel obstruction. *Ann Surg* 187:189–193, 1978.
   In only 5 pages the authors establish well-known truisms about small bowel obstruction in 238 patients.
3. Wangensteen OH: Understanding the bowel obstruction problem (Great Ideas in Surgery). *Am J Surg* 135:131–147, 1978.
   This article represents the lifetime experiences of a pioneer in the study of obstructive bowel disease.
4. Greenlee HB: Acute large bowel obstruction: an update. *Surg Ann* 14:253–276, 1982.
   Includes cancer, diverticulitis, volvulus, and other less common causes.
5. Sarr MG, Bulkley GB, Zuidema GD: Preoperative recognition of intestinal strangulation obstruction. Prospective evaluation of a diagnostic capacity. *Am J Surg* 145:176–182, 1983.
   A multivariate analysis of clinical and laboratory features.
6. Kurtz RJ, Heimann TM, Kurtz AB: Gallstone ileus: a diagnostic problem. *Am J Surg* 146:314–317, 1983.
   Uncommon but easily curable if recognized.
7. Ballantyne GH: Review of sigmoid volvulus. Clinical patterns and pathogenesis. *Dis Colon Rectum* 24:823–830, 1982.

Case 38
Fever and Confusion with Cirrhosis

PAUL CUTLER, M.D.

DATA A 50-year-old man, in whom Laennec's cirrhosis was proven by biopsy 2 years ago, was brought to the emergency room by his family because of fever and confusion for 24 hours. Even since this diagnosis was made, he continued to drink 1 pint of 86 proof whiskey daily as he had done for 30 years before. He never had a gastrointestinal (GI) hemorrhage and his ascites had been treated with attempted salt restriction and 100 mg of hydrochlorothiazide daily.

LOGIC Altered mentation in an alcoholic patient with known liver disease requires three sets of considerations. First, you think of hepatic or portal-systemic encephalopathy (PSE) as a likely explanation. But second, you must also consider other central nervous system disturbances in a patient with this background. These include acute alcoholic intoxication, other drug intoxication, acute hallucinosis, delirium tremens, Wernicke-Korsakoff encephalopathy, hypoglycemia, acute infections (meningitis, pneumonia, sepsis), and subdural hematoma from the head trauma that heavy drinkers often incur. And third, alcoholism does not exempt him from the cerebrovascular accidents that nondrinkers get. Each of these many diseases can present with similar behavior disorders, though the fever favors some more than others.

DATA Additional history obtained from the patient and his family confirmed that he had been drinking his usual amounts up to and including the very day of admission to the emergency room. He never experienced "the shakes," hallucinations, or delusions, and he had suffered no recent head trauma. Though he ate poorly, he had no nausea, vomiting, hematemesis, or known melena and has taken no other drugs.

LOGIC Since he has not stopped drinking and has not had the usual manifestations of

delirium tremens, alcohol withdrawal syndromes can probably be excluded. Similarly, the absence of a recent history of hematemesis, melena, and other drug ingestions make GI bleeding and drug intoxication unlikely.

DATA Physical examination disclosed an unkempt, poorly nourished man who looked much older than his age. The vital signs were T 39 C, P 106, BP 128/70, R 20; no orthostatic changes were present. He was slightly lethargic and disoriented to time and place, but he had no gross tremor, perseveration, confabulation, or ideas of reference. There were no signs of head trauma such as ecchymoses, hematomas, or lacerations; the sclerae were slightly icteric, ocular movements were normal, pupils reacted well, and the fundi were normal.

Muscular tone was somewhat increased so that neck stiffness and tests for Kernig and Brudzinski signs were uninterpretable. There was temporal muscle wasting, parotid enlargement, numerous spider angiomas, and palmar erythema, but no gynecomastia. His breath had a musty odor suggestive of fetor hepaticus. The heart and lungs were normal; but the abdomen was moderately distended and the umbilicus was effaced. Chest hair was present. There was no caput medusae, though some distended abdominal veins were present. The liver was ballottable 3 cm below the costal margin and its vertical percussion span was 15 cm in the midclavicular line; the splenic tip was palpable. No abdominal tenderness was noted, and bowel sounds were present though faint. The testes were normal in size, rectal examination was normal, and the stool was brown and negative for occult blood. The extremities showed palmar erythema and white fingernails but no clubbing or Dupuytren's contractures.

On neurologic examination, there were no

lateralizing signs and deep tendon reflexes were 3+ and symmetrical. Bilateral "hand flap" (asterixis) was present and the Babinski signs were absent. His signature was shaky and his performance of a number-connecting test was very slow.

LOGIC The history and physical examination were directed at trying to distinguish between the cited diagnostic possibilities. Based upon the presence of asterixis and fetor hepaticus in a patient with severe chronic liver disease (portal hypertension, ascites, and other stigmata), PSE is by far the most likely explanation for the patient's altered mental status. Although asterixis is a nonspecific sign that may be present in other forms of organic encephalopathy, fetor hepaticus appears to be specific for PSE when it is detected.

Note the presence of many physical signs that are characteristic of cirrhosis but the absence of some that are often present (testicular atrophy, gynecomastia, loss of chest hair). Also, in PSE the Babinski sign is often present.

Subdural hematoma is less likely without neurologic signs, but it is certainly not ruled out even in the absence of a clear-cut trauma history. Wernicke-Korsakoff psychosis is unlikely in the absence of ophthalmoplegia, confabulation, and polyneuritis, and there is no focalizing neurologic evidence of a stroke.

While PSE may occur in the course of decompensated liver disease, especially in the presence of portal hypertension with shunting, it is often precipitated by GI bleeding, other sources of increased enteric protein load, infection, hypokalemic metabolic alkalosis, or sedative/narcotic administration. This patient's fever is of special concern. Further studies are therefore directed at determining which of the precipitating factors may be present and at finding the cause of the fever itself.

DATA Chest x-ray and ECG were normal. Abdominal film showed diffuse haziness compatible with ascites; the liver and spleen were not clearly visualized. The nasogastric aspirate was clear and negative for occult blood. Except for 1+ bilirubin, the urinalysis was normal. Other emergency laboratory data included a hemoglobin/hematocrit of 8.6/30, unchanged from tests done 2 months prior. There were 20,000 white blood cells/mm^3 of which 75% were polymorphonuclear and 15% were band cells; the blood smear showed poikilocytosis and anisocytosis with a normal number of platelets. Blood chemistry determinations were: urea nitrogen 36 mg/dl, glucose 120 mg/dl, sodium 130 mEq/liter, potassium 2.5 mEq/liter, chloride 99 mEq/liter, and bicarbonate 34 mEq/liter. Serum and urine amylase were normal. Prothrombin time was 16 seconds (control 12), unchanged since last measured 2 months ago. Minimal intoxication was indicated by a blood alcohol level of 50 mg/dl. A toxic screen for sedatives and tranquilizers in the blood and urine was negative.

LOGIC GI bleeding is highly unlikely on the basis of a negative history of hematemesis or melena, the absence of detectable blood in the stool and gastric aspirate, and the stable though abnormal hematocrit. The cause of the anemia remains to be determined, but in patients with cirrhosis the usual cause is previously undetected episodes of GI bleeding from varices, ulcer, or gastritis. The low level of blood alcohol and the negative toxic screen make drug encephalopathy unlikely.

Mild azotemia may have resulted from diuretic-induced fluid losses. The elevated blood urea may contribute to encephalopathy by diffusing across the gut mucosa where bacterial ureases reduce it to absorbable ammonia.

Hypokalemia and elevated serum bicarbonate suggest a metabolic alkalosis. This may be caused by thiazide diuretics, lack of potassium supplementation, volume contraction, and the secondary hyperaldosteronism that sometimes occurs in patients with cirrhosis and ascites. Alkalosis also aggravates PSE by increasing the diffusion of ammonia into (central nervous system) cells where it may be trapped as ammonium ion resulting in disturbed oxidative metabolism.

While the EEG, arterial blood gases, arterial ammonia, and spinal fluid ammonia or glutamine determinations may help to confirm PSE, the clinical picture is reasonably complete and such additional studies are not likely to change your approach. Furthermore, the exact biochemical disturbance responsible for PSE has not yet been verified.

DATA Rehydration with 5% dextrose in water was guided by a central venous pressure monitor, and potassium chloride was carefully supplemented to correct possible excessive water loss and metabolic alkalosis. Dietary protein was withheld, tap water enemas were given, and oral lactulose was started—all counterencephalopathy measures—while the evaluation proceeded.

LOGIC You should be especially concerned about the unexplained fever and leukocytosis. Alcoholic cirrhotic patients are predisposed to tuberculosis (pulmonary, meningeal, peritoneal, and miliary), bacterial meningitis, pneumonia (aspiration), spontaneous bacterial peritonitis in the presence of ascites, and other sources of sepsis. Each can precipitate PSE but may also threaten life by the nature of the infection itself. Although alcoholic hepatitis may cause fever and leukocytosis all by itself, there is nothing in the data so far obtained to suggest a marked worsening of liver function or sudden increase in hepatic cell necrosis.

Pneumonia is excluded by the normal chest examination and negative chest x-ray, and urinary tract infection is unlikely with a normal urinalysis. However, the examination and culture of the cerebrospinal and peritoneal fluids are the most important tests, and these should be performed as emergency studies on the day of admission.

DATA A lumbar puncture yielded clear colorless fluid under normal pressure. The proteins, glucose, and cell count were normal. Fluorochrome stain, Gram stain, and India ink preparation were all negative. Cultures for various pathogens were begun.

Midline paracentesis below the umbilicus obtained 20 ml of straw-colored, slightly cloudy fluid. The specific gravity was 1.020, proteins 3.7 g/dl, glucose 40 mg/dl, and amylase was undetectable. There were 1800 white blood cells/mm^3, of which 90% were polymorphonuclear leukocytes. Gram stain showed gram-negative rods and fluorochrome stain was negative.

LOGIC The picture is now clear. Meningitis, septicemia, and tuberculosis are excluded. Most important, there is strong evidence that the patient has peritonitis which is no doubt the cause of his acute deterioration. The paracentesis fluid has the characteristics of an exudate; numerous polymorphonuclear leukocytes are counted and bacteria are present. This disorder may occur spontaneously in the complete absence of physical signs of peritonitis and in the absence of any obvious focus of intraabdominal suppuration. Gram-negative organisms, especially *Escherichia coli*, are the usual offenders.

DATA Ticarcillin and tobramycin were added to the intravenous fluids in an effort to treat this frequently catastrophic complication of cirrhosis and ascites. Other tests of liver function were sent to the laboratory. Skin tests for tuberculosis and fungi were also applied. Blood cultures were drawn.

Over the next 48 hours, evidence of PSE abated, urine output rose, the blood urea nitrogen fell to normal, the temperature dropped, and general improvement was noted. Culture of the blood and ascitic fluid yielded a heavy growth of *E. coli* sensitive to the antibiotics in use.

While the course of treatment continued, studies were done to seek out a focal infection. Abdominal plain films and repeated physical examinations failed to detect any suggestion of intraabdominal suppuration such as biliary, pancreatic, periappendiceal, or diverticular disease. Intermediate strength purified protein derivative and fungal tests were negative; mumps antigen was positive; total serum bilirubin was 4.6 mg/dl (3.0 mg direct); alkaline phosphatase was 280 IU/liter, SGOT 210 IU/liter, serum proteins 5 g/dl, and albumin 2.5 g/dl.

LOGIC Tuberculosis is ruled out by the skin test and lack of lymphocytes in the exudate. The liver tests are what you would expect with chronic liver disease and the modest SGOT is not in keeping with severe acute necrosis. There is no apparent source for the infected peritoneal fluid, so it is assumed to be spontaneous. A gallium isotope scan for intraabdominal suppuration was deemed unnecessary.

DATA The patient was discharged on completion of antibiotic treatment. In the meantime, his diuretic was changed to spironolactone given in doses adjusted to remove ½ lb of ascitic fluid/day. Attempts to have him curtail alcohol were considered hopeless. Arrangements were made to follow him at frequent intervals.

LOGIC When a patient with Laennec's cirrhosis takes a sudden downhill course, you must think of hepatoma, portal vein or hepatic vein thrombosis, peritonitis or other forms of infection, acute alcoholic hepatitis, marked electrolyte disturbances, and hepatorenal syndrome, as well as PSE and some of its causes.

While this patient clearly had alcoholic cirrhosis, it is wise to remember that cirrhosis may be caused by other disorders, and some of these, such as Wilson's disease, hemochromatosis, secondary biliary cirrhosis, and cirrhosis due to chronic active hepatitis may respond to treatment and should be sought.

Cirrhosis has many faces. Liver disease of itself has few symptoms. A large liver may be discovered in a patient who sees a physician for an unrelated problem. Other common presentations are those related to the associated alcoholism: acute alcoholic hepatitis, acute alcoholic intoxication, and delirium tremens. Last, the patient may not see a physican until he has noticed jaundice, has PSE, GI hemorrhage, ascites, or an infectious complication.

DATA *Problem list:*

1. alcoholism
2. portal cirrhosis
3. acute bacterial peritonitis
4. portal-systemic encephalopathy.

COMMENTS Disorientation in a patient with cirrhosis and alcoholism suggests many possibilities. But the presence of fever makes a small cluster which rapidly limits the diagnostic hypotheses, unless there are two independent processes going on. At any rate, pertinent negative clues helped rule out many possibilities, while highly specific decisive clues such as fetor hepaticus and the nature of the ascitic fluid confirmed the two diagnoses that were present.

This patient presented with many complications of cirrhosis—ascites, portal hypertension, hypokalemic alkalosis, peritonitis, and encephalopathy—each having adversely compounding effects on the others. Cause and effect relationships were multiple and complex. For example, cirrhosis, portal hypertension, and ascites laid the background for peritonitis. Portal hypertension with shunting, hypokalemic alkalosis, and peritonitis combined to precipitate PSE.

Given a patient with PSE and fever, the experienced clinician would have quickly sought out the main problem with a paracentesis, because that is where the answer is most apt to lie.

(P. C.)

Suggested Readings

1. Refer to **Case 64**, it details the causes for confusion that can occur in chronic alcoholic persons.
2. Conn HO: Cirrhosis. In Schiff L, Schiff ER (eds): *Diseases of the Liver*, ed 5. Philadelphia, Lippincott, 1982, pp 847–977.
   This beautifully written chapter takes you from an ancient Egyptian papyrus through the first description by Laennec and on into the 1980s. It tells you everything about the causes, types, clinical picture, diagnosis, and consequences of one of today's most common diseases. Physical signs are detailed as nowhere else. All aspects of Case 38 are discussed here.
3. Pimstone NR, French SW: Alcoholic liver disease. *Med Clin North Am* 68:39–56, 1984.
   Details the various pathologic liver states caused by alcohol.
4. James SP, Hoofnagle JH, Strober W, et al: NIH conference: Primary biliary cirrhosis: a model autoimmune disease. *Ann Intern Med* 99:500–512, 1983.
5. Grossley IR, William R: Progress in the treatment of chronic portasystemic encephalopathy. *Gut* 25:85–98, 1984.
   Explains the pathophysiology as well.
6. Jones EA: The enigma of hepatic encephalopathy. *Postgrad Med J* 59:42–54, 1983.
   A high-level review of the biochemical abnormalities including ammonia, γ-aminobutyric acid, and neurotransmitters.
7. Conn HO, Fessel JM: Spontaneous bacterial peritonitis in cirrhosis: variations on a theme. *Medicine* 50:161–197, 1971.

The wide spectrum of clinical presentations of spontaneous bacterial peritonitis in cirrhosis is delineated. Although more recent publications have added some details to this spectrum of "spontaneous" infections, this article stands as a landmark.

8. Pinzello G, Simonetti RG, Craxi A, et al: Spontaneous bacterial peritonitis: a prospective investigation in predominantly nonalcoholic cirrhotic patients. *Hepatology* 3:545–549, 1983.

Of 224 patients with ascites, 54 had positive cultures; only some had overt peritonitis.

9. Kao HW, Reynolds TB: The diagnosis of spontaneous bacterial peritonitis in alcoholic cirrhosis (letter). *Hepatology* 3:275–276, 1983.
Shows that the diagnosis is not so simple.

10. Atterbury CE: Prognosis in cirrhosis: disbelieving Cassandra. *J Clin Gastroenterol* 5:359–360, 1983.
The auther denies the credibility of the prophecy of others regarding the reversibility of cirrhosis.

Chapter 19

Renal Problems

"What is the kidney but an infinitely artful device for turning the sweet wines of Shiraz into urine?" It is natural that the filtrate of this process should reflect so much of what goes on in the kidney itself. Not surprisingly, the urinalysis often delivers the key clue in the patient with kidney disease. The presence of white blood cell (WBC) casts, red blood cell (RBC) casts, doubly refractile fat bodies, coarse granular casts, or bacteria tells us much of what is wrong. Significant bacteriuria denotes infection; WBC casts tell us the infection is in the tubule where casts are forming; and RBC casts say that the RBCs originate in the glomerulus and are incorporated into casts which are forming in the tubule. Whether or not all the wine is being turned into urine is measured by the blood urea nitrogen or serum creatinine—determinants of kidney function.

These simple laboratory examinations are essential in kidney disease and give much valuable information. Other than in the patient with chronic uremia, or in the patient with large palpable kidneys, the physical examination rarely offers key clues. The history, however, is another story. A few symptoms may put us directly on the diagnostic trail.

Bloody urine often augurs serious disease, but it does not locate or denote the pathologic process. Colicky pain usually indicates ureteric obstruction by a stone. Frequency and burning on urination suggest infection. A downhill course including nausea, weight loss, anorexia, and gastrointestinal and neurologic symptoms is indicative of chronic renal failure, though other diagnostic possibilities exist. Acute renal failure has no characteristic symptoms except perhaps for nausea, vomiting, and lack of urine formation; but this cluster usually occurs in the course of a disease whose severe nature (shock, sepsis) may obscure its renal effects. A progressively downhill course suggests cancer too; the kidney and prostate are frequent primary sites, and no other symptoms need be present. Other common presentations of patients with renal disease are peripheral edema in the nephrotic syndrome, flank pain and fever in acute pyelonephritis, and albuminuria found on routine examination.

Frequently a patient is not aware of kidney disease until renal failure, hypertension, and their complications occur—visual defects, stroke, heart failure, coronary thrombosis, or electrolyte disturbances.

Prostatic hypertrophy, prostatic cancer, and bladder cancer, though not kidney diseases, are mentioned in this chapter since they are so prevalent and often cause urinary tract symptoms similar to some of the renal disease presentations just described.

As has been noted for other disease systems, there are very many kidney diseases, far fewer modes of clinical presentation, and only a handful of commonly seen diseases. These include urinary tract infection, calculi, obstructive uropathy, acute and chronic renal failure, neoplasms, and the nephrotic syndrome. Know these and you know a substantial core.

It is important to note that kidney disease is often found coincidentally in the course

413

of another illness or may exist as part of a generalized disease. The patient with marginally compensated renal function may decompensate under the stress of pneumonia or congestive heart failure. Or an abnormal urinalysis or elevated blood urea nitrogen may be found during a routine insurance, military, or employment-related examination. Then too there are the large number of multisystem diseases which also affect the kidneys—myeloma, systemic lupus erythematosus, infective endocarditis, diabetes mellitus, and hepatic failure.

As for diagnostic clues derived from further studies, the past two decades have seen a host of new and valuable invasive and noninvasive techniques evolve for kidney disease, as well as for other organ systems. This armamentarium includes ultrasound, computed tomography, arteriography, and biopsy. The exact role of each remains to be delineated as we aim for specificity, sensitivity, economy, and safety.

The matter of renal vein thrombosis and the nephrotic syndrome—the chicken and the egg, and which comes first—seems to have been greatly clarified in the past few years. Not so the question of analgesic nephropathy! The issue of which analgesic, alone or in combination, causes interstitial nephritis is not yet crystal clear. Indeed, doubts are being raised that analgesics are as guilty as was once thought.

The common use of dialysis and renal transplantation, perhaps more than anything else, has added understanding to the pathophysiology of renal failure and has advanced and broadened the field of nephrology. These therapeutic modalities have been springboards for quantum leaps into many other fields—organ transplantation, immunology, and, unfortunately, infectious disease.

By creating a large population of immune-compromised hosts, we have unwillingly given birth to numerous nosocomial infections. There is an ever escalating conflict between new drugs and "funny bugs," and between new generation antibiotics and transformed microorganisms. Patients on dialysis and those with surrogate kidneys are good subjects for the investigation and demonstration of altered hormonal, electrolyte, and mineral disturbances, as well as drug-chemical interactions. A *textbook* of new problems exists in this subset of patients. (*P. C.*)

Case 39
Bloody Urine

MEYER D. LIFSCHITZ, M.D.

DATA The patient is a 57-year-old man whose urine has been intermittently red over the past few weeks. He has had no flank pain, abdominal pain, or pain referred to the groin or testis. But he has had a narrowed stream, increasing hesitancy, worsening urgency and frequency of urination, and nocturia two to three times nightly for the previous 6 months.

LOGIC Red urine usually means blood in the urine—hematuria. But red urine cannot be equated with blood nor does blood always make the urine red. Hemoglobin (excessive hemolysis), myoglobin (acute muscle necrosis), porphyrins, laxatives containing danthron or phenolphthalein, foods like red cabbage or beets, and drugs like rifampin and Pyridium can also make the urine red.

On the other hand, some of the above can make the urine smoky gray, dark brown, or even orange. "Cola-colored" urine usually refers to bilirubin. Blood may become dark gray or brown as the hemoglobin becomes oxidized.

Note too that the patient has symptoms which suggest lower urinary tract obstruction. Benign prostatic hypertrophy (BPH), stricture, bladder neck obstruction, and cancer of the prostate are all possible. The red urine and the obstructive symptoms could be causally related. Since you want to know what the chief complaint signifies, a urinalysis is done first.

DATA A freshly voided urine specimen is diffusely pink and cloudy and shows innumerable red blood cells (RBCs) and a trace of albumin. The last portion of the voiding was just as pink as the first. The specific gravity is 1.024, pH 6, and there is no glucose. Careful microscopic examination finds one white blood cell (WBC) and a few hyaline casts/high power field. No bacteria, crystals, or abnormal casts are seen.

LOGIC Much information is immediately available. The patient indeed has hematuria. The absence of much protein and RBC casts tends to rule out the glomerulus as the source of the RBCs. Lack of crystals makes stone less likely but does not rule it out; crystals can appear in showers. Infection is rendered unlikely by the absence of WBCs, WBC casts, and bacteria. A urine culture is not deemed necessary. The high specific gravity implies reasonably good kidney function.

Gross or microscopic hematuria must always be investigated except in women with symptoms of obvious severe cystitis. Always make sure the blood is not vaginal in origin.

If considerable albumin and especially RBC casts are present in the urine too, the source of bleeding lies in the nephron and a medical kidney disease is present. Depending on the patient's age and history, the cause may be analgesic nephropathy, immunoglobulin A nephropathy, acute poststreptococcal glomerulonephritis, membranoproliferative glomerulonephritis, Henoch-Schönlein purpura, or other immune-complex glomerulopathies. If such were the case, a renal biopsy might be needed since treatment differs for the various types.

Had no RBCs been found, either the patient had temporarily stopped bleeding (a common occurrence) or the discoloration was due to a cause other than hematuria. A further search would have been indicated. Note that there is no hurry to investigate hematuria. It takes very little blood to make the urine red. Exsanguination via the urinary tract is virtually impossible.

DATA　There have been no previous episodes of hematuria or history of stone disease. The patient has felt well, the systems review and past medical history are negative, and the family history is negative for kidney disease. He does not ingest large quantities of milk or alkali, takes no vitamin supplements, and has no gastrointestinal symptoms or known bone diseases.

LOGIC　The causes of hematuria are many and can be listed in anatomic sequence from the kidney down to the urethra. By and large, we are dealing mainly with *cancer, stone,* or *infection*. Starting with the kidney, there can be trauma, tumor, stone, polycystic disease, tuberculosis, infarct, pyelonephritis, or glomerulonephritis. Trauma is evident by history, stones are painful, and an infarct must postulate a source; the latter two can be ruled out by the absence of associated symptoms. The history gives no evidence for any of the causes of hypercalcemia and stones (milk-alkali, excessive vitamin D, etc).

Proceeding downward, the ureter may have cancer or stone. The bladder may be affected by cancer, stone, or inflammation. Cancer is often asymptomatic, stone is usually painful on urination if it is too large to pass, and inflammation is apparent by associated acute severe frequency, urgency, burning, and dysuria.

The prostate and urethra can be the source of hematuria too. BPH causes bleeding from venous distortions and varices, and prostatic cancer causes it by direct bladder wall invasion. Urethral malignancies are uncommon but do bleed too.

Do not forget the hemorrhagic disorders (overanticoagulation and thrombocytopenia) which may be manifested by hematuria or may unmask underlying silent neoplasms. Geography, sex, and age influence our logic. If in Egypt, the most common cause of hematuria is schistosomiasis of the bladder (Egyptian hematuria). Bladder stones are very common across North Africa and Central Asia. Men are prone to prostate problems, whereas women have a much higher incidence of hemorrhage cystitis.

Children are afflicted with acute glomerulonephritis, but cancer is more common in adults.

Many of the above diagnostic possibilities have already been ruled out. The most serious problem is still to be considered. Cancer (bladder or kidney) accounts for 25% of patients with hematuria. Stones account for almost 25% too but the absence of any type of pain, crystals, and an underlying cause refutes this possibility.

Another clue can help localize the source. If only the first portion of the urine sample is bloody, the bleeding is urethral. If the urine is diffusely bloody, the source is from the vesical neck up. Large clots suggest bleeding in the bladder. Wormy clots indicate bleeding from above the bladder.

DATA　Physical examination reveals a well-developed slim man who is in no acute distress and does not look sick. Two abnormalities are noted. The lower abdomen is full and tenderness, dullness, and urgency are noted on percussion. Rectal examination discloses a 3+ enlarged smooth, firm, nontender prostate; it contains no hard nodules. The stool is guaiac negative. There are no masses in the abdomen, no band keratopathy, and no tenderness over the kidneys.

LOGIC　Absence of band keratopathy is against prolonged severe hypercalcemia. Kidney cancer is not ruled out by the absence of palpable masses; kidneys themselves are rarely palpable and a mass would have to be quite large and in the lower pole to be felt. He does seem to have an enlarged prostate which is causing obstructive symptoms and urinary retention. Its effect on kidney function must be determined. Examination of the external urethra and prostate gland is vital in cases such as this.

DATA　Laboratory tests show a normal blood count. The urinalysis is repeated and the findings are the same as before. An 18-test blood chemistry profile is completely normal except for: blood urea nitrogen (BUN) 50 mg, creatinine 1.8 mg, calcium 11.1 mg/dl. The latter three are repeated and found to be correct. Alkaline and acid phosphatase are normal.

LOGIC Cancer of the kidney (hypernephroma) can secrete a parathormone-like substance which elevates the calcium and erythropoietin which causes polycythemia. Hypercalcemia is present; polycythemia is not. The absence of band keratopathy suggests the modest hypercalcemia is not longstanding. Renal malfunction with a disproportionately elevated BUN suggests pre- or postrenal azotemia. Prerenal azotemia is not likely because the physical examination is normal and there is no evidence for gastrointestinal bleeding (stool negative). The large prostate and bladder suggest that the azotemia is most likely the result of prostatic obstruction. A normal acid phosphatase is against prostatic cancer but does not rule it out.

DATA The chest x-ray, abdominal x-ray and ECG are normal except for apparent bladder distention. In particular, no metastatic lesions are noted in the lung (a favorite site for hypernephroma), the renal contours are not well visualized, and the ECG shows no evidence of hypercalcemia.

LOGIC So far, we have eliminated many possibilities but have not pinpointed the cause for the hematuria. Further studies are needed. First do an intravenous pyelogram (IVP), but only after determining lack of allergy to iodine and to any previously done IVP. The mild azotemia does not preclude doing an IVP because intrinsic renal disease and dysfunction are considered unlikely.

DATA An IVP was performed the next day. It demonstrated a normally functioning right kidney. The left kidney was somewhat enlarged and the upper pole, which was functioning poorly, appeared to have a distorted, thinned-out calyx and protruded beyond the rest of the renal contour. Both ureters visualized adequately and the ureters and collecting systems were moderately dilated. The bladder was enlarged and there was a postvoid residual volume of 200 to 300 ml. Intrusion of a large prostate into the

bladder base was visible. No stones were seen in this study.

LOGIC A left upper pole carcinoma is strongly suspected; 90% of stones are radiopaque, so this entity is virtually ruled out. The bilateral hydroureter, mild hydronephroses, and large residual volume are diagnostic of bladder outlet obstruction and are most likely due to the patient's enlarged prostate. Diminishing renal function no doubt results from the obstruction. The small loss of functioning renal tissue in the left upper pole could not possibly account for it. Prompt relief of the obstruction with an indwelling catheter is indicated.

DATA After the insertion of a Foley catheter, 3000 ml of urine were excreted in the first 24 hours. Three days later, the BUN and creatinine approached normal. Obstructive symptoms vanished.

LOGIC Were this the only problem, a prostatectomy would have been done. But the left upper pole lesion is the critical situation and must be diagnosed before kidney surgery is attempted.

The lesion in the upper pole is either a benign cyst or a malignant tumor and a distinction must be made by an ultrasound study or a computed tomographic (CT) scan. Both give essentially the same information but the former is less costly, less invasive, easier to do, and may have greater capacity for making the crucial differentiation between cyst and tumor.

DATA The next day an ultrasound study showed a lesion with irregular echogenicity, suggesting a solid rather than a cystic lesion. On the following day, a renal arteriogram was performed via the left femoral artery. This revealed a highly vascular tumor in the upper pole of the left kidney, a typical tumor blush, and abnormal vessels, but no aberrant or anomalous arteries. Films taken in the late venous filling phase showed no evidence of tumor infiltrating the renal vein.

LOGIC The diagnosis is now reasonably certain. The IVP distortion was not caused by a cyst. The patient has a carcinoma of the left kidney (hypernephroma) and there is no evidence of spread beyond the kidney. It is probably resectable and surgery is indicated. Careful attention must be given to adequate hydration so that the hypercalcemia gives no problems while it lasts. A catheter may be needed for a brief time to maintain normal renal function. Prostatectomy will be done at a future date if the kidney lesion is resectable and there are no evident metastases. If the initial ultrasound study had shown a *purely cystic* lesion, you might then have performed a guided needle aspiration with cytologic study, or perhaps done nothing referable to the cyst. Had the renal lesion been only partially cystic, aspiration first, followed by surgery if the fluid were bloody or contained neoplastic cells, would be the route for some—direct surgery for others.

Most physicians obtain a renal arteriogram before surgery in order to (*a*) define the renal vascular anatomy, (*b*) determine renal vein invasion, and (*c*) confirm the diagnosis.

Consider another scenario in this patient. The IVP is normal or shows a lesion that proves to be a benign cyst. In these circumstances you must hunt further for a hematuria-causing lesion. Cystoscopy is indicated. This procedure will detect a bladder neoplasm and note the degree of prostatic hypertrophy. In older people the search may end at this point even if nothing is found. If blood is seen coming from a ureteral orifice, retrograde pyelography may be done to find a rare ureteral tumor. Prostatic hypertrophy as a cause for hematuria is a diagnosis made by exclusion; renal and bladder cancer *must* be ruled out. In younger persons arteriography may detect an arteriovenous malformation.

If, as in this case, prostatic cancer may coexist, it may be diagnosed by newer more sensitive techniques for measuring the acid phosphatase, isotope bone scans for metastases, and aspiration biopsy. But since this patient will shortly need prostatic surgery too, further studies are deferred until then.

You might justifiably debate the necessity for all the diagnostic procedures done for this patient. Prior to the past 15 years, the IVP was enough; but this resulted in the removal of too many benign cysts and normal kidneys. Here, the IVP and sonogram were probably sufficient. But if the IVP and sonogram were equivocal, nobody would argue against doing a needle aspiration and/or an arteriogram. Where the diagnosis of tumor is reasonably certain, many would question the need for a risky invasive arteriogram to guide the surgeon and a sometimes-performed inferior vena cavagram to detect direct tumor invasion. The relative values of CT and ultrasound in the diagnosis of a renal mass are not yet established.

In a child with hematuria, suspect infection, immune-complex glomerulonephritis, sickle cell anemia, Wilms' tumor, or a congenital anomaly. This differential necessitates a careful urinalysis, urine culture, hemoglobin electrophoresis, an IVP, and a voiding cystourethrogram.

QUESTIONS

1. If this patient had shown a normal IVP, the next diagnostic maneuver would have been cystoscopy. Given the same clinical picture, what would have been the most likely finding?
   (a) cancer of the bladder
   (b) hemorrhagic cystitis
   (c) bladder stone
   (d) cancer of the urethra.
2. In a patient with obstructive uropathy, all of the following would be expected except one:
   (a) BUN:creatinine ratio greater than 20
   (b) no urine production for 24 hours
   (c) urine osmolality equal to plasma osmolality
   (d) urine pH 6.0.
3. A 56-year-old man has five to ten RBCs/high-power field in his urine on a routine insurance examination. Otherwise nothing abnormal was found. Which statement is correct?
   (a) It is only mild microscopic hematuria and can be ignored.
   (b) Even though mild, it should be rechecked in a month.
   (c) If no albumin or RBC casts are noted, it is not significant.
   (d) It should be immediately investigated.
4. Hematuria may be seen as a complication of all the below except one:
   (a) sickle cell trait
   (b) gentamicin therapy

(c) urethral caruncle
(d) myocardial infarction.
5. Hypernephromas are slow-growing, retroperitoneal, and rarely present as masses in the abdomen. However, they can present in a variety of ways other than hematuria. These include all but one of the following:
(a) fever of unknown origin
(b) pulmonary embolus
(c) bilateral leg edema
(d) pathologic fracture of the femur.

ANSWERS

1. **(a) is correct.** Cancer of the bladder is the most likely of the four. It usually gives no symptoms—just bleeding. Cystitis, on the other hand, whether caused by infection or drugs (cyclophosphamide), is associated with severe symptoms not present in this patient. Bladder stones cause bleeding, but an IVP would have detected this. In cancer of the urethra, blood would have been primarily in the initially voided portion of the specimen; the urine would not have been uniformly pink.

2. **(b) is correct.** Obstructive uropathy can be present for months to years and renal function deteriorate, yet urine formation continues. A BUN:creatinine ratio greater than 20 is common in obstructive uropathy presumably because of decreased tubular fluid flow rate leading to increased urea resorption and thus a higher BUN. A defect in renal concentrating ability and an inability to maximally acidify urine are common in obstructive uropathy, so that (c) and (d) result.

3. **(d) is correct.** Microscopic hematuria can have the same serious causes as gross hematuria. The presence of five to ten RBCs, confirmed by immediate recheck, is definitely abnormal. (a) and (b) are therefore obviously wrong courses to follow. The absence of albumin and RBC casts tends to rule out a glomerular source of the blood, but by no means rules out other serious diseases like cancer.

4. **(b) is correct.** Gentamicin is nephrotoxic and can lead to renal failure, but not to hematuria. Its major site of action is the tubule, although recent evidence suggests it may affect the glomerulus as well. Sickle cell trait may be associated with hematuria (gross or microscopic). In this condition, the red cells are thought to sickle in the medulla where there is lower oxygen tension. The vasa recta in this region become obstructed, burst, and bleed into the urine. Sickle cell disease is notorious in this regard. Hemoglobin electrophoresis and sickling preparations must be obtained if this disorder is suspected. Urethral caruncles at the distal end of female urethrae often bleed. Myocardial infarction itself does not cause hematuria, but anticoagulants used to treat it may do so. Also, a renal infarct from a mural thrombus can cause flank pain and hematuria.

5. **(d) is correct.** Hypernephromas do not metastasize like other tumors. They do not spread to long bones, so a pathologic fracture of the femur would be quite uncommon. However, they do grow into the renal vein and up the vena cava; tumor emboli to the lungs or partial vena cava obstruction with bilateral leg edema can result. Since the tumor often has necrotic tissue, fever of unknown origin may be a mode of presentation. Remember that polycythemia and hypercalcemia detected on a routine blood screen can also be initial presentations. These result from the production of hormone-like material: erythropoietin-like substance and parathyroid hormone-like substance (or even 1,25-dihydroxycholecalciferol, the active form of vitamin D).

COMMENT After a careful consideration of the overlap of red urine and bloody urine, hematuria was established as the key clue, and a list of diagnostic possibilities was formed. A urinalysis was the initially obtained portion of the data base—not the usual order.

Numerous possibilities were ruled out with pertinent negative clues. Bayes' probability theory was properly respected since only common possibilities were seriously considered; geography, age, and sex created various subsets of population in whom the probabilities differed. The presence of two genitourinary diseases, each of which can cause hematuria, established another Boolean overlap. While both BPH and cancer of the kidney can cause bloody urine, there were other features present which related to only one or the other (renal mass, urea retention, urine retention). Indeed, the cause for the hematuria was never clearly distinguished, but treatment for cancer took precedence.

A dendrogram approach to the solution would have been simple. Answer a series of questions: (*a*) Is it blood? (*b*) Is there any pain? (*c*) Are there symptoms of infection? (*d*) Is the prostate or bladder enlarged? (*e*) Is a renal mass palpable? And so forth. (*P. C.*)

PROBLEM-BASED LEARNING You have just learned a few things about a patient with hematuria. In order to have a well-rounded knowledge of the subject you should read and know all about:

1. the causes of hematuria
2. what else may make the urine red
3. the concomitant urine abnormalities that guide you
4. the significance of microscopic vs gross hematuria

5. hemorrhagic cystitis
6. carcinoma of the kidney, its pathologic types, varied clinical presentations, the role of excessive "erythropoietin," and the use of the IVP, CT scan, ultrasound, and arteriography in defining the lesion
7. how to distinguish renal cancer from renal cyst
8. polycystic kidneys
9. how hematologic disorders cause hematuria
10. benign prostatic hypertrophy and carcinoma of the prostate, their clinical pictures, how each may cause hematuria, and the value of the acid and alkaline phosphatase
11. the role of aspiration for renal cysts and prostatic cancer
12. how kidney stones cause hematuria, yet no pain
13. obstructive uropathy
14. carcinoma of the bladder and the role of cystoscopy and ultrasound in its diagnosis
15. the remaining limited use for retrograde pyelography.

Learn this, and you have added another 5% to your medical information base.

SELF-EVALUATION EXERCISES

(Answers appear after the last question.)

1. Draw an algorithm that starts with gross hematuria, utilizes three diagnostic procedures (IVP, CT scan, and cystoscopy), and has four possible endpoints (1. renal cancer, 2. renal cyst, 3. bladder cancer, and 4. no diagnosis).
2. You are deciding whether to drive into town and buy some shoes on sale or stay home and work in the garden. The weather bureau predicts a 50% chance of rain. If you stay home and it rains, you can't garden but can watch football on TV. If you go downtown and it rains, you will be discomforted, yet can buy the shoes. On weighing the relative benefits and costs, you estimate the pleasure of buying shoes at a bargain (+4), the pleasure of gardening (+2), and the pleasure of watching the football game (+1). The only possible source of displeasure (negative pleasure) is shopping in the rain (−2).

    Design a decision tree, insert values, perform the necessary calculations, and choose the course of action from which the most pleasure is derived.
3. An intravenous pyelogram discovers a round lesion in the upper pole of the left kidney in a patient who was noted to have microscopic hematuria. On the basis of the clinical picture you decide there is a 50-50 chance of cancer:cyst. Ordinarily you would not hesitate to request surgery, but the patient is not a good

operative risk. So you seek greater certainty with an expensive discomforting diagnostic procedure.

The test is 90% sensitive and 90% specific. If the patient has cancer, death will result if no treatment is given. The operative mortality is 10% and the mortality if cancer is present is 40%. This includes the 10% immediate surgical mortality and the subsequent 30% mortality from disease recurrence. At this time no attempt is made to compare the relative utilities of immediate death and subsequent death from recurrence.

(a) Construct a crude decision tree and calculate the risk of dying if nothing is done and the risk of dying if surgery is performed. (*See Figs. 8.1 to 8.3.*)
(b) Next add the test into the decision tree and calculate the mortality risk if all who test positive have surgery and those who test negative do not have surgery. (Add a branch to the decision tree.)
(c) Which is the best course to follow?
(d) If you were able to use a gold standard test with 100% sensitivity and 100% specificity as a basis for the "test and decide" strategy, what would the predicted mortality rate be?
(e) Assume that *no diagnostic test is available.* At what clinical estimate of cancer probability would the decision to operate or do nothing have equal outcomes?
(f) How would a decrease in the patient's operative risk alter the treatment threshold? (Assume no test is available.)

ANSWERS

1. First do an IVP. If positive for a mass do a CT scan; this distinguishes between cyst and tumor. If negative for a renal mass, do cystoscopy; this results in bladder cancer or no diagnosis.

2. Go to town and shop. Take your chances on rain. This choice will give you the most pleasure. If you go shopping and it rains you derive 2 units of pleasure (4 minus 2); if it doesn't rain you derive 4 units of pleasure. If you stay home and it rains, you acquire 1 unit of pleasure, but if it doesn't rain you acquire 2 units. The exact calculation of expected pleasure via the go-shopping route is: .50(2)+.50(4) which is equal to 3. The stay-home route is .50(1)+.50(2) which is equal to 1.5. This scenario is similar to Figure 8.2.

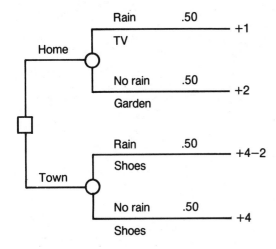

3. (a) .50 and .25. If nothing is done the risk of death is equal to the P(D) for cancer. If surgery is done the risk of death is .25 (.50 × .40 if cancer exists plus .50 × .10 if cancer does not exist).

   (b) The test, if applied to a cohort of 100 such individuals, will yield 45 TPs, 5 FPs, 5 FNs, and 45 FPs. If surgery is performed on all who test positive and not performed on all who test negative, it is clear that some patients *with no disease* (FP) are operated upon, and some patients *with disease* (FN) do not receive surgical treatment. The mortality using the "test and decide" strategy is .235 (.45 × .40 for those with cancer plus .05 × .10 for those who do not have cancer in the operated group—plus .05 × 1 in the untreated group who test falsely negative.

   (c) On the surface this seems to be a tossup since there is little difference between .25 and .235. But the "test and decide" strategy inevitably results in some cancer patients not being treated (FNs) and some noncancer patients having needless surgery (FPs). On the other hand, performing surgery without first testing creates many unnecessary operations and hospital costs escalate thereby. As always, the patient's

values regarding procedures and surgery help you decide.

   (d) A perfect test eliminates FPs and FNs. A single patient who tests positive has cancer, surgery, and a .40 mortality. A negative testee has no cancer, no surgery, and no mortality. Given a cohort of 100 patients with a cancer prevalence of .50, a perfect test accurately partitions those who do and those who do not require surgery. Indeed, the test performance reduces surgery by half. The overall mortality is an irreducible .20 (.50 × .40)—.40 for the 50 patients *with* cancer, and zero for the 50 patients *without* cancer. Thus an efficient test reduces needless surgery, cuts costs, minimizes moral-ethical issues, and saves lives.

   (e) .14. If the P(D) = .14 either strategy would have the same outcome. This is the "treatment threshold." It is calculated by letting x = P(D) and y = P($\bar{D}$). If either strategy is to have the same mortality rate, $1.0x = .4x + .1y$. Since $x + y = 1$, substitute and solve. The clinical significance of this calculation lies in the conclusion that if the probability of cancer is only .10 in this patient he should be spared surgery; if the P(D) is .20, surgery is best.

   (f) Intuitively you operate at a lower P(D) if the operative risk is lower; and you require greater diagnostic certainty if the operative risk is higher. This makes good clinical sense. Such medical logic is proven by performing a sensitivity analysis in which the two variables are the *treatment threshold* and the *operative mortality*. The treatment threshold is the P(D) where the two available options have equal expected outcomes.

   Let the immediate operative mortality be represented by m; since there is an additional 30% mortality from cancer recurrence or metastases, the overall mortality for cancer patients receiving surgery is $m + .30$. Those patients who have surgery, yet no cancer, have a mortality of m. All patients with cancer who do not have surgery will die.

   For any P(D) the mortality from doing nothing is equal to 1.0 P(D); similarly, the overall mortality from routinely performing surgery equals P(D) × ($m + .3$) plus P($\bar{D}$) × m. As an example, if the P(D) is .10, m equals .07. This conclusion is reached by constructing and solving the following equation in which the mortalities from both options are equal: $.10 = .10(m + .3) + .90m$. If you now calculate and graph the treatment thresholds and the corresponding operative mortalities that make each decision a tossup, you will note a direct linear relationship.

Suggested Readings

1. Smith RB: Evaluation of hematuria. In Bricker NS, Kirschenbaum MA (eds): *The Kidney: Diagnosis and Management.* New York, Wiley, 1984, pp 33–39.
   A concise textbook discussion of the causes.
2. Abuelo JG: Evaluation of hematuria. *Urology* 21:215–225, 1983.
   A diagnostic protocol designed to increase clinical acumen and minimize tests.
3. Nieh PT, Conant JC, Zablow BC, et al: Episodic flank pain and gross hematuria in a young woman (clinical conference). *J Urol* 121:99–102, 1984.
   While the patient turns out to have a rare disease, the problem-solving process for pain and hematuria is discussed.
4. Ng RC, Seto DS: Hematuria. A suggested workup strategy. *Postgrad Med* 75:139–144, 1984.
   A step-by-step plan is given.
5. Sufrin G: The challenges of renal adenocarcinoma. *Surg Clin North Am* 62:1101–1118, 1982.
   Surveys the types, diagnosis, staging, and management.
6. Gatenby RA: Diagnostic evaluation of a renal mass. *Semin Oncol* 10:402–412, 1983.
   Portrays the use of plain films, CT, ultrasound, arteriography, and nuclear magnetic resonance.
7. Coleman BG, Arger PH: Sonography of renal adenocarcinoma. *CRC Crit Rev Diagn Imaging* 19:203–255, 1983.
   Covers all diagnostic modes but mainly ultrasound.
8. Perrin RL, Poller WR: Computed tomography of renal mass lesions. *CRC Crit Rev Diagn Imaging* 20:191–214, 1983.
   Beautiful reproductions that demonstrate the value of CT scans for renal mass lesions.
9. Jewett HJ: Prostatic cancer: a personal view of the problem. *J Urol* 121:845–849, 1984.
   From the perspective of one of the world's most famous urologists.
10. Rickards D, Gowland M, Brooman P, et al: Computed tomography and transrectal ultrasound in the diagnosis of prostatic disease—a comparative study. *Br J Urol* 55:726–732, 1983.
    The use of high technology procedures is extended to the prostate gland, especially for cancer.
11. Lippman RW: *Urine and the Urinary Sediment,* ed 2. Springfield, IL, Charles C Thomas, 1977.
    A how-to-do-it book. Describes the techniques of urinalysis and aids in their interpretation.
12. Coe FL: Clinical and laboratory assessment of the patient with renal disease. In Brenner B, Rector R (eds): *The Kidney,* ed 3. Philadelphia, Saunders, 1985, chap 18.
    Outline of the appropriate maneuvers to assess various renal problems, including a logical sequence of steps for the evaluation of hematuria.
13. Berman LB: When the urine is red. *JAMA* 237:2753, 1977.
    Short discussion of the differential diagnosis of red urine. Includes not only hematurias but other processes leading to red urine.
14. Lange PH, Limas C: Molecular markers in the diagnosis and prognosis of bladder cancer. *Urology* 23 (4 suppl):46–54, 1984.
    A look into the future.

Case 40
Frequent and Painful Urination
MARVIN FORLAND, M.D.

DATA A 23-year-old woman sees you because of frequent and painful urination for 2 days. This had never happened before her marriage 6 months ago, but since then she has had four similar episodes. She has the impression they are related to sexual intercourse, though she cannot be sure. Fever, chills, gross hematuria, or back pain are never present. Twice she was treated with 1-week courses of sulfisoxazole and promptly got better. On the other occasions she got well without treatment.

There is a 19-year history of juvenile-onset diabetes mellitus (DM) which has been regulated with NPH insulin before breakfast and dinner. Urine glucoses are checked about twice daily and are either negative or trace-positive. She has been remarkably free of problems and symptoms related to her diabetes.

LOGIC The history is typical of recurrent lower urinary tract infections—urethritis-cystitis.

Among the most common problems seen in primary care are urinary tract infections. They occur in infants, children, men, and women; but the spectra of causes differ. It is notable that after age 60, 5 to 15% of men and women experience such infections.

The patient's diabetes seems well controlled according to urine tests and lack of polyuria and thirst. However, there are a number of factors which require more careful evaluation prior to merely giving another brief course of antibacterial therapy.

First, the organism causing these infections has never been identified. When bacteria are found, 95% are gram-negative bacilli (mostly *Escherichia coli*, some *Aerobacter-Klebsiella*); the remainder consists of gram-positive cocci, *Proteus*, *Pseudomonas*, and fungi. This may be related to the anal-urethral-bladder route of contamination. Specific local infections about the genitalia can also cause dysuria and frequency. These include gonorrhea, herpes progenitalis, *Monilia*, and *Trichomonas vaginalis*. The same symptoms commonly occur without evidence of infection, since half the women with these symptoms have no significant growth on routine urine culture. This is called the "urethral syndrome"; it may relate to a functional disorder of the bladder, or altered local urethral defenses with low-grade bacterial colonization, or infection with an organism not grown on routine culture preparations such as *Chlamydia trachomatis*.

Second, these episodes have recurred over a brief period of time. They may be marriage related, and may be of benign origin. However, recurrent urinary tract infection (UTI) under any circumstances is an indication for careful evaluation. You must look for congenital, anatomic, functional, or obstructive factors which can be the predisposing cause for infection. Obstruction to urine flow is a principal concern and it may be either functional or anatomic. Such abnormalities can exist at any level of the collecting system from the urethral meatus to the renal pelvis.

Here, sex and age are important clues. Youngsters with UTIs frequently have structural abnormalities and congenital defects such as ureterovesical reflux, bladder neck obstruction, ureteropelvic obstruction, horseshoe kidney, etc. These predispose to infection. For, as in other systems of the body, obstruction often leads to infection.

A 28-year-old sexually promiscuous male may have gonorrhea with a urethral stricture. Young and middle-aged men develop acute prostatitis with a typical picture of severe urinary symptoms, fever, and marked prostatic tenderness. They also commonly harbor chronic prostatitis which is usually asymptomatic but causes recurrent episodes of cystitis. *Bacteroides*, *Chlamydia*, and *Trichomonas* are frequent offenders.

In an older multigravid woman, think of a poorly emptying bladder caused by a large cystocele. And in the 65-year-old man, remember prostatic hypertrophy. It commonly causes retrograde infection.

A third important consideration here is diabetes. Increasing data suggest UTIs are more frequent in women with DM than in nondiabetic women, with a high prevalence of upper tract involvement in the former. Why this is not so in males remains speculative. But it is well established that serious complications like papillary necrosis and perinephric abscess are more common in DM. Another point to remember is that long-standing DM can cause neurogenic impairment of bladder emptying, thus predisposing to infection.

DATA More facts are obtained. The family history, review of systems, and previous medical history give no helpful information. Vital signs are normal, and the patient does not look sick. There are scattered microaneurysms and a few hard yellowish exudates in the fundi. No tenderness is noted over the kidneys or bladder, and Murphy's sign is negative. Other than decreased proprioception in the legs and absent Achilles tendon reflexes, the examination is normal. There is no discharge and the urethral meatus is normal in situation and appearance. A clean-catch midstream urine specimen is collected while the patient is in the lithotomy position.

LOGIC Several important bits of information are revealed. There is no evidence of a local specific infection such as moniliasis, frequent in poorly controlled diabetes. In addition, the absence of kidney tenderness and fever is important in separating upper UTI from lower UTI. Fever is the most valuable clue in the differentiation of the two. Note that the urine specimen was easily collected without adding the risk of introducing infection by catheterization. The fundi show specific evidence of diabetic retinopathy, and the neurologic abnormalities support the impression of early diabetic neuropathy.

DATA Preliminary data are available. The complete blood count is normal. The sterilely collected urine specimen was divided into three aliquots. One was used for immediate study, the second for routine culture and sensitivity, and the third for immunofluorescence study for antibody coating of bacteria. Routine urinalysis shows pH 5.5, protein 2+, glucose trace, 20 to 30 white blood cells (WBCs) with clumps/high-power field, and one to two hyaline casts with an occasional granular cast/low-power field. There are no WBC casts. Many bacteria are seen in the unspun specimen. A Gram stain of a dried smear shows gram-negative rods.

LOGIC Bacteria and WBCs in an unspun clean-catch specimen confirm a UTI of bacterial origin. The presence of bacteria correlates well with a culture growth of at least 100,000 colonies/ml and provides a useful screening method. In fact, more than ten WBCs/high-power field of centrifuged urine suggest that infection is present. More than one bacterium/oil-immersion field from a stained unspun specimen is predictive of 100,000 or more colonies/ml of urine and indicates an infectious process. Gram stain

helps identify the organism. Pyuria without bacteriuria might hint at tuberculosis. The proteinuria and casts suggest possible concomitant diabetic glomerulosclerosis in keeping with other evidences of microangiopathy noted. The absence of WBC casts and a normal peripheral WBC count are further evidence against kidney involvement by infection.

DATA Pending the results of culture, nitrofurantoin is given. The patient returns in 48 hours and the symptoms had cleared. Culture grew more than 100,000 colonies of *E. coli*, sensitive to all agents, but resistant to sulfonamides. The immunofluorescence study for antibody coating was negative. Repeat urinalysis showed persistent 2+ proteinuria and casts, but a rare WBC and no bacteria. Continuation of nitrofurantoin for a full 10-day course is recommended, and the patient is asked to collect a 24-hour urine sample for protein and creatinine. Blood is drawn for 18-test blood chemistry determination.

LOGIC Response to treatment was excellent. The absence of antibody coating usually indicates limitation of infection to the lower urinary tract. Immunoglobulin coating of bacteria is seen with renal parenchymal, prostatic, or complicated bladder infections. But it may be absent in some cases of classical acute pyelonephritis of rapid onset. X-ray studies were deferred pending evaluation of renal function. The greater risk of renal function complications associated with intravenous pyelography in diabetics is well known.

DATA Further studies return. Serum creatinine is 1.0 mg/dl and creatinine clearance is 85 ml/minute—both normal. Blood glucose is 128 mg/dl; other blood chemistry tests are normal. When she sees her physician the next week, an intravenous pyelogram and voiding cystourethrogram are ordered. Both are normal and there is no residual urine. The radiologist comments that the kidneys look slightly larger than normal for the patient's stature.

LOGIC While the patient may well have diabetic nephropathy based on the urine findings and the slightly enlarged kidneys, function is still normal. X-ray studies rule out anatomic, congenital, and obstructive abnormalities which could be responsible for the recurrent UTIs. Diabetic neuropathy with incomplete bladder emptying is excluded, and there is no evidence of reflux or undiagnosed papillary necrosis.

DATA A repeat urine culture is negative and the urinalysis stays the same. The patient is apprised of her diabetic status and reassured that the infections are not serious. Postcoital voiding and cleansing of the urethral meatus with a mild soap solution are recommended. She is to return promptly if symptoms recur.

LOGIC You realize that recurrence is common. But you are aware that the diagnosis of UTI is often plagued by silence. Chronic cystitis has a high prevalence, yet no symptoms. Chronic pyelonephritis may silently destroy the kidneys and cause renal failure.

On the other hand, acute infections speak out with signs and symptoms. Acute pyelonephritis usually presents a classic picture that subsides in several days. It did so even before the antibiotic era. Yet sometimes this infection may progress to renal abscess, perinephric abscess, necrotizing papillitis, or gram-negative sepsis. These serious and often life-threatening complications may be detected by gallium scan, computed tomographic scan, and blood culture—sometimes by simple pyelography.

Should your patient's next infection involve her kidneys too, you must be well aware of such complications because some are more apt to occur if DM is present.

QUESTIONS

1. The features most strongly suggesting renal parenchymal involvement in an acute UTI are:
    (a) suprapubic tenderness
    (b) clumps of WBCs in the urine
    (c) fever
    (d) WBC casts.
2. Acute pyelonephritis with flank pain, fever, chills, and pyuria can be seen in which of the following clinical settings?
    (a) colicky pain radiating to testis associated with hematuria
    (b) 6 months' pregnancy
    (c) cystoscopy with ureteral catheterization for diagnostic purposes
    (d) previous IVP showed marked hydronephrosis of one kidney.
3. Obstruction predisposes to infection. The site of obstruction may determine the clinical picture. Which of the following is untrue?
    (a) Large obstructing prostate glands may cause repeated episodes of cystitis or epididymo-orchitis.
    (b) Obstructing prostate glands can cause bladder hypertrophy, many symptoms, hydronephroses, and renal failure.
    (c) Urethral strictures in younger men, and congenital valves at the vesicourethral junction in male children can cause the same picture as in (b).
    (d) Bilateral ureteral obstruction can cause silent deteriorating renal function.
4. Match the following four conditions with the appropriate clinical setting:
    (a) a 68-year-old man with frequency, dribbling, and severe nocturia
    (b) a 48-year-old woman with a 25-year history of frequent severe migraine headaches
    (c) a 55-year-old woman with a long history of psychoneurosis and tension headaches
    (d) a 3-year-old girl with recurrent acute pyelonephritis

    (1) ureterovesical reflux
    (2) interstitial nephritis with papillary necrosis
    (3) hydronephroses secondary to retroperitoneal fibrosis
    (4) benign prostatic hypertrophy.

ANSWERS

1. **(c) and (d) are correct.** Fever is not seen with simple urethritis-cystitis. It indicates renal and sometimes prostatic involvement. WBC casts tell us the WBCs are in the tubules where casts form. Suprapubic tenderness goes with bladder inflammation. Clumps of WBCs are seen no matter where the UTI is.
2. **All are correct.** Situation (a) suggests a stone obstructing the ureter, and obstruction often leads to infection. Pregnant women are susceptible to kidney infection because pregnancy causes hydroureters and poor drainage. Instru-

mentation always carries a risk of introducing infection. The previous IVP in (d) suggests the presence of ureteropelvic obstruction by an anomalous renal artery.

3. **No answers are untrue.** This question is designed to demonstrate the various levels and types of obstructive uropathy and how obstruction at each level can cause serious problems. (d) can result from stones, strictures, cervical cancer, and retroperitoneal fibrosis.

4. **(a-4)** This is common and needs no explanation. **(b-3)** Methysergide, commonly used to prevent chronic vascular headache, can cause retroperitoneal fibrosis and ureteral obstruction. **(c-2)** This patient is prone to analgesic abuse, usually by phenacetin, a drug which can cause the named renal disease. **(d-1)** Ureterovesical reflux is an important and common cause of upper UTI in young children.

COMMENT   Diagnosis was no problem here. Diabetes was prominent in the author's thinking, both from the standpoint of overlapping complications (neuropathy, retinopathy, nephropathy) and because of its relation to UTIs through a variety of known and unknown mechanisms.

Many complex cause and effect relationships were present. For example, diabetes can cause infection in three ways. The first is direct and unknown; the second is via autonomic neuropathy; the third is by the presence of associated moniliasis. Diabetes, sexual intercourse, pregnancy, obstruction, congenital anomaly, poor drainage, and instrumentation can combine in various ways to cause infection.

Sex and age alter the statistical likelihoods of the underlying causes for UTI. So do the presence of other genitourinary diseases and the taking of certain immunity-altering drugs.

Upper and lower UTI were differentiated by a number of clues. Fever, WBC casts, and antibody coating are all highly specific and sensitive in this regard. That is to say—fever is reliable in distinguishing between upper and lower UTI, but not in distinguishing UTI from infection in another area. However, if all three clues are present, then the evidence for an upper UTI becomes overwhelming. (*P. C.*)

Suggested Readings

1. Rubin RH, Tolkoff-Rubin NE, Cotran RS: Urinary tract infection, pyelonephritis, and reflux nephrop-

athy. In Brenner BM, Rector FC Jr (eds): *The Kidney*, ed 3. Philadelphia, Saunders, 1985, chap 24.
   Textbook coverage of the entire subject.

2. *Am J Med* 75 (1B), July, 1983, pp 44–52, 53–58, 71–78, 79–84.
   Four excellent articles in this single journal relate the urine bacterial count and the degree of pyuria to confirmatory laboratory procedures.

3. Abraham E, Brenner BE, Simon RR: Cystitis and pyelonephritis. *Ann Emerg Med* 12:228–234, 1983.
   The clinical features of these two entities are detailed.

4. Sheldon CA, Gonzalez R: Differentiation of upper and lower urinary tract infections: how and when? *Med Clin North Am* 68:321–328, 1984.
   An important issue is tackled but not completely downed.

5. Forland M: Urinary tract infections. In Stein JH (ed): *Nephrology*. New York, Grune & Stratton, 1980, pp 223–235.

6. Forland M, Thomas V, Shelokov A: Urinary tract infections in patients with diabetes mellitus. *JAMA* 238:1924–1926, 1977.
   An epidemiologic study employing the immunofluorescence technique for antibody coating of bacteria.

7. Eknoyan G, Qunibi WY, Grisson RT, et al: Renal papillary necrosis: an update. *Medicine* 61:55–73, 1982.
   A review of a clinical entity with many aliases.

8. Shortliffe LM: Prostatitis: still a diagnostic and therapeutic dilemma. *West J Med* 139:542–544, 1983.
   This article adds some order to a disordered subject.

9. Wong ES, Stamm WE: Urethral infections in men and women. *Annu Rev Med* 34:337–358, 1983.
   Includes the gonococcus, *Chlamydia*, and *Ureaplasma* groups.

10. Ireton RC, Berger RE: Prostatitis and epididimitis. *Urol Clin North Am* 11:83–94, 1984.

11. Rayfield EJ, Ault MJ, Keusch GT, et al: Infection and diabetes: the case for glucose control. *Am J Med* 72:439–450, 1982.
    A clinical study demonstrating a striking direct correlation between the overall prevalence of infection and mean plasma glucose levels in a large group of patients with diabetes mellitus.

12. Berg AO, Heidrich FE, Fihn SD, et al: Establishing the cause of genitourinary symptoms in women in family practice. Comparison of clinical examination and comprehensive microbiology. *JAMA* 251:620–625, 1984.
    Considers the various causes of genitourinary tract infections and how to diagnose them. The use of laboratory procedures doubles the yield.

Case 41
Sharp Flank Pain

MEYER D. LIFSCHITZ, M.D.

DATA Excruciating waves of sharp left-sided abdominal pain radiating to the left groin bring a 38-year-old man to the emergency room. Over the past 10 years, he had three similar episodes and passed three kidney stones; once the pain was on the right side. There is no burning, urgency, or frequency of urination.

The diagnosis seems clear, so you inject 75 mg of meperidine hydrochloride, start intravenous fluids, and hospitalize the patient. He does not know the cause for his stones and never had a workup. A urinalysis done in the emergency room shows 20 to 30 red blood cells (RBCs)/high-power field and nothing else.

LOGIC Treatment takes temporary precedence over the complete study. But already there is evidence that the patient has recurrent stones involving both sides of the urinary tract, so a unilateral obstructive anomaly is unlikely. Also, there are no symptoms to suggest concurrent infection.

DATA The colicky pains subside in ½ hour. A plain x-ray film of the abdomen shows an 8-mm irregular radiopaque calculus lodged in what seems to be the upper third of the left ureter. The patient is instructed to void all urine specimens through a strainer, to save any debris, and to call the nurse if pain recurs. He goes to sleep, but not before blood samples are drawn and another urine specimen is obtained for analysis and culture.

LOGIC Now you begin to consider the various causes of stones. Many have a clear-cut pathophysiologic explanation; some do not. It is important to realize that most renal stones are single episodes and do not recur; their cause is unclear and little if any workup is needed. Concern exists mainly when the stones are recurrent and you suspect an underlying potentially curable or preventable disorder. The etiology and chemical composition of stones are often easily related (Table 19.1).

Triple phosphate stones occur in the presence of chronic urinary tract infection, usually with *Proteus* species, though sometimes with other gram-negative bacilli. This organism is a urea-splitter, creates an alkaline pH, and liberates much NH_4^+—an ideal situation for precipitation of such stones.

Uric acid stones occur from hyperuricemia and excessive uric acid excretion due to gout, chemotherapy for malignancies, and myeloproliferative disorders. They also occur when the serum uric acid is normal if the urine pH is persistently low, as in chronic diarrheal states and ileostomies.

Cystine stones result from an inherited disorder, begin to form in early childhood, and exist in other members of the family. Such patients usually die of renal failure at a young age.

Calcium stones are by far the most common, are radiopaque, and consist of oxalate, phosphate, or both. They have many causes. Twenty-five to 40% of calcium stone formers excrete excessive calcium in the urine, which in men is >300 mg/24 hours, and in women is >250 mg/24 hours. Of these, hyperparathyroidism causes 5%; sarcoidosis, milk-alkali syndrome, hypervitaminosis D, and prolonged immobilization cause a few more. But most are the result of *idiopathic*

Table 19.1.
Chemical Composition of Renal Stones

Composition	Percentage
Calcium oxalate, phosphate, or both	67
Triple phosphate or $MgNH_4$ phosphate	15
Uric acid	8
Cystine	4
Miscellaneous	6

hypercalciuria whose cause is not definitely known but may be related to increased absorption from the gut or increased excretion by a "leak" through the kidney. The latter group has a strong family history. In 20% of those with idiopathic hypercalciuria there is associated hyperuricemia resulting in mixed stones.

In a large percentage of stone formers (20 to 60%) no metabolic defect is ever found. Some have slightly high excretion of calcium and oxalate but levels which are still within upper normal limits. Further research and clarification are needed.

DATA   Your patient has awakened so you take his history. He does not ingest large quantities of milk and cheese or take absorbable alkali, vitamins, or drugs. There is no indigestion or heartburn, though he has recently been constipated; and he has had no joint pains or stiffness. Systems review is negative for additional data and the family history is not significant for stones.

LOGIC   The milk-alkali syndrome (excessive calcium intake) is excluded; so is vitamin D intoxication. He has no upper gastrointestinal symptoms to suggest hyperparathyroidism, though constipation is often seen with this disease. The lack of symptoms of urinary tract infection is against stone formation from that cause, though smouldering chronic renal infection can exist without symptoms. There are none of the joint complaints often seen in sarcoidosis. The negative family history rebuts inheritable stone-forming diseases such as cystinuria and xanthinuria.

Other items in the history may guide your judgment in evaluating renal stone disease. *Age* is one such factor. Hyperparathyroidism and idiopathic hypercalciuria are uncommon prior to puberty, while metabolic disorders which cause stones (cystinosis, primary hyperoxaluria, and renal tubular acidosis) start early in childhood. *Gender* is important too; the stones of idiopathic hypercalciuria are five times more frequent in males, while hyperparathyroid stones are twice as common in females. *Diet and drug*

history may reveal vitamin D fads, excessive milk and/or alkali, or large oxalate intake (rhubarb). *Geography* is a factor in that stones are far more common in the southeast United States, North Africa, and all across central Asia.

DATA   Physical examination discloses a well-nourished healthy-looking man who now looks comfortable. The vital signs are normal. Except for the heart, there are no positive findings. In particular, there are no masses in the neck, no band keratopathy, no lymph node enlargement, and no renal tenderness. The apex beat is in the fifth left intercostal space, 12 cm from the midline; there is a grade 3/6 high-pitched pansystolic murmur at the apex radiating to the left axilla. Otherwise the heart is normal and the lungs are clear.

LOGIC   There is no physical evidence of hyperparathyroidism, though parathyroid adenomas are only rarely palpable. The lack of renal tenderness is difficult to interpret. Cardiac findings are typical for an enlarged heart secondary to mitral regurgitation. This is most likely a result of rheumatic heart disease, though there is no history of an acute episode or previously heard heart murmur. At any rate, it is not related to his stone disease, and he is not in left ventricular failure.

DATA   He has two more brief episodes of pain not requiring a narcotic. Laboratory results return the next day. The urine is normal except for 20 to 30 RBCs/high-power field and some crystals of calcium oxalate. A nitroprusside test of the urine is negative for cystine and the Sulkowitch test shows 4+ calciuria. The serum calcium, phosphorus, alkaline phosphatase, creatinine, and uric acid are normal, as are the rest of the blood chemical tests. Urine culture is negative and the complete blood count is normal.

LOGIC   The RBCs are expected; calcium oxalate crystals in the urine are not diagnostic since they are omnipresent. Large quantities might have some significance. The strongly positive Sulkowitch test indicates hypercalciuria, yet the serum calcium is normal. This suggests idiopathic hypercalciuria. Renal function is normal and gout is unlikely in the absence of joint symptoms, tophi, and hyperuricemia. Hyperparathyroidism is now even more remote in the presence of normal calcium and phosphorus. With a negative culture, so is chronic renal infection.

DATA   Chest x-ray shows a moderately enlarged left ventricle but the lungs are clear and there are no enlarged nodes. The ECG indicates left ventricular hypertrophy. An intravenous pyelogram demonstrates a normal right kidney and ureter; the left renal pelvis and left ureter are slightly dilated above the calculus which is clearly within the ureter and is now in the lower third. There is no postvoid residual and no other stones are seen.

LOGIC   The fact that the stone has moved down and is less than 10 to 12 mm in size suggests it will pass by itself. Sarcoidosis can be excluded by the negative chest x-ray, absence of lymph nodes, normal proteins, and normal calcium. The heart studies corroborate the physical findings; for now and the immediate future no cardiac treatment is needed, though investigation for valve replacement may be in order later.

That evening you reprogram your fading memory by reading about nephrolithiasis because you have not encountered the problem for many months. You are reminded that the clinical pictures and presentations by patients with renal stones may vary. Stones may be silent, may cause only microscopic or gross hematuria, may give pain, may aggregate in the renal pelvis to form a staghorn calculus, may destroy kidney function, may predispose to infection, or may precipitate primarily in the distal nephron resulting in nephrocalcinosis. Staghorn stones have varying radiopacity, are usually made of struvite ($MgNH_4PO_4$) and are associated with chronic infections caused by *Proteus* organisms. Multiple papillary calcifications are notable in distal renal tubular acidosis; the malfunction in the distal nephron results in hyperchloremic acidosis and excessive calcium excretion, causing nephrocalcinosis and eventual renal failure.

Stones cause pain only when they obstruct or are migrating. As they pass down to the lower third of the ureter the pain which was in the flank radiates to the groin, thigh, or testicle. When the stone lodges in the intramural portion of the ureter at its junction with the bladder, frequency and urgency are added to the picture, thus simulating infection. Since the ureter is 10 to 12 mm wide, stones larger than 1 cm have difficulty passing and may cause great pain. Once the stone drops into the bladder it is easily passed since the urethra has a larger caliber. A clinking sound in the toilet bowl tells you that all is over—until the next episode which may be months or years away. Sometimes the stone lodges silently in a ureteral "alcove" for a long while. At other times it may silently cause obstructive changes in the ureter, pelvis, and calyces above it.

DATA   Next morning, the stone is passed and collected in a strainer. Analysis shows pure calcium oxalate. A 24-hour urine collection while on a low-calcium diet shows: creatinine clearance 120 ml/minute, phosphate tubular reabsorption 90%, uric acid 300 mg/24 hours, and calcium 400 mg/24 hours. All are normal except the calcium excretion which is markedly elevated. Repeat serum calcium and phosphorus are normal.

LOGIC   These findings are helpful. The stone composition tells you this is the most common type of stone; it is not basically uric acid which has precipitated a coat of calcium oxalate around it. Chemical studies of the urine offer further evidence against hyperparathyroidism and hyperuricosuria. The high amount of urinary calcium, even on a restricted calcium intake, suggests either hyperabsorption of calcium or a renal leak of calcium. In either event, hypercalciuria is the cause of the patient's stones.

Since most hospitals are not equipped to

distinguish between the two possible mechanisms of idiopathic hypercalciuria, the patient is started on hydrochlorothiazide 50 mg twice daily. This reduces urine calcium excretion and should diminish or eliminate renal calcium stone formation; serial urine and serum calcium determinations will be made. He is also advised to drink liberal amounts of fluid.

Recent treatment strategies that either diminish calcium absorption from the gut or decrease its excretion in the urine have their drawbacks. For the moment, the use of thiazides to decrease calcium excretion seems to offer less deleterious effects.

It might be well to mention that the aforementioned mechanisms of stone formation do not tell the entire story. Solubility products, matrix nucleation, saturation and supersaturation indices, precipitation, crystallization, and stone inhibition factors in the urine are more and more being recognized as playing important roles

Overriding many of these mechanisms is the balance between solute and solvent as well as the urine pH. A decrease in available solvent (water) or an increase in solute (calcium, oxalate, etc) may work separately or together to form stones. And last, the acidity or alkalinity of the urine is a potent force in determining which if any crystals may deposit.

The importance of capturing and analyzing the stone, and of performing a detailed urologic and metabolic workup at least once in the life of a stone former, cannot be overemphasized. Most have remediable metabolic disorders. Moreover, you must also be aware of the interrelationship and interactions between *stone*, *obstruction*, and *infection*, for often one causes the other.

But the entire stone story is still untold.

QUESTIONS

1. In reference to uric acid stones, which of the following statements is incorrect?
   (a) They are usually radiolucent.
   (b) They are often found in overexcreters of uric acid (>600 mg/24 hours).
   (c) They are often found in patients with persistently alkaline urine.

(d) They are often found in association with tophaceous deposits in the ear cartilage and recurrent episodes of acute monarticular arthritis.

2. Approximately 90% of stones are radiopaque. The rest are not visualized by ordinary x-rays; contrast methods or chemical tests must be used if stone is suspected yet not visible. Which of the following are radiopaque?
   (a) triple phosphates
   (b) cystine
   (c) oxalates
   (d) xanthines.

3. While calcium oxalate stones are common and the cause is usually an excess of calcium, in a small percentage of cases hyperoxaluria is the basic defect. This can occur in which of the following circumstances?
   (a) malabsorption syndrome
   (b) an inherited deficiency of d-glyceric dehydrogenase
   (c) pyridoxine deficiency
   (d) excessive rhubarb ingestion.

4. The clinical picture in a 48-year-old male diabetic patient suggests he is passing a stone. Plain film of the abdomen shows a 1.5-cm calcification in the left midabdomen. Which of the following statements may be true?
   (a) Intravenous urography visualizes both ureters and the calcified area is outside the ureter.
   (b) Intravenous urography reveals a radiolucent area in the left midureter; there is dye above it and the calcification is outside the ureter.
   (c) The pain continues and the patient develops fever and chills.
   (d) The serum uric acid is 10.4 mg/dl.

ANSWERS

1. **(c) is correct because it is wrong.** Uric acid stones tend to form in persistently acid urine because of their insolubility at a low pH; thus this type of stone may be caused by a defect in ammonia production so that the kidneys must excrete their net acid production each day in the form of titratable acid. In this way uric acid stones can form in the absence of hyperuricemia and hyperuricosuria. (a) is a true statement, but at times uric acid serves as a nidus for calcium deposition, and the stone becomes partially radiopaque. Excessive uric acid excretion is the principal cause of this type of stone; it occurs in most cases of gout, hematoproliferative disorders especially on beginning treatment, and the Lesch-Nyhan syndrome (an inborn error of metabolism characterized by an overproduction of uric acid). (d) is a classic clinical description of gout.

2. **(a), (b), and (c) are correct.** Triple phosphates contain calcium. Cystine is radiopaque because of its sulfur content. Oxalates are combined with calcium. Xanthine is radiolucent, as are uric acid stones and some small but not dense calcium-containing stones. Newer imaging techniques show versatility in detecting stones that were formerly not demonstrable by the usual methods.

3. **All are correct** and can cause stones because of excessive oxalate excretion in the urine. In the malabsorption syndrome which is associated with a variety of diseases, calcium is bound to fatty acid in the gut, thereby leaving oxalate free for absorption. Normally much oxalate is bound to calcium and excreted in the stool. Enteric disease is the most common cause of hyperoxaluria. (b) is a description of primary oxaluria where a deficiency of the stated enzyme interferes with normal metabolic pathways and results in hyperoxaluria. These children develop stones and calcifications early and usually die of uremia by age 20. Rarely, pyridoxine deficiency interferes with similar metabolic pathways, resulting in oxalate stones. Rhubarb contains much oxalate and can cause stones by hyperoxaluria too.

4. **All may be true.** The calcified area is probably a calcified mesenteric node and the stone, if present, may be radiolucent. The radiolucent area delineated by contrast in answer (b) may be a uric acid stone, a blood clot, a tumor, or a sloughed renal papilla. Diabetic patients are prone to severe infections of the kidney with renal papillary necrosis and sloughing. Anything that causes bleeding may cause the clot. An impacted stone may cause retrograde infection of the kidney—(c). And, of course, the patient may also have hyperuricemia, a condition that occurs more commonly in diabetics than in the rest of the population—much more often than a simple concurrence.

Suggested Readings

1. Coe FL, Favus MJ: Disorders of stone formation. In Brenner BM, Rector FC Jr (eds): *The Kidney*, ed 3. Philadelphia, Saunders, 1985. chap 32.
   A detailed textbook discussion of kidney stones.

2. Brickman AS: Stone disease and the kidney. In Bricker NS, Kirschenbaum MA (eds): *The Kidney. Diagnosis and Management*. New York, Wiley, 1984, pp 187–201.
   Stones succinctly covered.

3. Abraham PA, Smith CL: Medical evaluation and management of calcium nephrolithiasis. *Med Clin North Am* 68:281–299, 1984.
   An up-to-the-minute coverage of stone formation.

4. Smith CL: When should the stone patient be evaluated? Early evaluation of single stone formers. *Med Clin North Am* 68:455–459, 1984.

5. Erickson SB: When should the stone patient be evaluated? Limited evaluation of single stone formers. *Med Clin North Am* 68:461–468, 1984.
   These last two readings represent two sides of an ongoing controversy.

6. Menon M, Krishnan CS: Evaluation and medical management of the patient with calcium stone disease. *Urol Clin North Am* 10:595–615, 1983.
   A superb summary from two urologists.

7. Ng RH, Menon M, Ladenson JH: Collection and handling of 24-hour urine specimens for measurement of analytes related to renal calculi. *Clin Chem* 30:467–471, 1984.
   Measuring the urine concentrations to diagnose the stone chemistry.

8. Robertson WG, Peacock M, Marshall RW, et al: Saturation-inhibition index as a measure of the risk of calcium oxalate stone formation in the urinary tract. *N Engl J Med* 294:249–252, 1976.
   This article introduces the concepts of saturation of urine with solute and the presence in the urine of natural inhibitors to stone formation.

9. Pak CYC, Waters O, Arnold L, et al: Mechanisms for calcium urolithiasis among patients with hyperuricosuria. *J Clin Invest* 59:426–431, 1977.
   A possible explanation for this recently recognized cause for renal stones.

10. Pak CYC: The definition of the mechanisms of hypercalciuria is necessary for the treatment of recurrent stone formers. *Contrib Nephrol* 33:136–151, 1982.
    An opposing view is given on pp 152–162 of the same issue.

11. Fowler JE Jr: Bacteriology of branched renal calculi and accompanying urinary tract infection. *J Urol* 131:213–215, 1984.
    Documents the relation between struvite stones and bacterial infection.

12. Resnick MI, Kursh ED, Cohen AN: Use of computerized tomography in the delineation of uric acid calculi. *J Urol* 121:9–10, 1984.
    These stones are radiolucent but CT dense; their dissolution can be monitored.

Case 42
Swelling of Face and Legs
MARVIN FORLAND, M.D.

DATA A 32-year-old housewife consults her physician because of intermittent swelling of her face, hands, and legs for 1 month. Though she felt well, she became increasingly aware of periorbital puffiness on awakening, tightening of her rings, and ankle swelling toward the end of the day. More recently, her legs were also swollen on awakening. Despite no change in her normally good appetite or in her usual food intake, she noted a gradual 10-lb weight gain.

LOGIC This woman has generalized edema as noted by gain in weight and swelling of the face, legs, and hands. When fluid retention and edema occur (expansion of the interstitial component of the extracellular fluid volume), three possibilities immediately come to mind: *congestive heart failure* (CHF), *cirrhosis of the liver*, and the *nephrotic syndrome*. Less likely considerations are idiopathic cyclic edema, often characterized by abrupt weight changes correlating with the menstrual cycle, and hypothyroidism where brawny swelling can be mistaken for pitting edema. Venous or lymphatic obstruction in the legs can be ruled out by the presence of facial and hand edema too.

Constrictive pericarditis is an unusual and dramatic cause of edema though curable if discovered. Protein-losing enteropathy is another rare cause; suspect it if edema occurs in the absence of heart, liver, or kidney disease and the serum protein is low. Localized edema of the face and eyelids may be caused by trichinosis, and edema occurs on the paralyzed side in hemiplegia. In children, acute post-streptococcal glomerulonephritis may cause edema, but this disease has other obvious hallmarks—hypertension, hematuria, rising antistreptolysin titer, etc.

In each of the three main considerations, decreased renal blood flow (RBF) invokes the renin-angiotensin-aldosterone system.

This results in sodium and water retention in an effort to preserve effective arterial blood volume. But other mechanisms are at work too. In CHF, edema is caused by increased capillary pressure as well as by decreased cardiac output and diminished RBF. Cirrhosis causes edema in many ways. Hypoalbuminemia, portal hypertension, intrahepatic lymphatic obstruction, and inability to destroy antidiuretic hormone and aldosterone contribute to sequestration of fluid in the abdomen and elsewhere. Then a decreased RBF initiates the renal mechanism for salt and water retention. The sequence of events in nephrosis is: glomerular defect, massive proteinuria, hypoalbuminemia, edema, decreased RBF, renal retention of salt and water, and more edema. Adding to this sequence is an increased fractional catabolism of the decreased serum albumin pool, most likely related to increased destruction of filtered proteins by the renal tubular cells.

DATA Further history reveals excellent previous health and two uneventful full-term pregnancies 8 and 5 years ago. She takes no medication, does not smoke, and averages one alcoholic drink each week. There is no history of hepatitis or jaundice. She tolerates activity and exercise quite well, does not get dyspneic or fatigued on exertion, is comfortable in cold weather wearing no more clothes than others, and has normal bowel habits and an unchanged menstrual pattern. Recently she has had nocturia once or twice nightly, and has noticed some "foaminess" in the toilet bowl after completing urination. The edema is unrelated to her menstrual cycle.

LOGIC Good exercise tolerance and lack of dyspnea or fatigue on exertion tend to exclude CHF. Furthermore, there is no history of congenital heart disease, acute rheumatic fever, hypertension, or murmurs, which might be expected in a young woman with CHF. Absence of drug or alcohol abuse and no history of jaundice make severe liver disease unlikely. Tolerance to cold, normal bowel habits, and absence of other related symptoms refute thyroid hypofunction; cyclic premenstrual edema is denied by the history. Nocturia is a common manifestation of edema from any cause and relates to more effective renal perfusion in the reclining position. Foamy urine occurs in patients with massive proteinuria. So far, then, the evidence points to the kidney as the source of her illness.

DATA Physical examination reveals a well-nourished patient. Vital signs are BP 110/70, P 80 and regular, R 12, and T 36.6 C. No jaundice or pallor is noted. The neck veins are not distended and the examination of the heart and lungs is normal. There are no rales, flatness, dullness, or altered fremitus, and breath sounds are normal (no evidence for congestion or effusion). The apex beat is normally located, heart sounds are normal, and there are no S_3, S_4, or murmurs noted. Spleen and liver are not palpable, and ascites cannot be detected. None of the stigmata of cirrhosis is present. No definite facial edema is noted at this time, though the legs show 2+ pitting edema to the midcalf. Several fingernails display whitish arcuate bands parallel to the lunulae. The remainder of the examination is normal.

LOGIC Cirrhosis can now be ruled out by the absence of historical or physical evidence. CHF is also excluded by the normal cardiac and pulmonary findings. Myxedema, only a remote consideration, is eliminated by the absence of its facial features, the type of edema, and normal reflexes. Constrictive pericarditis can be excluded by the absence of cardiac abnormalities, distended neck veins, Kussmaul's sign, prominent y descents in the jugular veins, and the presence of leg edema without hepatomegaly and ascites. The only abnormal findings are edema of the legs and a clue to its cause. The whitish bands in the nailbeds are called

Muehrcke's lines; they develop during periods of severe hypoalbuminemia (less than 2.0 g/dl). The nephrotic syndrome is strongly suspected. There is clinical evidence of *edema, hypoalbuminemia,* and *severe proteinuria* (foamy urine)—a highly suggestive cluster.

DATA Initial laboratory tests are now returning: the hemoglobin, hematocrit, and white blood cell count are normal. Urinalysis shows: pH 6.0, glucose—trace, urobilinogen and bilirubin negative, protein 4+ (by sulfosalicylic acid method); one white blood cell and one red blood cell/high-power field; and two to four hyaline casts with occasional fatty inclusions and one oval fat body/low-power field.

LOGIC The heavy proteinuria, casts with fatty inclusions, and fat bodies add further strength to the diagnosis of a nephrotic syndrome. Advanced renal insufficiency is probably not present with a normal hemoglobin. The few red blood cells and white blood cells on urine examination suggest we are not dealing with a typical glomerular inflammatory process. A trace of glucose in the urine may suggest diabetes mellitus, a possible cause for the nephrotic syndrome, but mild glycosuria is often present with massive albuminuria as an apparent consequence of impaired proximal tubular function.

In general, the proteinuria of renal-caused nephrotic syndromes consists mainly of albumin since it is the smallest of the major protein molecules. A loss of over 3.5 g/1.73 m^2/24 hours is considered a prerequisite for the diagnosis. But κ and λ chains slip through in multiple myeloma. Other proteins may be lost too. A low T_4 and increased T_3 resin uptake may result from leakage of thyroid-binding globulin, loss of transferrin can cause hypochromic microcytic anemia, and loss of antithrombin III can result in a hypercoagulable state (iliofemoral or renal vein thrombosis).

For unknown reasons the liver in the nephrotic syndrome is stimulated to synthesize lipids. This results in hyperlipidemia, an increase in low-density lipoproteins and cholesterol, and the presence of lipid bodies in the urine (fatty casts, oval fat bodies, and doubly refractile maltese crosses). The lipid abnormalities are not always present in the nephrotic syndrome.

The physician now orders a series of laboratory studies which fall into three major categories:

1. To confirm the diagnosis of nephrotic syndrome, he orders a serum protein electrophoresis, total serum proteins, serum cholesterol, and 24-hour urinary protein.
2. To evaluate the status of renal function, he orders a serum creatinine and requests a urine creatinine level on the 24-hour urine collection.
3. To seek a cause for the nephrotic syndrome, he orders a 2-hour postprandial blood glucose, antinuclear antibody (ANA) test, and serum C′3 complement level.

This series may only initiate the search.

DATA   Serum protein electrophoresis shows a decrease in albumin and α_1-/ and γ-globulins, with a mild increase in α_2- and β_1-globulins; total proteins are 5.1 g/dl (albumin 2.1 g and globulin 3.0 g). Twenty-four-hour urine protein excretion is 6.4 g. Serum cholesterol is 390 mg/dl. Serum creatinine is 0.9 mg/dl and creatinine clearance is 94 ml/minute. The 2-hour postprandial blood glucose is 98 mg/dl; ANA is negative and serum complement is normal. The rest of the 18-test chemistry profile (including liver function tests) and the Venereal Disease Research Laboratory test are normal or negative.

LOGIC   The cluster needed to establish the existence of the nephrotic syndrome is clearly present: (*a*) edema, (*b*) proteinuria (usually but not necessarily more than 3 g/24 hours), and (*c*) hypoalbuminemia (less than 3 g/dl). Increased blood cholesterol is often though not necessarily found. Kidney function is normal, and there is no evidence for diabetes or systemic lupus erythematosus

(SLE)—two common causes for the syndrome under discussion.

Pause a moment and consider the sequence of events resulting in the nephrotic syndrome before searching further for a cause. Whatever the etiology—streptococcal infection, diabetes, or blood vessel disease—the common denominator is glomerular injury. This allows for protein leakage and increased urinary protein. Loss of protein in the urine (plus other factors, such as increased fractional catabolism) leads to decreased serum protein, decreased colloid osmotic pressure, and edema. This in turn causes decreased blood volume and then decreased RBF which activates the renin-angiotensin-aldosterone sequence and perhaps other renal mechanisms. Thus, salt and water are retained and edema is compounded.

Diabetic glomerulosclerosis is ruled out by the absence of diabetes. SLE can be dismissed by the absence of cardinal clinical features (rash, arthritis, pleuritis, etc) and the absence of immunologic abnormalities (ANA and complement testing). But a list of all the other causes of the nephrotic syndrome could fill a page. Included are various types of idiopathic glomerulonephritis, amyloidosis, multiple myeloma, other connective tissue diseases, allergens, drugs, and acute infections. Bilateral renal vein thrombosis, often thought to be a cause of the nephrotic syndrome, now appears to be a result of it. Thrombosis of one or both renal veins is seen especially in membranous nephropathy, membranoproliferative glomerulonephritis, and amyloidosis.

As the physician considers the extensive list of disease processes which may result in altered glomerular permeability and massive proteinuria, he must carefully regard age, sex, and geography. In some still developing areas, amyloidosis related to tuberculosis may be the leading cause. In the tropics, quartan malaria provides the antigen for an immune complex form of nephrotic syndrome. Lipoid nephrosis (minimal change lesion) is responsible for 80% of all cases in children. SLE and other collagen diseases would be prominent considerations in our patient—a young woman—though from the evidence acquired so far, these diseases are not present. If the patient were older, primary amyloidosis, multiple myeloma, or underlying malignancy might deserve more attention.

Exposure to penicillamine, Tridione, Paradione, probenecid, captopril, gold, mercury, and bismuth is easily ruled out, as are bee stings, poison oak, and poison ivy—all possible causes of the nephrotic syndrome.

It is interesting to note how many other primarily extrarenal diseases, by known and unknown mechanisms, may affect the kidneys and produce a nephrotic syndrome. These include infections such as endocarditis and secondary syphilis; neoplastic diseases like lymphomas, Hodgkin's disease, leukemia, and carcinomas; and some general disorders such as sarcoidosis, diffuse vasculitis, sickle cell anemia, and others which have already been mentioned.

We have considered and excluded the many generalized diseases that affect the kidney and thus cause the nephrotic syndrome. At this point, one of the varieties of glomerulonephritis must be highly suspect, since this group is indeed the most common cause for the nephrotic syndrome in adults. What was called "Bright's disease" or chronic glomerulonephritis only two decades ago is now known to consist of many different entities. All are associated with glomerular disease, autoimmune processes, and basement membrane deposits—but the histopathologic changes may be proliferative, membranous, or both; focal or diffuse. And so we inherit a host of long-named diseases that differ mostly in their microscopic appearance. But the histologic type must be identified, for it helps determine the natural course of the disease, the prognosis, and the treatment.

Therefore a renal biopsy must be done. *Minimal change disease* (nil lesion, lipoid nephrosis, foot process disease) is the predominant cause of nephrotic syndrome in children but it also occurs in adults. Its names derive from the fact that ordinary light microscopy reveals nothing abnormal; electron microscopy shows effacement of the epithelial foot processes. In most other instances, the histologic findings provide us with diagnoses of mesangial proliferative glomerulonephritis, focal and segmental glomerulonephritis, membranous glomerulopathy, membranoproliferative glomerulonephritis, and other unclassified lesions.

The various renal diseases just mentioned may for the most part eventually lead to what was and still is known as chronic glomerulonephritis with its associated hypertension, symmetrically contracted kidneys, and renal failure.

DATA After consultation with the patient and her husband, the patient is admitted to the hospital for a renal biopsy. Preliminary intravenous pyelography demonstrates normal kidney size, function, and location; no tumors, cysts, or hydronephrosis are seen. A urine culture shows no growth. A bleeding disorder is ruled out by normal platelet count, prothrombin time, and partial thromboplastin time. Percutaneous renal biopsy is obtained and the specimen is sectioned for light, electron, and immunofluorescence microscopy. There are no complications. Characteristic lesions of membranous glomerulopathy, an immune complex form of glomerulonephritis, are found on the three forms of microscopy.

Finding the cause was easy. The difficult problem is treatment.

QUESTIONS

1. The same patient is seen 3 years later. She has been treated intermittently with steroids, immunosuppressives, and diuretics without beneficial effect. Massive edema is now present. You would not be surprised to find any of the following except:
   (a) hypertension
   (b) serum creatinine 4.0 mg/dl
   (c) ascites and pleural effusion
   (d) urine 24-hour albumin = 0.5 g.
2. The level of serum albumin below which edema invariably occurs is:
   (a) 3.0 g/dl
   (b) 2.5 g/dl
   (c) 2.0 g/dl
   (d) none of the above.

3. The nephrotic syndrome could be related to each of the following clinical circumstances except:
   (a) patient receiving phenytoin for epilepsy
   (b) patient with recently diagnosed carcinoembryonic antigen-positive colon adenocarcinoma
   (c) patient with large tongue, malabsorption, orthostatic hypotension, and cardiac hypertrophy without apparent cause
   (d) patient under treatment for rheumatoid arthritis.

4. You see a 62-year-old woman with the recent onset of severe edema of the legs. There is no edema apparent elsewhere. Examination is otherwise completely normal. The urinalysis shows +3 glucose and a trace of albumin. Serum albumin is 3.5 g/dl. Which of the following statements is/are true?
   (a) She may have diabetes which is causing a nephrotic syndrome.
   (b) CHF may be causing her swollen legs.
   (c) She may have diabetes but it is not causing her swollen legs.
   (d) Her edema may be caused by venous or lymphatic obstruction in the legs or pelvis; a pelvic examination may supply the answer.

5. A full-blown nephrotic syndrome is found in a 3-year-old child. Which one of the following statements is incorrect?
   (a) Renal biopsy will most likely show normal renal morphology by light microscopy.
   (b) Polarized light microscopy of the urine will show doubly refractile fat bodies, often shaped like maltese crosses, within casts and cells.
   (c) This is a benign condition called "nil disease" and the patients invariably recover if let alone.
   (d) Fever and diffuse tenderness of the abdomen may occur.

ANSWERS

1. **(d) is correct,** because a marked decrease in albuminuria would not be expected. However, progressive renal failure with elevated creatinine, and worsening fluid retention with ascites and pleural effusion occur in the natural course of the disease, often in spite of treatment. As with renal failure from most causes, hypertension is common.

2. **(d) is the correct answer.** No distinct level can be drawn. Edema can be seen at 3.0 g and may not be seen at 2.0 g. Other factors, such as salt intake, posture of the patient, aldosterone activity, use of diuretics, and timing of the menstrual cycle, are related.

3. **(a) is correct,** because Tridione and Paradione used for petit mal can cause nephrosis. Phenytoin does not. Patient (b) probably has an immune complex nephropathy. Patient (c) has manifestations of primary amyloidosis and patient (d) might have renal amyloidosis secondary to rheumatoid arthritis, or a nephrotic syndrome from treatment with gold injections or penicillamine. Therefore (b), (c), and (d) can definitely be associated with a nephrotic syndrome.

4. **(c) and (d) are correct.** Heavy glycosuria suggests diabetes mellitus, but she has no nephrotic syndrome for diabetes to cause. Nephrotic syndrome is negated by the urine and serum protein values. A large pelvic mass or neoplasm could cause swollen legs by obstruction of veins or lymphatics. Bilateral thrombophlebitis could exist too. (a) is wrong for the same reason that (c) is correct. (b) is impossible in the presence of an otherwise normal physical examination.

5. **(c) is the only incorrect statement.** Nil disease (or lipoid nephrosis) is so named because light microscopy of the biopsy may show nothing abnormal. It is far from a benign disease and may last for years, but rarely results in death. The urine shows lipiduria as described in (b). Peritonitis may complicate ascites secondary to nephrotic syndrome.

COMMENT   The time-conscious physician would immediately consider the few major causes of generalized edema and use a stepwise approach. Liver disease and CHF are ruled out with a few questions, a look at the patient, and a listen to the heart and lungs. Serum proteins and urinalysis would prove the cluster to be caused by kidney disease—the nephrotic syndrome. The specific etiology would be suspected by considering probabilities as they relate to commonness, age, sex, and geography. History or associated physical findings might offer the decisive clue, though renal biopsy is often the ultimate diagnostic study with the highest specificity and sensitivity in this arena.   *(P. C.)*

Suggested Readings

1. Earley LE, Forland M: The nephrotic syndrome. In Earley LE, Gottschalk C (eds): *Strauss and Welt's Diseases of the Kidney,* ed 3. Boston, Little, Brown, 1979, pp 765–800.
   A detailed consideration of the nephrotic syndrome with emphasis on its pathophysiology and multiple etiologic factors.
2. Cogan MG: Nephrotic syndrome. *West J Med* 136:411–417, 1982.
   A Grand Rounds discussion from San Francisco; focuses on the features and glomerular changes.
3. Tejani A, Nicastri AD: Mesangial IgM nephropathy. *Nephron* 35:1–5, 1983.
   Relates to presentations with proteinuria, hematuria, or the nephrotic syndrome.

4. Sullivan MJ, Hough DR, Agodoa CY: Peripheral arterial thrombosis due to the nephrotic syndrome: clinical spectrum. *South Med J* 76:1011–1016, 1983.
   Dwells on the hypercoagulable state seen in the nephrotic syndrome.

5. Cameron JS: Pathogenesis and treatment of membranous nephropathy. *Kidney Int* 15:88–103, 1979.
   A clinical case discussion which provides an excellent review of this common cause of nephrotic syndrome in the adult.

6. Trew PA, Biava CG, Jacobs RP, et al: Renal vein thrombosis in membranous glomerulonephropathy: incidence and association. *Medicine* 57:69–82, 1978.

7. Eagen JW, Lewis EJ: Glomerulopathies of neoplasia. *Kidney Int* 11:297–303, 1977.

8. Pru C, Kjellstrand CM, Cohn RA, et al: Late recurrence of minimal lesion nephrotic syndrome. *Ann Intern Med* 100:69–72, 1984.
   Childhood illness that recurred 4 to 25 years later in 16 patients.

9. Kassirer JP: Is renal biopsy necessary for optimal management of the idiopathic nephrotic syndrome? *Kidney Int* 24:561–575, 1983.
   The author uses "decision analysis" to help him decide.

Case 43
Unconsciousness
HENRY J. REINECK, M.D.

DATA A 64-year-old man was brought to the emergency room after having been found comatose in his room. He was seen by a neurologist and a neurosurgeon who diagnosed a cerebral vascular accident after a computed tomographic scan demonstrated infarction of a large area supplied by the left middle cerebral artery. A lumbar puncture disclosed no cellular elements. He was then admitted to the medical intensive care unit.

On the evening of his admission, routine blood chemistry tests done earlier in the day revealed: blood urea nitrogen (BUN) 60 mg, creatinine 7.2 mg, glucose 85 mg/dl; Na^+ 142, K^+ 6.0, Cl^- 92, CO_2 17 mEq/liter; Ca^{++} 8.0, phosphate 5.0, uric acid 19.3 mg/dl; hemoglobin/hematocrit 17.3/52, white blood cell (WBC) count 11,400, platelets 420,000/mm³.

LOGIC At this point, the only certainties are that the patient has renal insufficiency and has suffered a cerebral vascular accident. Though most of our thoughts and efforts center about his stroke, we are curious about his azotemia. First determine whether the renal failure is acute or chronic in nature. The history may be helpful in making this decision.

DATA The patient was brought to the hospital by his landlady who discovered him unresponsive after not having seen him for 2 days. She knew little of his medical problems except that he was on a low-salt diet because of high blood pressure and had suffered a stroke 2 years previously, but he had no apparent residual neurologic impairment.

LOGIC Although this history does not document any chronic renal disease, the prior history of high blood pressure is consistent with underlying renal disease, e.g. chronic glomerulonephritis. Likewise, it is possible that he had long-standing hypertension with nephrosclerosis resulting in renal insufficiency. On the other hand, the elevation in BUN and creatinine may be acute. A closer look at his laboratory values may be informative.

The absence of anemia strongly suggests that the renal insufficiency is an acute problem. The electrolytes are typical of those found with chronic renal failure of this degree, though the K^+ is usually not this high with chronic disease of this severity. Patients with chronic renal failure are able to increase tubular secretion of potassium to compensate for their diminished renal mass. The Ca^{++} and phosphate are not helpful, as the former will fall and the latter rise within 48 hours of the onset of acute renal failure (ARF). The markedly abnormal uric acid is strongly suggestive of acute disease as this compound is generally only mildly elevated in the chronic setting (9 to 12 mg/dl). Thus, these data, especially the lack of anemia and the severe hyperuricemia, are indications of ARF.

A sudden severe decrease in renal function in association with a decreased glomerular filtration rate, rapidly rising azotemia, and oliguria indicates the presence of ARF. Less than 400 ml of urine/24 hours is insufficient for elimination of the normal load of waste products; this condition is called "oliguria." *Anuria* refers to 100 ml of urine or less/24 hours.

While the patient's stroke is of principal concern, ARF is close behind since it may cause complications and death. The common causes of such renal deterioration quickly confront you. Immediately you discard the 60% of cases that are due to surgery or trauma and consider the 40% that arise from other causes—renal ischemia, renal damage, or renal obstruction.

An x-ray of the abdomen to determine renal size may be helpful.

DATA   A flat film of the abdomen is obtained and the vertical renal size is normal, measuring 14 cm bilaterally.

LOGIC   Bilaterally small kidneys suggest a chronic process like chronic glomerulonephritis or pyelonephritis. Acute processes do not generally have much effect on kidney size. Patients with polycystic disease, amyloidosis, and diabetic glomerulosclerosis in chronic renal failure usually have enlarged kidneys.

The next question to confront is the cause of the acute renal failure. In general, you should first consider the possibilities in the broadest terms, i.e. prerenal azotemia, parenchymal renal disease, and postrenal (or obstructive) uropathy.

Prerenal azotemia results from decreased effective renal blood flow and decreased renal perfusion resulting in a lowered glomerular filteration rate. Aside from the shock and blood loss of surgery, anesthesia, or trauma, it may be caused by extracellular volume depletion, septic shock, cardiogenic shock, or "third space" loss (bowel obstruction, peritonitis, etc).

Postrenal defects are caused mainly by obstructive uropathy from an enlarged prostate; uncommonly, bilateral ureteral obstruction from retroperitoneal fibrosis occurs. Whether crystal, heme, or myeloma deposits in the tubules represent a renal or a postrenal problem is a moot point.

There are many renal parenchymal problems that can cause ARF. Essentially they result from a prolonged period of renal hypoperfusion, severe kidney infection, or acute tubular necrosis from renotoxic drugs or chemical compounds.

It is important to remember that often multiple causes are operative at the same time.

The physical examination and, again, the laboratory are helpful in these differentiations.

DATA   Physical examination reveals: BP 140/80 supine, 110/50 tilted to 40°; pulse 100 and regular when supine, 140 tilted. Skin turgor is poor, there is tenting, and the mucous membranes are dry. Ophthalmoscopy reveals only moderate arteriolar narrowing. There is no jugular venous distention at 45°. His right lower extremity is cool, discolored, and markedly swollen; because of the edema, pulses could not be verified as absent or present. There is no edema elsewhere and pulses are palpable in the left leg.

LOGIC   The etiology of the abnormal swollen leg is not certain. His landlady reported that when he was found in his room, his right knee was flexed and the leg positioned under his trunk and thigh.

The BP and pulse findings are consistent with a decreased effective extracellular fluid volume, possibly due to sequestration of fluid in the markedly edematous right leg. Thus, prerenal azotemia is a real possibility. However, parenchymal renal disease and obstructive uropathy are not excluded.

DATA   Further physical findings pertinent to his renal failure include a moderately enlarged smooth prostate but no suprapubic distention. The rest of the examination is normal except for evidence of a complete right hemiplegia.

LOGIC   In this age group, the most likely cause of obstructive uropathy is benign prostatic hypertrophy. In a stroke victim, however, urinary retention due to an atonic bladder can also occur. At any rate, the bladder is not enlarged, so marked retention is not likely.

DATA   A Foley catheter is inserted into the bladder and only 30 ml of dark brown urine are obtained. The laboratory reports a urine Na^+ concentration of 60 mEq/liter and an osmolality of 320 mOsm/kg of H_2O.

LOGIC   The small urine volume rules out urinary retention with obstructive uropathy at the level of the prostate gland.

When in doubt it is sometimes necessary to do other procedures to exclude obstruction higher up. Techniques to visualize the calices, renal pelvis, and ureters include visualization by computed tomographic scan, ultrasound, or retrograde pyelography. Intravenous pyelography for this purpose is potentially dangerous and may not even visualize the kidneys, though it is sometimes used. If prerenal events (e.g. dehydration) were the cause of the azotemia, one would predict a urine sodium concentration of less than 10 mEq/liter and a urine osmolality of greater than 500 mOsm/kg of H_2O. Additionally, you will recall that the BUN is 60 and creatinine 7.2. The normal ratio of BUN:creatinine is approximately 15:1. With azotemia due to either prerenal or postrenal causes, one expects the BUN to be elevated out of proportion to the elevation in creatinine. This is due to the flow-dependent nature of urea reabsorption along the nephron; i.e. at low flow rates seen with prerenal and postrenal azotemia, urea reabsorption is enhanced. Thus, the high urinary Na^+ concentration, the low urine osmolality, the relatively low BUN:creatinine ratio, and the absence of obstructive findings have virtually excluded both prerenal and postrenal causes

of renal insufficiency. Our differential diagnosis has therefore narrowed to those causes of ARF associated with renal parenchymal disease as listed in Table 19.2.

DATA   Urinalysis: color, brown; specific gravity 1.012; pH 6; glucose negative; protein 2+; occult blood 3+; microscopic: many coarse granular pigmented casts; one to four renal tubular epithelial cells/high-power field; an occasional WBC; no red blood cells (RBCs) or RBC casts.

LOGIC   The urinalysis is extremely helpful in narrowing the list. Acute glomerulonephritis is effectively excluded by the absence of RBCs and RBC casts. Furthermore, the previously noted urine sodium concentration of 60 mEq/liter dissuades this diagnosis since avid salt retention with a urine sodium concentration less than 10 mEq/liter is characteristic. As with acute glomerulonephritis, microscopic or gross hematuria is characteristic of ARF secondary to vascular disease or arterial emboli. Additionally, vasculitic diseases such as systemic lupus erythematosus or polyarteritis nodosa are usually manifest by a skin rash and often by ophthalmoscopic abnormalities (cytoid bodies). There is no evidence for malignant nephrosclerosis in light of the normal blood pres-

Table 19.2.
Causes of Acute Renal Failure Associated with Renal Parenchymal Disease

A. Glomerular disease—acute glomerulonephritis
B. Vascular disease
  1. Vasculitis
  2. Arterial or venous obstruction
  3. Malignant nephrosclerosis
C. Tubulointerstitial disease
  1. Tubular precipitation
    a. Urates
    b. "Myeloma kidney"
  2. Papillary necrosis
  3. Acute interstitial nephritis
  4. "Acute tubular necrosis"
    a. Postischemia
      1) Hypotension
      2) Sepsis
    b. Nephrotoxins
    c. Heme-pigments

sure and relatively benign ophthalmoscopic findings.

This patient was noted to have severe hyperuricemia, and tubular precipitation of uric acid may be a cause of oliguric ARF. However, this situation is limited almost exclusively to patients with myelo- or lymphoproliferative diseases, especially after undergoing either radiation or chemotherapy. With treatment of these diseases, cell lysis releases into the circulation a large quantity of purine nucleotides which are metabolized to uric acid. We have no evidence, however, that this patient has such a disease or that he is undergoing such treatment. Finally, in such cases the urine sediment contains large amounts of precipitated uric acid; none was observed in this patient.

Papillary necrosis, when bilateral, may cause ARF. This disease is often associated with infection, the urinalysis usually reveals heavy pyuria, and it occurs mostly in patients with diabetes mellitus, sickle cell anemia, obstructive uropathy, or analgesic abuse. There is no evidence of any of these entities in this patient, though we cannot exclude the latter possibility.

Acute interstitial nephritis is generally related to a drug reaction (e.g. penicillin and its analogues) and is often accompanied by eosinophilia. In addition, acute inflammatory cells are frequently found in the urine sediment. There is no evidence for this diagnosis.

Acute tubular necrosis is the most common cause of ARF. A partial list of nephrotoxins includes various antibiotics (especially aminoglycosides), nonsteroidal antiinflammatory drugs, heavy metals, chlorinated hydrocarbons, and anesthetic agents. We have no knowledge of exposure to any known nephrotoxic agent; however, we cannot exclude this possibility. ARF is often observed in association with renal ischemia or vasoconstriction secondary to an acute myocardial infarction, burn, hemorrhage, or sepsis. The patient presented here did not have a documented episode of hypotension, but it should be emphasized that acute tubular necrosis can occur due to renal ischemia without *overt* hypotension or shock. Yet burns, myocardial infarction, hemorrhage, and sepsis can be virtually excluded by inspection, ECG, normal blood count, and negative blood cultures.

DATA An ECG showed only nonspecific ST-T changes; the chest x-ray was normal. Blood cultures drawn the day before were negative. No evidence or cause for sepsis could be found. As for the stroke, nursing and supportive care were given; the patient became more lucid. The cause of the ARF and right leg findings remained obscure. Marked oliguria persisted.

LOGIC However, the patient was noted to have one additional significant finding: dark brown urine. Pigments, specifically hemoglobin and myoglobin, are well-recognized causes of oliguric ARF. Recall that the urinalysis was positive for "occult blood," but no RBCs were noted. The "dipsticks" commonly used for occult blood utilize orthotolidine which gives a positive reaction with both hemoglobin and myoglobin. Thus in the absence of RBCs this finding suggests either hemoglobinuria or myoglobinuria. In view of the normal complete blood count (i.e. no evidence for hemolysis), myoglobinuria appears to be present.

As pointed out, the patient was noted to have a discolored, markedly swollen right extremity. It is likely that as a result of his cerebral vascular accident the patient fell and his position caused compression and ischemia of this lower extremity, resulting in muscle necrosis (rhabdomyolysis), myoglobinuria, and finally ARF.

Muscle necrosis as a cause of ARF is becoming more widely recognized. Prolonged pressure from coma caused by stroke or drug overdose, crush injuries, and sudden vascular occlusion to large muscles may cause muscle necrosis, along with the release of myoglobin and measurable large quantities of aldolase and creatine phosphokinase. The mechanism by which myoglobin damages the kidney is unknown.

It should be noted that the stroke, rather than the uremia, was the probable cause of the patient's unconsciousness. But if not for the stroke, there would have been nausea, vomiting, somnolence, and stupor—the usual symptoms of ARF.

DATA After several days consciousness returned but the hemiplegia and aphasia persisted. Azotemia and oliguria continued for several weeks and then gradually improved. Special care was given to prevent problems such as thrombophlebitis, water and salt overload, hyperkalemia, infection, and other complications explained in question 2 which follows.

QUESTIONS

1. Necrosis of muscle tissue occurs under many circumstances. It is common in comatose patients who compress muscles for long periods of time. Rhabdomyolysis and myoglobinuria with ARF are associated with all the following except:
   (a) BUN:creatinine ratio <10
   (b) hypophosphatemia
   (c) hypercalcemia
   (d) hyperuricemia.
2. The chief cause of death in patients with ARF is:
   (a) hyperkalemia
   (b) severe acidosis
   (c) infection
   (d) pericarditis.
3. Which of the following procedures is not helpful in excluding obstructive uropathy as the cause of ARF?
   (a) intravenous pyelography
   (b) retrograde pyelography
   (c) mannitol infusion
   (d) urine electrolyte determination.
4. Following ARF, the kidney may secrete large quantities of dilute urine, yet azotemia may persist. Which of the following statements concerning this diuretic phase of ARF is true?
   (a) The risk of pericarditis is low.
   (b) The likelihood of hyperkalemia is reduced.
   (c) Sodium restriction should be continued.
   (d) Dialysis is never necessary.

ANSWERS

1. **(b) is correct.** Hypophosphatemia does not occur with rhabdomyolysis. The soft tissue necrosis may release large amounts of phosphate into the extracellular fluid space. This endogenous phosphate load coupled with renal failure causes marked and rapid hyperphosphatemia. A low BUN:creatinine ratio (a) may be seen with rhabdomyolysis due to the release of the muscle enzyme, creatine, which

is metabolized to creatinine. Hypercalcemia (c) may occur late in the course of ARF in this setting. This is thought to be due to the release of deposited calcium from damaged muscle tissue. Finally, hyperuricemia (d) in the 20 to 30 mg/dl range may occur in this entity and is probably due to the release of purines from damaged muscle.

2. **(c) is correct.** Infection with resultant sepsis remains the primary cause of death in ARF. The remaining choices are life-threatening complications of ARF, but these can be avoided or promptly treated as they occur.

3. **(c) is correct.** An infusion of mannitol is often helpful in excluding prerenal causes of azotemia but not obstruction. The intravenous pyelogram (a) may reveal a nephrogram even with oliguria; dilated calices will be detected as filling defects in obstructive uropathy. Unilateral retrograde pyelography is occasionally necessary to assure patency of at least one collecting system. A lower urinary sodium concentration (d) is characteristic of acute obstruction. However, in cases of chronic urinary tract obstruction, the urinary sodium concentration is elevated (similar to "acute tubular necrosis"). Today many physicians prefer ultrasound or computed tomographic scan to detect obstructive uropathy.

4. **(b) is correct.** Since potassium excretion is at least in part flow-dependent, urinary potassium excretion increases with an increase in urine output. Pericarditis (a) may occur at any time during the course of ARF and dialysis (d) may continue to be necessary since the glomerular filtration rate often remains severely compromised even during the diuretic phase of the illness. It may be necessary to liberalize sodium intake (c) since the urinary sodium concentration may remain elevated and thus extracellular fluid volume depletion may occur if sodium restriction is continued.

Suggested Readings

1. Brezis M, Rosen S, Epstein FH: Acute renal failure. In Brenner BM, Rector FJ Jr (eds): *The Kidney*, ed 3. Philadelphia, Saunders, 1985, chap 19.
   A detailed textbook analysis of the subject.
2. Dougherty JC: Acute renal failure. In Forland M (ed): *Nephrology—A Concise Textbook*, ed 2. New Hyde Park, NY, Medical Examination, 1983, pp 168–189.
   A complex subject simply explained.
3. Schrier RW: Acute renal failure. *JAMA* 247:2518–2525, 1982.
   A brief excellent overview with an algorithmic diagnostic approach.
4. Smolens P, Stein JH: Pathophysiology of acute renal failure. *Am J Med* 70:479–482, 1981.
   Covers the ischemic and nephrotoxic insults.
5. Berkseth RO: Radiologic contrast-induced nephropathy. *Med Clin North Am* 68:351–370, 1984.

Outlines the renal considerations that must always be given when doing any type of contrast study.

6. Sherman RA, Byun KJ: Nuclear medicine in acute and chronic renal failure. *Semin Nucl Med* 12:265–279, 1982.

Isotopes are still of considerable diagnostic aid in a variety of clinical settings.

7. Cohen DJ, Sherman WH, Osserman EF, et al: Acute renal failure in patients with multiple myeloma. *Am J Med* 76:247–256, 1984.

Explains the many reasons why patients with multiple myeloma lose renal function.

8. Ron D, Taitelman U, Michaelson M, et al: Prevention of acute renal failure in traumatic rhabdomyolysis. *Arch Intern Med* 144:277–280, 1984.

The myoglobin-ARF relationship in seven crush victims is presented.

9. Haapanen E, Pellinen D, Partanen J: Acute renal failure caused by alcohol-induced rhabdomyolysis. *Nephron* 36:191–193, 1984.

Nontraumatic myoglobinuria occurs too.

Case 44
Nausea, Weakness, Confusion

PAUL CUTLER, M.D.

DATA The patient is a 58-year-old man who has not felt well for over a year but has refused to see a physician. He was brought to the emergency room in a semistuporous confused state. A close friend provided the history. The patient has had progressive lassitude, weakness, confusion, depression, and torpor for many months.

LOGIC At this point many possibilities enter your mind. A progressive downhill course in a person this age suggests uremia, brain tumor, carcinomatosis, cirrhosis, chronic brain syndrome, drug abuse, or diabetic ketoacidosis.

DATA In the past month he had anorexia, nausea, vomiting, and weight loss. More recently, itching and scratching of the skin, twitching motions about the face, and deep rapid breathing were noted. No further history is available.

LOGIC The possibilities are narrowing. In carcinoma, you would expect the gastrointestinal symptoms to precede or coincide with the downhill course; the reverse occurred here. The absence of both excessive thirst and frequent urination would refute diabetic ketoacidosis, though those symptoms might have been present but unnoticed by the friend.

Itching of the skin could be caused by: jaundice, uremia, skin diseases, drug allergy, diabetes, and psychogenic disorders. Jaundice would be apparent and could be related to cancer or cirrhosis. The other causes would become evident as information is gathered.

Twitching facial movements sound like hypocalcemia, though a focal irritative brain lesion could cause them too. The heavy breathing is also not specific. It could result from uremic acidosis, diabetic ketoacidosis, superimposed pleural effusion, pneumonia, or congestive heart failure. Weight loss is no mystery when there is anorexia, nausea, and vomiting.

So far, then, we have a patient with a 1-year downhill course, whose seven symptoms have appeared in the following order: weakness, confusion, nausea and vomiting, weight loss, itching, twitching, and heavy breathing. While uremia seems to be the most likely common denominator, other possibilities must be ruled out.

The basic problem in chronic renal failure and resultant uremia is *loss of nephrons*. Two million nephrons at birth diminish to 1 million by age 50 to 60. When kidney disease reduces nephron mass to 400,000 or less, the glomerular filtration rate and creatinine clearance fall to approximately one-fourth to one-third of normal. At this point, the adaptive mechanisms of the kidney can no longer maintain homeostasis, and the clinical picture of uremia begins.

Simply put, the purpose of the kidneys is to (a) eliminate metabolic waste products (30 g of solute/day); (b) secrete hormones (erythropoietin, renin, vitamin D analogue, prostaglandins, kallikrein-kinins); (*c*) maintain blood osmolality and blood volume; (*d*) regulate the concentration of electrolytes; and (*e*) govern acid-base balance.

When these regulatory functions are compromised or lost, most body organs are affected and profound changes occur. First there is retention of nitrogen wastes and toxins. Blood volume expands but is easily depletable. Sodium concentration can fall; potassium may decrease or terminally increase; phosphates and acids are retained; metabolic acidosis with Kussmaul breathing may ensue. As phosphates are retained, serum calcium decreases, resulting in excessive secretion of parathyroid hormone (secondary hyperparathyroidism) and renal osteodystrophy. This is abetted by decreased absorption of calcium from the gut resulting from the inability of the kidney to convert vitamin D to 1,25-dihydroxyvitamin D_3, its active analogue.

Other derangements occur. Anemia results from bone marrow toxic depression, diminished erythropoietin, shortened red blood cell survival (hemolysis), and frequent gastrointestinal bleeding; the anemia is usually normochromic and normocytic. Hypertension is almost universal; congestive heart failure and pericarditis may occur too. Carbohydrate tolerance diminishes, and the liver produces increased triglycerides. In the central nervous system we see lethargy, impaired mentation, asterixis, seizures, and coma. The skin demonstrates pallor, urochrome pigment deposition, uremic frost, pruritus, and ecchymoses (from a coagulopathy). Anorexia, nausea, vomiting, ulcers, and bleeding are manifestations of gastrointestinal tract affliction. The breath is ammoniacal. Peripheral neuropathies are common and the chest x-ray often shows "uremic lungs" (perihilar hazy congestion) and cardiac hypertrophy.

These are the origins of the symptoms, signs, and paraclinical findings in chronic renal failure. And as you proceed to gather more information about the patient, the entire gamut of metabolic derangements must be kept in mind.

DATA Physical examination reveals a dehydrated, pale, cachectic, unresponsive man. Longitudinal scratch marks are noted all over the skin of the arms, legs, and anterior trunk. There is no jaundice, but the skin has a slightly yellow waxy cast. The BP is 220/120, P 88, R 24 and deep, T 37 C.

LOGIC Dehydration would be expected in a patient with vomiting and stupor who has no access to fluids. The scratch marks are only on accessible areas. Severe hypertension is present. The deep, somewhat rapid breathing suggests Kussmaul respirations seen in severe acidosis from any cause. Retained chromogens cause the yellowish skin. Uremia becomes more likely.

DATA The breath has a strong ammoniacal odor and white powdery material is noted over the face and hair roots. Tapping of the facial nerve in front of the tragus causes twitching movements of the corner of the mouth and adjacent cheek. The conjunctiva and skin are very pale.

LOGIC The uremic syndrome now appears definite. Uremic frost is present; it represents excretion by the skin of those waste products which are normally eliminated by the kidneys. The odor of the breath is unmistakable. A positive Chvostek sign in this instance represents probable hypocalcemia, even though this sign can be seen in alkalosis and occasionally in normal persons. But you would not expect alkalosis in this clinical situation. Furthermore, the pallor is also part of the picture of renal failure.

It is important to note that tetany and a positive Chvostek sign are *uncommon* in uremia even though the serum calcium is low. The critical factor for these signs is the amount of *ionized* calcium. Acidosis favors ionization and alkalosis retards it. Thus, in other situations, you may see tetany with a normal serum calcium if alkalosis is present, and there may be no tetany even in the presence of a low serum calcium if acidosis exists. Uremics develop tetany mainly if they are given large amounts of base to correct the acidosis.

DATA   Cervical veins are distended to the angles of the jaw with the patient lying at 45°. Fine, moist end-inspiratory rales are heard at both bases. The apical impulse, strong and diffuse, is felt in the sixth intercostal space at the anterior axillary line. A grade 2/6 systolic ejection murmur is heard at the base of the heart, S_2 is loud, and a low-pitched sound is heard at the apex with the bell attachment about 0.15 second after S_2. Examination of the abdomen, rectum, genitalia, and extremities is normal.

LOGIC   These findings indicate cardiac enlargement, left ventricular failure (loud S_2, S_3, and rales), and beginning right ventricular failure (distended neck veins). The failure results from hypertension which may be caused by renal disease. Both cardiac and renal failure contribute to the deep rapid breathing. Valuable negative information is obtained. Liver disease is ruled out; the fact that the kidneys and prostate are not palpably enlarged will help to determine the cause for the patient's renal failure; the absence of hepatomegaly and leg edema tells us that right ventricular failure has only just begun. Note that congestive heart failure (CHF) can occur in the presence of dehydration.

DATA   Studies are as follows: hemoglobin 8.5 g/dl, red blood cells (RBC) count 3 million/mm³, hematocrit 25%, white blood cell (WBC) count 5800/mm³, normal differential; urinalysis shows specific gravity 1.010, albumin +4, glucose and acetone negative, many fine and coarse granular casts, no RBCs, no WBCs; urine culture negative; blood urea nitrogen 230, creatinine 16, glucose 148 mg/dl; sodium 128, potassium 3.6, chloride 85, bicarbonate 12 mEq/liter; pH 7.2; calcium 5.4, phosphorus 5.6 mg/dl; ECG shows left ventricular hypertrophy with prolongation of the QT interval and ST segment; chest x-ray shows cardiac enlargement and pulmonary congestion.

LOGIC   The ECG and chest film are what you would expect in a patient with uremia, hypertension, and CHF. The heart is enlarged and strained, the lungs are congested, and there is ECG evidence of hypocalcemia.

Retention of phosphates by the kidneys plus decreased absorption of calcium from the gut cause the low serum calcium. Normochromic anemia results in part from bilateral renal disease which depresses RBC production because of lack of erythropoietin. The blood urea nitrogen and creatinine are proportionately markedly elevated and confirm the main problem.

Urine abnormalities indicate severe renal disease affecting the glomerulus and tubule. Low sodium stems from diminished intake, excessive vomiting, and defective tubular reabsorption. In other patients, injudicious salt restriction by the physician may be a contributing factor. Acidosis in chronic renal failure is caused by an impaired tubular mechanism for the excretion of acids, retention of sulfates and phosphates, loss of bicarbonate, and inability to form ammonia and conserve sodium. The elevated glucose should be rechecked.

So far there are four problems:

1. chronic renal failure
2. hypertension (secondary to 1)
3. CHF (secondary to 2)
4. hyperglycemia.

Uremia is well established by the symptoms, signs, and laboratory tests. Still to be determined is the specific renal disease causing renal failure. First, the hypertension and CHF need immediate treatment; digitalis, diuretics, and antihypertensive drugs must be especially carefully administered in the presence of uremia. Fluids and electrolytes need judicious juggling since the patient has dehydration and hyponatremia side by side with CHF; dialysis may be needed.

Once treatment of CHF is begun, further thought can be given to the cause of renal failure. In this age group, we must consider: chronic pyelonephritis, chronic glomerulonephritis, prostatic hypertrophy with hydronephroses, arteriolar nephrosclerosis, polycystic renal disease, and analgesic abuse.

DATA   Repeat studies confirm all the previous blood chemistry tests except for several glucose determinations which are now normal. Plain film of the abdomen shows easily defined kidney shadows which are much smaller than normal for this man's size; no calculi are seen. So far as can be determined by history, discussion with friends, and checking the patient's apartment, there has been no analgesic abuse.

LOGIC The patient does not have diabetes, but it is interesting to note that mild glucose intolerance is commonly seen in advanced uremia. Conversely, if a known diabetic develops renal failure his glucose intolerance may improve. Small kidneys rule out polycystic disease and hydronephroses but point to chronic glomerulonephritis or chronic pyelonephritis. The negative urine culture and the absence of WBC's and WBC casts in the urine rebut pyelonephritis. Systemic lupus erythematosus and diabetes are not considered causes for renal failure in this patient because tests disprove diabetes and other clinical features of systemic lupus erythematosus are not present. Since chronic glomerulonephritis (the likely diagnosis in this case) consists of a diverse group of diseases, some of which may benefit from steroids, a renal biopsy might be considered. But in the presence of markedly contracted kidneys, this degree of renal insufficiency with a chronic course, and the associated heart failure, a biopsy is not advisable in this case. While arteriolar nephrosclerosis from long-standing hypertension is a viable diagnosis, a biopsy will not alter management. The possibility of finding a renal lesion which would respond to therapy is negligible in this setting and the microscopic appearance of an end-stage kidney may not permit etiologic definition.

QUESTIONS

1. Other physical findings commonly observed in end-stage kidney disease include all the following except one:
   (a) hyperactive reflexes
   (b) ecchymoses
   (c) abnormal fundi
   (d) pericardial friction rub.
2. Which analgesic drug is most noted for causing renal failure?
   (a) aspirin
   (b) codeine
   (c) phenacetin
   (d) acetaminophen.

3. If the abdominal film had shown large kidneys, all the following possibilities would have needed consideration except:
   (a) polycystic kidneys
   (b) hydronephroses caused by prostatic obstruction
   (c) hydronephroses caused by retroperitoneal fibrosis
   (d) acute tubular necrosis.
4. The severe hypertension so often seen in patients with advanced bilateral kidney disease is:
   (a) caused by the kidney disease
   (b) the cause of the kidney disease
   (c) the result of hyperreninemia
   (d) the result of abnormal sodium and water retention.

ANSWERS

1. **(a) is not found.** Uremics may develop a peripheral neuropathy, first sensory and later motor; reflexes may be diminished. (b), (c), and (d) could be expected since bleeding tendencies are common in uremia; the fundi usually show evidence of hypertension and renal disease (exudates, hemorrhages, arteriolar narrowing, and arteriovenous nicking); and a fibrinous pericarditis producing a friction rub is common.
2. **(c) Phenacetin is generally regarded as the principal offender.** But it is contained in so many proprietary analgesic mixtures that we are not sure whether it acts alone or in conjunction with aspirin to damage the kidney. It causes an interstitial nephritis which may be reversible if detected in time and the drug is stopped. (a) alone, (b), and (d) do not cause renal damage. But this entire subject is still unsettled (see Suggested Readings).
3. **(d) is correct** because it does not fit the picture. This is an acute disease characterized by nausea, vomiting, and oliguria or anuria. It has a recognizable cause (e.g. shock, sepsis, poison, or toxin), is rapid in onset, and does not cause large kidneys. The other answers are all possible. Prostatic obstruction with big kidneys can exist in the presence of a large median lobe which may not be palpable on rectal examination, but the patient would also have symptoms of prostatic obstruction. Periureteral retroperitoneal fibrosis with hydronephroses usually has no demonstrable cause, though methysergide, used for vascular headaches, is a known offender.
4. **All are correct.** Long-standing severe hypertension can cause arteriolar nephrosclerosis. The reverse is also true; chronic kidney disease may cause hypertension. When it does, it is by either of two methods. Eighty per cent of patients with end-stage renal disease have volume-dependent hypertension that is related to

abnormal sodium and water retention. The remaining 20% have hyperreninemia.

COMMENT The presentation was not specific. It was necessary to cull the body systems for diseases which present with a downhill course plus cerebral and gastrointestinal manifestations. Pattern building established a cluster which indicated uremia, and thus the diseased organ was quickly pinpointed. The sequence whereby the downhill course preceded the other features tended to rule out primary brain or gastrointestinal disease.

The presence of CHF complicated the picture somewhat. A vicious circle of cause and effect was established whereby chronic renal failure (CRF) caused hypertension which caused CHF which worsened the renal failure by decreasing the renal blood flow. Furthermore, CRF caused nausea and vomiting which worsened the CRF by virtue of dehydration and decreased renal blood flow. Simpler cause and effect relationships were profusely used to explain the various findings in uremia.

The common causes for CRF in this age group were considered and most were easily excluded on a clinical basis. While a biopsy (essentially 100% sensitive and 100% specific) might define the precise histopathology, it is not considered necessary or valuable in this instance. Indeed, it might very well reveal a multiplicity of pathologic processes going on at the same time.

Statistics for the causes of CRF vary, but for practical purposes the following estimates are acceptable. One-fourth are caused by interstitial-tubular diseases (analgesics, pyelonephritis, polycystic disease, urate deposits, and obstructive uropathy); one-fourth by vascular disease (nephrosclerosis); one-fifth by systemic disease (diabetes, systemic lupus erythematosus, multiple myeloma, etc); one-fifth by forms of glomerulonephritis; and the rest have unknown causes. Remember that in many instances a biopsy or autopsy in CRF shows mixed disease. For example, a diabetic patient with CRF may exhibit intercapillary glomerulosclerosis, arteriolar nephrosclerosis, arterial nephrosclerosis, and chronic pyelonephritis on microscopic examination. So too for other situations.

The mode of presentation for patients with CRF must be mentioned. Often evidence of diminished renal function is accidentally detected by routine screening of patients who have other primary problems. In some instances the patient sees the doctor for the early symptoms of CRF—e.g. fatigue, weakness, pruritus, nausea and vomiting, hiccoughs, etc. On occasion the function of barely compensating kidneys is markedly worsened by an intercurrent event such as myocardial infarction, CHF, pneumonia, or some other infection. It is uncommon for patients to present with florid uremia as this patient did.

Earlier treatment usually alters the course and the picture. (*P. C.*)

Suggested Readings

1. Dougherty JC: Chronic renal failure. In Forland M (ed): *Nephrology—a Concise Textbook*, ed 2. New Hyde Park, NY, Medical Examination, 1983, pp 190–221.
   Thirty pages of an easy-to-read current book cover the entire field—pathophysiology, causes, manifestations, treatment.
2. Kurtzman NA: The pathophysiology of uremia. In Brenner BM, Rector FC Jr (eds): *The Kidney*, ed 3. Philadelphia, Saunders, 1985, chap 37.
   This is a 50-page detailed textbook analysis. Subsequent Chapters 38, 39, and 40 cover the hematologic, osteodystrophic, and neurologic complications of renal failure.
3. Frocht A, Fillet H: Renal disease in the geriatric patient. *J Am Geriatr Soc* 32:28–43, 1984.
   Covers the renal failure diseases that affect the elderly—infection, tumor, obstruction, vascular problems, and "aging."
4. Tu WH, Petitti DB, Biava CG, et al: Membranous nephropathy: predictors of terminal renal failure. *Nephron* 36:118–124, 1984.
   A multifactorial analysis of predictors for serious outcomes.
5. Dahlberg PJ, Keimowitz RM: Renal disease and multiple myeloma. *Wis Med J* 83:20–28, 1984.
   A short excellent review of a highly prevalent relationship.
6. McCrary RF, Pitts TO, Puschett JB: Diabetic nephropathy: natural course, survivorship, and therapy. *Am J Nephrol* 1:206–218, 1981.
7. Kotler MN, Segal BL: Cardiovascular problems in chronic renal failure. *Geriatrics* 39:69–84, 1984.
   Most deaths in patients with CRF are cardiovascular. The authors explain why.
8. Case records of the Massachusetts General Hospital. Weekly clinicopathological exercises. Case 18—1984. A 32-year-old woman with proteinuria and impaired renal function. *N Engl J Med* 310:1176–1181, 1984.
   A good exercise in the logic of problem solving.
9. Danovitch GM, Nissenson AR: The role of renal biopsy in determining therapy and prognosis in renal disease. *Am J Nephrol* 2:179–184, 1982.
10. Gault HM, Muehrcke RC: Renal biopsy: current views and controversies. *Nephron* 34:1–34, 1983.
    A decision analysis—to biopsy or not.
11. McAnally JF, Winchester JF, Schreiner GE: Analgesic nephropathy. An uncommon cause of end-stage renal disease. *Arch Intern Med* 143:1897–1899, 1983.
    Gives a percentage breakdown for all causes of chronic renal failure while noting the *rarity* of analgesic abuse as a cause.
12. Hartman GW, Torres VE, Leago GF, et al: Analgesic-associated nephropathy. *JAMA* 251:1734–1738, 1984.
    Cites specific radiologic features of a *common* cause of end-stage renal failure; describes the pathogenesis.
13. Analgesic-associated kidney disease. A consensus conference sponsored by NIH. *JAMA* 251:3123–3125, 1984.
    The joint views of a large panel of experts.

Chapter 20

Electrolyte Problems

It is with reservations that a separate chapter is devoted to electrolyte disorders, since these are not diseases in themselves. They are syndromic manifestations of endocrine, renal, gastrointestinal, or brain diseases, or the result of injudicious treatment of cardiac, renal, or liver diseases.

Yet derangements of electrolytes cause profound clinical disturbances—even death. When an electrolyte disturbance occurs and is detected, finding its cause often requires careful investigation, and problem solving enters the picture.

These are usually complex situations, since an electrolyte disturbance depends on a balance between intake and output, the ratio of the total body electrolyte to total body water, numerous control mechanisms (antidiuretic hormone, renal function, aldosterone), iatrogenic factors (e.g. salt-restricted diets and potent diuretics), and so forth.

Water balance (dehydration and overhydration) and blood pH (acidosis and alkalosis) are integral parts of the subject of electrolyte disorders, since they often go hand in hand. Sodium and water disorders usually accompany each other; sodium depletion is always relative to the amount of water on board. Serum sodium concentration reflects the relative proportions of sodium and water in the serum, not the absolute amount of sodium in the body. The same can be said for potassium. Thus either hyponatremia, hypernatremia, hypokalemia, or hyperkalemia can occur when the total body sodium or potassium content is decreased, normal, or increased.

Calcium, sodium potassium, and magnesium are the principal cations, while phosphate, chloride, and bicarbonate are the anions associated with metabolic electrolyte disturbances. Of these, decreased or increased serum concentrations of calcium, sodium, and potassium give us the most concern. You must bear in mind the fact that these disorders are frequently unnoticed; they occur in the course of other diseases and may be overshadowed by the prime problem. Furthermore, the manifestations of the electrolyte disturbance are often not very different from what you would expect in the natural course of the underlying disease. Hypopotassemia causes weakness, neuromuscular disturbances, cardiac arrhythmias, and death—what you might expect in a terminal cardiac patient who did not have a low serum potassium induced by potent diuresis. In addition, since the patient is taking digitalis, he is even more susceptible to arrhythmias. A situation is created whereby low serum potassium directly causes arrhythmias, and also indirectly causes them by making the myocardium more susceptible to digitalis intoxication.

The patient with severe advanced congestive heart failure may die seemingly from his heart disease unless severe hyponatremia can be distinguished and extracted from a backdrop of cardiac findings. Similarly, the patient with cancer of the kidney may die of uremia caused not by the malignancy but by an associated hypercalcemia. After all, wouldn't you expect a cancer patient to die with nausea, vomiting, obtundation, and uremia?—all manifestations of hypercalcemia too!

Unless the physician is alert, an electrolyte disturbance may deliver the coup de grace—nobody being the wiser even at the autopsy table. If you are aware of the possibilities, then the ECG, serum and urine concentrations, and serum and urine osmolality are accurate measuring tools. Even if you are not alert, the common use of batteries of chemical studies may call these problems to your attention—provided you carefully read the laboratory reports.   (*P. C.*)

Case 45
Fatigue and Abnormal ECG
PAUL CUTLER, M.D.

DATA You have been asked to cover another physician's practice for the weekend. Upon arriving at his office on Friday evening, you are given an ECG to evaluate. The patient from whom the ECG was obtained, a 24-year-old woman, has just been admitted to the hospital complaining of overwhelming fatigue and weakness so severe she could hardly move. Her physician felt that the complaint had a psychoneurotic basis but in order to be certain he wanted to observe the patient in the hospital.

As you review the ECG, you notice that it is unremarkable except for depression of the ST segments, lowering of the amplitude of the T waves, and a marked increase in the U waves, particularly in V_2 and V_3. The QT is markedly prolonged (0.56 second), and the heart rate is 72 beats/minute.

LOGIC The amplitude of the U wave may be increased by certain drugs such as epinephrine or digitalis, or in patients with ventricular hypertrophy, bradycardia, or hyperthyroidism. But its association with hypokalemia is most noteworthy, especially in the absence of ECG evidence for the other conditions mentioned. The heart rate is neither abnormally fast nor slow. At this point, further historical information and data from the physical examination and plasma electrolytes must be obtained.

DATA The patient appears to be quite nervous and occasionally cries, and it is difficult to obtain a reliable history. She claims to have been in reasonably good health until 2 weeks prior to admission when she noted that she was tiring more easily than usual. In addition, she has had sleep disturbance and bouts of spontanenous weeping.

LOGIC At this point, inasmuch as you expect her to have hypokalemia, history regarding entities causing hypokalemia should be obtained. Table 20.1 classifies hypokalemic disorders and separates them into those caused by inadequate intake, excessive renal loss, extrarenal loss, and intracellular shift.

Knowledge of these disorders cannot be completely obtained by history. Yet information about a number of them can be derived, particularly those relating to gastrointestinal losses of potassium and the use of diuretics. Some common causes of hypokalemia include gastrointestinal losses, vigorous diuretic treatment, and the presence of mineralocorticoid excess. The universal use of diuretics for hypertension and congestive heart failure probably represents by far the most common cause of this electrolyte disturbance.

Frequently the manifestations of an electrolyte disorder are not well defined, and you become aware of a disturbance only after obtaining routine electrolyte determinations. Yet certain clinical entities are so frequently the cause of electrolyte disturbances that one must constantly bear the possibility in mind when these clinical situations are encountered.

DATA Further careful questioning of the patient was fruitless. She denied any gastrointestinal disturbance, drug usage, or hypertension. The remainder of the review of systems was likewise negative. Her social history indicated that she had moved to the city from a small town in order to obtain a job, and she lived alone in a one-bedroom apartment. She neither drank nor smoked. Her family history was noncontributory.

The physical examination revealed an overweight young woman (60 inches tall, 154 lb) who, although not in acute distress, was crying intermittently. Vital signs were: BP 110/70 mm Hg without postural change; pulse 70/minute; respirations 16/minute;

Table 20.1.
Classification of Hypokalemia Disorders

I. Inadequate dietary intake
II. Renal losses
  A. Diuretics
  B. Mineralocorticoid excess
    1. Primary aldosteronism
      a. Adenoma
      b. Bilateral hyperplasia
    2. Cushing's syndrome or disease
      a. Primary adrenal disease
      b. Pituitary tumor
      c. Secondary to nonendocrine tumor
      d. Exogenous steroid administration
    3. Accelerated hypertension
    4. Renal vascular hypertension
    5. Renin-producing tumor
    6. Adrenogenital syndrome
    7. Licorice excess
  C. Bartter's syndrome
  D. Liddle's syndrome
  E. Renal tubular acidosis
  F. Metabolic alkalosis
  G. Acute hyperventilation
  H. Starvation
  I. Ureterosigmoidostomy
  J. Antibiotics—carbenicillin, amphotericin, gentamicin
  K. Diabetic ketoacidosis
  L. Acute leukemia
III. Extrarenal losses
  A. Vomiting
  B. Diarrhea from various causes
  C. Chronic laxative abuse
  D. Villous adenoma
  E. Enterocutaneous fistulae
  F. Biliary fistulae
  G. Profuse sweating
IV. Cellular shift
  A. Alkalosis
  B. Periodic paralysis
  C. Barium poisoning
  D. Insulin administration

temperature 37 C. Examination of the head, eyes, ears, nose, throat, chest, heart, abdomen, rectum, and pelvis was normal or negative. Muscle strength was possibly diminished although there was some question as to her cooperation. The neurologic examination was normal. She was oriented to time, place, and person and has had no hallucinations or paranoid ideation.

LOGIC We are provided little positive information by the patient, but important neg-

ative data have been obtained. Her weight excludes starvation as a cause of the suspected hypokalemia. Likewise, she was not clinically hyperventilating and did not have hypertension. These negative clues are important because alkalosis causes potassium loss into the cells and out in the urine, and hypertensive diseases caused by corticoid excess have low potassium levels. Reflexes may be diminished or normal in hypokalemia.

While waiting for the blood electrolyte profile to return, you ponder the pathophysiology of hypokalemia. Potassium homeostatic mechanisms maintain a normal serum level between 3.8 and 5.0 mEq/liter. These regulatory tools consist mainly of aldosterone and renal function, though insulin, glucagon, and the sympathetic nervous system play minor roles. As for potassium, the human body contains 50 to 55 mEq/kg; most is intracellular and only 2% is extracellular; daily dietary intake is 50 to 100 mEq. Generally speaking, the amount absorbed each day equals the amount excreted by the kidney. Losses in the sweat and stool are small. Unfortunately, the renal mechanism for *conserving* potassium is inefficient and severe gastrointestinal potassium loss may therefore rapidly produce serious hypokalemia. Between 200 and 300 mEq of loss lowers the serum potassium by 1 mEq/liter.

DATA The laboratory data have returned. The plasma electrolytes are (in mEq/liter) Na^+ 131; Cl^- 90; HCO_3^- 33; K^+ 2.1. Normal values are Na^+ 135 to 145; Cl^- 98 to 106; HCO_3^- 21 to 28; K^+ 3.5 to 5.0. She has marked hypokalemia, the plasma Na^+ concentration is modestly depressed, and the plasma HCO_3^- level is elevated. The blood pH is 7.50. A complete blood count and urinalysis are both normal.

LOGIC These data confirm your initial impression of hypokalemia. The cause is still unknown. Consider the scheme shown in Figure 20.1 as a means to aid in your diagnosis.

We have already excluded those conditions associated with both hypokalemia and

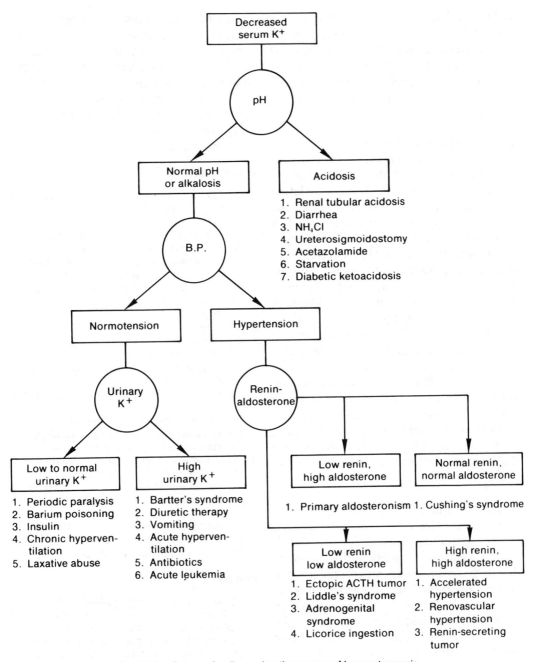

Fig. 20.1. Scheme for diagnosing the causes of hypopotassemia.

hypertension because the patient is normotensive. The slightly alkalotic blood pH and elevated plasma HCO_3^- are consistent with a metabolic alkalosis. As shown in Figure 20.1, a 24-hour urine for K^+ determination would be helpful. If K^+ excretion exceeds 20 to 30 mEq/24 hours with this degree of hypokalemia, renal losses are excessive and a search should be made for more factors which accelerate renal K^+ loss.* If less, then the hypokalemia is due to other mechanisms listed in the table.

---

* Depending upon the duration of the hypokalemia, excessive renal loss is suggested by a spot urine sample with a K^+ concentration greater than 20 mEq/liter.

DATA A 24-hour urine collection is sent to the laboratory for determination of the K^+ concentration and the result is returned to you 1 day later: 120 mEq/day. During her stay in the hospital no vomiting or diarrhea has been noted, although she has not eaten well.

LOGIC This urinary K^+ excretion is excessively high. Returning once again to our schematic outline, six diagnoses are to be seriously considered with this constellation of findings. Bartter's syndrome is historically unlikely although not definitely excluded. A diagnosis of acute hyperventilation is inconsistent with the plasma HCO_3^- concentration. Acute leukemia seems unlikely on the basis of available physical and laboratory data. Its mechanism is unknown. Although prolonged vomiting remains a consideration, it was not observed during her hospital stay. Certain antibiotics and acute leukemia may cause hypokalemia. Surreptitious drug usage seems a likely consideration. All the antibiotics listed in Table 20.1 are administered parenterally and are therefore unlikely candidates. Diuretic therapy seems more likely; she may still be taking it, but even if she is not, its effect may continue for 48 hours.

DATA The patient was again questioned regarding possible causes for hypokalemia. When confronted with the findings which suggested excessive urinary K^+ loss, possibly due to diuretics, she admitted that she had begun diuretic use 2 months ago in an effort to lose weight. She had a job as a waitress in a pharmacy and had access to the drug. She had become lonely since she left home and was hoping to make herself more attractive by losing weight. The patient was begun on KCl therapy and a psychiatric consultation was requested.

LOGIC Hypokalemia may have a number of adverse consequences. For example, cardiac effects include electrocardiac changes indicating abnormal repolarization, predisposition to digitalis toxicity, arrhythmias, and, in sudden severe cases, cardiac arrest.

Profound skeletal muscle weakness may be present and sometimes results in paralysis. Renal functional impairment is frequently seen as a *result* of hypokalemia; a decrease in concentrating ability is the most common finding. The potassium level at which disturbances occur is variable, but levels of 2.5 mEq/liter or below are dangerous and require attention.

QUESTIONS

1. The two major causes of hypokalemia in the patient with persistent vomiting are:
   (a) loss of potassium in the vomitus
   (b) movement of potassium into cells
   (c) loss of potassium in the urine
   (d) inadequate dietary intake of potassium because of the persistent vomiting.
2. Which of the following are important consequences of hypokalemia?
   (a) hypoglycemia
   (b) intestinal hypomotility
   (c) glucose intolerance
   (d) muscle weakness.
3. Prevention of hypokalemia is particularly essential for patients:
   (a) receiving drugs which accelerate potassium loss
   (b) receiving digitalis compounds
   (c) receiving antialdosterone medication
   (d) receiving triamterene for diuresis.
4. Hyperkalemia is even more dangerous than hypokalemia. It can result from:
   (a) the terminal phase of chronic renal failure
   (b) use of oral potassium in the presence of renal failure
   (c) Addison's disease
   (d) immediate use of intravenous potassium in a patient with diabetic coma.

ANSWERS

1. **(b) and (c) are correct.** Although the patient with persistent vomiting loses potassium in gastric juices, the shift of potassium into cells and urinary loss of potassium both caused by the associated metabolic alkalosis, are the major causes of hypokalemia in this circumstance.
2. **(b), (c), and (d) are correct.** Intestinal hypomotility and muscle weakness are both well-known effects of hypokalemia on the smooth and skeletal muscle, respectively. Despite much investigation, the cause is still unclear. Glucose intolerance in the hypokalemic patient results from an impairment in insulin release. Hypoglycemia does not occur.
3. **(a) and (b) are correct.** Diuretics commonly cause hypokalemia in patients with congestive

heart failure and cirrhosis of the liver, but not so commonly in ordinary hypertensives. Thus supplementary potassium is sometimes used in the former. Patients taking digitalis should be watched closely because hypokalemia enhances the potential for digitalis intoxication. Antialdosterone medications induce potassium retention, as does triamterene (and amiloride too).

4. **All are correct.** Terminal anuria will cause potassium to rise. Oral potassium in renal failure may be dangerous; the regulation of potassium excretion does not take place quickly enough. Addison's disease is a hypocorticoid state in which sodium is lost and potassium retained. In diabetic coma, even though the total body potassium is depleted, the serum potassium may be low, normal, or high. Potassium supplementation, if given immediately, may be lethal. Wait until treatment is well under way and potassium is reentering the cells. Then give it orally.

COMMENT A broad knowledge of pathophysiology and an understanding of cause and effect relationships were needed to solve this one. The key clue (hypopotassemia) was recognized from the beginning, and the author pursued a self-constructed flow chart as he gathered bits of evidence and arrived at only one possible conclusion. Note that only a few decision points (pH, blood pressure, potassium excretion) were needed to direct him to the terminal branch, where the final twig (diuretic abuse) was found. The author probably had a hunch about what was wrong. This was a healthy but unhappy obese patient who had easy access to oral drugs. *(P. C.)*

PROBLEM-BASED LEARNING Self-education referable to disorders of potassium homeostasis obliges you to cross many modular boundaries. Potassium disturbances occur in gastrointestinal, renal, endocrine, cardiac, and pulmonary diseases—and indeed in any disease requiring treatment with drugs that can affect potassium kinetics. You should learn about:

1. potassium metabolism: its intake, output, distribution, and regulatory mechanisms
2. the broad classification of disorders causing disturbances in potassium homeostasis (Table 20.1)
3. the clinical features of each disease in that table
4. the special roles of diuretics, diabetic ketoacidosis, and diarrheal states

5. the effect of steroids and high-steroid states
6. how alkalosis and acidosis affect potassium distribution
7. Cushing's syndrome, Conn's syndrome, Bartter's syndrome, and Liddle's syndrome
8. symptoms and signs of hypokalemia
9. ECG manifestations of both hypo- and hyperkalemia
10. disastrous effects of extremely low or high serum potassium
11. causes of hyperkalemia
12. when to anticipate and how to manage hypokalemia and hyperkalemia.

Suggested Readings

1. Kirschenbaum MA: Abnormalities of potassium metabolism. In Bricker NS, Kirschenbaum MA (eds): *The Kidney: Diagnosis and Management.* New York, Wiley, 1984, pp 149–164.
   The physiology and pathophysiology of hypokalemic and hyperkalemic disorders are concisely and completely presented.
2. Sebastian A, Hernandez RE, Schambelan M: Disorders of potassium homeostasis. In Brenner BM, Rector FJ Jr (eds): *The Kidney*, ed 3. Philadelphia, Saunders, 1985, chap 14.
   A good standard textbook presentation that covers both hypokalemic and hyperkalemic states.
3. Tannen RL: Potassium homeostasis. *Kidney Int* 11:389–515, 1977.
   Though not recent, still an excellent series of articles concerning clinical and nonclinical aspects of potassium metabolism.
4. Knockel JP: Neuromuscular manifestations of electrolyte disorders. *Am J Med* 72:521–533, 1982.
   Hypokalemia is emphasized though the role of other ions is included.
5. Johansson BW, Larsson C: A hypokalemic index ECG as a predictor of hypokalemia. *Acta Med Scand* 212:29–31, 1982.
   Demonstrates a method of correlating the ECG changes with hypokalemia in the presence of other influencing factors.
6. Costello J, Bourke E: Bartter's syndrome—the case for a primary potassium-losing tubulopathy: discussion paper. *J R Soc Med* 76:53–56, 1983.
   Shows the complexity of a still not clearly defined syndrome.
7. Carmine Z, Ettore B, Curatola G, et al: The renal-tubular defect of Bartter's syndrome. *Nephron* 32:140–148, 1982.
   Explores the role of prostaglandins in counteracting excessive aldosterone.
8. Narins RG, Jones ER, Strom MC, et al: Diagnostic strategies in disorders of fluid, electrolyte, and acid-base homeostasis. *Am J Med* 72:496–520, 1982.
   A fine paper that discusses all common disorders of potassium, sodium, calcium, magnesium, phosphate, and bicarbonate concentrations. This is good reading for Cases 45 and 47.

Case 46
Hypercalcemia
RALPH S. GOLDSMITH, M.D.

DATA During his routine annual health examination, the 48-year old vice-president of Strato Airways was found to have a serum calcium concentration of 11.5 mg/dl.

LOGIC High serum calcium values have been among the most frequent abnormalities detected on routine laboratory screening procedures. Although there is some variation in the normal ranges found in various laboratories, a serum calcium of 11.5 mg/dl in the presence of normal serum albumin undoubtedly would be classified as definite, albeit modest, hypercalcemia.

Until recently, measurement of serum calcium was relatively difficult and subject to substantial laboratory error. The ready availability of atomic absorption spectroscopy and automated colorimetric procedures has reduced error to a very acceptable 2% or so (1% under ideal circumstances). As a result, it is now recognized that the normal range for serum calcium is much narrower than had been previously thought. One such study found that the normal range (95% confidence limits) for women aged 20 to 80 was 8.9 to 10.1 mg/dl, while that for men progressively declined with age, from 9.1 to 10.3 mg/dl at age 20 to 30—to 8.8 to 9.9 mg/dl at age 70 to 80. (This is to be contrasted with values sometimes published in textbooks or laboratory guides as 8.5 to 11.0 mg/dl.)

The more common causes of hypercalcemia in the general adult population, in approximate order of frequency, are:
1. Cancer, including multiple myeloma, lymphomas, leukemia, and various solid tumors with or without skeletal metastases
2. Primary hyperparathyroidism
3. Sarcoidosis
4. Hyperthyroidism
5. Use of thiazide diuretics
6. Milk-alkali syndrome

7. Vitamin D intoxication
8. Immobilization-induced acute bone atrophy.

To this list of diseases must be added spurious hypercalcemia, which is relatively uncommon and easily eliminated from consideration. This is a result of:
1. Blood drawn after leaving a tourniquet in place for an excessively long time. This may be avoided, even in the patient with "difficult" veins, by removing the tourniquet after venipuncture and allowed reestablishment of normal blood flow before withdrawing the sample.
2. Contact of the blood or serum with cork. Cork is rarely used as a test tube closure in chemistry laboratories today and should no longer be a source of contamination.
3. Laboratory error. Relatively small errors are present with most procedures for calcium measurement in common use today. Repeat analysis should suffice to rule out this problem.

DATA History taken from the patient failed to disclose any recent illnesses, obvious symptoms, or medications. He denied any unusual food habits.

LOGIC It is reasonable to exclude milk-alkali syndrome, thiazide diuretics, and intoxication with vitamin D. Incidentally, some health food faddists may ingest excessive amounts of vitamin D (and/or A, which may also cause hypercalcemia). In addition, the fact that our patient has not been ill obviously eliminates immobilization-induced acute bone atrophy. Despite the apparent absence of symptoms, none of the other listed diseases can be ruled out.

Hypercalcemia occurs in about one-sixth of all patients with hyperthyroidism as a direct effect of thyroid hormone's increasing bone resorption, but it is not often symptomatic or clinically troublesome. The absence of any of the usual symptoms aids in eliminating the diagnosis of hyperthyroidism, but it may be relatively asymptomatic and appropriate laboratory tests should be performed. In most cases, a serum thyroxine (T_4) and a T_3 resin uptake should be sufficient. (Results were normal in this patient.)

DATA A more comprehensive and detailed history disclosed some pertinent information. The patient had passed three kidney stones during the past 10 years, but had hesitated to admit to his employer that he was ill for fear it might jeopardize his career. Two of the episodes were associated with pain in the left flank, and one with pain in the right. These stones had passed spontaneously and were not saved for examination, although the patient thought that they were tan or brownish in color. In addition, the patient reluctantly admitted that he regularly used an electric cart on the golf course because for the last 2 years or so he had noticed lethargy and easy fatigability. Some years earlier he had been the "boy wonder" of Strato Airways, with boundless energy and enthusiasm. Recently, however, he just did not have his old pep and had been passed over for the presidency of the company as a result of his apparent inability to make important decisions quickly.

LOGIC Now we are beginning to get somewhere. Although there are many causes of renal calculi, such a long history (10 years) in association with current hypercalcemia leads one to think of primary hyperparathyroidism (HPT). The passage of stones from both kidneys helps rule out a congenital or acquired ureteral lesion that might predispose to stone formation by obstructing normal urine flow. The absence of symptoms of acute urinary tract infection, however, does not eliminate the possibility of chronic pyelonephritis as a predisposing factor, since the latter may be totally silent while destroying the kidneys. It would have been helpful to examine and analyze the stones; they are usually calcium oxalate, apatite, or brushite in primary HPT. Magnesium ammonium phosphate stones, on the other hand, would indicate infection. The tan to brownish appearance of the stones is not necessarily helpful, because this coloration might have represented small amounts of blood collected on the surface of the stones as they passed with difficulty through the ureters.

There are many causes of kidney stones, any one of which could have a chance association with any of the causes of hypercalcemia. It is worth noting, however, that renal stone has been one of the most frequent presenting features of primary HPT and may continue for many years before detection of hypercalcemia. It has been estimated that 5 to 10% of patients with urolithiasis have primary HPT. Incidentally, patients with HPT who have stones usually do not have clinically significant nephrocalcinosis.

The characteristic symptoms of mild hypercalcemia are lethargy, easy fatigability, weakness, loss of energy, and aprosexia (inability to concentrate). These symptoms are often so gradual in onset that the patient may be unaware of their presence. Furthermore, they are so nonspecific as to be of little diagnostic value. With increasing severity of hypercalcemia, symptoms may include anorexia, constipation, and drowsiness or stupor. Polyuria and nocturia may be noted because hypercalcemia antagonizes the action of antidiuretic hormone and thus leads to a loss of renal concentrating ability.

DATA On physical examination, the patient appears to be healthy. The only abnormal physical findings were mild hypertension and some granular deposits in the cornea bilaterally, just medial to the limbus. Subsequent examination by slit lamp confirmed band keratopathy.

LOGIC There are no physical findings characteristic or pathognomonic of primary HPT. Only rarely can even a large parathyroid adenoma be felt. The fact that the patient appeared well is compatible with that diagnosis, however, and does not support the possibility of an advanced malignancy.

Hypertension has come to be recognized as a fairly common finding in patients with primary HPT. But because of the frequency with which it occurs in the general population, its presence is of little or no diagnostic value. Hypertension may occur in any form of hypercalcemia and has even been observed during infusion of calcium lasting only a few hours.

Detectable band keratopathy with only modest hypercalcemia suggests that hypercalcemia has been present for a long time and helps further to make the diagnosis of cancer less likely. Band keratopathy is the deposition of calcium salts in the cornea, sclera, and conjunctiva. It is sometimes appreciated by the patient as an irritation of the eyes or conjunctivitis. More often it is asymptomatic and appears as fine white granules in the cornea and sclera just medial and lateral to the limbus and usually separated slightly from it. On casual inspection it may be mistaken for arcus senilis. Two features distinguish band keratopathy, however: granularity and absence of deposits from the superior and inferior aspects of the eye. Band keratopathy can appear slowly in patients with long-standing but minimal to moderate elevations of serum calcium; or it can develop rapidly in patients with severe hypercalcemia.

DATA   Examination of other routine laboratory data disclosed the following pertinent results:

Normal: hemoglobin, hematocrit, leukocyte count, differential; erythrocyte sedimentation rate; urinalysis; serum creatinine and urea nitrogen; serum protein electrophoresis; serum sodium, potassium, bicarbonate; and liver function tests.

Abnormal: serum phosphorus (inorganic phosphate) 2.3 mg/dl; serum chloride 109 mEq/liter; serum uric acid 9 mg/dl; serum alkaline phosphatase 100 IU/liter; and urinary calcium excretion 320 mg/24 hours.

LOGIC   It is always reassuring to find normal values for hemoglobin, hematocrit, leukocyte count, sedimentation rate, urinalysis, and the serum protein electrophoresis, since they virtually rule out a host of malignant diseases: myeloma, lymphoma, leukemia, and widespread carcinomatosis. Admittedly, a relatively small and inconspicuous malignant tumor (such as a hypernephroma or bronchogenic carcinoma) could produce enough of its hypercalcemic hormone to cause hypercalcemia without otherwise appearing to affect the patient. In fact, at this time the tumor may be resectable. Therefore, some investigators suggest that hypercalcemia and other hormonal effects be used as tumor markers to identify early malignant disease.

The abnormal laboratory values shown are quite typical for primary HPT. But such values could also result from a malignant tumor that secretes parathyroid hormone or a closely related peptide. This situation is sometimes called ectopic hyperparathyroidism or pseudohyperparathyroidism for obvious reasons. Some studies have indicated that a relatively high serum chloride (107 mEq/liter) or a high ratio of chloride: phosphorus (30) strongly favors the diagnosis of primary HPT, whereas the reverse favors malignancy. Hyperuricemia is a common accompaniment of primary HPT but may occur coincidentally in any hypercalcemic disorder. Minimal elevation of the serum alkaline phosphatase is often seen in primary HPT and suggests that x-ray evidence of osteitis fibrosa may be found. It may also be increased in malignant disease due to bone involvement or hepatic metastases. Chemical distinction between alkaline phosphatases of skeletal and hepatic origin can be made in some laboratories and may be helpful.

Urinary excretion of calcium is particularly likely to aid in distinguishing primary HPT from sarcoidosis and vitamin D intoxication. In the latter diseases, secretion of parathyroid hormone is greatly decreased, so long as there is no significant impairment of renal function (or at least of the glomerular filtration rate). The hypercalcemia of vitamin D intoxication, and probably of sarcoidosis as well, is due to the effects of a high blood concentration of one or more active metabolites of vitamin D. When the serum blood calcium increases, secretion of parathyroid hormone is inhibited. Since parathyroid hormone is a potent factor in the renal tubular reabsorption of calcium, its relative absence would be expected to permit urinary excretion of a higher fraction of filtered calcium. Because the filtered load of calcium is the product of plasma ultrafiltrable calcium (about 55 to 60% of the total) and the glomerular filtration rate, urinary excretion of calcium is higher (at any given level of serum calcium) in sarcoidosis and vitamin D intoxication than in HPT, at least when renal function is normal. Urinary calcium rarely exceeds 500 mg/day in HPT; it often does so in the other two diseases.

One must be particularly wary in milk-alkali syndrome, which is usually due to excessive ingestion of milk and calcium carbonate. As orginally described, this syndrome consists of hypercalcemia, normophosphatemia, azotemia, normocalciuria, and often alkalosis. The normophosphatemia and normocalciuria, however, are probably a result of renal insufficiency and therefore could occur in HPT complicated by renal insufficiency. In fact, milk-alkali syndrome may be superimposed upon HPT, as was the case in several patients of the initially reported series, presumably due to overzealous treatment of peptic ulcer (symptoms of which are common in primary HPT).

DATA   X-rays of the skull, hand, clavicles, pelvic, spine, and long bones were obtained. There were no lytic lesions suggestive of metastases or myeloma. The skull was thought to show a finely stippled pattern suggestive of numerous minute areas of bone resorption. The radial aspects of several fingers showed cortical thinning, small intracortical cysts and tunneling, and subperiosteal resorption. The cortex of the distal third of each clavicle was very thin, producing an almost cystic appearance. Both bony margins of the acromioclavicular joint, but especially the clavicle, were irregular and frayed.

LOGIC   These findings are characteristic of osteitis fibrosa, the skeletal lesion of HPT.

Only rarely will a patient with ectopic HPT be found to have the characteristic x-ray features of osteitis fibrosa, presumably because the course of the disease is usually too rapid for the bone disease to become manifest. Even though our patient did not have any "brown tumors" (osteoclastomas) or cysts, enough x-ray evidence of bone disease was present to make the presumptive diagnosis of osteitis fibrosa.

At this point, therefore, the diagnosis of primary HPT seems most likely, with cancer becoming more remote. Sarcoidosis seems equally well ruled out by the normal chest x-ray, absence of lymphadenopathy, absence of characteristic cystic changes in the phalanges, normal serum protein electrophoresis, normal liver function tests, and normal renal function. High serum concentrations of 1,25-dihydroxyvitamin D, the most potent natural metabolite of vitamin D, have been found in hypercalcemic patients with sarcoidosis or other granulomatous diseases. This suggests the possibility that the granulomas are in some way responsible for uncontrolled synthesis of this metabolite. However, measurement of this metabolite is not necessarily of diagnostic value since it is sometimes elevated in patients with primary HPT. On the other hand, the combination of a high 1,25-dihydroxyvitamin D and low parathyroid hormone would be very supportive of sarcoidosis or another granulomatous disease.

DATA   For added assurance, it was considered advisable to obtain measurement of serum parathyroid hormone concentration; this was elevated, confirming the diagnosis of primary HPT. Surgery was thought to be indicated. On careful dissection, a pea-sized adenoma of the parathyroid gland was found behind the right lobe of the thyroid.

LOGIC   Measurement of the serum concentration of parathyroid hormone is not always required for the diagnosis, but it is often helpful in less clear-cut situations than the present one. Since antisera used in this radioimmunoassay have not been standardized, there is some variability in the relative diagnostic utility of various assays. For that reason, some endocrinologists have found that measurement of total urinary excretion of cyclic adenosine monophosphate (cyclic AMP), or of the nephrogenous portion only, is easier to interpret with consistency. Excretion of this substance generally parallels the serum concentration of parathyroid hormone; therefore it is high in HPT and low in patients with cancer.

In this patient, the need for surgical removal of the parathyroid adenoma was clear. In addition to modest hypercalcemia, the patient had radiographic evidence of osteitis fibrosa. Some authors have suggested, however, that "chemical" HPT, i.e. HPT without clinically apparent involvement of target organs such as bone and kidney, need not be treated surgically and needs only periodic confirmation that no change has occurred. This seems a rather risky position, since a hypercalcemic crisis can occur quite unexpectedly in these patients, and the development of bone disease or kidney impairment cannot be predicted. In fact, it has been reported as a result of a 10-year prospective study that it was impossible in retrospect to find any clues that would indicate which patients would subsequently require surgery. Especially with the exciting new capability of locating even rather small adenomas before surgery through the use of high-resolution ultrasonography, there seems to be little justification for withholding definitive cure.

Quite a different case can be made for *familial hypocalciuric hypercalcemia*, a syndrome of still unknown dimension that may be confused with HPT. It has a strong familial occurrence with autosomal dominant transmission. There are few symptoms and signs, no morbidity, and no clear-cut cause. This newly described entity needs further clarification. But it must be considered when hypercalcemia is found.

COMMENT   Another lanthanic presentation! Or so it seemed until a history of urinary calculi, lack of energy, and inability to concentrate was ferreted out. Many patients with bilateral renal stones have hyperparathyroidism, so this clue is important. The other two symptoms were non-specific though fairly sensitive. Band keratopathy is a highly specific clue; so is the parathyroid hormone assay if properly done. The vagaries of the serum calcium, alkaline phosphatase, and urine calcium excretion were also discussed.

The solution to this problem was achieved with a delightful demonstration of "*think along with me.*" The author used lots of logic and few data; he formed a complete list of causes for hypercalcemia and systematically eliminated all but one, which he proceeded to prove.

This is another instance where a dendrogram or self-generated flow chart would be useful, since there are only a few critical decision points and branches to be taken.

In other cases, cancer may merit strong consideration. Especially common causes of hypercalcemia are multiple myeloma, lymphoma, and cancer of the breast, lung, and kidney. The hypercalcemia may occur without bone metastases in lung and kidney cancers which elaborate a parathyroid-like hormone, and in neoplasms that invade and destroy bone by in part elaborating an osteoclast-activating factor. This complex subject is detailed in Suggested Reading 12.   (*P. C.*)

Suggested Readings

1. Aurbach GD, Marx SJ, Spiegel AM: Parathyroid hormone, calcitonin, and calciferols. In Williams RH (ed): *Textbook of Endocrinology*, ed 6. Philadelphia, Saunders, 1981, pp 922–1031.
   Complete discussion of parathyroid physiology and disease.
2. Brennan MF: Primary hyperparathyroidism. *Adv Surg* 16:25–47, 1983.
   Covers the prevalence, diagnosis, location of tumor, and surgery.
3. Heath H III, Hodgson SF, Kennedy MA: Primary hyperparathyroidism. Incidence, morbidity, and potential economic impact in a community. *N Engl J Med* 302:189–193, 1980.
4. Scholz DA, Purnell DC: Asymptomatic primary hyperparathyroidism—10 year prospective study. *Mayo Clin Proc* 56:473–478, 1981.
   Important follow-up data on the only prospective study of its kind.
5. Gaz RD, Wang C: Management of asymptomatic hyperparathyroidism. *Am J Surg* 147:498–502, 1984.
   Surgeons conclude that mild asymptomatic hypercalcemia can be watched and does not need immediate surgery.
6. Marx SJ: New insights into primary hyperparathyroidism. *Hosp Pract (Off)* 19:55–63, 1984.
   Weighs the risk of watching or treating asymptomatic HPT.
7. Link K, Centor R, Buchsbaum D, et al: Why physicians don't pursue abnormal laboratory tests: an investigation of hypercalcemia and the follow-up of abnormal test results. *Hum Pathol* 15:75–78, 1984.
   Chides the clinician for ignoring important laboratory test abnormalities.

8. Clark OH, Gooding GW, Ljung BM: Locating a parathyroid adenoma by ultrasonography and aspiration biopsy cytology. *West J Med* 135:154–158, 1981.
   One of the first reports of this excellent technique.
9. Parr JH, Tarkunde I, Ramsay I: The use of ultrasound in the localization of parathyroid glands in parathyroid disorders. *Clin Radiol* 34:395–400, 1983.
10. Carroll PR, Clark OH: Milk-alkali syndrome: does it exist and can it be differentiated from primary hyperparathyroidism? *Ann Surg* 197:427–433, 1983.

It exists and the distinction is possible though difficult.
11. Marx SJ, Spiegel AM, Levine MA, et al: Familial hypocalciuric hypercalcemia. The relation to primary parathyroid hyperplasia. *N Engl J Med* 307:416–426, 1982.
   Excellent review of a still poorly understood syndrome.
12. Mundy GR, Ibbotson KJ, D'Souza SM, et al: The hypercalcemia of cancer. Clinical implications and pathogenic mechanisms. *N Engl J Med* 310:1718–1727, 1984.
   Details the humoral and cellular mechanisms for hypercalcemia in different malignancies.

Case 47
Weakness and Disorientation

PAUL CUTLER, M.D.

DATA A 68-year-old man was brought to the emergency room by his wife because he had become disoriented. Although he had always been in excellent health, for the last month or so he had experienced persistent diffuse muscle weakness, lassitude, and "wasn't himself." Further careful questioning by the intern failed to reveal any significant additional pieces of information. He had had no previous hospitalizations and had recently retired from his position as an accountant. He denied the use of tobacco, had only an occasional drink of alcohol, and took no drugs except for a daily multivitamin tablet. The family history was noncontributory.

On physical examination, the patient appeared his stated age, was well nourished, and was in no obvious distress. Vital signs were: BP 120/82 mm Hg with no postural change; P 82; T 37 C; R 16. The skin was free of any lesions and normal in appearance. Examination of the head, eyes, ears, nose, and throat was normal. The chest was clear to auscultation and percussion. The cardiac, abdominal, and genital examinations were normal. No evidence of clubbing, cyanosis, or edema was demonstrable. There was no apparent muscle atrophy or tenderness. The neurologic examination was unremarkable except for the suggestion of generalized weakness.

LOGIC The intern was puzzled by the chief complaint and the apparent absence of any clues which might suggest a fruitful area to investigate. Because of the history, he thought in terms of a small nonfocalizing cerebral thrombosis, subdural hematoma, brain tumor, generalized cancer, diabetes, uremia, or chronic brain syndrome, but there was nothing in the examination to confirm any of these. He requested laboratory tests to aid in his evaluation.

DATA One hour later the following laboratory results were received: hemoglobin 13 g/dl; hematocrit 41%; white blood cell count 9500; differential normal; blood glucose 90 mg/dl; electrolytes in mEq/liter—Na^+ 115, Cl^- 79, HCO_3^- 22, K^+ 3.2; blood urea nitrogen 8 mg/dl. Chest x-ray, ECG, and sedimentation rate were normal.

LOGIC These studies give strong evidence against the various possibilities which first occurred to the intern. Uremia and diabetes may be disregarded in view of the normal data thus far derived. Metastatic cancer appears unlikely.

But the laboratory data are particularly notable for the marked hyponatremia and hypochloremia, mean normal values being Na$^+$ 140 and Cl$^-$ 100 mEq/liter. Is the degree of hyponatremia consistent with muscle weakness, fatigue, and disorientation? The symptoms and signs of hyponatremia are dependent upon the cause, magnitude, and acuteness of the condition. Table 20.2 lists the signs and symptoms which may be associated with hyponatremia. The neurologic manifestations usually do not appear until the plasma Na$^+$ is below 125 mEq/liter.

The diagnostic approach to the patient with hyponatremia should be undertaken with an understanding of the physiology of the urinary concentrating and diluting mechanisms and of those factors which affect their function. In addition, the clinical conditions in which one observes hyponatremia should be appreciated. Table 20.3 lists clinical circumstances which may be associated with hyponatremia and a general comment regarding etiology.

It is important to note that the average human body contains 2000 mEq of sodium; that the normal serum sodium concentration varies from 138 to 144 mEq/liter; that sodium and its associated anions contribute over 90% of serum osmolality; that normal serum osmolality is 285 to 295 mOsm/kg H$_2$O; and that hyponatremia is one of the most commonly encountered electrolyte problems.

Table 20.2.
Signs and Symptoms That May Be Associated with Hyponatremia*

Symptoms	Signs
Lethargy, apathy	Abnormal sensorium
Disorientation	Depressed deep tendon
Muscle cramps	reflexes
Anorexia, nausea	Cheyne-Stokes respiration
Agitation	Hypothermia
	Pathologic reflexes
	Pseudobulbar palsy
	Seizures

* From Berl T, Anderson RJ, McDonald KM, et al: Clinical disorders of water metabolism. *Kidney Int* 10:117–132, 1976, with permission.

Table 20.3.
Classification of Hyponatremic States*

I. Free water intake in excess of normal excretory ability: primary polydipsia
II. Free water intake in excess of depressed excretory ability
   A. Decreased delivery to diluting segments
      1. Decreased glomerular filtration rate
      2. Volume depletion
      3. Congestive heart failure
      4. Hepatic cirrhosis with ascites
      5. Nephrotic syndrome
      6. Glucocorticoid deficiency
      7. Myxedema?
   B. Decreased solute absorption by diluting segments
      1. Diuretics
      2. Bartter's syndrome
   C. Increased water permeability of diluting segments—vasopressin absent
      1. Glucocorticoid deficiency
   D. Increased water permeability of diluting segments—vasopressin present
      1. Ectopic antidiuretic hormone (ADH) production
      2. Increased cerebral ADH production due to nonosmotic stimuli
      3. Increased cerebral ADH production due to pharmaceuticals

* From Hays RM, Levine SD: Pathophysiology of water metabolism. In Brenner BM, Rector FC (eds): *The Kidney*, ed 2. Philadelphia, Saunders, 1981.

More important, the serum sodium concentration and serum osmolality are governed by a delicate interplay between thirst, diaphoresis, osmoreceptors that control the hypothalamic-posterior pituitary antidiuretic hormone axis, and the renal medullary countercurrent system that regulates sodium and water excretion and reabsorption. The management of sodium and water by the kidney depends mainly upon the concentration of antidiuretic hormone, sodium intake, extrarenal sodium loss, corticosteroids, and the kidney's functional integrity.

What laboratory tests might be of benefit? *Pseudohyponatremia* may be present when a fall in plasma sodium concentration is not accompanied by a decrease in plasma osmolality. When this occurs, some molecule which does not diffuse freely across the cell membranes is present in the plasma in high concentrations. Glucose is most often responsible, although occasionally lipids and proteins also contribute. Thus, a measurement of the plasma osmolality may be of considerable value. In addition, insight into the state of the renal concentrating and diluting mechanism can be gained by measurement of the urinary osmolality. Finally, as part of the initial evaluation, serum creatinine and urinary sodium concentrations are helpful, as will be discussed below.

DATA   The following laboratory results were obtained: plasma osmolality 240 mOsm/kg H_2O; urinary osmolality 425 mOsm/kg; blood urea nitrogen (above); creatinine 1.0 mg/dl, and urinary sodium concentration 45 mEq/liter.

LOGIC   These values tell us that (*a*) the patient does not have pseudohyponatremia, (*b*) the urinary osmolality is inappropriately concentrated for the level of plasma osmolality, and (*c*) the urine sodium concentration does not suggest an active salt-retaining state.

DATA   Let us again return to the patient. How might we most profitably undertake an evaluation which will lead us to the correct diagnosis? With the use of the scheme shown in Figure 20.2 we can evaluate the patient with true hyponatremia.

LOGIC   As you proceed from the observation of the presence of hyponatremia, the chart shown in Figure 20.2 then separates the disorders into various categories depending upon the relative state of the extracellular fluid (ECF) volume. The categorization of a particular patient depends upon information derived from the history and physical examination and certain critical laboratory tests which were previously mentioned. The patient did not have renal insufficiency nor was he in a sodium-retaining state. Furthermore, he was not edematous nor was any suggestion of ECF volume depletion noted, e.g. postural hypotension or tachycardia. Thus he would seem to fall into the middle category, i.e. those patients who may

have modest ECF volume excess but who are not edematous.

Several of the diagnostic considerations in this group can be reasonably excluded by the data currently available. No suggestion of hypothyroidism or altered emotional state was manifest by the patient's history or physical examination. Pain seems unlikely and, as mentioned, except for multivitamins, he denied the use of drugs. Chlorpropamide, clofibrate, vincristine, thiazides, and tricyclic antidepressants may cause clinical pictures which fit this category. Although glucocorticoid deficiency (Addison's disease) cannot be definitely excluded, it seems unlikely without some of the usual stigmata, such as cutaneous and mucosal hyperpigmentation, arterial hypotension, and gastrointestinal complaints. Absolute exclusion of this possibility, however, would depend upon appropriate measurement of steroid production.

Seemingly this patient would fit into the group of patients with a disorder known as the syndrome of inappropriate antidiuretic hormone production (SIADH). This syndrome, which can be diagnosed only in the presence of an otherwise intact diluting mechanism, is characterized by:

1. hyponatremia and plasma hypoosmolality
2. urine which is less than appropriately dilute
3. urine sodium excretion which parallels sodium intake
4. absence of other causes of hyponatremia.

Table 20.4 lists the causes of this syndrome. Diagnostic considerations should include those studies required to investigate the various possibilities. The relationship between SIADH and most of the causes listed is not entirely clear.

DATA   The patient was treated with fluid restriction and his serum sodium rose to normal levels. In the meantime, a search was made for a cause. A small retrocardiac pulmonary mass, overlooked on the pre-

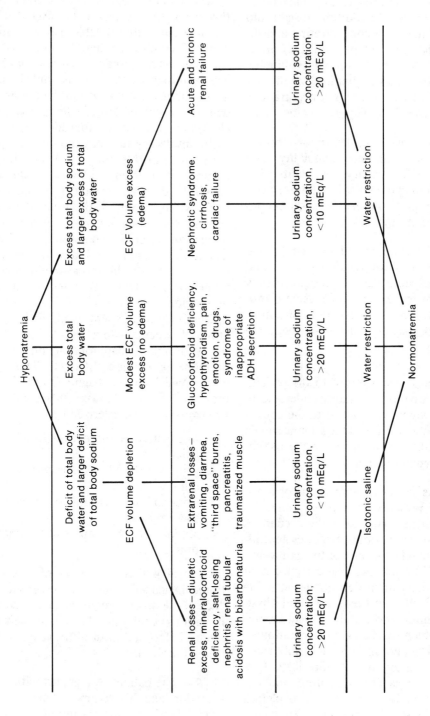

Fig. 20.2 Clinical approach to the patient with hyponatremia. (From Berl T, Anderson RJ, McDonald KM et al: Clinical disorders of water metabolism. *Kidney Int* 10:117–132, 1976, with permission.)

Table 20.4.
Causes of the Syndrome of Inappropriate
Antidiuretic Hormone Production (SIADH)*

I. Malignancies
   A. Bronchogenic carcinoma
   B. Adenocarcinoma of pancreas and duodenum
   C. Carcinoma of ureter
   D. Lymphoma
   E. Thymoma
II. Pulmonary diseases
   A. Tuberculosis
   B. Pneumonia
   C. Aspergillosis with cavitation
   D. Lung abscess
   E. Chronic chest infection
III. Diseases of the central nervous system
   A. Acute psychoses
   B. Infections, e.g. encephalitis, meningitis, brain abscess
   C. Trauma
   D. Subarachnoid or subdural hemorrhage
   E. Guillain-Barré syndrome
   F. Brain tumor
   G. Systemic lupus erythematosus
   H. Acute intermittent porphyria
   I. Stroke

* From Hays RM, Levine SD: Pathophysiology of water metabolism. In Brenner BM, Rector FC (eds): *The Kidney*, ed 2. Philadelphia, Saunders, 1981.

vious chest x-ray, was found. There were no evidences of metastases. It was resected and the histology disclosed an oat cell carcinoma of the lung. This cell type is known to secrete antidiuretic hormone-like substances, so the SIADH should disappear.

However, the prognosis for oat cell carcinoma is not good. Most oncologists consider this a medical problem requiring chemotherapy. The disease is already widespread at the time of detection, and surgical resection is generally not curative.

But only time will tell. . . .

QUESTIONS

1. A patient with severe congestive heart failure who is actively retaining sodium and who is hyponatremic (Na^+ = 128 mEq/liter) would be expected to have:
   (a) urine appropriately hypoosmotic
   (b) urine hyperosmotic relative to plasma osmolality
   (c) no reasonable conclusions drawn from the data
   (d) a normal total body sodium.

2. Hyponatremia will develop in the patient with SIADH:
   (a) because the amount of antidiuretic hormone present will result in renal sodium wasting
   (b) but is unusual unless sodium is restricted in the diet
   (c) and is due to a marked increase in total body water and sodium, the amount of water retained being greater than the amount of sodium
   (d) provided the patient has access to adequate amounts of water.

3. The plasma osmolality in a patient with a plasma sodium concentration of 143 mEq/liter and a glucose of 1800 mg/dl is approximately:
   (a) 285 mEq/liter
   (b) 385 mEq/liter
   (c) 520 mEq/liter
   (d) 257 mEq/liter.

4. A 38-year-old diabetic was taking an oral hypoglycemic for control of his hyperglycemia. Routine plasma electrolytes revealed a sodium of 120 mEq/liter. The blood sugar was normal and the plasma was not grossly lipemic. Which of the following is most likely?
   (a) The patient has been ingesting too much water.
   (b) The patient very likely has diabetic nephropathy with an inability to appropriately dilute his urine.
   (c) The patient may be ingesting a hypoglycemic agent, chlorpropamide, which can cause water retention.
   (d) Diabetics are known to be profound salt wasters and sodium depletion may contribute to the hyponatremia.

ANSWERS

1. **(b) is correct.** For a number of reasons, patients with congestive heart failure and avid sodium retention cannot appropriately dilute their urine. Thus the urine will be hypertonic to plasma. The presence of edema essentially always indicates an increase in total body sodium, regardless of the serum sodium level.

2. **(d) is correct.** Hyponatremia will occur only if the amount of water ingested exceeds insensible losses and the obligatory amount required to excrete the urinary solute load. If combined water loss equals the amount of water ingested, hyponatremia will not occur. Sodium excretion, retention, and ingestion are not related to the action of antidiuretic hormone or the SIADH.

3. **(b) is the correct answer with the information provided.** The osmolality can be estimated as 2 times the sodium concentration plus the contribution of the glucose. The latter can be

determined by dividing the number of milligrams of glucose per liter by the molecular weight of glucose which is 180. Thus, 18,000 ÷ 180 = 100 mOsm/kg H_2O. It is obvious that the glucose in milligrams per deciliter divided by 18 will provide the same answer. This patient is hyperosmolar.

4. **(c) is the most logical choice** although others, particularly (a) and (b), deserve a second look. Chlorpropamide, like a number of other drugs, may impair the renal excretion of water. (d) is not typical of diabetic patients.

COMMENT   This presentation could have been caused by many different pathologic states, but a battery of laboratory tests led to the key clue– hyponatremia. A very few additional clinical findings and decision points limited the possible diagnoses to a small handful. SIADH became the obvious underlying pathophysiologic mechanism. A further search disclosed the cause of this syndrome—often not an easy task because of the strange assortment of unrelated diseases in which this syndrome is inexplicably found.   (*P. C.*)

Suggested Readings

1. Robertson G, Berl T: Pathophysiology of water metabolism. In Brenner BM, Rector FJ Jr (eds): *The Kidney*, ed 3. Philadelphia, Saunders, 1985, chap 11.
   A detailed textbook explanation of disorders of osmolality and sodium homeostasis, including SIADH.
2. Bartter FC, Schwartz WB: The syndrome of inappropriate secretion of antidiuretic hormone. *Am J Med* 42:790–806, 1967.
   One of the initial but still valid and excellent descriptions of the syndrome.
3. Hamilton RW, Buckalew VM: Sodium, water, and congestive heart failure (editorial). *Ann Intern Med* 100:902–903, 1984.
   Discusses the hyponatremia seen in congestive heart failure and alludes to two articles on the subject in the same issue (pp 777–781 and pp 782–789).
4. Rush DR, Hamburger S: Hyponatremia. *South Med J* 77:565–575, 1984.
   A practical and schematic approach to the entire subject with special emphasis on SIADH.
5. Booker JA: Severe symptomatic hyponatremia in elderly outpatients: the role of thiazide therapy and stress. *J Am Geriatr Soc* 32:108–113, 1984.
   The danger from diuretics is in the first week.
6. Bear RA, Neil GA: A clinical approach to common electrolyte problems. Hyponatremia. *Can Med Assoc J* 128:1171–1174, 1983.
   A common-sense diagnostic discussion.
7. Hainsworth JD, Workman R, Grecco FA: Management of the syndrome of inappropriate antidiuretic hormone secretion in small cell lung cancer. *Cancer* 51:161–165, 1983.
   Study of 18 patients with these two related disorders.
8. Roberge R, Gernsheimer J, Sparano R, et al: Psychogenic polydipsia—an unusual cause of hyponatremic coma and seizure. *Ann Emerg Med* 13:274–276, 1984.
   How compulsive water drinking can cause coma.

Chapter 21

Gynecologic Problems

The gynecologist is faced not only with problems peculiar to his own field but with all the problems of women. That is because he has developed the kind of interpersonal relationship which encourages his patient to consult him for all matters—medical, family, social, and sexual.

After all, he was the one who performed the first pelvic examination, discussed contraception, and delivered the children, so it is only natural that he should become the primary care physician for many women concerning any matter relating to their emotional or physical health. Such is the confidence and confidentiality which has ideally developed! Consequently his knowledge base must and does rise far above the pelvis.

Since the field of gynecology revolves mainly about the reproductive organs, sex, pregnancy, and relationships with children and husband, it is logical that psychosomatic factors often play a large role in modifying or even being the reason for the patient's complaints.

Commonly seen problems are those relating to vaginal discharge, acute and chronic pelvic pain, menstrual abnormalities, vaginal bleeding, pregnancy, sexual intercourse, contraception, and menopause. In the case of bleeding, it may be because menses are late, absent, or long. As for pregnancy, the patient consults her physician because she is pregnant, because she fears she is pregnant, or because she is unable to become so. Various symptoms which may or may not be menopause-related can be the cause for the visit. Sexual problems may consist of painful intercourse, frigidity or the opposite state, inability to have an orgasm, or incompatibility.

Perhaps one of the most common reasons for visiting a gynecologist is the periodic checkup for cancer. This usually includes a pelvic and rectal examination, Pap smear, examination of the breasts, and sometimes a complete physical examination including x-rays and laboratory tests. Indeed, if the gynecologist is the only physician the patient sees, all these procedures are in order.

While vaginal discharge is one of the most frequent problems encountered, it requires only simple problem-solving skills. The answer should be obtainable by a pelvic examination, Pap smear, gonococcus smear and culture, and KOH and wet drop preparations. New techniques may identify more recently recognized agents.

As for problem solving in general, the pelvic examination usually provides the answer. However, since there is so often an overlap with endocrinologic problems whereby pelvic organ disease can cause systemic endocrine effects and endocrine disease can cause gynecologic symptoms, the examination must often be more generalized.

Three more points! History taking is not routine and easy; tact, diplomacy, warmth, privacy, and confidentiality are crucial. Second, it is necessary to know what is "*normal.*" This is particularly true for such items as vaginal discharge, the amount of pain with the menses, the amount of blood loss with each menstrual flow, the frequency of intercourse, and the duration of menopause. Last, the physician must always be alert for the presence of the most serious pelvic disease: cancer (cervix, endometrium, or ovary)—especially in women beyond the age of 30. (*P. C.*)

Case 48
A Missed Menstrual Period
PAUL C. WEINBERG, M.D.

DATA A 42-year-old woman is concerned because her menstrual period is 3 weeks late. She had two full-term pregnancies with normal deliveries at ages 20 and 23. Until 3 years ago, she had successfully used oral contraceptives. At that time she was advised to use an alternative method because of beginning mild hypertension (148/90). She chose a diaphragm and jelly contraceptive which she had used early in her marriage, and now wears her diaphragm regularly with each coital encounter.

The patient's menses began at age 13, were always regular, and lasted 3 to 4 days without dysmenorrhea. The onset of amenorrhea was abrupt, was not preceded by a gradual decrease in amount or frequency of menstrual bleeding, and had never happened before.

Further history discloses recent insomnia, "more nervousness than usual," nighttime perspiration, and occasional flushed feelings during the day. These symptoms have been pronounced since she missed her period, but she is unsure when they actually began. She takes no drugs or medications.

LOGIC When you first hear the chief complaint, a number of common possibilities immediately surface from your knowledge base. But before considering them you remember that absolute menstrual regularity is a rarity. Also, you know from experience that an occasional irregular or missed period usually has no significance, though it may cause profound anxiety.

Patients who are accustomed to absolute regularity may visit you if their menstruation is only 2 weeks late. Others who often miss one or more menstrual periods are not so readily concerned.

For starters, you consider pregnancy, premature menopause, persistent corpus luteum, and psychogenic amenorrhea. Secondary amenorrhea is defined as the cessation of menses after they have already started. One swallow does not make a summer, nor does one missed period fulfill the definition of secondary amenorrhea. Wait a few months and see.

In spite of the regular use of and prior success with mechanical contraception, pregnancy must still be a consideration. It is too early for symptoms or even for confirmation by pelvic examination (unless the pregnancy is tubal). However, newer pregnancy tests that measure β-human chorionic gonadotropin would now be positive if the patient were pregnant.

Psychogenic factors are extremely common. In some unknown way, they affect the hypothalamus which regulates the release of gonadotropic hormones. Menstrual flow can begin prematurely or not at all. Acute psychologic stress, major or seemingly trivial, can temporarily alter menstrual regularity. Going away to college, getting married, an emotional upset, or mental distress of any sort can be implicated, though sometimes no obvious stress factor can be elicited. An acute transient organic illness may also cause a temporary menstrual derangement. Anorexia nervosa may halt the menses too. In our patient, the symptoms could be psychophysiologic but so far there is no positive evidence for a psychogenic problem and further questioning about the patient's psychosocial situation is indicated.

Although this patient takes no drugs, it is important to be aware of the fact that amenorrhea may be caused by major tranquilizers, psychotropics, heroin, possibly marijuana, cancer chemotherapy, and the cessation of oral contraceptives.

Premature menopause is less likely. The symptoms fit, but they came on rather suddenly and could be manifestations of anxiety. Also, in menopause the menses usually alter gradually in flow and frequency. They do not suddenly stop. And last, though premature menopause is not unheard of, it is unusual. The average age in our western civilization is 51. If hard pressed for a diagnosis, you might obtain a follicle-stimulating hormone level (FSH), since it is elevated with the onset of menopause. But time and patience will tell the story. Persistent corpus luteum (Halban's syndrome) is another possibility. The pelvic examination should detect an adnexal mass, though a mass could also be a tubal pregnancy. In this instance, ultrasonography may add precision by determining whether the ovarian mass is cystic or solid.

DATA   Physical examination shows a normal-sized uterus and ovaries, no evidence of vaginal atrophy, no adenexal masses, and no cervical discoloration. The breasts are normal and do not show increased vascularity, engorgement, or Montgomery glands around the nipples. A careful search fails to find galactorrhea. In fact, the entire examination is normal. The blood pressure is now 118/60, so her prior pill-induced hypertension is resolved.

LOGIC   There is no objective evidence of pregnancy or menopause, though it may be too early to see such evidence even if those conditions existed. A persistent corpus luteum cyst might be palpable.

The patient did not complain of a milky discharge from the nipples. But had it been elicited on examination, consideration of the amenorrhea-galactorrhea syndrome would be indicated. This invokes a search for a prolactinoma as in the mini-case in Chapter 13.

DATA   Careful delicate questioning reveals that she has recently been involved in an extramarital affair for the first time in her 24-year marriage. She states that she has used her diaphragm and contraceptive jelly regularly, but is upset about this continuing relationship and does not know how it will resolve vis-à-vis her marriage. While you were gathering your data base, your assistant has performed a pregnancy test. It is negative.

LOGIC   You now have positive data to support a psychogenic reason for the missed period. Pregnancy is ruled out with reasonable certainty. The lack of physical evidence is against pregnancy, and a negative pregnancy test at this time would be especially reliable if the urine is concentrated. Menopause, still a distant possibility, can be ruled out with time or an FSH level. This latter test requires a week for results.

DATA   After a frank but tactful discussion with the patient, she is still not satisfied she is not pregnant. So you collect a sample of blood for FSH determination. You also give the patient an injection of 150 mg of progesterone in oil, though you could have given her 5 days of orally active progesterone. Several days later, she develops a bleeding episode similar to normal menstruation.

LOGIC   This simple test induces progestin withdrawal and precludes pregnancy. But it is important to know that the "progesterone challenge test" may be used only after the possibility of pregnancy has been excluded. The test may cause congenital defects if a fetus is present; therefore the Food and Drug Administration prohibits its use as a test for pregnancy.

In this case the test was used to convince a patient who needed reassurance; the physician was already sure. But in other instances the test can serve as an algorithmic divider in difficult diagnostic situations. Amenorrheic patients who respond with vaginal bleeding have adequate ovarian estrogen function; those who don't respond have poor ovarian estrogen production. Then proceed toward the diagnostic possibilities from this pathophysiologic separator.

DATA   The FSH test has returned and shows normal levels. Your assistant repeats the pregnancy test and it is again negative.

LOGIC   Since the FSH level is high in early menopause, this possibility is excluded. Both you and your patient are now satisfied that the diagnosis is psychogenic amenorrhea. You have solved her problem. She hasn't . . . .

QUESTIONS

1. Suppose the same patient sees you for the first time after having missed six consecutive menstrual periods. She has no other symptoms and her abdomen has not enlarged. Each of the following is possible except one:
   (a) pseudocyesis (false pregnancy)
   (b) Stein-Leventhal syndrome
   (c) hypopituitarism
   (d) potent psychogenic factors.
2. Pseudocyesis may be a form of psychogenic amenorrhea. It occurs in women who firmly believe themselves to be pregnant, and develop most of the signs and symptoms. Only one of the following statements is incorrect:
   (a) The abdomen enlarges, the breasts become full, and morning nausea is present.
   (b) Amenorrhea is the rule for 9 months (sometimes longer).
   (c) It is seen in women who desperately do or do not want to become pregnant.
   (d) The uterus enlarges, as in true pregnancy.
3. The patient in the protocol developed hypertension from birth control pills. This was reversible. There are other possible complications of birth control pills which include all of the following except one:
   (a) increased tendency to develop thromboembolic complications
   (b) enlarged breasts with galactorrhea
   (c) increased incidence of carcinoma of the breast
   (d) increased incidence of carcinoma of the uterus.
4. Consider a reverse situation. You see a 64-year-old woman who had her menopause 10 years ago. She is taking estrogen pills for backache and postmenopausal osteoporosis because her physician thinks this may help. Suddenly she has what seems to be a menstrual period. Your course of action should be:
   (a) stop estrogen pills and see what happens
   (b) do nothing and see what happens
   (c) hunt carefully for cancer of the uterus
   (d) change to an estrogen-testosterone combination.
5. An anxious mother brings you her 15-year-old daughter who has not yet begun to menstruate. The girl looks normal and feels well. Her breasts are well developed and she has pubic hair. Which of the following statements is/are false?
   (a) Pregnancy is excluded.
   (b) The hymen may be imperforate or she may not have a uterus or vagina.
   (c) There may be a chromosomal disorder.
   (d) She may simply be a "late starter."

ANSWERS

1. **(a) is correct** because it is not possible. Pseudocyesis is characterized by all the outward signs and symptoms of pregnancy including enlargement of the abdomen. The Stein-Leventhal syndrome is caused by polycystic bilateral ovarian enlargement resulting in primary hypogonadism. In 80% of cases the ovaries are palpably enlarged on pelvic examination; hirsutism may be present. Hypopituitarism can be caused by postpartum infarction of the pituitary (Sheehan's syndrome), a chromophobe adenoma, craniopharyngioma, or infiltrative disease destroying the pituitary. No menses following childbirth is the hallmark of Sheehan's syndrome. In any event, the gonadotropic hormones are the first to be affected. There is no clinical evidence for a pituitary disorder in this patient. Many cases of secondary amenorrhea are caused by a persistent corpus luteum (Halban's syndrome)—not included on the list in this case. (d) is correct for long periods of amenorrhea as well as for a single missed period. Such a profound psychologic disturbance may be found in schizophrenia. It is interesting to note that the onset of simple severe obesity or severe starvation (as in concentration camps) may be associated with cessation of menses. More recently amenorrhea has been frequently noted in women who jog or train vigorously for distance running or serious ballet careers. This is thought to be due to a shift in lean:fat body mass ratios.
2. **(d) is the only incorrect statement.** (a) occurs for postural, psychologic, and unknown reasons. Ninety per cent of patients with pseudocyesis stop having menstrual periods. (c) is an obvious truth as potent psychologic factors are invoked. The uterus does not enlarge, nor does the pregnancy test become positive.
3. **(c) is correct.** Some of the issues mentioned in this question are still controversial. At the moment, breast cancer is not considered to be a consequence of the pill, though epidemiologic studies do seem to prove an increased incidence of carcinoma of the uterus and thromboembolic phenomena. The latter include strokes, leg vein thromboses, and pulmonary emboli. Enlarged breasts do occur and galactorrhea may be discomforting.
4. **(c) is correct.** Regardless of hormone therapy, cancer must be your prime consideration at this age. Do a Pap smear, cervical biopsy, and diagnostic curettage if considered necessary to rule out cancer of the cervix or endometrium. While estrogen may indeed cause bleeding, it usually does so after the medication is stopped. A "wait and see" attitude would be dangerous. Changing to another preparation, even though

it contains testosterone, would also be ill advised at this point since you must look for cancer anyway. Furthermore, there is much doubt that sex hormones do anything to prevent postmenopausal osteoporosis in this age group.

5. **(a) and (d) are false.** Pregnancy cannot be excluded even if she has never menstruated. While the average menarche is at 12½ years, the normal range is 9 to 16, so this might simply have been a delayed onset were it not for the breasts and pubic hair. The presence of secondary sex characteristics may require the consideration of abnormal sex chromosome mosaics and warrants a buccal smear. As for answer (b) the physician may be subsequently embarrassed to learn that the hymen is closed as the uterus continues to enlarge, or that no uterus exists; a rectal examination may be indicated. In the *absence* of secondary sex characteristics, a search for a hypothalamic-pituitary disorder is indicated or (d) may exist.

COMMENT   A physician would easily solve the problem of a missed period by a brief stepwise approach: first, a short menstrual, sexual, and psychosocial history; next, an examination of the pelvis and breasts; third, a pregnancy test. Based on these three easily gathered bits of information, a reasonably certain conclusion could be reached. If necessary, an FSH level and a short period of observation would establish the diagnosis. Other problem-solving methods used in this case presentation were (*a*) frequent use of cause and effect relationships; (*b*) diagnosis by exclusion; (*c*) attention to specificity and sensitivity of clues—e.g. early pregnancy test, FSH level, palpability of ovaries in Stein-Leventhal syndrome; (*d*) regard for absence of clues which would be pertinent if other diagnoses existed; and (*e*) statistical likelihoods. Consider pregnancy as the cause of secondary amenorrhea until proven otherwise.

(*P. C.*)

PROBLEM-BASED LEARNING   On the surface, this is simply a case of a missed menstrual period—common enough. But the reader should learn all about:

1. the complex physiology of the menstrual cycle
2. the causes of primary amenorrhea
3. the causes of secondary amenorrhea
4. the early signs of pregnancy
5. the menopause
6. pregnancy tests
7. the effects of birth control pills
8. the mystery of pseudocyesis
9. psychogenic aspects of menstrual disturbances
10. the effects of certain drugs
11. endocrinopathies that cause amenorrhea (pituitary tumors; thyroid, ovarian, and adrenal dysfunctions)
12. newer concepts of prolactinomas, Stein-Leventhal syndrome (polycystic ovaries), and hyperthecosis.

There's a lot of gynecology in this one!

Suggested Readings

1. Speroff L, Glass RH, Kase NC: *Clinical Gynecologic Endocrinology and Infertility*, ed 3. Baltimore, Williams & Wilkins, 1983, pp 141–179.
   This chapter deals with both primary and secondary amenorrhea.It affords an excellent overview and practical discussion of the problem solving involved in amenorrhea, including Halban's syndrome, and some of the less common causes such as pituitary adenomas and Asherman's syndrome.

2. Gold JJ: *Gynecologic Endocrinology*, ed 2. Hagerstown, MD, Harper & Row, 1975, pp 191–212.
   The causes, descriptions, and diagnosis of the various amenorrheas are covered in this detailed chapter.

3. Little AB, Goldfarb J: Abnormalities of menstruation and gynecologic disorders. In Danforth DN (ed): *Obstetrics and Gynecology*, ed 4. Philadelphia, Harper & Row, 1982.
   pp 912–924 discuss amenorrhea from all causes, especially the endocrine disorders.

4. Jones HW Jr, Jones GS (eds): *Novak's Textbook of Gynecology*, ed 10. Baltimore, Williams & Wilkins, 1981.
   pp 733–775 discuss neurogenic, psychogenic, and endocrine causes of amenorrhea.

5. Rowe TC: The action of clomiphene in stress-induced amenorrhea. *Am J Obstet Gynecol* 148:613–616, 1984.

6. Hughesdon PE: Morphology and morphogenesis of the Stein-Leventhal syndrome and of so-called "hyperthecosis." *Obstet Gynecol Surv* 37:59–77, 1982.
   Shows how these two entities may be related.

Case 49
Acute Pelvic Pain
PAUL C. WEINBERG, M.D.

DATA A 19-year-old girl visits the emergency room with the sudden onset of constant moderately severe lower abdominal and pelvic pain which she has had for the past 8 hours. She has a vaginal discharge but says it is no different than usual.

LOGIC The patient's age, sex, and complaint lead us to many possibilities. Pain is the main clue. We do not know the significance of the discharge since it is usually there. The considerations include acute appendicitis, regional enteritis, urinary tract infection, ureteral stone, ovarian cyst (twisted, ruptured, or sudden enlargement), ectopic pregnancy, threatened abortion, and acute pelvic inflammatory disease (PID). More information is needed.

DATA Two years ago a pregnancy was terminated by suction abortion. Menses have since been normal and regular. She has continued to be sexually active with different partners and irregularly uses foam contraception. One week ago she had a more scant menstrual period than usual, and she has had some spotting of blood with the present onset of pain. Requestioning confirms the fact that the pain is constant and not crampy. There has been no nausea, anorexia, vomiting, epigastric pain, dysuria, urgency, frequency, visible hematuria, burning on urination, or other previous surgery.

LOGIC The type and location of pain, slight menstrual disturbance, and unprotected sexual activity lean us toward a gynecologic disorder. Ectopic pregnancy, ovarian cyst, and PID head the list, but other possibilities have by no means been ruled out. The constancy of the pain is against ureteral colic and threatened abortion. Absence of urinary tract symptoms tends to exclude urinary infection and is against ureteral calculus. The lack of preceding nausea, anorexia, and epigastric pain are points against appendicitis. Ileitis can present in many ways, though this would be an unusual presentation and there is no previous evidence for the disease.

Can she be pregnant, yet have menstrual periods? Rarely so, but possible. Can she have an ectopic pregnancy? She did not miss any period, but the last one was abnormal for her and she is spotting. So it is definitely possible. Venereal disease always hovers in the background of such a setting. Foam kills sperm, not the gonococcus.

DATA Her temperature is 38.7 C, pulse 80, respirations 22, and blood pressure 116/74 in the reclining, sitting, and standing positions. The head and neck, breasts, lungs, and heart are normal. There is no pallor. The abdomen is not distended. Direct and referred tenderness, rebound tenderness, and muscle guarding are present in both lower quadrants. Bowel sounds are normally active. The costovertebral angles are not tender. Pelvic examination reveals normal external genitalia, a well-epithelialized cervix with no lesions, and a mucopurulent discharge coming from the cervical os. This is sampled for Gram stain and cultured on Thayer-Martin media. Marked bilateral tenderness and tenderness with cervical motion is noted on bimanual and rectovaginal examination. The uterus is normal in size, shape, and position, and there are no palpable adnexal masses. Culdocentesis yields 5 ml of seropurulent material. This is also prepared for Gram stain, smear, and culture.

LOGIC The diagnostic possibilities are narrowing. Localization of the findings to the lower abdomen and pelvis further supports pelvic pathology as the major consideration. Acute appendicitis becomes even more remote in view of the bilaterality of signs. Even a pelvic appendix would give unilateral signs, unless it had ruptured and an abscess or peritonitis were present.

Several findings would preclude ectopic or tubal pregnancy: moderately high fever, bilaterality, no evidence of hypovolemia, mucopurulent endocervical discharge, and seropurulent culdocentesis material rather than unclotted blood. Also, no adnexal mass is palpated. Against hypovolemia are the absence of pallor and no orthostatic blood pressure changes. Normal pregnancy and threatened abortion are not likely in the presence of a normal-colored cervix and normal-sized uterus.

On the other hand, the data support an inflammatory condition as the most likely diagnosis. The cluster favoring inflammation consists of pain, tenderness, guarding, fever, and purulent discharge. Acute PID should be foremost in our minds.

DATA Laboratory studies immediately available show: hematocrit 42%, hemoglobin 12.5 g/dl, white blood cell (WBC) count 12,300/mm^3 with 86% neutrophils. Urinalysis is normal except for a few WBCs/high-power field. A Gram stain of both the cervical discharge and the culdocentesis material shows numerous WBCs, some of which contain gram-negative intracellular diplococci. X-rays of the chest and abdomen are normal. The 18-test blood chemistry profile, ordered routinely on admission, is completely normal as expected. (It was really not necessary.)

LOGIC The diagnosis of acute gonorrheal PID is clearly established by the clinical picture and confirmed by the positive Gram stains and leukocytosis. The normal red blood cell count and hematocrit further rule out ruptured ectopic pregnancy with hemoperitoneum. The urinalysis is against stone and infection, and you are not surprised to see a few WBCs in the presence of an internal genital infection. Procaine penicillin and probenecid were given and the patient improved markedly in 48 hours. At that time the cultures returned positive for *Neisseria gonorrhoeae*.

Subsequent review of the situation impresses you with the fact that venereal disease must always receive prime consideration in a sexually active nonprotected individual having relations with many partners. You still cannot fully explain the scant menstrual period and spotting unless they were related to already existing pelvic inflammation. Though the gonococcus was the proven felon in this case, *Chlamydia trachomatis* may cause the same picture.

On questioning the patient again, you learn that her chronic vaginal discharge did change in quantity and nature at about the time she became ill. It was more profuse and had become more creamy and foul-smelling. She had douched before coming to see you.

QUESTIONS

1. The most specific clue in making this patient's diagnosis was:
   (a) leukocytosis
   (b) vaginal discharge
   (c) the sexual history
   (d) presence of the gonococcus.
2. Suppose that pelvic examination had disclosed a tender 8-cm round mass in the right adnexal area, and no laboratory work had yet been done. Pain and tenderness were limited to the right side and there was no fever. The most likely diagnosis would have been:
   (a) tubal pregnancy
   (b) acute appendicitis
   (c) ovarian cyst
   (d) tubo-ovarian abscess.
3. Change the clinical picture a bit. The patient is 28, married, and professes to have only one sexual partner: her husband. He is a traveling salesman and is frequently away from home. The same acute clinical episode happens to the patient while her husband is briefly away. The rest of the history and examination are the same. In addition, you can palpate both ovaries; they are tender though not enlarged. Your leading impression prior to laboratory work is:
   (a) ruptured ectopic pregnancy
   (b) acute PID
   (c) twisted ovarian cyst
   (d) bilateral oophoritis.
4. Another 28-year-old patient sees you for a dull nagging pain in the right lower quadrant which she has had for several days. She missed her last period and is spotting. On the way to the hospital she fainted several times. The blood

pressure is 118/80, dropping to 90/60 when she stands up. Even before doing your examination, you have a pretty good idea that she has:

(a) gastrointestinal bleeding
(b) pregnancy plus anxiety
(c) tubal pregnancy
(d) acute appendicitis

5. Get back to your 19-year-old patient with gonococcal PID. She receives the necessary penicillin treatment but leaves town immediately. Her culture returns later, but the gonococcus strain is sensitive to spectinomycin and not to penicillin. Three months later she returns complaining of a dull aching pain in the pelvic area. Her discharge has gradually disappeared and she feels well except for her chief complaint. Pelvic examination shows bilateral sausage-shaped masses in both adnexal areas. She has:

(a) bilateral tubal pregnancies
(b) redundant filled colon
(c) bilateral hydrosalpinx
(d) anxiety state.

ANSWERS

1. **(d) is correct.** All the other clues could be and very frequently are present without the patient's necessarily having acute PID. Indeed, the gonococcus can be found in asymptomatic patients, but the presence of the venereal organism in the cervix and peritoneal aspirate is positive evidence for the diagnosis in this clinical setting.

2. **(c) is correct.** An ovarian cyst may be twisted on its pedicle and give the acute picture. Tubal pregnancy would not be so large. Acute appendicitis would cause fever and a tender area, but not a large mass in the pelvis. A tubo-ovarian abscess would not be round, and there would probably be some findings on the left side too.

3. **(b) is correct.** Acute PID is still the diagnosis of choice and gonorrhea is a prime suspect. She may be truthful about having a single sex partner, but her husband may be the promiscuous one. Oophoritis is only a part of generalized PID. Diagnoses (a) and (c) are ruled out by the clinical picture just as in the case presentation.

4. **(c) is correct.** The tube is ruptured, and she has already lost considerable blood into the abdomen. The orthostatic blood pressure changes and history of syncope indicate reduced blood volume. A missed period, spotting, and nagging pain all point to a tubal pregnancy rather than gastrointestinal bleeding as the cause for her blood loss. Orthostatic changes are not seen in normal pregnancy or acute appendicitis.

5. **(c) is correct.** She was inadequately treated. Her acute infection gradually subsided, but she was left with bilateral hydrosalpinx. Distended colon may exist but does not give pain and the weight of evidence is in favor of (c). Bilateral tubal pregnancies would be a statistical impossibility and the masses would not be that large anyway. She has good cause for concern, since surgery is imminent.

COMMENT Acute pelvic pain is a common emergency situation that requires a prompt decision regarding medical treatment vs hospitalization and surgery. The array of diagnostic possibilities in a sexually active female is not large. Selected bits of information in the history and examination may often pinpoint the cause. Aside from the blood count, cervical smear, and pregnancy test, the laboratory has little to offer. A pelvic examination may be painful, difficult, and only sometimes fruitful.

But an ultrasound examination of the pelvis, often available in the emergency room, may offer an excellent and highly reliable means for help in the important decision needed here. It may reveal ectopic pregnancy, ovarian cyst, tubo-ovarian abscess, abortion in progress, etc, with such a high degree of accuracy that the need for laparoscopy is often eliminated (see Suggested Readings 7 and 8). (*P. C.*)

Suggested Readings

1. Green TH: *Gynecology*, ed 3. Boston, Little, Brown, 1977, pp 247–256.
   A succinct presentation of gynecologic pelvic inflammatory disease.
2. Jones HW Jr, Jones GS (eds): *Novak's Textbook of Gynecology*, ed 10. Baltimore, Williams & Wilkins, 1981.
   pp 462–475: acute PID and its differential diagnosis
   pp 564–565: torsion and rupture of ovarian cysts
   pp 658–689: gestational trophoblastic diseases
   pp 636–658: the clinical picture of ectopic pregnancy wherein the methods of diagnosis are highlighted
   All these entities cause acute pelvic pain.
3. Barnes AB: Ectopic pregnancy: incidence and review of determinant factors. *Obstet Gynecol Surv* 38:345–356, 1983.
4. Patrick JD: Ectopic pregnancy—a brief review. *Ann Emerg Med* 11:576–581, 1982.
5. Adler MW: ABC of sexually transmitted diseases. *Br Med J (Clin Res)* 288:383–385, 1984.
6. Gibbs RS: Sexually transmitted diseases in the female. *Med Clin North Am* 67:221–234, 1983.
7. Vine SH, Birnholz JC: Ultrasound evaluation of pelvic pain. *JAMA* 244:2540–2542, 1980.
8. Voss SC: Ultrasound and the pelvic mass. *J. Reprod Med* 28:833–837, 1983.
9. Tam MR, Stamm WE, Handsfield HH, et al: Culture-independent diagnosis of *Chlamydia trachomatis* using monoclonal antibodies. *N Engl J Med* 310:1146–1150, 1984.

Case 50
Abnormal Vaginal Bleeding

ROBERT W. HUFF, M.D.

DATA A 47-year-old woman comes to the emergency room because of abnormal vaginal bleeding. She has not seen a physician since the birth of her last child 5 years ago.

LOGIC There are numerous causes of abnormal bleeding. The data base you collect should include her past menstrual history, her method of contraception, and a precise description of the abnormal bleeding. Table 21.1 defines some terms used to describe abnormal bleeding.

DATA History reveals she is gravida 7, para 6, ab 1. Her first child was placed for adoption when she was 16 years old. Her current husband (fourth) had a vasectomy after her last delivery, so she is using no other contraception. Menarche was at age 13 and menstrual cycles have occurred every 25 to 30 days until 4 months ago when she missed two menstrual periods. Two months ago she bled heavily for 8 days followed by intermenstrual bleeding of varying degrees. She bled heavily again last week but stopped 2 days ago. She has experienced cramps with the bleeding and passed large clots which "left her weak" after passage. She says the blood was bright red.

LOGIC You can now define the problem more precisely as hypermenorrhea and intermenstrual bleeding (menometrorrhagia) in a 47-year-old woman following 2 months of amenorrhea. You have excluded few diagnostic possibilities except contraceptive complications. The presence of clots in the menstrual flow indicates brisk bleeding. Passage of clots is frequently associated with cramping and is of no particular significance in her history. The color of menstrual blood is frequently reported by patients but has little diagnostic importance.

Now that you have some estimate of the blood loss and the relationship to normal menstruation, additional historical information should be obtained. Is the bleeding associated with body function such as coitus, urination, or defecation? Is there abdominal or back pain? How does the abnormal bleeding bother her? Additionally, a review of systems, family history, and medication history should be recorded.

DATA The patient states her bleeding is not related to bodily functions and she has no pain except with the passage of clots. When she initially missed two menstrual periods she thought she might be pregnant or "going through the change of life" so she took some of her neighbor's "hormone pills" for a few weeks to see if she could induce menstrual bleeding. The first heavy bleeding episode ensued so she quit taking the hormones. Abnormal bleeding continued. She is afraid she has cancer because her mother died of cervical carcinoma which was detected because of abnormal bleeding. She is quite anxious and asks you for some "nerve pills." The remainder of her history is unremarkable.

LOGIC There are grounds for her fear of cervical carcinoma since she had an early age of first coitus, has had multiple sexual partners, has had no recent cytologic evaluation, and is 47 years old—the peak age of incidence for cervical carcinoma. Her bleeding history is not characteristic for cervical carcinoma, for she has had no postcoital bleeding. If she does have invasive cervical carcinoma, there should be a gross lesion visible on pelvic examination. You should now proceed to physical examination in order to try to identify the cause of her abnormal bleeding.

DATA Weight 140 lb, pulse 96, BP 130/70. She does not appear pale but seems quite anxious. She has no evidence of jaundice,

Table 21.1.
Terms Used to Describe Abnormal Bleeding

A.	Menstrual cycle	normally 21–35 days
	1. Polymenorrhea	menstrual cycles more frequent than 21 days
	2. Oligomenorrhea	menstrual cycles less frequent than 35 days
B.	Duration of menstrual bleeding	normally 2–7 days
	1. Shortened menses	less than 2 days
	2. Prolonged menses	more than 7 days
C.	Menstrual blood loss	normally 30–150 ml
	1. Hypomenorrhea	less than normal blood loss
	2. Menorrhagia or hypermenorrhea	greater than normal blood loss
D.	Metrorrhagia or intermenstrual bleeding	bleeding between menses
E.	Spotting	light bleeding
F.	Postcoital bleeding	bleeding after intercourse
G.	Postmenopausal bleeding	bleeding 1 year after menopause
H.	Perimenopausal bleeding	bleeding within 1 year of presumed menopause

petechiae, or easy bruisability. Her thyroid is not palpable, there are not heart murmurs, and no abdominal organs can be felt. The breasts are normal.

Pelvic examination reveals normal external genitalia. Her vagina is supple, pink, and rugated. No blood is seen. She has a small cystocele and urethrocele. The cervix appears parous and has a small ectropion with numerous nabothian cysts. There is no bleeding when cervical cytology is obtained. The uterus is axial and does not seem enlarged or irregular in contour. It is mobile, firm, and nontender. The adnexa are nontender and the ovaries are barely palpable. Rectal examination is normal and the stool is brown and guaiac negative.

LOGIC Most abnormal vaginal bleeding is uterine in origin. Vaginal sources of abnormal bleeding are easily seen during examination and none were detected in this woman. Occasionally, patients are unsure whether blood is coming from the vagina, urethra, or rectum, so examination should be performed while they are bleeding. Such is not the case with this patient.

After the clinical data base has been collected, patients with abnormal bleeding may be grouped into one of four categories for further evaluation and treatment (Table 21.2).

Hyperpolymenorrhea of adolescence can be excluded. Abnormal uterine bleeding usually does not complicate systemic illness until the illness is overt. She has no signs of systemic illness but a complete blood count, T_4, and T_3 resin uptake might be performed for completeness. She has no indication of pregnancy and no other diagnosable causes of abnormal bleeding. Cervical carcinoma, uterine leiomyomas, and ovarian tumor can be reasonably excluded by the normal examination.

Her bleeding abnormality suggests a time of anovulation with continued estrogenic stimulation of the endometrium which was worsened by the hormone pills (probably estrogen). Although abnormal bleeding is commonly encountered near the menopause, it should never be considered normal and should be completely investigated for possible endometrial adenocarcinoma. Certainly, hormone therapy should never be given without a tissue diagnosis of the disease process.

This patient would be classified as having no demonstrable disease, but her history is suspicious for cancer. Minimum evaluation at present should consist of a complete blood count, urinalysis, cervical cytology, and an endometrial biopsy. The biopsy could be diagnostic of endometrial carcinoma. A diagnostic dilation and curettage (D&C) should also be scheduled in several weeks, after the assumed time of ovulation.

DATA Hemoglobin 12.4 g/dl; hematocrit 37%; white blood cell count 7,800/mm³ with a normal differential; platelets 240,000/

Table 21.2.
Categories of Patients with Abnormal Uterine Bleeding

Group I. Adolescents with Hyperpolymenorrhea: Usually due to anovulation
Group II. Women with Detectable Disease:
  A. Systemic illnesses—thyroid disease, liver disease, immunologic thrombocytopenic purpura, leukemia, von Willebrand's disease, etc
  B. Pregnancy complications—abortion, ectopic pregnancy, hydatidiform mole
  C. Gross cervical lesions—polyps, carcinoma, some ectropions
  D. Uterine leiomyomas
  E. Other pelvic pathology—functioning ovarian tumors, endometriosis, chronic salpingitis
Group III. No Detectable Disease—History Confusing, Short Duration, or Uncertain—Not Suspicious for Cancer:
  A. Minor variations from normal
  B. Related to contraception
Group IV. No Detectable Disease—History of Persistent Abnormality or Suspicious for Cancer:
  A. Patient over age 40
  B. Abnormality recurrent or present for more than 3 months
  C. Postcoital bleeding

---

mm^3. Urinalysis is unremarkable. T_4 and T_3 resin uptake are normal. Endometrial biopsy is reported as showing focal adenomatous hyperplasia, and cervical cytology is normal. When the woman returns for these reports, she asks why she needs a D&C and whether or not you will give her hormones.

LOGIC A D&C is necessary to exclude the possibility of endometrial adenocarcinoma which could coexist with adenomatous hyperplasia. Estrogenic hormones would certainly not be used with this patient.

DATA At the time of D&C the patient is anesthetized and pelvic examination is unchanged from 3 weeks previously. The uterus is sounded to 8 cm and the curettage performed without complications. Pathologic report is still focal adenomatous hyperplasia.

LOGIC Your impression of anovulatory bleeding near the menopause has been confirmed. There are now several methods of management for this patient. Many women have no further abnormal bleeding after a D&C so a time of observation could be recommended. Progestins could also be utilized to induce regular bleeding episodes and minimize the chance for recurrent hyperplasia. She is not a candidate for estrogens.

QUESTIONS

1. Suppose you decided not to treat the patient with progestins. She returns 8 months later and says she had no bleeding for 6 months after the D&C, but for the last 2 months she has again had heavy and irregular bleeding. Proper management now would be:
   (a) hysterectomy
   (b) estrogenic hormones
   (c) progestins
   (d) D&C.
2. You see a 26-year-old nullipara who has episodes of amenorrhea followed by hyperpolymenorrhea. She is slightly hirsute and her ovaries are easily palpable. D&C is done in the expected luteal phase and the pathologic report is endometrial hyperplasia. Correct management is:
   (a) observe for future abnormal bleeding
   (b) induce ovulation with clomiphene
   (c) give cyclic progestins to induce regular menses
   (d) give combination estrogen-progestin oral contraceptives.
3. A 56-year-old woman who has been taking estrogen since her menopause comes to see you because of "spotting" for 2 weeks. Her vagina appears well estrogenized and the remainder of the pelvic examination is normal. Proper management includes:
   (a) stopping estrogen replacement
   (b) continuing estrogen replacement and adding progesterone
   (c) cervical cytology
   (d) D&C.
4. A 24-year-old mother of three comes to see you because her menses have increased in

length and flow and she has had cramps and some intermenstrual spotting since she was fitted for an intrauterine device (IUD) 2 months ago. Pelvic examination is normal. Proper management is:

(a) remove the IUD
(b) remove the IUD and do a D&C
(c) remove the IUD and give oral contraceptives
(d) reassure her that her symptoms are not uncommon and will probably abate.

5. An 18-year-old girl comes to the emergency room with a history of 3 months of amenorrhea followed by 3 weeks of daily vaginal bleeding. A mass arises from the pelvis to the umbilicus. A fetal heart cannot be heard. Her BP is 160/100. The most likely diagnosis is:

(a) uterine leiomyoma
(b) ovarian tumor
(c) hydatidiform mole
(d) threatened abortion.

ANSWERS

1. **(d) is correct.** The woman has perimenopausal menometrorrhagia which is probably still the result of anovulation, but some women with adenomatous hyperplasia progress to endometrial adenocarcinoma. A diagnosis should be made prior to treatment. Hysterectomy is not indicated. Estrogens are contraindicated. Cyclic progestin therapy is warranted if her pathologic diagnosis is still endometrial hyperplasia.

2. **(b), (c), or (d) is correct.** This patient is anovulatory and most likely has polycystic ovary disease. She is at high risk to develop endometrial cancer since her endometrium is being exposed to estrogen and not to progesterone. Her chance for endometrial cancer can be reduced by providing progesterone and this can be accomplished by inducing ovulation if she seeks pregnancy or by providing progestins alone or in oral contraceptives.

3. **(a), (c), and (d) are correct.** (a) and (c) should of course be done, but a D&C is mandatory. Prolonged estrogen administration may be associated with an increased risk of endometrial adenocarcinoma and this is best diagnosed by a D&C. Abnormal bleeding is the early warning of endometrial cancer and this possibility must always be considered whenever postmenopausal bleeding occurs. (b) is unacceptable and perilous.

4. **(d) is correct.** Many women have hypermenorrhea and occasionally intermenstrual spotting for the first few months they have an IUD. If symptoms persist or are distressing, the device can be removed. A D&C is unnecessary as her cancer risk is quite low.

5. **(c) is correct.** Hydatidiform moles are frequently associated with a uterus larger than expected for the duration of amenorrhea. In addition, most patients with moles have abnormal bleeding and many develop preeclampsia as suggested by her blood pressure. A leiomyoma of this size would be quite uncommon in a girl her age. Most abortions occur in the first 12 weeks of pregnancy. An ovarian tumor is always a possibility but the story presented is more characteristic for a mole. Sonography could give the correct diagnosis in a matter of minutes. Pregnancy complications must always be considered in the patient with abnormal uterine bleeding.

COMMENT After a detailed analysis of the types of abnormal vaginal bleeding, the author pursues a branched pattern of problem solving based on a systematic list of causes for bleeding. Only a few decision points are needed: the age of the patient, the use of contraceptives, the presence of apparent systemic disease, the pelvic examination, cytologic studies, endometrial biopsy, and D&C. Questions and answers take the reader through different pathways of logic as varied settings for abnormal bleeding are presented.

High-yield questions in patients with vaginal bleeding focus on the taking of hormones and the possibility of pregnancy.

The patient's age often alters diagnostic likelihoods. Abnormal vaginal bleeding in teen-agers results mainly from hormonal imbalances (dysfunctional uterine bleeding), though complications of pregnancy and ovarian tumors must be considered. From 20 to 40, bleeding problems relate mainly to birth control devices and pills, but pregnancy, polycystic ovaries, and hormonal imbalances are important here too. From 40 on, and perhaps even earlier, carcinoma of the cervix and endometrium is your principal concern. The few years around the menopause are where the interplay between anovulatory bleeding, endometrial hyperplasia, and endometrial carcinoma exists; alteration of the normal menstrual pattern, taking estrogens for symptom relief, and the high incidence of cancer are three factors that may cause confusion, anxiety, and mistakes at this age.

Remember that idiopathic thrombocytopenic purpura and other coagulopathies often first manifest themselves in young to middle-aged women with profuse menstrual bleeding. A platelet count may be indicated. Other diagnostic studies that may be of value in selected instances are hormone assays, Pap smears, D&C, ultrasonography, and laparoscopy.

It must be recognized that abortions, polyps, carcinomas, and other pathologic processes account for roughly one-quarter of all cases of abnormal vaginal bleeding. The rest are the result of the hormonal imbalances that stem from the complex hypothalamus-pituitary-ovary relationships responsible for the menstrual cycle, and whoever wishes to understand such problems must know the physiology of all the loops and feedbacks involved.   (*P. C.*)

Suggested Readings

1. Jones HW, Jr, Jones GS (eds): *Novak's Textbook of Gynecology*, ed 10. Baltimore, Williams & Wilkins, 1981, pp 777–796.

    A standard textbook which discusses many common aspects of abnormal uterine bleeding, including polyps, leiomyomas, cancer, ovarian disorders, anovulatory bleeding, etc.

2. Pauerstein CJ, Huff RW: *Physiology and Pathophysiology of Reproduction.* New York, Wiley, 1979, pp 132–147.

    Much of this logic session's approach to abnormal bleeding is taken from the chapter, "Changes in Menstruation."

3. Speroff L, Glass RH, Kase NC: *Clinical Gynecologic Endocrinology and Infertility*, ed 3. Baltimore, Williams & Wilkins, 1983.

    Abnormal bleeding is discussed in several areas in this short, very enjoyable book.

4. Goldfarb JM, Little AB: Abnormal vaginal bleeding. *N Engl J. Med* 302:666–669, 1980.

5. Gross BH: Computed tomography of gynecologic diseases. *AJR* 141:765–773, 1983.

Chapter 22

Musculoskeletal Problems

Here, a symbiotic relationship often exists between the rheumatologist and the orthopaedic surgeon. However, in most cases there is no overlap, and the problem lies clearly in one field or the other.

The orthopaedic surgeon is usually faced with problems related to trauma, deformities, bone tumors, or pain syndromes. Backache, neck pain, and shoulder pain are common situations with which he must deal. A branch of the history and physical examination is usually sufficient. What he sees by retinal multicolor or by radiographic chiaroscuro is what he usually diagnoses. A few additional physical maneuvers may be necessary. But sometimes the problems are much more complicated (e.g. backache) and extensive studies are needed. Visceral diseases may first manifest themselves with what appears to be an orthopaedic complaint. Aneurysms cause backache and lung cancer can cause a painful shoulder. Or the seeming orthopaedic problem may really be part of a systemic medical disease (e.g. metastases, Paget's disease, atherosclerosis).

Front-line diagnostic advances in orthopaedic surgery include the *computed tomographic scan* for disk delineation; high-resolution radiographic techniques for the study of bone disease by *densitometry; radioisotope scans* for bone inflammations and metastases; *arthroscopy* for looking directly inside joints; and *arthrography* for radiocontrast study of the joint contents. Total joint replacement must be mentioned, for it represents a miraculous advance in the management of joint diseases. Diagnostic certainty must exist before such interventions are undertaken.

With the advent of "Olympianism" for all ages and both genders, almost everybody plays tennis, golf, cycles, skis, jogs, or performs aerobics or isometrics. This creates a swarm of diagnostic problems—proudly called "athletic injuries"—in both athletes and amateur exercisers. one wonders whether such activity is more costly than beneficial.

Arthritis can affect one or many joints, can be acute, subacute, or chronic, or can be part of a systemic disease like systemic lupus erythematosus (SLE), sarcoidosis, gout, or rheumatoid variants. For every case of SLE seen by the primary care physician, there will probably be 15 cases of rheumatoid arthritis, 30 cases of gout, 100 cases of degenerative osteoarthritis, and far more cases of aches and pains of unknown cause. Such is the approximate relative frequency of joint diseases.

But certainly the realm of the rheumatologist extends far beyond the synovial cavity. Joint diseases are most often part of multisystem disorders with far-reaching immunologic significance and consequences. Hundreds of scientists labor to unravel the mysteries of antigen-antibody complexes with only modest success.

As we approach the end of the 1980s, the quest for specific diagnostic markers and clusters continues. Rheumatoid arthritis, rheumatoid variants, and SLE still overlap and are often difficult to define and diagnose. None has a known cause or cure, and their manifestations are body-wide. The unknown still clouds the pathophysiology of one of the world's oldest recorded diseases—gout—and the reasons for its acute episodes are still not understood.

Immunologic disorders of connective tissue overlap and often coexist with similar diseases of the liver and kidney. The burgeoning field of immunology keeps broadening as it engulfs many other organs within its domain—brain, heart, lung, liver, kidney, gastrointestinal tract, endocrine glands, blood, lymph nodes, etc.

The existence of fibrositis or fibromyositis, alleged by some to be the most common cause of diffuse aches and pains, is still in dispute and considered a myth by many. Drugs continue to be incriminated in the causation of more and more diseases, especially the collagen-vascular disorders.

On the success side of the ledger are the better and broader use of joint fluid for diagnosis and the recognition of newer entities like Lyme disease and apatite arthritis—yet another crystal-induced arthropathy. (*P. C.*)

Case 51
Painful Swollen Joint
PAUL CUTLER, M.D.

A third-year medical student presents the following case to her attending physician on ward rounds. The method of presentation closely parallels the sequence of problem solving used.

MS III: Last night we admitted an unmarried 34-year-old traveling salesman who had just returned from a convention in Las Vegas with a very painful hot swollen right knee. The joint was extremely tender and inflexible, and he couldn't bear any weight on it; the skin over and around the joint looked purplish-red and inflamed. This came on rather suddenly.

MD: Were you sure the inflammation was in the joint itself rather than in the periarticular tissue?

MS III: Yes. We considered various extraarticular inflammations such as cellulitis, bursitis, tendonitis, and an inflamed Baker's cyst. But the clinical picture was typical for arthritis. Furthermore, he had pain on both active and passively assisted motion, so we were sure the trouble was within the joint.

MD: Sounds like typical acute gout! Why did you admit him to the hospital?

MS III: There were some other features that worried us. He felt chilly, had a temperature of 38 C, and told us he had had a chronic recurrent urethral discharge for several years for which he had many times received penicillin. His occupation, unmarried status, and trip to Las Vegas may have influenced us too much.

MD: So what were your provisional hypotheses?

MS III: I thought mainly in terms of gout and acute suppurative arthritis, probably gonococcal.

MD: What data did you then get to substantiate or disprove your hypotheses?

MS III: As for gout, he never had any similar joint problem; his father and older brother do have gout but they get it in their big toes. Also, he never passed any kidney stones and doesn't have any tophi in his

ears. The blood studies haven't returned yet so I don't know the serum uric acid. Yesterday, before the acute joint episode started, he had a tremendous dinner: a 1-lb steak and a whole bottle of wine.

MD: Well, so far you've given me several important clues for gout: the meal preceding the attack, the family history, and the appearance of the joint. But you've presented some negative clues too. What speaks for or against a suppurative joint?

MS III: First I milked his urethra and found no discharge. His throat wasn't sore and his anorectal examination was normal. He has no other infectious foci; I looked carefully for skin pustules. He had no high fever or frank chills. He denied having had sexual intercourse in the previous 2 weeks. The leukocyte count was 13,000 with 84% polymorphonuclear leukocytes (PMNs), and the urinalysis showed five to ten white blood cells (WBCs)/high-power field but was otherwise normal.

MD: Of course, the absence of observable discharge at the moment doesn't rule out urethritis or prostatitis. But the point you make about absence of high fever and chills is a good one. He certainly has an excess of WBCs in the urine, and the blood leukocytosis could go with either condition. The clues you gave were mainly negative and against infection. But if the gonococcus is suspected, a look is not enough. Cultures of the urethra, anus, blood, throat, skin vesicles if present, and the cervix in women will be positive from at least one site in 95% of cases. The synovial fluid culture is only 50% sensitive.

And speaking of bacteria, the gonococcus is not the only villain. Septic joints are usually associated with fever and chills and often infection elsewhere. *Staphylococcus aureus* and *Staphylococcus pyogenes* are probably the most common organisms causing suppurative arthritis in such instances. In children, *Haemophilus influenzae* is usually at fault; the staphylococcus favors intravenous drug users and gram-negative bacilli predominate in immunosuppressed persons.

Tell me, did you consider other possibilities like pseudogout and Reiter's syndrome?

MS III: Yes, we did, but not for long. Pseudogout occurs in older people and doesn't come on with such explosiveness. Reiter's syndrome usually involves two or more joints and is associated either with active nongonococcal urethritis or with diarrhea, as well as with conjunctivitis and mucocutaneous lesions. Except for possible urethritis, these features are not present here.

MD: So the location of joint involvement and the number of joints involved influenced your reasoning?

MS III: Yes, to some extent. Gout usually involves only one joint. The gonococcus and other bacteria which invade the bloodstream often cause multiple mild transitory joint involvement, but then settle down in one, two, or sometimes several joints. Pseudogout is not a strong consideration here because of the patient's age.

Gout can affect any joint, but the first metatarsophalangeal joint is most common (75%); the ankles and knees may be affected early too. Bacteria are not too particular, though the knees and hips are common sites. Pseudogout favors the knee.

An important thing I learned is that gout can involve the soft tissues near a joint and can simulate cellulitis. So many a patient with gout mistakenly receives penicillin.

MD: I note that the patient seems quite comfortable today, his temperature is normal, and his knee doesn't look so bad. What happened?

MS III: We aspirated some fluid from the knee shortly after he was admitted last night. It was cloudy yellow and had a decreased viscosity and poor mucin clot. There were 20,000 WBCs/mm^3, most of which were PMNs. We're waiting for the fluid glucose determination. A culture was begun at the bedside, and a Gram stain showed many PMNs but no bacteria. Under polarized light microscopy, negatively birefringent needle-shaped crystals, 2 to 10 μm in length, were found free in the synovial fluid and inside leukocytes.

MD: That proves the diagnosis of gout, doesn't it? The presence of typical monosodium urate crystals tells you the patient has a crystal-induced arthritis. The calcium pyrophosphate dihydrate crystals of pseudogout are rod-like or rhomboid in shape and are weakly positive birefringent.

There's a third uncommon crystal-induced arthritis. Calcium hydroxyapatite crystals can be found in some cases of arthritis. These crystals are too small to be seen with the ordinary light microscope; they can be identified by electron microscopy or x-ray diffraction studies.

Why did you proceed with synovial aspiration even before the serum uric acid returned?

MS III: The uric acid wouldn't have been conclusive. First of all, the patient might have hyperuricemia, yet have an unrelated suppurative joint. Next, he might have gout, yet the uric acid be within normal limits. In addition, the definitive diagnosis of infectious arthritis can be made by identifying the organism in the synovial fluid. So we decided to go ahead.

MD: An excellent thought! Approximately 5% of patients with gout have serum values below the upper limit of normal (7.0 mg/dl ± 0.2 mg) as demonstrated by population studies. Furthermore, 20% of patients with pseudogout have hyperuricemia, and large numbers of patients with hyperuricemia never develop gout. Remember too that the presence of urate crystals in the joint fluid does not necessarily exclude the added presence of another articular disease.

MS III: Here come the results of the blood chemistry tests ordered last night. Everything is normal except the serum uric acid, which is 12.2 mg/dl. The blood glucose is 100 mg/dl, while the synovial fluid glucose is 70 mg/dl. We have already started treatment with colchicine and the patient is improved this morning.

MD: I'm glad to see you ordered an old but effective remedy even though your diagnostic techniques are very modern. Hippocrates described gout 2500 years ago, Galen noted tophi, and 3500 years ago the Ebers Papyrus mentioned a drug which was probably colchicine; it was brought to this country by Benjamin Franklin who suffered with gout. Can you tell me about the pathophysiology of gout?

MS III: Yes. I had time to do some reading during the night. It is caused by monosodium urate crystals and is associated with *hyperuricemia*. This results from an overproduction of uric acid in some patients with primary or familial gout; many of these have a disturbance in urate excretion by the kidney as well. But defective elimination by the kidney is solely responsible for *most* cases of gout.

Myeloproliferative states including leukemia, lymphoma, multiple myeloma, pernicious anemia, and polycythemia vera—especially under treatment—release large amounts of nucleoprotein which is degraded to uric acid. This may cause gout too. I suppose I should mention drugs that may cause hyperuricemia and precipitate an acute gouty attack, especially in gout-prone individuals. These include diuretics, ethambutol, nicotinic acid, pyrazinamide, and alcohol.

The exact cause for acute arthritis in most hyperuricemic patients is not clear, though it often seems to be precipitated by surgery, trauma, emotional upset, dietary excess, or alcohol. Often there is no clear-cut trigger event.

MD: You haven't mentioned an x-ray of the joint. Wasn't it done?

MS III: Yes, but it didn't help much. It showed some soft tissue swelling but no bone changes. The fact that there was no calcium in the cartilage, chondrocalcinosis, is against pseudogout, though I wasn't inclined toward that diagnosis anyway.

MD: I note that the glucoses have returned. This joint fluid is clearly a group II fluid. Do you know the classification?

MS III: I believe there are three groups: I, II, and III—depending on the cell count, synovial:serum glucose ratio, viscosity, and the presence of bacteria by Gram stain or culture. Group I fluids are noninflammatory, have less than 5,000 WBCs/mm^3, glucose ratio > 0.90, high viscosity, and no bacteria. Group II fluids are aseptic inflammatory, have 5,000 to 50,000 cells/mm^3, glucose ratio > 0.50, low viscosity, and no bacteria. Group III fluids are septic inflammatory, have 20,000 to 200,000 cells/mm^3, glucose ratio < 0.50, low viscosity, and are positive for bacteria on Gram stain or culture. In groups II and III fluids the cells are mostly PMNs, except for tuberculosis where lymphocytes predominate. A fasting blood glucose is used for comparison.

Group I fluids are found in normal joints and in hypertrophic osteoarthritis; group II fluids are seen in gout, pseudogout, Reiter's syndrome, acute rheumatic fever, rheumatoid arthritis, and systemic lupus erythematosus; group III fluids occur in septic and tuberculous joints.

MD: Very good! I got more than I expected.

A point about the study of joint fluids! Don't hesitate to aspirate if in doubt. If carefully done, it's simple, without risk, and yields quality information. You may be surprised. Chronic gout mimics rheumatoid arthritis. Patients with known gout or degenerative joint disease may develop a suppurative joint. Gout and pseudogout may coexist. At least once in the lifetime of an arthritic patient, a joint must be aspirated. And even in a previously diagnosed case, arthrocentesis may again be indicated if symptoms persist in spite of good treatment.

Suppose you saw a 65-year-old woman with a painful stiff knee for 3 years. What would you consider, and what would you do?

MS III: I would think more in terms of hypertrophic osteoarthritis or degenerative joint disease since it is so common, especially in this age group. Tuberculosis would be a far less likely possibility. The x-ray and joint fluid for each would be characteristic.

MD: Do gender and age enter very much into the logic of determining the type of arthritis?

MS III: Very much so! More than 90%

of gout and ankylosing spondylitis is seen in men. Pseudogout is more common in men. Sjögren's syndrome, rheumatoid arthritis, and systemic lupus erythematosus are far more common in women.

MD: I agree with your evaluation of pseudogout. But it merits more discussion. It is usually asymptomatic and is simply an x-ray finding. Calcification of cartilage is seen in x-rays of the knees, symphysis pubis, wrists, elbows, hip, spinal disks, etc. Clinically the disease may be manifested by an acute or subacute monarticular or polyarticular arthritis. It can thus mimic any of the common joint diseases—gout, rheumatoid arthritis, or degenerative joint disease. Aspiration reveals positively birefringent calcium pyrophosphate dihydrate crystals seen by polarized microscopy. This disease process is closely related to aging. But when found, it is sometimes associated with hyperparathyroidism or hemochromatosis.

One last item. You've mentioned those clues that were pertinently positive or negative to your provisional hypotheses. What about the rest of the examination?

MS III: After the prime diagnosis was established and treatment was begun, the rest of the history and physical examination were completed. Except for obesity and hypertension, no other problems were uncovered.

MD: An excellent job! Remember that a patient may have hyperuricemia for years without ever developing symptoms, that he may have uric acid stones instead of or before arthritis, and that he may progress into the stage of chronic tophaceous gout. This severe form of chronic destructive and deforming arthritis is unusual with today's forms of good treatment. We also see less tophi today for the same reason. These urate aggregates were formerly common and were seen in the helix, antihelix, extensor surface of the forearms, and around any involved joints. Sometimes they eroded the skin and exuded a milky or chalky material. When seen they are diagnostic.

Gout is such a fascinating disease! A few more points are worth mentioning. Careful questioning uncovers a family history in 70% of patients. The natural history of the disease is notable. The first attack of gouty arthritis comes after many years of hyperuricemia; in 90% of cases it affects one joint first, but it may affect several. Ultimately almost all patients experience podagra—involvement of the first metatarsophalangeal joint. Don't confuse this with an inflamed bunion!

Recurrent attacks occur in 1 to 10 years. Between episodes all is well except for the ongoing ravages of hyperuricemia. Eventually the attacks get longer, more severe, and polyarticular, and the disease becomes chronic and persistent. Good treatment should circumvent the latter situation.

The related problems are many. *Nephropathy* occurs in 90% of patients. Its mechanism is controversial, but it is associated with urate deposits in the interstitial tissue and tubules. This may be manifested simply by albuminuria or by serious obstructive and inflammatory nephropathy leading to renal failure. *Nephrolithiasis* is frequent. The stones consist of uric acid but sometimes calcium stones are seen; perhaps the uric acid crystals act as a nidus for calcium deposition. Obesity, hypertriglyceridemia, diabetes mellitus, and hypertension are commonly associated with gout.

Don't forget to look after this patient's obesity and hypertension!

COMMENT In the first minute of patient contact, this capable student generated several initial hypotheses. Then she immediately sought specific clues to reject or confirm her hypotheses just as the experienced clinician does. As if guided by radar, she "hit the bull's-eye" with confirmatory irrefutable tests. And last, after diagnosis and treatment were well established, she filled in the rest of the data base. Note that statistical likelihoods, overlap, coincidence, test specificity and sensitivity, gender, age, and the number and location of involved joints all entered into her very mature logical approach.

The problem of monarticular arthritis is generally best solved by an algorithmic or flow chart application of logic. Only basic skills and two or three tests are needed. On the basis of the clinical picture you can be reasonably sure of the diagnosis. But arthrocentesis and detailed fluid examination are almost invariably indicated and should produce a definite diagnosis. If not, a therapeutic trial with colchicine or antibiotics may be indicated if the joint is "hot." Otherwise a "wait-and-see" strategy followed by a synovial biopsy in 4 to 6 weeks is indicated for the "cold" chronic undiagnosed joint. This may uncover a granulomatous disease or pigmented villonodular synovitis. (*P. C.*)

PROBLEM-BASED LEARNING The student who presented and discussed this case had obviously learned very much about the patient, his disorder, and related disorders before the presentation. Her performance was excellent. To do likewise, you must learn about:

1. gout and its pathophysiology, symptoms and signs, differential diagnosis, precise diagnosis, and complications
2. gouty nephropathy in particular
3. asymptomatic hyperuricemia and what to do about it
4. acute suppurative arthritis, its features, and its microbiology
5. gonorrhea, where to look for it and how it affects joints
6. pseudogout and apatite-induced arthropathy
7. causes of secondary gout (diseases and drugs)
8. synovial fluid aspiration, the three general types of fluids and their features, and the type of fluid that characterizes various diseases
9. polarized light microscopy for crystal identification
10. Reiter's syndrome
11. radiographic features of various joint diseases.

Suggested Readings

1. McCarty DJ (ed): *Arthritis and Allied Conditions: A Textbook of Rheumatology*, ed 10, Philadelphia, Lea & Febiger, 1985.
    Chapters 3, 4, 91, 93, 94, 100, and 101 of this excellent very recent edition tell you about the signs and symptoms, synovial fluid, crystal depositions, and infections in joint diseases.
2. Dieppe P, Doherty M, Macfarlane D: Symposium on crystal-related arthropathies. *Ann Rheum Dis* 42 (suppl 1):1–114, 1983.
    This entire supplement consists of 52 gemstone articles from Bristol, England, in only 114 pages. It includes all you might wish to know about gout, pseudogout, apatite deposition, their manifestations, and diagnostic details.
3. Freed JF, Nies KM, Boyer RS, et al: Acute monarticular arthritis. A diagnostic approach. *JAMA* 243:2314–2316, 1980.
    Analyzes the results obtained by studying 59 patients and formulates a diagnostic protocol.
4. Eisenberg JM, Schumacher HR, Davidson PK, et al: Usefulness of synovial fluid analysis in the evaluation of joint effusions. *Arch Intern Med* 144:715–719, 1984.
    The authors use threshold analysis and likelihood ratios to assess a diagnostic test and answer the question: Does synovial fluid analysis really help?
5. Hart FD: Diagnosis and management of gout. *Practitioner* 227:1089–1099, 1983.
6. Berg E: The acutely swollen joint. First impressions may mislead. *Postgrad Med* 75:62–75 passim, 1984.
    Discusses the diagnostic pitfalls and how to avoid them.
7. Forrester DM, Hensel AL, Brown JC: The use of gallium-67 citrate to distinguish between infectious and non-infectious arthritis. *Clin Rheum Dis* 9:333–345, 1983.
    A useful diagnostic tool where the clinical distinction is often difficult.
8. Nakayama DA, Barthelmy C, Carrera G, et al: Tophaceous gout: a clinical and radiographic assessment. *Arthritis Rheum* 27:468–471, 1984.
    Discusses why patients can justifiably reach the advanced stage.

Case 52
Shoulder Pain

JAMES D. HECKMAN, M.D.

DATA A 53-year-old left-handed carpenter comes to your office complaining of left shoulder pain for 3 months. At first the pain was intermittent but now it is persistent and so severe that he is unable to work.

LOGIC Carpenters and certain other heavy laborers are prone to early degenerative changes in the joints of the dominant extremity. The patient's job and hobbies often give clues to the cause of musculoskeletal pain.

Most episodes of shoulder pain are the result of local inflammatory changes in the shoulder joint complex (subdeltoid bursitis, bicipital tendonitis, rotator cuff injury, calcific tendonitis, osteoarthritis, rheumatoid arthritis, fracture, subluxation or dislocation, tumor, impingement syndrome, gout, and septic arthritis). On occasion, pain can be referred to the shoulder from a distant lesion (cervical radiculopathy, coronary artery disease, carpal tunnel syndrome, lung cancer, subdiaphragmatic abscess). Our first goal is to localize the pain.

DATA The pain is constant and aching in nature. It is fairly well localized to the anterior portion of the shoulder and deltoid muscle, and it occasionally runs down the arm to the elbow. The pain is aggravated by any shoulder motion but particularly by abduction and forward flexion. Partial relief is obtained by resting the arm in a sling and taking aspirin. Hot packs applied to the shoulder give temporary relief.

LOGIC The additional data indicate that the pain is the result of local inflammation in and around the shoulder joint complex. "Bursitis" is a term used to describe this local inflammation. There are several different causes of shoulder bursitis. Inflammation in the tendon of the rotator cuff is usually secondary to compression of the tendon between the humeral head and the undersurface of the acromion process (the impingement syndrome). This results in calcification of the tendon (calcific tendonitis) and inflammation of the bursa which lies between the acromion and the rotator cuff (subdeltoid bursitis). With prolonged impingement and inflammation, the rotator cuff ruptures, producing weakness of abduction and atrophy of the cuff muscles. After rupture of the cuff, there is a permanent communication between the shoulder joint and the subdeltoid bursa.

The biceps tendon runs through the shoulder joint, just deep to the rotator cuff. Repetitive activity of the biceps may produce inflammation in the tendon, resulting in

pain in the same area. Thus, this whole group of problems is involved in "bursitis" of the shoulder. Shoulder pain is increased in all of them by motion of the joint; limitation of motion and local application of heat decrease the pain.

DATA The patient denies any recent injury to the shoulder or neck. He does remember one episode of acute shoulder pain 5 years ago after pitching baseball. This lasted about 2 weeks and then completely resolved. He has no pain in any other joints. There is no numbness, paresthesia, or weakness in the left upper extremity.

LOGIC It is very important to know if there has been trauma to the shoulder. Fracture, subluxation, and dislocation are frequent causes of local joint pain. No history of injury virtually eliminates trauma as a possible cause in this case. Conversely, if the patient had remembered an episode of forceful abduction and external rotation of the shoulder in the past, recurrent subluxation or dislocation of the shoulder would be a definite possibility. The incident of transient pain 5 years ago, after moderate shoulder activity, supports the pattern of a local recurrent inflammatory process in that area.

The fact that the patient has not had pain, heat, or swelling in other joints now or in the past allows us to think less in terms of polyarticular diseases (rheumatoid arthritis, gout, pseudogout, degenerative arthritis). While some of these diseases can initially exhibit monarticular complaints, it is unusual for them to do so in the shoulder.

The absence of neck pain and no history of neck injury are very important. Remember that diseases of the cervical spine, especially osteoarthritis with radiculitis, often present with pain in the shoulder, particularly over the area of the trapezius muscle. But careful questioning usually elicits a radicular distribution of the pain with some associated numbness or weakness of the involved limb.

Carpal tunnel syndrome may sometimes start as a pain radiating to the shoulder from the wrist. Numbness and weakness in the median nerve distribution will usually be prominent complaints as well. This syndrome is caused by compression of the median nerve in the rigid and narrow carpal tunnel. It is frequently seen after wrist fracture but can occur in hypothyroidism and rheumatoid arthritis.

DATA The patient has been self-employed for 32 years and has four children, two of whom are still in college. Because he has been in "great" health, he has not seen a physician in years. He has smoked two packs of cigarettes/day for 35 years but has no other bad habits. He specifically denies any chest pain, fatigue, shortness of breath, anorexia, or weight loss; however, he does have a morning cough which produces a small amount of clear phlegm. This has not changed over the last year and there has been no hemoptysis.

LOGIC With musculoskeletal problems it is especially important to assess the patient's motivation regarding his job. Very often a significant amount of secondary gain can be derived from physical impairment. As our patient is self-employed and has burdensome family financial obligations, it is doubtful that he is seeking disability compensation.

Cardiopulmonary disease may cause shoulder pain, especially in this age group. But if the patient had angina, he would have episodic chest pain radiating to the left shoulder which comes on exertion and may be accompanied by fatigue and/or dyspnea. This is not the case here. However, his smoking history should raise a red flag. Shoulder pain is a common presentation of lung carcinoma arising in the medial part of the apex (Pancoast tumor). The mild chronic cough is probably from smoking but must be checked. He has no hemoptysis, weight loss, anorexia, or fatigue to suggest cancer. It is important to note that shoulder pain of visceral origin (lung cancer, heart disease, diaphragmatic disease) is not worsened by shoulder movement. Thus far we have a healthy middle-aged man with disabling pain in his dominant shoulder which probably has a local cause.

DATA Physical examination is performed. The patient appears healthy, has good color, and is muscular and slightly overweight. Complete examination is normal except for the findings in the shoulder area. The cervical spine shows no deformity or difficulty with full flexion, extension, rotation, and left and right side bending. There is no pain on axial compression of the cervical spine or tenderness to palpation.

LOGIC The absence of abnormalities in the heart and lungs reinforces the absence of major symptoms there. Inspection, palpation, and the performance of range of motion of the cervical spine require less than 1 minute. After this normal examination we can be virtually certain that the origin of the pain is not in the cervical spine.

DATA On inspection of the shoulder there is wasting of the muscles of the supraspinous and infraspinous fossae. Otherwise the shoulder is normal in appearance without swelling, erythema, or deformity. Comparison with the normal shoulder demonstrates no other discrepancy in appearance.

LOGIC The limbs are paired organs, and one limb should always be compared to its opposite member which is usually a normal mirror image. All of the examinations (inspection, palpation, range of motion, strength, and even x-rays) should be performed on both limbs using the opposite normal limb as a control. Wasting of the muscles of the rotator cuff (supraspinatus, infraspinatus, teres minor, and subscapularis) indicates probable tear of part or all of the cuff and reinforces our impression that the problem lies within the shoulder joint. Paralysis of the suprascapular nerve or a C5-C6 nerve root lesion could produce this positive finding, but this is rare without trauma and without positive cervical spine findings.

DATA   On palpation there is slight tenderness over the distal clavicle and acromioclavicular joint. Exquisite point tenderness is noted over the anterolateral acromion and mild tenderness over the biceps tendon, but there is no tenderness on the posterior or lateral aspects of the shoulder.

LOGIC   Point tenderness is the single most helpful diagnostic finding in evaluation of musculoskeletal problems. Careful gentle palpation of the bony landmarks in the area of pain will usually demonstrate one point of maximal tenderness. By knowing what musculotendinous or ligamentous structures pass over, around, or insert into these landmarks, the physician can pinpoint the involved structure.

In this case, the point of maximal tenderness is the inferior edge of the anterior and lateral acromion. This is the location of the subacromial bursa, and tenderness there points to inflammation in the bursa and probably a lesion of the underlying rotator cuff.

DATA   Range of motion of the shoulder shows extension to 30°, external rotation 30°, internal rotation 60°. On passive forward flexion there is severe pain in the shoulder, especially from 45° to 90°. Actively the patient can flex to only 60° because of severe pain. Abduction is limited to 60° actively and passively. Strength is excellent throughout except for mild weakness of abduction.

LOGIC   Normal active and passive range of motion would be a good indication of the absence of disease within and about the joint, but this patient has significant limitation of range of motion. He demonstrates the classical findings of the impingement syndrome: pain on forward flexion due to impingement of the humeral head on the undersurface of the acromion. This coincides with our findings on inspection of a probable rotator cuff tear (the rotator cuff is caught between the humeral head and acromion and has gradually worn away, nar-

rowing the acromiohumeral space and allowing the head to impinge on the acromion in forward flexion).

DATA   The remainder of the limb is examined and no deformity is seen or palpated. There is a full range of motion of the other joints. Circulation, sensation, and motor function are normal.

LOGIC   Completion of the upper extremity examination shows no other disease process (multiple joint disease, cervical radiculopathy, or carpal tunnel syndrome).

DATA   X-rays in the anteroposterior and lateral projections of the shoulders show no evidence of fracture or dislocation. There is mild degenerative arthritis of the acromioclavicular joint and marked narrowing of the space between the acromion and the humeral head on the left side. There are no osteolytic or osteoblastic lesions present. The glenohumeral joints appear normal. Chest x-rays, including apical lordotic view, are normal.

LOGIC   The radiographs of the shoulder support the physical findings (remember the importance of always obtaining x-rays in two planes at right angles to one another). The patient has early degenerative arthritis of the acromioclavicular joint which explains the moderate tenderness in that area. Narrowing of the acromiohumeral space results from the old tear of the rotator cuff— the spacer effect is lost—and from osteophytic proliferation of the acromion. The absence of other bony lesions reassures us that there is no bone tumor. Such a tumor most likely would have been a metastatic lesion. In the middle-aged and older individual this possibility must always be remembered. Similarly, the chest x-rays rule out a Pancoast tumor. Although rare, the grave consequences of such tumors require that we search diligently for them.

The diagnoses of impingement syndrome, old rotator cuff tear, and subacromial bursitis are now virtually certain. A final simultaneously diagnostic and therapeutic step can be made.

DATA   Arthrocentesis of the shoulder joint is performed. Ten milliliters of clear yellow joint fluid with fair viscosity are aspirated. The shoulder joint is injected with 10 ml of 1% lidocaine and 40 mg triamcinolone. Following injection, the patient has complete relief of pain and a full passive range of motion of the shoulder. Laboratory evaluation of the joint fluid shows: aerobic and anaerobic cultures—no growth; white blood cell count 5000/mm³, 50% polymorphonuclear leukocytes and 50% lymphocytes; glucose 108 mg/dl; rheumatoid factor negative; antinuclear antibody negative; examination for crystals—no monosodium urate, no calcium pyrophosphate.

LOGIC   Arthrocentesis provides us with the best material for examination in a patient with joint pain. The cultures demonstrate the absence of septic arthritis. This is supported by the low white blood cell count and the normal glucose. The absence of crystals rules out gout and pseudogout, and a negative rheumatoid factor and antinuclear antibody make the possibility of collagen disease very remote.

The ability to relieve joint pain by instillation of a local anesthetic confirms our suspicion that the source of the pain is inflammation in the shoulder joint. By careful questioning and precise examination, we have been able to localize the source of the patient's pain. Trauma, systemic disease, and tumor have been eliminated. Inflammation of the subdeltoid bursa due to chronic impingement of the humeral head on the acromion process with rupture of the rotator cuff is the most likely diagnosis.

QUESTIONS

1. The usual cause of acute shoulder pain in a 20-year-old man who sustains an abduction and external rotation stress to the joint is:
(a) impingement syndrome
(b) subluxation or dislocation of the shoulder
(c) shoulder separation
(d) shoulder-hand syndrome.
2. The tumor most apt to cause shoulder pain in a 60-year-old woman is:
(a) osteogenic sarcoma
(b) synovial sarcoma
(c) metastatic carcinoma
(d) enchondroma.
3. A 39-year-old woman presents with a 6-day history of right shoulder pain after a car wreck. On examination she demonstrates weakness of grip strength and decreased sensation in the little and ring fingers of the right hand. It is likely that we will find additional abnormalities on further examination of the:
(a) chest
(b) cervical spine
(c) shoulder
(d) wrist.
4. A 64-year-old woman has shoulder pain after falling on her outstretched hand. The probable diagnosis is:
(a) acute rotator cuff tear
(b) rupture of the biceps tendon
(c) fracture of the surgical neck of the humerus
(d) dislocation of the shoulder.

ANSWERS

1. **(b) is correct.** Anterior dislocation and subluxation of the shoulder occur very commonly in this age group and the mechanism of injury is almost always abduction and external rotation stress. Impingement syndrome occurs in older individuals after years of repeated stress, particularly of forward flexion. Shoulder separation means acromioclavicular separation and, while common in this age group, it usually occurs from a direct blow to the point of the shoulder. The shoulder-hand syndrome is a chronic problem usually not related to acute injury; it frequently follows myocardial infarction.
2. **(c) is correct.** The most likely tumor in the older woman is a metastatic lesion to the proximal humerus. The metastasis usually comes from the breast, lung, kidney, or gastrointestinal tract. An enchondroma is a benign, usually asymptomatic, tumor. Osteogenic sarcoma is rare in adults unless the patient has underlying Paget's disease. Synovial sarcoma is also rare, especially in the shoulder joint.
3. **(b) is correct.** The cervical spine is very frequently injured in car wrecks and a nerve root injury in the neck often presents with shoulder pain and a neurologic deficit in the limb. Shoulder injury with damage to the brachial

plexus might cause these findings, but injury of the brachial plexus is uncommon.

4. **(c) is correct.** The prevalence of osteoporosis among elderly women makes fracture the most likely result of trauma to the shoulder. The muscles and supporting ligaments are much less likely to be injured in a fall.

COMMENT On the basis of a key clue, various possibilities were considered. Bayes' theorem established periarticular inflammation as the most likely possibility. All others were ruled out and the most likely one was proven. False positive symptoms (cough, cigarettes) were present. The type of pain, relation to shoulder motion, and occupation were important additional clues. Cause and effect relationship was frequently invoked. An anatomic approach was used in the physical examination. The diagnosis was reasonably certain, but an invasive diagnostic procedure (arthrocentesis) was done to clinch the diagnosis and employ a therapeutic trial at the same time. A decision tree could easily have been used here. A few selected questions and examination techniques, x-rays, and joint aspiration, and the problem would have been very rapidly solved. Age, sex, and history of injury weighted our thinking in the questions and answers. (*P. C.*)

Suggested Readings

1. Bateman JE: *The Shoulder and Neck*, ed 2. Philadelphia, Saunders, 1978, pp 242–372.
   A textbook which explores the pathophysiology, diagnosis, and treatment of all shoulder problems in depth.
2. Booth RE, Marvel JP Jr: Differential diagnosis of shoulder pain. *Orthop Clin North Am* 6:353–379, 1975.
   Short review of the multiple causes of shoulder pain and the techniques for differentiating them.
3. Penny JN, Welsh RP: Shoulder impingement syndromes in athletes and their surgical management. *Am J Sports Med* 9:11–15, 1981.
   A review of the impingement syndrome as it presents in the athlete, stressing the differential diagnoses in these patients.
4. Rothman RH, Marvel JP Jr, Heppenstall RB: Anatomic considerations in the glenohumeral joint. *Orthop Clin North Am* 6:341–352, 1975.
   This short article provides a good review of anatomy of the shoulder joint complex and demonstrates the intricate relationships between its various components.
5. Brashear JR Jr, Ramey RB Sr (eds): *Shand's Handbook of Orthopaedic Surgery*, ed 9. St Louis, Mosby, 1978, pp 436–447.
   Fine textbook coverage of afflictions of the shoulder.
6. Resnick D: Shoulder pain. *Orthop Clin North Am* 14:81–97, 1983.
7. Cofield RH, Simonet WT: The shoulder in sports. *Mayo Clin Proc* 59:157–164, 1984.

Case 53
Painful Stiff Joints

PAUL CUTLER, M.D.

DATA Difficulty in performing the duties of her occupation brings a 37-year-old secretary to your office. For the past 3 years she has had intermittent episodes of pain, stiffness, warmth, and swelling of the hands and wrists. Each bout lasted for several months and then subsided. Now she has similar symptoms in her knees and elbows too. The present illness began 2 weeks ago, and she not only finds it impossible to type but can hardly get out of bed and do her morning chores.

LOGIC Symmetrical polyarthritis brings to mind many diseases: rheumatoid arthritis

(RA), systemic lupus erythematosus (SLE), acute rheumatic fever, Reiter's syndrome, other connective tissue diseases like scleroderma and dermatomyositis, and sarcoidosis.

Rheumatic fever can be eliminated almost immediately because of the length of the illness and the frequency of recurrences; it is an acute febrile illness lasting only 6 to 8 weeks. Sarcoidosis presents with different complaints (lymphadenopathy, dyspnea), and most of the other diseases mentioned are not nearly so prevalent as RA and SLE. RA is the most common, has its peak incidence in women of this age, behaves in precisely this way, and thus becomes your first provisional hypothesis. Next in order of likelihood is SLE. It too has a predilection for the same population subset and usually begins in the same manner, but it is only one-twentieth as common as RA.

With the information already on hand, you lean toward RA. But in thinking of RA you realize that this disease, whose main features are in the synovial cavities, has widespread extraarticular manifestations. It may be associated with inflammations of various layers of the eyeball; diffuse vasculitis; generalized amyloidosis; cardiac manifestations (pericarditis, coronary arteritis, valvulitis); pulmonary indicators (effusion, nodules, fibrosis); hematologic omens (normocytic anemia of chronic disease, hypochromic anemia from aspirin-induced blood loss); splenomegaly (Felty's syndrome); renal abnormalities signaled by proteinuria (vasculitis, amyloidosis, proliferative glomerulonephritis, treatment with gold, penicillamine, and nonsteroidal antiinflammatory drugs, and papillary necrosis from analgesics); and carpal tunnel syndrome.

DATA   The patient has seen various physicians in the past, each of whom treated her for "arthritis," although no type was ever specified. She had received pills, tablets, injections, and physiotherapy with partial benefit. Between the last few episodes, she did not become symptom-free as before, but continued having some residual pain and stiffness, especially on awakening.

LOGIC   Degenerative joint disease, or hypertrophic osteoarthritis, is by far the most common form of arthritis. It too may affect multiple joints, but it occurs in older age groups, is not usually associated with inflammation or constitutional symptoms, and tends not to be so episodic.

Crystal-induced arthritis was not considered from the start. Gout is unusual in young premenopausal women, it tends not to affect the small joints of the hands at first, nor is it so symmetrically polyarticular. Pseudo-

gout involves mostly large joints and is seen in older individuals.

The patient has had a variety of treatments, some of which may have helped, but it is difficult to judge this by her history. Note that she is no longer symptom-free between bouts of arthritis. Further inquiry must aim toward proving or disproving one of the two principal hypotheses. The difficulty in doing this lies in the fact that both diseases (RA and SLE) present similarly and both have systemic manifestations and laboratory abnormalities in which there is great overlap.

The American Rheumatism Association (ARA) has adopted criteria for the diagnosis of and distinction between RA and SLE. These criteria also help differentiate RA and SLE from other arthritic diseases that may resemble them. Table 22.1 lists the criteria for RA and Table 22.2 lists the criteria for SLE. Note the number of criteria considered to be diagnostic when present in concert.

Sad to say, the criteria for RA may not be reliable in all cases, especially the early, the atypical, or the complicated ones. There can be overlap with other diseases bearing a family resemblance. Therefore the sensitivity and specificity of this supposedly diagnostic set are not spectacular.

Textbook cases of SLE are simple to diagnose. For example, visualize a young woman with fever, polyarthritis, serositis,

Table 22.1.
American Rheumatism Association Revised 1982 Criteria for Rheumatoid Arthritis*

1. Morning stiffness
2. Pain on motion or tenderness (at least one joint)
3. Swelling (at least one joint)
4. Swelling of one other joint within 3 months
5. Symmetric joint involvement
6. Subcutaneous nodules
7. Typical x-ray findings
8. Positive latex test (rheumatoid factor)
9. Poor mucin clot in synovial fluid
10. Synovia or nodules show characteristic histology

* The presence of any five supports a "definite diagnosis." Seven indicate the presence of "classic rheumatoid arthritis."

Table 22.2.
**American Rheumatism Association Revised
1982 Criteria for Systemic Lupus
Erythematosus***

1. Malar rash
2. Discoid rash
3. Photosensitivity
4. Oral or nasal ulcers
5. Arthritis (two joints)
6. Serositis (pleuritis, pericarditis)
7. Renal disorder—proteinuria or abnormal casts
8. Seizures or psychosis
9. Hematologic disorder—hemolytic anemia, or leukopenia, or lymphopenia, or thrombocytopenia
10. Immunologic disorder—positive LE cell preparation, or high anti-DNA titer, or false positive serologic test for syphilis
11. ANA titer abnormal

* If four or more criteria are present simultaneously or serially, the diagnosis is established.

malar rash, marked albuminuria, and a high titer antinuclear antibody (ANA) test. Often, however, the case is not so typical and it has features that overlap with other autoimmune disorders. Only *some* earmarks may be present. The newly adopted 1982 ARA criteria try to simplify the diagnosis and require the presence of any four salient points. But this attempt to establish paradigms doesn't work. It, too, overlooks early atypical cases, and some patients whose symptoms seem to fit don't have the disease. So these criteria also are not only insensitive, but they are not even specific.

DATA   Over the past year, she has noted malaise, weakness, and easy fatigability. For the past 2 weeks she has not felt well and thinks she has had some fever. She has never noted any color changes in the fingertips on immersing them in cold water. There has been no diarrhea, blood in the stool, abdominal cramps, rashes of any kind including any on the face, cough, sharp chest pain, shortness of breath, convulsions, mental changes, eye problems, dryness of the mouth and eyes, loss of hair, or cutaneous sensitivity to sunlight. Other than aspirin for her arthritis, she now takes no medication.

LOGIC   The constitutional symptoms of fever, weakness, and malaise are common to both diseases. Raynaud's phenomenon is not present; it is seen in 20% of SLE patients and sometimes in RA. Arthritis which is occasionally associated with inflammatory bowel diseases (ulcerative colitis, regional ileitis) can be ruled out by the lack of gastrointestinal symptoms. Absence of a facial rash and no evidence of cerebral disease are against SLE since each occurs in one-quarter to one-half of the cases. Neither is there a history of patchy alopecia or sunlight sensitivity, which are peculiar to SLE. No symptomatic evidence is present for lung or pleuropericardial disease; these are more common in SLE but can be found in both diseases. There is nothing in the history to suggest uveitis, keratoconjunctivitis, or sicca syndrome—each sometimes seen in RA.

Moreover, the patient takes no medication other than aspirin; hydralazine, procainamide, certain antiepileptics, and, rarely, other drugs can cause pictures identical to SLE.

So far there are no distinguishing clues, but the absence of those frequently found in SLE (rash, cerebral symptoms, and pleuropericardial disease) makes this diagnosis even less likely.

Physical examination in the patient with joint disease often discloses an abundance of findings. These vary with the type of arthritis and have different diagnostic significance. Look for alopecia, photosensitivity, sicca syndrome, Sjögren's syndrome, eye inflammations, temporal arteritis, heliotrope of the eyelids, oral or nasal ulcers, psoriasis, Raynaud's phenomenon, vasculitic lesions, decreased neck and spinal flexion, nodules over the elbow, erythema nodosum, the special rashes of SLE and Lyme disease, carpal tunnel syndrome, anemia, splenomegaly, and of course abnormalities of the joints themselves. Don't forget the CREST syndrome seen in scleroderma, a disease that often produces a polyarthritis. This acronymic syndrome consists of calcinosis, Raynaud's phenomenon, esophageal abnormalities, sclerodactyly, and telangiectasia.

DATA   The patient seems a bit pale and the temperature is 38.2 C. There is swelling, tenderness, slight redness, and warmth of most proximal interphalangeal joints, the metacarpophalangeal joints, the wrists, knees, and elbows. She can hardly walk, cannot shake hands, and has great difficulty getting in and out of a chair.

Her eyes appear normal and there is no rash across the cheeks nor nodules on the extensor surfaces of the elbows and hands. The blood pressure, heart, and lungs are normal; in particular, there is no evidence of pleural effusion, and no friction rubs or murmurs are heard. The rest of the examination is normal too.

LOGIC   Pallor, fever, and symmetrical subacute polyarthritis are present. These are nondiscriminatory. While it may be too early to see the characteristic hand deformities of RA, if these deformities are present RA becomes likely, since SLE is less often the cause of subluxations and ulnar deviation of the fingers. The absence of findings in the head and chest corroborates the lack of symptoms there and does nothing to alter likelihoods. Subcutaneous nodules commonly seen in RA (20%) are not present. The absence of a heart murmur is of no help; systolic murmurs are common in SLE and rare in RA.

While found in 10% of cases in both diseases, splenomegaly is not noted here. Neither is lymphadenopathy. An important discerning clue will be the presence or absence of renal disease since it is rare in RA (amyloidosis) and common (50%) in SLE. The laboratory may help.

So far, SLE has not been proven since only one criterion—arthritis without deformity—is noted to be present.

An abundance of tests helps in the differential diagnosis. Each must be interpreted with caution since sensitivity and specificity are variable. A *blood count* usually discloses anemia; if there is leukopenia too, suspect Felty's syndrome and search again for an enlarged spleen. The *sedimentation rate* is very rapid in polymyalgia rheumatica (tem-

poral arteritis), moderately rapid in any active inflammatory arthritis, and normal in degenerative joint disease. A 1:160 *ANA titer* is over 90% sensitive for SLE, but the test may be positive in RA too. The *anti-DNA antibody* test correlates well with SLE and is fairly specific. However, the *rheumatoid factor* (RF) (latex test), while positive in 75% of RA cases, is not very specific; it is positive in 5% of normals and 20% of the elderly, and is often positive in other types of arthropathy. Be wary of a diagnosis in an older patient with diffuse aches and pains who happens to have a positive latex test. The *LE cell preparation* is 80% sensitive for SLE but is also positive in 10 to 20% of patients with RA. *Serum complement* is decreased in active SLE but normal in RA (Table 22.3).

The radiograph is not so valuable as you might think. In early cases it shows nothing. In late cases where the x-ray is helpful, the diagnosis has long since been made by other clinical features.

DATA   The following studies are done: Complete blood count shows mild "anemia of chronic disease," normal white blood cell count and differential, and adequate platelets; urinalysis is normal; erythrocyte sedimentation rate is rapid (40 mm/hour); serologic test for syphilis is negative; the 18-test blood chemistry profile is normal.

LOGIC   Anemia is common to both diseases, but hemolytic anemia and cytopenia are frequent in SLE. The normal urinalysis speaks for RA; had there been much protein and cellular casts present, SLE might have moved into the first position. Also, 15% of patients with SLE have a false positive serologic test for syphilis. The rapid erythro-

Table 22.3.
Incidence of Positive Antibody Tests

Test	RA (%)	SLE (%)
ANA	10–25	99
Anti-DNA	5	>50
LE cells	10–20	60–80
Hypocomplementemia	0–10	75
RF	>75	20

cyte sedimentation rate is almost always present in both conditions. Kidney function is normal.

Autoimmune processes exist in both diseases, but there are many more demonstrable antibodies in SLE. Further tests are needed.

DATA The ANA test is positive; anti-DNA is negative; LE cells are not present; serum complement is normal; RF as measured by latex agglutination is positive. Creatine phosphokinase and serum glutamic-oxaloacetic transaminase are normal. (Note that the test for LE cells is no longer commonly done, since it has been replaced by more specific antibody tests.)

LOGIC There is much overlap in most of these tests regarding both diseases. In fact, some tests are occasionally positive in other diseases or in nondisease. The problem is evident as shown in Table 22.3. However, even without using formulas and Bayesian equations, it can be seen that these test results lean more heavily toward RA. Had the ANA been negative, there would have been no question about the diagnosis of RA, since this test is very highly sensitive for SLE. Also, had serum complement been low, RA would have been rendered most unlikely. Normal muscle enzymes rule out the already unlikely rare disease, dermatomyositis.

No discussion of joint diseases can exclude one of the newest members of the family—Lyme disease. This spirochetal disease is transmitted by the tick, *Ixodes damminni* and was first noted in the area of Lyme, Connecticut. It affects mainly the young and is characterized by erythema chronicum migrans and recurrent arthritis. Notably, 25% of those with arthritis don't have skin lesions, and arthritis is seen in only 50% of cases.

DATA To complete the workup: a chest x-ray is normal, x-rays of the involved joints show only periarticular swelling and bone demineralization, and the ECG is normal.

LOGIC The chest x-ray lays to rest any

possibility of lung or pleural disease. A normal ECG does not aid in diagnosis though sometimes a conduction abnormality caused by a critically located rheumatoid nodule is seen in RA. The joint x-rays at this stage are the same for both diseases, and synovial fluid aspiration would have shown a group II fluid in both instances. With all the evidence on the scales, RA weighs in the heavier.

DATA The patient is told she has rheumatoid arthritis and is placed on a carefully prescribed regimen of high-dose aspirin, rest, and physiotherapy.

COMMENT Because RA and SLE have different complications, prognoses, and treatments, it is advisable to be sure which of these two closely related diseases is present.

The overlap of criteria and the incomplete sensitivity and specificity of tests and procedures used to diagnose these two diseases make their distinction all the more difficult. However, on the basis of criteria set up by the ARA, this differentiation may often be possible.

While provisional hypotheses were formed early, it was difficult to prove one or the other decisively, even with all the clues at hand. Statistical probability gives RA the overwhelming Bayesian likelihood, though the clinical picture is inconclusive; the laboratory tests lean more toward RA. The patient's future course may mandate a change in diagnosis and perhaps in treatment too. No wonder her previous physicians would only label this disease as "arthritis." This writer is not so sure either.... (*P. C.*)

Suggested Readings

1. McCarty DM (ed): *Arthritis and Allied Conditions: A Textbook of Rheumatology*, ed 10. Philadelphia, Lea & Febiger, 1985.
   This new book has excellent chapters (38, 39, 40, 53, 54, 55, 61, 62) that very nicely cover RA, its variants, ankylosing spondylitis, and SLE.
2. *Clin Rheum Dis* 8, Apr 1982.
   An entire issue is devoted to SLE. Various articles detail the immunologic aspects, drug-induced lupus, the clotting defects, renal disease, and the central nervous system, cardiovascular, and dermatologic abnormalities so frequently seen.
3. Klemperer P, Pollack AD, Baehr G: Landmark article, May 23, 1942: Diffuse collagen disease. Acute disseminated lupus erythematosus and diffuse scleroderma. *JAMA* 251:1593–1594, 1984.
   This article opened the era of collagen diseases.
4. Tan EM, Cohen AS, Fried JF, et al: The 1982 revised criteria for the classification of systemic lupus erythematosus. *Arthritis Rheum* 25:1271–

1277, 1982.

    The struggle to establish criteria goes on. These are the ones adopted by the ARA.

5. Clough JD, Ebrezak M, Calabrese LH, et al: Weighted criteria for the diagnosis of systemic lupus erythematosus. *Arch Intern Med* 144:281–285, 1984.

    Devises a system to increase the sensitivity and specificity of the ARA criteria.

6. Meyerhoff J: SLE: making the diagnosis. *Md State Med J* 33:42–45, 1984.

    Elaborates on the sensitivity and specificity of clinical features.

7. Leib RC: Lupus nephritis: the dogma deliberated. *South Med J* 76:490–493, 1983.

    What to do about the renal complication.

8. Smith CD, Marino C, Rothfield NF: The clinical utility of the lupus band test. *Arthritis Rheum* 27:382–387, 1984.

    The presence of abnormal proteins at the dermal-epidermal junction may be a specific test.

9. Steinberg AD, Raveché ES, Laskin CA, et al: Systemic lupus erythematosus: insights from animal models. *Ann Intern Med* 100:714–727, 1984.

    The immunologic aspects are richly detailed.

10. West SG, McMahon M, Portanova JP: Quinidine-induced lupus. *Ann Intern Med* 100:840–842, 1984.

    Discusses drug-induced lupus in general.

11. Mowat AG: Rheumatoid arthritis: presentation, diagnosis, and management. *Practitioner* 227: 1103–1116, 1983.

12. Keat A: Reiter's syndrome and reactive arthritis in perspective. *N Engl J Med* 309:1606–1615, 1983.

    Gives greater understanding of this bizarre combination of arthritic, gastrointestinal, genital, and ocular manifestations.

13. Bowen GS, Griffin M, Hayne C, et al: Clinical manifestations and descriptive epidemiology of Lyme disease in New Jersey 1978 to 1982. *JAMA* 251:2236–2240, 1984.

    This disease exists elsewhere than Connecticut; its features are discussed.

Case 54

Backache

ARVO NEIDRE, M.D.

DATA   A 52-year-old man comes walking slowly into your office, stooped over and holding his hand to his back. He puts his hands on the arms of a chair, slowly lowers himself into the chair and exclaims, "Doctor, I've had this terrible back pain that shoots down my hip and into my leg for the past 2 weeks!"

LOGIC   Back pain is one of the most common symptoms seen in practice. Epidemiologic studies show that 80% of people in North America will experience some extent of back pain during their active lifetime. In industrial workers the yearly incidence of back pain is 50/1000 workers.

    When faced with the above scenario, you immediately recall the many different causes of back pain: (*a*) viscerogenic, (*b*) vascular, (*c*) neurogenic, (*d*) psychogenic, and (*e*) spondylogenic. The last category is by far the largest. It includes all those cases of backache which are directly related to the spinal column and its many components: bone, muscle, tendons, ligaments, fascia, disks, and nerves. The anatomy and biomechanical features of the back must be understood.

    To solve this problem, three important issues must be quickly settled: the exact location of the pain, the presence or absence of radiation down a leg, and the relation of back and leg activity to the pain. Pain down the leg is called "sciatica" since it tends to follow the course of the sciatic nerve. It usually starts in the low back or buttock, and then radiates down the posterior thigh into the calf and plantar aspect of the foot. Sometimes it can radiate from the posterior thigh into the anterior compartment and dorsum of the foot.

    Viscerogenic back pain is caused by penetrating ulcers or pancreatic or renal disease, is localized near the area of the disease, does not radiate down the leg, is not worsened by back motion, and is almost always accompanied by other manifestations of the disease. Kidney pain is in the flank or costovertebral angle, off to a side, while pancreatic or ulcer pain is high in the midback. Prostate or uterine disease can cause low back pain but, again, no radiation or worsening by movement—unless the disease is metastatic carcinoma to the spine.

Vascular causes include abdominal aortic aneurysms which cause boring pain where they exist, and peripheral vascular disease which causes pain in the lower extremity. The latter disease can be confusing in that the leg pain can include hip and buttock pain too, but it is easily distinguishable because pain is brought on by walking, relieved by stopping, and is not related to bending or lifting.

Spinal canal tumors can present with sciatic pain, but often the pain is at night and activity is required for relief. True sciatic neuritis can be caused by diabetes mellitus. Pure psychogenic pain is uncommon, but organic pain patterns can be confused by psychogenic overtones.

DATA   As the patient enters your office, you skim over your notes of his previous visits. He is a self-employed businessman running a shoe store, and he has been having financial problems. His wife has threatened to leave him. Ulcer symptoms have been intermittently present for 10 years, though x-rays done twice were inconclusive. He has been overweight for years. Recently he consulted a urologist for hesitancy and increasing frequency of urination. Cystourethroscopy was done, but he does not know the results; he was unable to keep his reappointment because of back pain. His mother had diabetes which she got in her sixties. Also, he had three previous visits because of back pain in the past few years. Each episode occurred after heavy gardening, radiated to the right gluteal area, and resolved with rest.

LOGIC   We have been barraged with a series of clues which may be relevant to his back pain. Psychosomatic components may be present. Malingering is unlikely since, being self-employed, he has nothing to gain

financially from his illness. However, back pain could be a means of getting sympathy or an excuse for business failure.

While he may have an ulcer, it could not cause pains such as he has. The urologic problem worries you. Prostatic cancer with metastasis is possible. And cystoscopy can cause vertebral osteomyelitis via Batson's venous plexus. The family history of diabetes is a concern; diabetic neuropathy can present as sciatic neuritis, though back pain would be absent.

Many backaches seen in the primary care physician's office are transient and caused by a back strain or "sprain." This may relate to an injury of ligament, tendon, or muscle caused by a specific activity like lifting, bending, or twisting. But remember that this minor episode may be the first manifestation of discogenic disease. The potential for such minor injuries can be increased by conditions which put extra strain on the spine. These include obesity, severe spinal deformity (scoliosis, kyphosis, lordosis), poor body posture, and, occasionally, significant leg length differences. Some say that the latter conditions alone can cause backache, but this is debatable. At any rate, these predisposing conditions can be readily detected on examination.

Osteoarthritis of the spine can and does cause backache. But osteoarthritis is such a common x-ray finding in people without backaches that its presence is difficult to assess. Bony overgrowth can entrap nerve roots in the intervertebral foramina and produce pain radiating down the leg. It is difficult to be sure the x-ray findings correlate with the clinical picture.

Even though it is uncommon, be alert for tuberculosis of the spine. And persistent back pain can be a sign of a more common disease—metastatic cancer. X-ray and isotope scan may be needed. The entity of "muscular rheumatism" (fibrositis or fibromyositis) has not been proven to exist, though the term is frequently used to describe short-lived pain about the back; it remains a subject for dispute.

This patient has backache with sciatica.

Disk degeneration is the most common cause of this type of pain. His previous episodes of back pain could all be classified as mechanical or spondylogenic in that they were relieved with rest and aggravated with activity. They could be described as "lumbosacral strains" in that they resolved quickly with rest, but they may also suggest an ongoing process of degenerative disk disease. Shrinkage and degeneration of the disk itself allow abnormal disk motion and microtears in the annulus; eventual disk protrusion into the spinal canal takes place.

DATA The present episode started 2 weeks ago when he was lifting a tire from his trunk. A short while later he felt midline low back pain, which then radiated to his right buttock and down the posterior thigh into the anterior portion of his calf to the dorsum of his foot. He went to bed and has been quite comfortable lying down. The pain returns when he stands to resume his activities. If he coughs or strains, the same pain shoots down his right leg.

Examination of the vital signs, head, neck, chest, and abdomen is normal. He points to the lower lumbar spine as the site of his pain. There is slight curvature of the back and markedly decreased range of motion. By flexing the back, he can only reach his knees with his fingertips. This action aggravates the pain. He can toe walk, but on heel walking he finds it impossible to lift up his right foot. Straight leg raising is limited to 20° as compared to 80° on the left. Lasègue's sign is positive on the right. There is tenderness along the course of the right sciatic nerve in the buttock and popliteal space. He has markedly decreased power in the dorsiflexors of the ankle and the extensor hallucis longus, with hypesthesia to pinprick over the lower anterolateral calf and dorsum of the right foot. Patellar and achilles reflexes are normal. Good pulses are felt in both legs and feet.

LOGIC There is a foot-drop on the right with signs of sciatic nerve irritation and L5 nerve root compression as shown by the neurologic abnormalities, nerve tenderness, limitation of straight leg raising, and positive Lasègue's sign. Sensory abnormalities conform to the L5 dermatome too. The reflexes remain normal because the knee-jerk is an L2-L3-L4 reflex arc, and the ankle-jerk is an S1-S2 reflex arc.

Psychogenic causes are clearly ruled out. No vascular disease is detected in the abdomen or extremities. A herniated disk between L4 and L5 with L5 nerve root compression is almost certain. A spinal canal tumor can cause the same symptoms and the initial trauma history could be coincidental. The prostate and diabetes are yet to be evaluated.

DATA X-rays of the lumbar spine show a narrowing of the L5-S1 disk space with osteophyte formation. No osteolytic or osteoblastic lesions are seen. Fasting and 2-hour postprandial glucoses are normal. Erythrocyte sedimentation rate, acid and alkaline phosphatase, calcium, phosphorus, protein electrophoresis, blood count, and urinalysis are normal.

LOGIC The osteoarthritis seen on x-ray does not correspond to the site of the known neurologic lesion. Disease between L5 and S1 would affect the first sacral nerve root and give a different picture. The normal complete blood count, erythrocyte sedimentation rate, and x-rays tend to rule out vertebral osteomyelitis, though it is a little early to be sure of the x-rays. Normal proteins essentially preclude multiple myeloma and normal phosphatases are against any bone-destroying lesion. The normal acid phosphatase does not rule out prostatic cancer.

DATA A rectal examination should have been done earlier. It shows a diffusely enlarged, smooth prostate gland. No nodules are felt. A telephone call to the urologist confirms the impression of benign prostatic hypertrophy based on cystoscopy.

LOGIC You are now more secure since 90% of carcinomas of the prostate are detectable on digital examination. The urologist helps allay your concern too. There is still the possibility of spinal canal tumor.

DATA   The patient is told he probably has a herniated lumbar disk. He is advised to rest in bed at home and is given an analgesic and muscle relaxant. An electromyogram and computed tomographic (CT) scan are performed on an outpatient basis.

The CT scan shows normal disk space at the L3-L4 and L5-S1 levels. At the L4-L5 disk level there is a diffuse bulge of the disk with focal herniation on the right side. This pushes against the dural sac on the right and obliterates the epidural fat planes.

Electromyography shows spontaneous fibrillations in the muscles supplied by the L5 nerve root as well as positive sharp waves at rest. There is also a decrease in the number and amplitude of action potentials on voluntary activity.

LOGIC   The CT scan confirms the clinical impression of disk herniation. It precisely locates and delineates the extent of the lesion. A radionuclide bone scan of the lumbar area for prostatic metastases is deemed unnecessary. The electromyogram merely confirms what you already know; under the circumstances some physicians might consider it equally unnecessary.

DATA   He does not improve with 2 weeks of bed rest at home, so he is hospitalized. A myelogram is performed. It shows an indentation of the dye column with probable impingement on the L5 nerve root on the right side at the L4-L5 level. On running the dye proximally and distally, no other lesions are seen.

LOGIC   Since he did not improve at home, hospitalization with enforced/supervised bed rest is initiated. The myelogram confirms the single lesion and excludes other concomitant lesions. Most patients improve on a conservative regime. He is given an H_2-receptor antagonist for the heartburn which began to recur a week ago. Now you wait and hope for signs of improvement.

The possibility of being the buffer between the patient, his family, the hospital administrator, and those who supervise the Diagnosis Related Groups system occurs to you. So you reach for some cimetidine for yourself.

QUESTIONS

1. Suppose the man in the case just discussed were to present with a history of severe back pain and bilateral leg pain. He is unable to void and has not had a bowel movement for 1 week. Examination reveals a patulous anal sphincter with an absent bulbocavernosus reflex. Your most likely diagnosis would be:
   (a) abdominal aneurysm
   (b) central disk herniation
   (c) benign prostatic hypertrophy with urinary obstruction
   (d) spinal cord tumor.
2. Which of the following tests would be of most benefit in confirming your diagnosis?
   (a) x-rays of the lumbar spine
   (b) cystometrogram
   (c) myelogram
   (d) lumbar puncture with manometrics.
3. A 28-year-old construction worker complains of low back pain which does not radiate. It has been slowly increasing in severity over the past year. Examination shows no neurologic abnormality, slight decrease in range of movement of the back, and decreased chest expansion. Based on these findings, you would consider the diagnosis of:
   (a) degenerative osteoarthritis
   (b) lumbar strain
   (c) ankylosing spondylitis
   (d) Scheuermann's disease.
4. A 12-year-old girl presents with back pain of 1 week's duration. No neurologic defect can be demonstrated, but she has marked loss of lumbar lordosis with tight hamstring muscles. Straight leg raising can be done to only 20° bilaterally. In your differential diagnosis at this time you would consider:
   (a) disk herniation
   (b) spondylolisthesis
   (c) vertebral osteomyelitis
   (d) idiopathic scoliosis.

ANSWERS

1. **(b) is correct.** A central disk herniation can produce compression of the sacral nerves with bowel and bladder dysfunction in addition to the pain described. We are dealing with a surgical emergency. The sacral nerves are mainly unmyelinated parasympathetic fibers which are very susceptible to pressure. Per-

manent dysfunction can result. (d) should also be considered because a spinal cord tumor can present exactly as described. However, one would expect more night pain and not so much mechanical pain. (a) and (c) can be ruled out because of the leg pain as well as the neurologic abnormalities.

2. **(c) is correct.** Myelography is the most valuable test in this situation. It will help rule out a spinal cord tumor, provide x-rays of the lumbar spine, show the level of the disk lesion prior to surgery, and allow access to cerebrospinal fluid. X-rays of the lumbar spine would not give you any more information than the clinical examination. (b) only confirms your clinical diagnosis: You would see a neurogenic bladder. (d) gives limited information which can all be obtained from myelography. A CT scan is helpful in such a situation too.

3. **(c) is correct.** Measurement of chest expansion is an important part of the back examination. With decreased chest expansion in a young man, the possibility of ankylosing spondylitis should always be considered. This disease process starts in the sacroiliac joints, presents with back pain, and spreads to the costovertebral joints, producing stiffness and decreased chest expansion. An erythrocyte sedimentation rate and x-rays of the sacroiliac joints would help confirm the diagnosis. The HLA-B27 test may also be of help. (a) does not occur at the age of 28. (b) is an acute event which tends to settle down over a short period of time and not linger for a year. Also, the decreased chest expansion would not be expected with a lumbar strain. (d) is a gradually progressive thoracic kyphosis found in adolescents. It may produce thoracic pain, but the pain generally abates by the end of spinal growth and this patient's age would rule it out.

4. **(a), (b), and (c) are all correct.** Idiopathic scoliosis or lateral curvature of the spine usually starts to present around the age of 10 and progresses during spinal growth. This condition, however, is rarely associated with pain. Children with (a), (b), and (c) tend to present in the above fashion, irrespective of the cause of the pain. Disk herniation can occur and has been reported in patients as young as 10 years old. The presence of a neurologic deficit would

be more suggestive, but in its absence disk herniation still cannot be ruled out. Spondylolisthesis, where there is slippage of one vertebral body under one below, usually presents exactly as described above. This can be identified by doing oblique x-rays of the lumbar spine to show a defect in the pars interarticularis as well as a standing lateral x-ray to show the degree of slippage. Vertebral osteomyelitis can also present in this manner; fever, leukocytosis, and rapid sedimentation rate would be present. A radionuclide bone scan may help in the first 2 weeks; conventional x-rays become positive later.

Suggested Readings

1. Macnab I: *Backache.* Baltimore, Williams & Wilkins, 1977.
   The author, a world-acknowledged expert, covers the whole problem of back pain in a clear and easily readable manner. He provides a logical approach and philosophy for the diagnosis of back pain.
2. Rothman RH, Simeone FA: Lumbar disc disease. In *The Spine.* Philadelphia, Saunders, 1982, pp 508–646.
   This is a well-illustrated in-depth review of the disk problem; all aspects of diagnosis are included.
3. Kirkaldy-Willis WH, Hill RG: A more precise diagnosis for low back pain. *Spine* 4:102–109, 1979.
4. Brashear HR Jr, Ramey RB Sr (eds): *Shand's Handbook of Orthopaedic Surgery,* ed 9. St Louis, Mosby, 1978.
   Afflictions of the low back are excellently covered on pp 333–355.
5. Burton CV: High resolution CT scanning: the present and future. *Orthop Clin North Am* 14:539–551, 1983.
   The value of CT scans in disk disease.
6. Kieffer SA, Cacayorin ED, Sherry RG: The radiological diagnosis of herniated intervertebral disc. A current controversy. *JAMA* 251:1192–1195, 1984.
   Myelography versus CT scan.
7. McCulloch JA, Macnab I: *Sciatica and Chymopapain.* Baltimore, Williams & Wilkins, 1983.
   An entire short valuable book on the disk and its controversial treatments.
8. Roland MO: The natural history of back pain. *Practitioner* 227:1119–1122, 1983.
9. Waddell G, Hamblen DL: The differential diagnosis of backache. *Practitioner* 227:1167–1175, 1983.

Chapter 23

Neurologic Problems

When a toastmaster says "our guest for tonight needs no introduction," he usually proceeds to give the guest speaker's full biography. It would seem on the surface that neurologic problem solving needs no introduction either, for nowhere in medicine are the signs and symptoms so clearly and understandably related to the underlying neuroanatomic alterations. Topical diagnosis is well established. Certain findings may limit the disease to an entire level of the spinal cord; in other instances you can be sure the disease process is in the right frontal lobe.

But locating the disease site is not tantamount to naming the disease process. Different diseases can affect the sites just mentioned. The transverse myelitis syndrome can be caused by trauma, tumor, viral infection, or vascular occlusion, whereas cerebral thrombosis, brain tumor, or brain abscess can affect the right frontal lobe. And "there's the rub!"

The relative importance of presenting neurologic problems and the amount of emphasis on teaching them, as in most other organ systems, depends on their frequency, seriousness, and treatability. It is better to find a rare serious disease that is amenable to treatment than to exhaust your diagnostic acumen in labeling a rare, relatively benign disease for which no treatment exists.

But, as in other systems, a few common problems account for most of what the primary physician sees. Statistics show the most frequently presenting issues are headaches, dizziness, pain syndromes (e.g. backache), alterations in consciousness or mentation, strokes, seizures, neuropathies, and Parkinson's disease. Situations needing urgent care include coma, meningitis, status epilepticus, and head trauma. The most readily treatable problems include seizures, transient ischemic attacks, migraine, subdural hematoma, Parkinson's disease, and meningitis.

Neurologic problems may be solved at a glance (Parkinson's disease, stroke), by pattern recognition (transient ischemic attacks, meningitis, multiple sclerosis), or by a stepwise approach with early hypothesis generation and testing (coma, polyneuropathy, brain tumor); or they may require a detailed data base (obscure atypical headaches).

Often a diagnostic procedure such as cerebral arteriography, radionuclide brain scan, computed tomography (CT), ultrasound, or lumbar puncture furnishes the ultimate clue.

The introduction of high technology has altered the diagnostic process in neurologic diseases perhaps more than in any other disease category. For example, CT scanning, though expensive, is a cost-saving procedure that saves days and has almost phased out radionuclide scans, ultrasound, pneumoencephalograms, etc. Nuclear magnetic resonance (NMR scans) and positron emission tomography (PET scans) may soon compete with CT scans for diagnostic dominance. CT scans define anatomic detail; NMR scans primarily describe anatomy but offer some information about brain function too; PET scans yield physiologic and biochemical data and are much more research-oriented at this time.

For the moment, a CT scan (with dye) is

the procedure par excellence in many instances. It should *not* be used for the routine workup of simple headaches, minor head trauma, syncope, dizziness, or every garden-variety typical cerebral thrombosis. But it *is* especially valuable for *severe head trauma* and *suspected neoplasm*. It can distinguish hemorrhage from edema, subarachnoid aneurysmal leak from intracerebral bleed, and cerebral hemorrhage from cerebral thrombosis. In so doing, lumbar puncture may not be needed and decisions on anticoagulation can be made. Furthermore, the CT scan detects subdural hematoma, intracranial aneurysm, tumor, abscess, and arteriovenous malformations. It is usually requested when an adult experiences an unexplained seizure, be it generalized, partial, or focal. (*P. C.*)

Case 55
Headache
HERSCHEL L. DOUGLAS, M.D.

DATA You see a 22-year-old woman in your office who complains of headache for 6 months. Actually she had had occasional dull headaches for several years; these began in the occiput and progressed into a band-like constriction of the head, were stress related, and occurred in the early evening.

For the last 6 months, however, the nature of the headaches changed. They consist of severe left temporal throbbing pain which starts in the morning, and are preceded by a few minutes of feeling "strange in the head." After several hours, the pain loses its throbbing character and becomes more generalized though still severe. She requires rest in a quiet, dark room, is usually nauseated, and often vomits. These headaches occur at irregular and unpredictable intervals of 2 to 14 days.

LOGIC Headache is one of the most frequent symptoms seen in office practice. It is humanity's most common pain and occurs, in one form or another, in more than 90% of people. You should be familiar with its usual causes and their clinical manifestations. The diagnosis is often easily established on the basis of history alone, though physical examination and, rarely, diagnostic procedures must be done before initiating treatment.

First, let us eliminate the headaches that almost everybody gets occasionally: the "ice cream headache" from rapid swallowing of cold food, the headache from too much noise, the one from an emotionally upsetting situation, the "hangover" or "morning after" headache—in short, headaches with obvious causes.

Posttraumatic headaches can mimic any type of chronic recurrent headache. They may continue for months to years after the initial trauma, and their intensity and duration cannot be correlated with the degree or severity of the initial trauma. Indeed,

headaches may follow seemingly trivial injury and their mechanisms are usually unexplainable.

Solving the headache problem may involve a consideration of many factors: age and gender; duration of the problem; statistical incidence of the various types of headache; duration of each individual headache; presence of tenderness, aura, or psychosocial factors; time of day and day of the week on which the headache occurs; and the presence or absence of visual symptoms, gastrointestinal symptoms, photophobia, or pulsatile pain.

Patients with mild recurrent headaches for many years do not commonly consult the physician; they take analgesics for relief. Those with a sudden-onset severe, single headache usually *do* see the physician; they may have an acute problem such as meningitis, any febrile illness, subdural hematoma, acute suppurative sinusitis, brain abscess, subarachnoid hemorrhage, acute glaucoma, etc. Their problems are readily recognized by the associated symptoms and physical signs.

Too often there is a tendency to blame headaches on mild coincidental hypertension, "eye strain," "bad teeth," or "sinuses" when such is not the case. Also, momentary head pains lasting 1 or 2 seconds are ubiquitous, meaningless, and without known cause.

However, you must be concerned about the 60-year-old patient who has had severe headaches for days to weeks (possible polymyalgia rheumatica or temporal arteritis); the patient whose headaches are of recent vintage, are getting worse, and are associated with morning vomiting (expanding intracranial lesion); and the patient who has recent focal neurologic abnormalities together with headache.

In the world of chronic recurrent headaches the great majority (almost 80%) are muscle contraction-tension headaches. About 20% are vascular in origin—migraine or cluster; these people *do* visit the doctor since their headaches are often excruciating and disabling. The remaining small percentage results from brain tumors, sinusitis, and ocular disorders. The eyes cause headaches when there is glaucoma, hypermetropia, astigmatism, or difficulty with convergence. Sinus headaches are not so common as television commercials lead you to believe.

Therefore, chronic recurrent headaches present a spectrum of diagnoses and causes that include:

1. Muscle contraction-tension headaches
2. Vascular headaches: (*a*) classic migraine, (*b*) common migraine, and (*c*) cluster headaches (Horton's headache, histamine cephalalgia)
3. Combination of 1 and 2
4. Psychogenic headaches
5. Diseases of the sinuses, eyes, or teeth
6. Hypertension
7. Temporal arteritis
8. Cervical osteoarthritis.

Again, note that well over 90% of chronic recurrent headaches are caused by items 1 and 2. In fact, elements of 1 and 2 often compound each other. It is not surprising to see the headache patient wander from one specialist to another for each places the headache outside his domain. Headaches related to special senses are uncommon but should be simple to recognize.

DATA Closer questioning elicits the story that the patient's second type of headache began shortly after her marriage. At that time a CU-7 intrauterine device was inserted and this was contrary to her religious convictions. Her headaches are worse prior to menses and her mother had similar "sick headaches" from the time she was a young woman until after the menopause. The recent courtship and marriage have been happy and without emotional disturbance, significant worries, or stress. There are no complaints of nervousness, anxiety, insomnia, crying spells, loss of libido, loss of self-

esteem, or feeling blue. She does not smoke or drink alcohol, drinks no coffee, and takes no medicines regularly.

LOGIC The very common tension headache is related to sustained contraction of the occipitofrontalis muscle and causes the type of pain which this patient had for several years before the headaches changed in character. Often it is described as head-tightness, a band-like or vise-like feeling, a drawing sensation, or soreness. It may be over the entire head, the front, back, or either side, but it is nonpulsatile, not associated with nausea, and likely to be relieved by analgesics, heat, and massage. Nervous headache, psychogenic headache, and tension headache are probably synonyms. They occur against the backdrop of an aggressive, frustrated, anxious, or depressed person who is confronted by an emotional tension state.

Psychogenic headaches (item 4) may overlap with muscular tension headaches. Even if 1 and 4 are separate varieties, they have similar symptoms and are related to concurrent stigmata of anxiety, tension, depression, or conversion.

While we cannot be certain that her original headaches could be listed under item 1 or 4 or both, we do know that the headaches the patient has had for the past 6 months are vascular in origin. The description is characteristic of common migraine, which accounts for 90% of vascular headaches. The onset is usually near important milestones in life's responsibilities—e.g. puberty, college, marriage, menopause. It is most often unilateral, with no (or vague) premonitory sensations, is pulsatile and throbbing, and progresses to a steady ache with nausea. The pain can be excruciating and disabling. The family history is 60 to 80% positive.

All of these elements are positive in your patient and you now have a well-substantiated working diagnosis. Other forms of vascular headache have not yet been eliminated, nor have certain organic diseases been ruled out. Invasive, expensive, time-consuming tests are not needed. First complete the history with a systems review, and do a physical and neurologic examination.

DATA The systems review discloses the absence of: unrelenting progression of headache, gait disturbance, vertigo, memory loss, visual changes, diplopia, paresthesias, and motor weakness—before, during, after, or between headaches. Physical and neurologic examinations are entirely normal, including the blood pressure and fundi. No bruits are heard over the eyeballs or cranium. Complete blood count, urinalysis, and sedimentation rate are normal.

LOGIC Armed with this additional information, you are now in a position to rule out various previously mentioned causes of headache:

a. *Intracranial tumor.* Here the headache is generally progressive and unrelenting, but not necessarily continuous. After 6 months you would expect additional symptoms, some neurologic abnormalities, or even abnormal fundi.

b. *Chronic subdural hematoma.* This may be preceded by a history of head trauma, though the trauma may be minor or forgotten and no history may be obtainable. Alcoholism or drug obtundation is often associated with injuries to the head. The pain is deep-seated and steady. By this time, other symptoms and signs like dizziness, altered sensorium, and hemiparesis might be expected.

c. *Brain abscess, meningitis, and encephalitis.* These are acute illnesses with a single constant headache, fever, meningeal irritation, a "sick" patient, and progression of symptoms and signs.

d. *Subarachnoid hemorrhage.* Sudden onset of severe headache followed by unconsciousness is a completely different story from the one in our patient. Aneurysms or other vascular malformations may cause this acute critical illness.

e. *Temporal arteritis* (polymyalgia rheumatica). This rarely occurs under age 50, is associated with a tender, palpable temporal artery, episodes of homolateral blindness, and signs and symptoms of diffuse arteritis—e.g. fever, malaise, anemia, muscle aching and tenderness, and a very rapid sedimentation rate.

f. *Hypertension.* Your patient is normotensive and has no history of hypertension. But remember that even though headaches are more common in hypertensive persons, there is little or no correlation between blood pressure levels and the presence or severity of headache.

g. *Cervical osteoarthritis.* This disorder not uncommonly causes occipital headaches that radiate to one side or the other and are usually related to motion of the head and neck. They are more common in middle age and in the elderly.

From the easily obtainable data base you conclude the patient has vascular headaches—common migraine. The next step would be a prophylactic diagnostic and therapeutic trial with an ergot preparation. Since the pathophysiology of migraine invokes intracranial arterial dilatation plus humoral mechanisms, a vasoconstrictor and serotonin inhibitor is used for prevention. If this drug causes a diminution of severity and frequency of headaches, your conclusion will be further confirmed. But with any long-term follow-up, be alert for changes in pattern of symptoms or new symptoms which could herald new problems or hint that the original diagnosis may have been wrong. Remember that ergot preparations may have serious side effects and the patient will need careful supervision. A decision is made to reserve propranolol for future use if treatment is not effective.

DATA You discuss the entire situation with the patient, tell her your conclusions, and begin to explore some of the psychodynamics, when she suddenly asks: "Are you sure there's nothing wrong with my eyes or sinuses? My sister gets sinus headaches and my 58-year-old mother gets headaches when she reads."

LOGIC The patient seems reluctant to accept a psychophysiologic diagnosis. Perhaps she is properly skeptical. Many diseases of the special senses can cause headaches. But these are much less common than patients or many physicians believe.

Glaucoma or an error in refraction can cause ocular headaches. In the first instance, the fundi may show cupping of the disc and tonometry should be done. In the latter, headaches are brought on by strain of the muscles of accommodation during reading.

Sinus headaches are usually located near the involved sinus, though the pain may radiate to another part of the cranium. They occur mostly in the morning and are altered by head position, and evidence of sinus disease is present on examination, e.g. swollen turbinates, mucopurulent nasal discharge, tenderness over the sinus, and x-ray evidence of a fluid-filled sinus, sometimes with an air-fluid level.

Headaches from a tooth abscess or disease of the temporomandibular joint are easily detected by simple examination techniques.

You recall that specific foods may act as trigger mechanisms for migraine headaches and make a verbal note to ask the patient about such a possibility.

DATA On questioning her, you learn she has already been informed of this concept; she has kept a careful food diary and has been unable to correlate the headaches with any particular food.

To reassure both the patient and yourself, you recheck the fundi, test ocular tension with a tonometer, and check for visual acuity. Then you carefully inspect the inside of the nose, elicit no tenderness over the sinuses, and transilluminate them in a dark room. The patient opens her mouth, and you inspect and tap the teeth, look at the gums, and feel and listen over the temporomandibular joints. All of these maneuvers give normal results. So you again explain the diagnosis to the patient. She seems more reassured, but states: "My neighbor gets migraine headaches and they're not like mine."

LOGIC Your interpersonal skills are being further tested. Many patients with migraine are rigid, ambitious, perfectionistic, and have self-conflicts, frustrations, and anxieties. They need extra attention, care and patience.

You explain that there are three types of vascular headache. The one she has is *common migraine.*

In *classic migraine* (the type she hasn't), constriction of a cerebral vessel causes transient contralateral neurologic manifestations for approximately ½ hour before subsequent vasodilatation results in homolateral headache. The initial vasoconstriction may be associated with scintillating scotomata, flashing lights, shining spots, zigzag lines, geometric apparitions, nasal congestion, lacrimation, and transient oculomotor ophthalmoplegia, hemianesthesia, hemiplegia, or hemianopsia. About 15 to 30 minutes later, the vessel dilates and causes throbbing headache in the hemicranium (mi-graine) on the side of the vascular disturbance— usually opposite from the neurologic signs or symptoms. Systemic complaints such as nausea, vomiting, and diarrhea are common ("sick headaches"). Serotonin, catecholamines, 5-hydroxyindoleacetic acid, prostaglandins, kallikreins, and bradykinins may be implicated in the vascular episode, but their roles are not clear.

It is the frequently associated neurologic symptoms and signs that often stampede the physician into hunting for a nonexistent intracranial lesion or epilepsy. This is especially true when the postspasm headache is mild or hardly noticed. In rare instances the patient with classic migraine develops a stroke or is found to have an arteriovenous malformation.

In classic migraine, the headache is more often unilateral and briefer than in common migraine. Many times there is a childhood history of motion sickness and frequent nausea. In both types of migraine, the family history is usually positive and the incidence is greater in women.

DATA The patient is still not satisfied. She says her neighbor is a 45-year-old man, and his headaches are not like either of the migraines you described.

LOGIC You hypothesize that the man may have cluster headaches (Horton's headache, histamine cephalalgia)—the third type of vascular headache. These almost always occur in middle-aged men. The patient is suddenly awakened at night by severe supraorbital pain, eye pain, tearing, and nasal congestion. The pain is excruciating, but lasts only a short time—perhaps up to 2 hours—goes away, and returns the next night. It may recur for a few to many consecutive nights, and then not reappear for months to years. That is why it is called "cluster" headache.

DATA When this situation is explained to the patient, she realizes that her neighbor indeed has cluster headaches and not migraine. She is now convinced, and you begin preventive therapy.

LOGIC Fortunately for both of you, she did not ask you to rule out a brain tumor. You had already done so in your own mind, but had she inquired, you might have been tempted to practice "defensive medicine" and request a skull x-ray, electroencephalogram, radionuclide brain scan, computed tomography, or even cerebral angiography—against your better judgment.

You think about elusive "migraine equivalents" and are glad they do not exist in your patient. These consist of a variety of intermittent recurrent syndromes that are allegedly also manifestations of migraine. Included are episodic nausea, vomiting, diarrhea, and abdominal pain; periodic thoracic, pelvic, or extremity pain; bouts of fever; paroxysmal vertigo; and recurrent psychic equivalents, such as episodic confusion.

Try explaining these to a patient—or to yourself.

COMMENT This problem was reasonably easy to solve. The author tracked one key clue, considered all the possibilities, and then, on the basis of a careful history, arrived at a tentative solution. This probability was further confirmed by age, gender, and statistical likelihood. Recognition of the total migraine pattern helped too. Other possibilities were ruled out by historical and physical features which were pertinently negative or absent. No paraclinical tests were needed.

The same conclusion—common migraine—could have been reached by constructing a diagnostic tree or flow chart, asking some appropriate questions, and performing a few simple physical examination maneuvers. Examples of such decision points are: (*a*) Are the headaches constant or intermittent? (*b*) Is there nausea, photophobia, lacrimation, or throbbing? (*c*) Are there other neurologic symptoms? (*d*) Do the headaches occur on awakening, on reading, in the evening, or during sleep? (*e*) Describe the fundi and blood pressure. The answer to each question decides which branch to follow toward the answer. (*P. C.*)

PROBLEM-BASED LEARNING To understand all about headaches, you must have a broad knowledge of the conditions that may cause them. Even though the great majority are benign, you cannot afford to overlook the unusual instance where the problem is serious and potentially either fatal or curable.

Therefore you must learn all about:

1. relative prevalence of different types of headaches
2. muscle contraction-tension headaches
3. psychogenic factors related thereto
4. vascular headaches including classic migraine, common migraine, and cluster headaches
5. headaches related to cerebrovascular accidents (hemorrhage, thrombosis, embolus, subarachnoid hemorrhage) and the clinical pictures of these illnesses
6. how afflictions of the ears, eyes, nose, sinuses, teeth, and cervical spine cause headaches, and their associated clues
7. temporal arteritis (polymyalgia rheumatica)
8. posttraumatic headaches including subdural hematoma, its clinical characteristics and diagnosis, plus other less definite varieties of headache resulting from head trauma
9. manifestations of brain tumors and other expanding intracranial lesions
10. evidences for meningeal irritation or infection
11. ophthalmoscopic signs of glaucoma and increased intracranial pressure
12. how to test the visual fields and extraocular motions, perform tonometry, and indeed do a complete neurologic examination
13. technologic procedures used to diagnose intracranial disease
14. effects of analgesics, ergotamine preparations, and, in particular, methysergide.

Although such a broad base of knowledge is not needed for the management of most patients with headaches, better physicians (and students) know all that has just been stated. Their patients with tension headaches won't be given ergot preparations or β blockers, migraine patients won't have CT scans performed, and the rare brain tumor won't be overlooked.   (*P. C.*)

Suggested Readings

1. Adams RD, Victor M (eds): *Principles of Neurology*, ed 2. New York, McGraw-Hill, 1981, pp 117–131.
      All types of headache are described in detail.
2. Friedman AP: Headache. In Baker AB, Baker LH (eds): *Clinical Neurology*. Philadelphia, Harper & Row, 1984, Chapter 13.
      Fifty pages offer complete textbook coverage; the author is one of the world's experts on headache.
3. Farrell DF: Headache. In Swanson PD (ed): *Signs and Symptoms in Neurology*. Philadelphia, Lippincott, 1984, pp 211–230.
      An excellent concise description of tension, migraine, cluster, and all forms of headache.
4. Vijayan N, Watson C: Headaches. In Blacklow RS (ed): *MacBryde's Signs and Symptoms*, ed 6. Philadelphia, Lippincott, 1983, pp 61–84.
      Headaches are completely covered in this symptom-oriented textbook.
5. Follender AB: Chronic headache. A realistic approach to management. *Postgrad Med* 74:249–255, 1983.
      Migraine and cluster headaches are well described.
6. Ziegler DK: An overview of the classification, causes, and treatment of headache. *Hosp Community Psychiatry* 35:263–267, 1984.
      All headaches in one neat package.
7. Drummond PD, Lance JW: Clinical diagnosis and computer analysis of headache symptoms. *J Neurol Neurosurg Psychiatry* 47:128–133, 1984.
      The input from 600 patients was programmed into clearly defined diagnostic patterns.
8. Thompson JK, Adams HC: Psychophysiological characteristics of headache patients. *Pain* 18:41–52, 1984.
9. Martin MJ: Muscle contraction (tension) headaches. *Psychosomatics* 24:319–324, 1983.
      All about the most common cause of headache.
10. Bartleson JD: Transient and persistent neurological manifestations of migraine. *Stroke* 15:383–386, 1984.
      Some fascinating aspects of migraine.
11. Bollet AJ: Polymyalgia rheumatica and giant cell arteritis. *Conn Med* 47:743–748, 1983.
      Headache is a common initial symptom of this serious disease.

Case 56
Convulsions

PAUL CUTLER, M.D.

DATA   Just after finishing lunch, a 50-year-old unmarried woman suddenly became unconscious, fell to the floor, and was noted to be making severe jerking movements of her entire body. She was taken to the hospital by the emergency rescue squad.

LOGIC   Unless the patient has known idiopathic epilepsy, hospitalization is advised after sudden and unexpected loss of consciousness in an adult, especially when it is accompanied by seizure activity. Only rarely does a doctor observe the patient's seizure, and reliance must be placed on a description by others. The patient, however, may give evidence of a bitten tongue, a broken tooth, and incontinence. These are good indicators of what transpired. Such an episode may indicate the presence of a serious disease and can have a variety of causes:

1. Withdrawal from drugs (alcohol, sedatives, narcotics)
2. Effect of medication and toxins (excessive heroin, stimulants, lead, arsenic)
3. Transient insufficiency of cerebral blood flow (transient ischemic attacks, cardiac arrhythmias)
4. Appearance of an anatomic lesion in the intracranial cavity (tumor, abscess, hematoma, infarct, metastasis)
5. Biochemical derangement secondary to systemic disease (hypoglycemia, hypocalcemia, hyponatremia, uremia)
6. Idiopathic epilepsy
7. Infection (meningitis, encephalitis)
8. Previous head trauma.

Therefore, the first questions asked of the patient (or those close to the patient) are directed at these eight categories to see which is at fault so that proper early treatment and more definitive evaluation can proceed.

DATA The patient had been behaving normally prior to lunch and had been having a routine day up to that point. She had the reputation of being a very stable and healthy person. Her appetite was good. She was not known to be using any drugs—prescribed, over-the-counter, or illicit. Furthermore, she never smoked, drank only decaffeinated coffee, had alcoholic beverages sparingly on festive occasions, and had never in her life been observed to be intoxicated. There was no known incident of head trauma.

The shaking spell lasted 3 minutes, she was unresponsive for 15 minutes, and at the hospital 30 minutes later she was conversing normally and felt well. There had never been a similar episode.

LOGIC The technology of our times has produced a proliferation of substances which can affect brain function, and it produces them in such abundance that they are readily available. The stresses of our times have created a perceived need for such drugs. Alcohol may be taken daily to allay anxiety and produce euphoria. The dose may escalate to one or two fifths of liquor daily over the years. A sudden discontinuation can cause a seizure. Sedative drugs such as barbiturates, benzodiazepines, chloral hydrate, glutethimide, methaqualone, and opium derivatives act similarly when suddenly discontinued. Stimulants such as cocaine, ephedrine, methedrine, and the like can also cause convulsions when taken in excess. The patient's history negates any drug-related seizures.

A temporary reduction in blood flow can cause syncope, convulsions, or other neurologic manifestations. This possibility would be rendered more plausible if there were a history of palpitations immediately preceding the attack or if there were a background for cerebral arteriosclerosis as evidenced by hypertension, arterial bruits, or additional brain symptoms.

Other cardiovascular causes for cerebral ischemia include acute myocardial infarction, episodic complete heart block from various causes, extracranial vascular stenosis with transient ischemic attacks, atrial fibrillation, and mitral stenosis. Each of these conditions can cause temporary decreases in cerebral blood flow or cerebral emboli. A physical examination usually detects these problems.

The possibility of an intracranial anatomic lesion still exists and we need further data. A stroke is unlikely since everything returned to normal in short order. But the possibility of a space-taking lesion is still present. After 50 years of age, *cerebrovascular diseases and tumors*, either primary or metastatic, assume greater prevalence in the list of causes for seizures.

Medication and toxic substances like lead or arsenic usually cause behavioral changes much before the seizure, and their effects are present for a considerable time afterward. This patient's excellent condition both before and after the attack precludes these causes. Lead intoxication can cause an unexpected seizure in an adult, but it also causes wrist-drop, foot-drop, emotional changes, and anemia. Arsenic gives a characteristic picture too. The effects of toxic substances are usually widespread and produce a clinical template which should suggest the possibility to the clinician. But if the cause for a seizure is not discovered promptly, laboratory tests for common toxic substances in the blood and urine are necessary. In fact, these tests should be requested as soon as the patient is seen.

Idiopathic epilepsy begins in childhood, and its onset at 50 would be most unlikely. If present, the electroencephalogram (EEG) would be positive in over half the cases, and a family history is common. The EEG in the subset of *all* patients with idiopathic epilepsy is positive in 70% of cases during the interictal phase; it is almost always abnormal during a seizure. It is noteworthy that some patients who do not have epilepsy have falsely positive abnormal EEGs.

Seizures can come on within 2 years after head trauma but there is no such history here. Other causes must be sought.

DATA   In the emergency room a fresh bite mark was noted on her tongue, but there was no evidence of urinary or fecal incontinence. She had skipped breakfast that morning because she was too busy, but she had skipped meals on many previous occasions and never felt any ill effects. There were no preceding palpitations or cardiac awareness, but she did tell of a "funny feeling" in the epigastrium which "came up" (here she gestured with her hand to show an epigastric sensation rising up to the level of her throat), at which time she "blacked out." At the same time, "my foot began to shake" (. . . the right foot only!). She was amnesic for the next 30 minutes and does not recall the ride to the hospital.

LOGIC   Rapidly developing hypoglycemia can cause a seizure. This can occur from insulin administration, an insulin-secreting tumor, or an alcoholic binge. None is likely here. Insulinomas cause convulsions which are preceded by milder manifestations of hypoglycemia; these attacks come after a missed meal or during the night, not immediately after a meal. Reactive or functional hypoglycemia causes mild sympathomimetic and not cerebral manifestations. The patient describes what sounds like a preseizure aura, and shaking of the right foot sounds like a key clue.

Focal or partial seizures usually imply focal pathology such as tumor, scar, or vascular malformation. Generalized seizures are usually idiopathic, toxic, or metabolic. But since partial seizures can eventually march into generalized convulsions, it is important to inquire for evidence of a focal onset.

DATA   She recalled that her right foot was shaking at the onset of the seizure. As this question was pursued, she further related that she seems to have had a weak feeling in the right foot for 5 months, though it functioned quite well. Then it began to tremble occasionally and in the past 2 months she

had actually developed clonic motions of the foot and ankle (as she described them); during the same period she could not walk on the right foot as well as she felt she should. This was attributed to "neuralgia." Review of systems brought out the fact that she had been experiencing mild brief headaches recently; these were episodic, a little worse in the morning, but, as with the foot, she tended to ignore them.

LOGIC   An important aspect of gathering data about a seizure is the sequence of events leading up to it. In this instance, you can be suspicious about the part of the brain controlling the right foot. The seizures seem to originate in a focal area of the brain—the parasagittal area of the left frontal lobe's precentral gyrus. Transient ischemia with such localization is unlikely. Metastases would give a more progressive picture. Abscess is unlikely in the absence of a demonstrable source and it too would not be so chronic and stable. Meningitis and encephalitis are acute infectious diseases in which the patient is sick—not so here. A brain tumor looms high on the list of possibilities. It is estimated that 16 to 20% of adults who have their first seizure after the age of 35 will demonstrate a mass lesion.

DATA   The general physical examination was normal. In particular, there were no "running" ears, extracranial arterial bruits, evidences of meningeal irritation, or primary tumor sites (thyroid, breast, etc). The neurologic examination was entirely normal except for the right leg; there the reflexes were hyperactive and there was weakness of dorsiflexion of the toes and foot, faint ankle clonus, and a Babinski sign. There were no sensory disturbances. The head jolt test was moderately positive on both sides and she localized the sensation to the front of her head.

LOGIC   The findings tended to confirm what was already suspected from the history: an intracranial lesion over the foot area of the left motor cortex. Further study is indicated.

DATA   The skull x-rays were almost normal; there were no fractures or evidence of increased intracranial pressure. While there was no enlargement of venous channels or the middle meningeal artery channel, this is not always a reliable negative finding in patients with meningiomas, a common type of brain tumor. However, there was a faint hyperostosis in the parasagittal area where we now suspect an intracranial lesion to be.

Chest x-ray and ECG were normal. The fasting blood glucose, 5-hour glucose tolerance test, complete blood count, urinalysis, blood urea nitrogen, serum calcium and sodium, and antinuclear antibody test were normal or negative. The urine and blood tests were negative for toxic substances.

LOGIC   Hypoglycemia, hypocalcemia, hyponatremia, and uremia might already have been disregarded since each should have had an accompanying indicative clinical picture. Vasculitis and collagen disorders are unlikely too without added clues. The cerebrospinal fluid was not studied because a lumbar puncture is dangerous if a mass lesion is suspected.

Some of the studies already done and some that you are about to do are for confirmation purposes only, since you are now reasonably certain of the diagnosis. The faint hyperostosis seen on the skull films bolsters your conviction. Three studies are still under consideration: an EEG, cerebral arteriography, and a computed tomographic scan of the head. The EEG is done first; it is the least expensive and not invasive.

DATA   The EEG shows bursts of rhythmic sharp waves over the left frontal vertex. In this area there was suppression of normal β activity whereas a small amount of β activity was seen on the right hemisphere. When the patient hyperventilated on command, there was a focal increase of θ waves only over the left frontal vertex.

LOGIC   Disturbances of electrical activity over the cited area reinforce the impression of a lesion in the left motor strip.

DATA   Computed tomography demonstrated a 5- to 6-cm mass on the screen. It was solitary and there were no satellite lesions. By virtue of the shape, location, and history, it was thought to be a meningioma. An arteriogram was also done.

LOGIC   No doubt the meningeal tumor pressing on the motor cortex is the cause of the seizure. In retrospect, she had been having brief partial seizures of the right foot for at least 2 months but was stoic and did not seek medical advice. The arteriogram was done to assess the vascularity of the lesion, its major feeder, and draining vessels; this too demonstrated a blood supply typical for a meningioma.

DATA   Surgery and histologic study confirmed the diagnosis. The tumor was successfully removed. The patient has some residual weakness in the right foot, but still walks well and is free of seizures while using anticonvulsant medication.

COMMENT   A single key clue—a convulsive seizure—had to be fleshed out by the author as he elicited information from the complete history which the patient thought was not important or significant. These were the symptoms referable to the right foot.

But first he formed a list of possibilities and quickly eliminated the absurd, the impossible, and the improbable. Left with a cluster of a seizure and involvement of the upper motor neuron supply to the right foot, the diagnosis became fairly evident. The one hypothesis which was most likely, most serious, and for which most can be done was chosen and then proven by carefully selected studies.

Nowadays, a 50-year-old healthy woman with a single seizure has a CT brain scan done promptly. If positive for tumor, the problem is solved. If negative, you must proceed through the traditional diagnostic sequence described in this case. Even though the CT scan is expensive, it often supplies the answer quickly, avoids other studies, and is therefore cost- and time-efficient. (*P. C.*)

Test Your Judgment by matching each of the following 10 clinical pictures with a lettered diagnosis that *explains convulsions*. Name the *single diagnostic measure* needed to prove each situation.

Diagnoses

(a) meningitis   (f) cerebral ischemia
(b) insulinoma   (g) brain tumor
(c) metabolic acidosis   (h) stroke
(d) epilepsy   (i) subdural hematoma
(e) hyponatremia   (j) drug withdrawal

1. 24-year-old heavyweight boxer complains of severe headaches for 3 days and gradually lapses into stupor
2. 58-year-old woman with chronic insomnia, emotional problems, and frequent visits to different physicians
3. 22-year-old army recruit with sore throat, headache, and macular rash
4. 68-year-old man with diabetes and hypertension
5. obese patient with good appetite and weak sweaty spells
6. 52-year-old woman who had a mastectomy 1 year ago
7. 56-year-old man with recent acute myocardial infarction, whose pulse intermittently drops to 20/minute
8. 16-year-old girl with gingival hyperplasia and the same kind of spells her mother had
9. 56-year-old male who smokes heavily and has a chronic cough, muscle cramps, anorexia, nausea, and agitation
10. 42-year-old woman with polyarthritis, a facial rash, nausea, anorexia, and drowsiness.

ANSWERS

1. **(i).** Head injury and subdural hematoma are likely; CT scan is indicated.
2. **(j).** It is likely she takes sedation from different sources but ran out of medication and has drug withdrawal; a history should suffice.
3. **(a).** Meningococcal meningitis is seen in army recruit camps. The patient probably has evidence of meningeal irritation too. A lumbar puncture is indicated.
4. **(h).** The man's age and background make him a candidate for cerebral thrombosis which may have its onset with a convulsion. A neurologic examination may provide help.
5. **(b).** The picture suggests hypoglycemia from a β cell tumor. A fasting blood glucose and simultaneous insulin immunoassay should tell the tale.
6. **(g).** A brain metastasis is likely; a CT scan will detect it.
7. **(f).** Stokes-Adams attacks occur under these circumstances. An ECG offers proof and a pacemaker is needed.
8. **(d).** Idiopathic epilepsy is likely in view of the family history. The phenytoin she takes causes gingival hyperplasia. In 70% of cases the EEG is corroborative.
9. **(e).** Hyponatremia resulting from inappropriate antidiuretic hormone secretion is sug-

gested by the symptoms; an oat cell lung carcinoma is likely. Order a chest radiograph.
10. **(c).** The picture suggests systemic lupus erythematosus with an immune-complex glomerulopathy resulting in uremia. A positive antinuclear antibody test is expected; so is an elevated creatinine.

Note: In a few instances, the answer is justifiably debatable since your logic may properly provide a different diagnosis. Such disagreements were deliberately introduced to encourage you to think.

Suggested Readings

1. Foster FM, Booker HE. The epilepsies and convulsive disorders. In Baker AB, Baker LH (eds): *Clinical Neurology.* Philadelphia, Harper & Row, 1984, chap 31.
   This short chapter of an outstanding textbook covers all types of seizures.
2. Crill WE, Swanson PD: Seizures. In Swanson PD (ed): *Signs and Symptoms in Neurology.* Philadelphia, Lippincott, 1984, pp 26–30.
   A symptom analysis in only 5 pages.
3. Adams RD, Victor M (eds): *Principles of Neurology,* ed 2. New York, McGraw-Hill, 1981, pp 211–230.
   Epilepsy and its variants are detailed.
4. Leppik IE: Seizures and epilepsy. Understanding the mechanisms, achieving control. *Postgrad Med* 75:229–234, 1984.
   Much is packed into only 6 pages.
5. Delgado-Escueta AV, Treiman DM, Walsh GO: The treatable epilepsies (2 parts). *N Engl J Med* 308:1508–1514, 1576–1584, 1983.
   Describes the various types of epilepsy and their treatment.
6. Snead OC III: On the sacred disease: the neurochemistry of epilepsy. *Int Rev Neurobiol* 24:93–130, 1983.
   Explores the role of neurotransmitters in a disease called "sacred" by Hippocrates and which afflicted many famous people.
7. Voskuil PH: The epilepsy of Fyodor Mikhailovitch Dostoevsky (1821–1881). *Epilepsia* 24:658–667, 1983.
   A beautifully written paper that interlaces the clinical features of the illness with the life of a famous novelist who had the disorder.
8. Schomer DL: Current concepts in neurology. Partial epilepsy. *N Engl J Med* 309:536–539, 1983.
9. Prescott JE, Johnson JE, Dice WH: Polyarteritis nodosa presenting as seizures. *Ann Emerg Med* 12:642–644, 1983.
10. Russo LS Jr, Goldstein KH: The diagnostic assessment of single seizures. Is cranial computed tomography necessary? *Arch Neurol* 40:744–746, 1983.
    The conclusion of this story is a surprise.
11. Spencer DD, Spencer SS, Mattson RH, et al: Intracerebral masses in patients with intractable partial epilepsy. *Neurology (NY)* 34:432–436, 1984.
    Twenty-five to 40% of patients had brain tumors in this series.
12. Gupta K: Epilepsy in the elderly. How far to investigate? *Br J Clin Pract* 37:249–252, 1983.
    This study is at odds with the previous one.

Case 57
Dizziness
PAUL CUTLER, M.D.

DATA   Leaning on her daughter, a 64-year-old woman totters into your office and tells you she has been troubled with recurrent episodes of "severe dizziness." When these occur, the room suddenly seems to spin around, and she must hold onto things to steady herself. She feels as if she is about to be "thrown to the floor" and on occasion the ground seems to rise up or suddenly quiver. The sensations are terribly unpleasant and frightening and are sometimes accompanied by nausea and vomiting; she must lie down for several hours or more until they pass away. Such an episode is just subsiding and she wants you to see her during one. Another physician told her she had "hardening of the arteries," but she is not satisfied with this diagnosis.

LOGIC   There are three principal questions to be resolved: Is this truly vertigo? Where is the lesion? What is causing it?

Vertigo is defined as a hallucination of movement of the surroundings or the person himself. It must be distinguished from light-headedness, confusion, absence seizures and partial complex seizures, feelings of unreality, presyncope or syncope, and incoordination and loss of position sense, for each of these symptoms conjures up a different list of diagnostic possibilities. For example, loss of position sense can be caused by posterior column disease or peripheral neuropathy wherein movements are incoordinated and the patient feels unsteady, but vertigo is not present. Lightheaded feelings or presyncope may occur in the cardiac patient with transient decreases in cardiac output. And nonspecific gait disturbances that can be confused with vertigo are common in the elderly. By description, the proposita does have true vertigo.

It is more difficult to locate this lesion because vertigo can be caused by diseases of the middle ear, inner ear, eighth nerve, vestibular nuclei, cerebellum, forebrain, eyes, or arteries. Each anatomic site can be afflicted with a variety of illnesses (Table 23.1).

Each of these lesions has its own special characteristics. To locate the site and determine the cause, it is often helpful to know whether the vertigo occurred once or many times, whether it is continuous or intermittent, and whether it is accompanied by headaches, nausea and vomiting, hearing loss and tinnitus, nystagmus, or other neurologic defects.

Before proceeding, a brief sketch of some diagnostic possibilities is in order:

Benign positional vertigo is extremely common; it lasts 1 to 5 minutes and is associated with changes in position. But momentary 1-second episodes of dizziness on bending over or straightening up occur in many people and are meaningless.

Vestibular neuronitis is suggested by several episodes of vertigo, each lasting about 1 week, recurring over a period of a year, unaccompanied by other symptoms, and allegedly caused by a virus. This entity is a common cause of vertigo.

Sudden complete unilateral deafness plus vertigo suggests an *acute labyrinthitis* of bacterial, viral, or vaso-occlusive origin. This is uncommon.

Disabling positional vertigo is a newly described entity. It occurs when the patient is up and about, and, as the name implies, it is quite incapacitating. No causes can be found. In such instances, the problem is thought to arise from compression of the eighth cranial nerve by arteries or veins, and microsurgical decompression is curative. But wait a few more years before final judgment is passed on this newly described disease and its cure.

In elderly patients, think especially about vascular disease, tumors, transient decreases

Table 23.1.
Causes of Vertigo Classified by Anatomic Site and Lesion

Site	Lesion
Middle ear	Suppurative otitis Cholesteatoma
Labyrinth	Acute vestibular neuronitis Benign positional vertigo Ménière's disease Acute labrinthitis
Eighth nerve	Acoustic neuroma Drugs (quinine, quinidine, salicylates, aminoglycosides) Disabling positional vertigo
Vestibular nuclei	Tumor, stroke, ischemia, multiple sclerosis
Cerebellum	Tumors or vascular lesions with associated vestibular nuclei involvement
Forebrain	Certain tumors, migraine, epilepsy (especially in the temporal lobe), psychogenic causes
Eyes	Ocular nerve palsy, adjusting to bifocals
Arteries	Vertebrobasilar transient ischemic attacks (TIAs)

in cardiac output, anemia, and medications. Seemingly trivial items such as slow adaptation to new shoes, new eyeglasses, or a new cane may cause disturbances in equilibrium which the patient equates with dizziness. Sedatives and hypnotics such as phenobarbital and diazepam may cause sensations that may also be interpreted as dizziness.

Vertebrobasilar ischemia should be suspected when episodes of dizziness occur in conjunction with diplopia, dysarthria, dysphagia, "drop attacks," or transient focal motor or sensory loss.

DATA The symptoms have been present for a month. They seem to develop suddenly, last from minutes to hours, and then subside. On at least one occasion, the patient's speech was transiently slurred. She

has had no aural discharge, headaches, seizures, blackouts, visual changes, impairment of hearing, tinnitus, weakness, or paresthesias. In fact she emphasizes that she felt absolutely well prior to 1 month ago, and she takes no medications.

LOGIC One positive and several negative clues may be helpful. Slurred speech suggests the possibility of a transient lesion in the brain stem involving the motor nerves as well as the vestibular nuclei. Ménière's disease is characterized by recurrent bouts of vertigo in a patient who already has impaired hearing and tinnitus; the absence of the latter two are strong points against this diagnosis. An acoustic neuroma (cerebellopontine angle tumor) is unlikely without associated hearing loss. The absence of headaches, seizures, and aural discharge is against migraine, epilepsy, and ear infection. Multiple sclerosis is unlikely without evidence of demyelination in other areas of the brain too, but sometimes dizziness may be the first and solitary manifestation.

DATA Past history is positive for intermittent hypertension which is not currently being treated. At age 14 she had a minor concussion following a fall from her father's ice wagon, and she had a hysterectomy 20 years ago. The family history is not remarkable and on eliciting a systems review, she gives a history of transient episodes of bilateral leg weakness in the past 6 months. She attributed this to her age. These short spells nearly resulted in falls, but the patient always regained strength immediately.

LOGIC The hypertension may be meaningful in that it hastens cerebrovascular disease. Too much time has elapsed for the childhood concussion to relate to the vertigo. But the spells she describes are alarming and could result from transient ischemia in the posterior circulation.

DATA Before beginning the history you checked her for nystagmus; it was present then but seems to be subsiding now. In fact, she is feeling much better. The entire physical and neurologic examinations are normal except for the blood pressure which is 180/ 100 in both arms. There is no cerumen in the auditory canals, the eardrums are normal, hearing is normal, and there are normal responses to the Weber and Rinne tests. The Romberg test is negative with both open and shut eyes; rapid alternating movements, tandem gait, finger-to-nose, and heel-to-shin tests are normal. No bruits are heard in the carotid, supraclavicular, or occipital regions, and the carotid pulses are equal and full. The heart is not enlarged and exhibits no murmurs or abnormal rhythm. There is no dysarthria, dysphonia, or cranial nerve palsies. Peripheral sensation, reflexes, and motor function are normal.

LOGIC Nystagmus is seen with many forms of vertigo and is only slightly discriminatory. It may result from lesions of the inner ear, vestibular nerve, brain stem, or cerebellum. There are many kinds of nystagmus—jerky, pendular, end-position, oblique, rotatory, vertical, horizontal, and positional; each has different significance in locating the lesion and identifying the cause. An analysis of this subject is too detailed for this book. But it is good to remember that not all nystagmus is pathologic; end-position horizontal nonsustained nystagmus is usually a normal finding.

The absence of bruits is against significant extracranial cerebrovascular disease. No neurologic deficit was noted in the brain stem. Normal cerebellar function and position and vibration sense are against disease in the cerebellum and posterior columns; these cause dysequilibrium rather than vertigo anyway. Equal blood pressure in both arms and the absence of a supraclavicular bruit are against the subclavian steal syndrome, a form of transient ischemia in the vertebrobasilar system.

DATA Because the diagnosis is uncertain and serious possibilities exist, the patient is admitted to the hospital. Complete blood count, 18-test chemistry profile, Venereal Disease Research Laboratory test, urinalysis, chest x-ray, and ECG are normal. A 24-hour

Holter monitor is applied and no arrhythmias are found. A skull x-ray with special Stenver's view to delineate the internal auditory canals is negative. The electroencephalogram (EEG) shows minor background slowing which is not believed to be significant; no paroxysmal features are seen. Computed tomographic (CT) scan is normal. A lumbar puncture reveals normal cerebrospinal fluid including a normal protein electrophoresis.

LOGIC The Holter monitor results are against paroxysmal cardiac arrhythmias that might cause transient cerebral ischemia. Normal spinal fluid protein is against multiple sclerosis. A normal CT scan is very strong evidence against an intracranial neoplasm. The CT scan probably makes both the skull x-ray and the isotope scan obsolete in cases of this sort because it is far more reliable. You might also question the need for a lumbar puncture.

Since several features point to transient ischemic attacks resulting from arteriosclerosis and marked insufficiency in the posterior cerebral circulation, arteriography is scheduled for the next day.

DATA Two hours before the scheduled test, the patient complains of dizziness and difficulty with speaking and swallowing. Examination reveals a marked change. There is now right and left gaze nystagmus and slight upward nystagmus as well. She has uncontrollable hiccups. The right pupil is constricted. Pinprick is poorly appreciated in the right lower face, while it is not perceived in the left arm and leg. Yet the strength and reflexes are normal and plantar response is bilaterally flexor. Gait is slightly ataxic and the patient sways from side to side on Romberg testing without falling in either direction

LOGIC These findings are typical of sudden involvement of the lateral portion of the right side of the medulla and signify vascular occlusion of the right posterior inferior cerebellar artery (Wallenberg's syndrome). The descending fibers of the fifth nerve nucleus, the vestibular nuclei, cerebellar tracts, and motor nerves originating in the medulla have been affected on the side of the lesion. Also, involvement of descending sympathetic fibers is causing a homolateral Horner's syndrome. There is damage to the spinal lemniscus which has already crossed over, thus giving sensory impairment on the contralateral half of the body.

A brain stem stroke has occured. You may now surmise that the episodes of vertigo, attacks of weakness ("drop attacks"), and incidents of slurred speech were the results of transient ischemia in the posterior circulation.

DATA   An arteriogram shows 50% occlusion of the basilar and left vertebral arteries with 100% occlusion of the right posterior inferior cerebellar artery—as expected. Occlusion of a vertebral artery may produce a similar picture.

LOGIC   Periods of transient ischemia preceded the eventual infarction of the lateral medulla. The degree of neurologic deficit and the prognosis depend in some measure on the amount of collateral circulation shunted to the affected area by the anterior cerebral circulation via the circle of Willis.

It is imperative to point out that vascular disease is not the most common cause of vertigo, even in the elderly. Primary vestibular dysfunction (neuronitis) is far more common. While relatively benign, its symptoms are very severe, the cause is unknown, and no other neurologic deficits are present. Ménière's disease is common too. And in the twenties, thirties, and forties, think also in terms of multiple sclerosis, but, in that event look for evidence of associated neurologic lesions.

COMMENT   Vertigo is a common key clue. As with many neurologic diseases or symptoms, the first task is to locate the lesion by associated clues. The second is to determine the pathology by more clues and further studies.

The specificity and sensitivity of diagnostic studies and the importance of age as a factor in the logical process are many times woven into the discussion.

While a complete data base was obtained, the author clearly had two principal provisional hypotheses: a medullary lesion and vestibular neuronitis. He leaned toward the former because of the possible existence of other symptoms of medullary origin (slurred speech). But with the large number of other possibilities, he chose to gather a complete data base rather than pursue individual hypotheses separately. It was wise to do so, since he discovered a very important clue in the systems review: imminent "drop attacks."

You may justifiably question the wisdom of the diagnostic procedural sequence in this case. Episodic vertigo, an episode of slurred speech, and several imminent "drop attacks" suggest a vascular lesion in the posterior cerebral circulation that is threatening to occlude completely. Under these circumstances, a Holter monitor, skull x-ray, EEG, and CT scan are considered superfluous by most clinicians. An arteriogram performed at the preocclusive stage may also be considered askance. It is risky and its results may not appreciably alter management. If a threatening vascular lesion *is* found by arteriography, or if the clinical picture suggests its existence, anticoagulants or anti-platelet-aggregation agents may be used; however, their efficacy is under scrutiny, especially in women.

Certainly the wisdom of doing a post-stroke arteriogram (as was done in this case) is highly questionable. The diagnosis was already established, and the procedure, expensive and dangerous under the circumstances, gave no additional useful information.

In fact, in almost all cases of vertigo, biochemical tests, EEG, radionuclide scans, CT scans, and angiography are either of no help or only rarely of value. The CT scan has its prime value if a cerebellopontine angle tumor is suspected. But remember that only 10% of those with acoustic neuromas have vertigo; their hallmarks are usually deafness and tinnitus.

In most cases the primary care physician can identify the cause for vertigo. Anxiety, vestibular neuronitis, benign postural vertigo, drug toxicity, Ménière's disease, etc are easily diagnosed. But in doubtful or possibly serious cases electronystagmography (including caloric stimulation) and audiometric tests are indicated. It may be wise to refer the dizzy patient to an otoneurologist if the diagnosis is in doubt, if there is need for further tests, or if there is suspicion of tumor or impending stroke.   (*P. C.*)

Suggested Readings

1. Ruff RL: Vestibular disturbances. In Swanson PD (ed): *Signs and Symptoms in Neurology.* Philadelphia, Lippincott, 1984, pp 119–131.
   A textbook coverage of vertigo.
2. Adams RD, Victor M (eds): *Principles of Neurology*, ed 2. New York, McGraw-Hill, 1981, pp 200–

207.
   A symptom analysis of dizziness and vertigo.
3. Weiss AD: Vertigo and dizziness—disorders of static and dynamic equilibrium. In Blacklow RS (ed): *MacBryde's Signs and Symptoms*, ed 6. Philadelphia, Lippincott, 1983, pp 707–724.
   The underlying neuropathology and all causes of vertigo and their closely related features are presented in an orderly logical manner.
4. Hybels RL: History taking in dizziness. The most important diagnostic step. *Postgrad Med* 75:41–43, 1984.
   Demonstrates that talking to the patient is more important than technology.
5. Davis LE, Johnsson L: Viral infections of the inner ear: clinical virologic and pathologic studies in humans and animals. *Am J Otolaryngol* 4:347–362, 1983.
   A well-done study that sheds light on a misunderstood subject.
6. Vonofakos D, Marcu H, Hacker H: CT diagnosis of basilar artery occlusion. *AJNR* 4:525–528, 1983.
   Shows how this diagnosis can be confirmed if suspected; pertinent to this case study.

7. Kerr AG: A symptomatic approach to vertigo. *J Laryngol Otol* 97:813–815, 1983.
   A laconic yet good description.
8. Hart RG, Gardner DP, Howieson J: Acoustic tumors: atypical features and recent diagnostic tests. *Neurology (NY)* 33:211–221, 1983.
9. Cashman MZ, Rossman RN, Nedzelski JM: Cerebellopontine angle lesions: an audiological test protocol. *J Otolaryngol* 12:180–186, 1983.
   A not-to-be forgotten cause of vertigo.
10. Curtin HD: CT of acoustic neuroma and other tumors of the ear. *Radiol Clin North Am* 22:77–105, 1984.
   An excellent demonstration of the value of CT scans.
11. Rogers JH: Romberg and his test. *J Laryngol Otol* 94:1401–1404, 1980.
   This 140-year-old test is more accurately described and its significance established; dispels confusion that exists today.
12. Jannetta PJ, Moller MB, Moller AR: Disabling positional vertigo. *N Engl J Med* 310:1700–1705, 1984.
   A new clinical entity is described.

Case 58
Paralysis
PAUL CUTLER, M.D.

DATA   Over a period of 48 hours, a 68-year-old right-handed woman gradually developed paralysis of the left side of her face and her left arm and leg. The arm, face, and leg became weak and then paralyzed in that order.

She was brought to the hospital where she was found to have left-sided hyperreflexia, a Babinski sign, and inability to move her left arm, leg, and the lower two-thirds of her face. There was no loss of consciousness or disturbance in sensation, and the other cranial nerves were intact. Speech was preserved.

LOGIC   This appears to be a "garden variety" stroke of the lacunar type involving the right lenticulostriate artery which supplies the corticobulbar and corticospinal tracts in the internal capsule. Since only the lower part of the face, arm, and leg (and sometimes the tongue) have unicortical innervation, the classical picture is as presented.

One feature of the stroke is disturbing. It evolved slowly. While the odds still favor a cerebral thrombosis, the slow evolution persuades you to consider other possibilities such as brain tumor, abscess, metastasis, or hematoma. Furthermore, a stroke can be caused by thrombosis, hemorrhage, or embolus, for which treatment may vary.

DATA   Additional history revealed a draining left middle ear infection for 20 years, treated hypertension for 15 years, diabetes mellitus controlled by diet for 10 years, recent trouble with an irregular heartbeat, and a mastectomy 2 years ago. She smokes 30 cigarettes daily and has a chronic cough which is often productive of purulent sputum. The rest of the systems review, family history, and patient profile added nothing significant.

LOGIC   The additional history raises many possibilities. Chronic suppurative otitis media is a good source for a brain abscess. So are the bronchitis and bronchiectasis which she may very well have. Hypertension and diabetes accelerate cerebrovascular disease and may predispose to thrombosis, and hypertension can certainly cause a cerebral hemorrhage. The irregular heartbeat makes you consider a cerebral embolus from a clot in the heart. Both the chronic cough and the mastectomy raise the specter of a metastatic brain lesion from the lung or breast. This case may not be so simple as it first appeared.

It is important to remember that a stroke may evolve slowly as this one did, and that, although present for a while, a space-taking lesion may suddenly give symptoms by occluding an adjacent vessel or developing bleeding within itself. However, if a neurologic picture appears very slowly, an expanding lesion must be your prime consideration, especially if the picture seems to involve only one location in the brain. Strokes usually appear suddenly, as their name implies.

However, special terms are often applied to their clinical course. A *transient ischemic attack* (TIA) represents an acute neurologic deficit that clears completely in 24 hours. A *reversible ischemic neurologic deficit* (RIND) clears fully in 3 weeks. A *stroke in evolution* develops in a stuttering slow mode over a period of hours rather than minutes or seconds. A *stroke* represents the acute onset of a neurologic deficit that is vascular in origin and clears very slowly if at all.

DATA Physical examination shows a conscious alert apprehensive patient. The vital signs are T 37 C, R 18, P 106 and irregular, BP 190/110 in both arms. There is a purulent discharge from the right ear. No bruits are heard in the neck and no attempt is made to feel the carotid arteries. The fundi show grade 2 hypertensive and arteriosclerotic changes. A right radical mastectomy scar is noted, but there are no nodes or masses palpable anywhere in the axillae, scar, other breast, or supraclavicular areas. There are coarse inspiratory rales and fine expiratory wheezes at both lung bases. The apex beat is strong and displaced downward and to the left. There are no murmurs or

gallops, but the apical rate is irregularly irregular and there is a pulse deficit of 12 beats/minute. The fingers show beginning clubbing, but the rest of the examination is normal.

LOGIC Additional diseases are present. The patient has otitis media with chronic ear drainage; probable bronchiectasis based on the history, rales, wheezes, and clubbing; and hypertensive cardiovascular disease with atrial fibrillation. There is no evidence of recurrent cancer. Each of these problems could relate to her stroke. While there is no history of trauma, subdural hematoma is a possibility to be reckoned with.

Hematomas generally cause headache and disturbed sensorium prior to or coincident with paralysis. Fever and leukocytosis accompany brain abscess 50% of the times.

In order to assess the situation immediately, a CT brain scan is ordered. This procedure will visualize a tumor, abscess, or subdural hematoma if present. If, on the other hand, the CT brain scan shows no mass lesion, then a vascular episode must exist. Under the latter circumstance, the scan shows evidence of hemorrhage but it may be too soon for cerebral infarction, whether caused by embolus or thrombosis, to be apparent.

DATA A CT scan is performed with dye enhancement. It is normal. Or almost normal! While there is no indication of a mass lesion and the pineal gland is in the midline, the radiologist reports a small lucent area in the left cerebrum. This is not compatible with the clinical picture, but a repeat study in the near future is suggested.

The chest x-ray shows cardiac enlargement and a few questionably enlarged nodes in the left hilum, but it is otherwise normal. A complete blood count, urinalysis, and 18-test blood chemistry profile are all normal except for a blood glucose of 190 mg/dl. The ECG shows left ventricular hypertrophy and atrial fibrillation.

LOGIC Although the neurologic picture unfolded slowly, there is no mass lesion present. The blood glucose is in keeping with the history of diabetes mellitus and the ECG abnormalities result from long-standing hypertension. Atrial fibrillation concerns you, for it raises the possibility of cerebral embolization which may recur. But the clinical picture overwhelmingly suggests cerebral thrombosis, so, for this reason and because of the hypertension, you decide against the use of anticoagulants.

The questionably enlarged hilar nodes and the seemingly inconsequential finding noted on the CT scan are put on the back burner for a few days. These studies will be repeated later. You elect not to do a lumbar puncture since the only reason for doing so is if hemorrhage or meningitis is suspected—not the case here. Furthermore, there is no need for an isotope scan, electroencephalogram, or cerebral arteriography. The picture seems clear-cut except for some questionable abnormalities noted on radiography.

As for vascular accidents, thrombosis is more common than other causes and tends to give the clinical picture seen in this patient. Recent figures show that the approximate incidence of thrombosis:embolus:hemorrhage is 3:1:1. Hemorrhages are usually more severe, more devastating, and more progressive; often the patient is unconscious. In recent years, emboli have been recognized to be much more common than was once thought. There is often indecision about whether the stroke is caused by thrombosis or embolus—an important distinction upon which treatment choices are based.

Atheroma formation and sclerosis with ulceration and partial obstruction occur at the bifurcation of the common carotid artery, the origin of the internal carotid artery, the carotid siphon, and the origins of the anterior and middle cerebral arteries—especially in atheroma-prone individuals. It is notable that in patients with cerebral thrombosis 60% have hypertension, 25% have diabetes mellitus, and 50% have clinically evident vascular disease elsewhere (heart or legs).

Patients with cerebral thrombosis often have minor prodromes. If severe narrowing already exists, an infarct may be precipitated by thrombosis at the atheroma site, an embolus, or a low flow state, especially if there is associated poor collateralization around the circle of Willis. A low flow state may be caused by a decreased cardiac output, a more proximal arterial narrowing, a drop in blood pressure, sleep, or certain body or neck positions.

In fact, sclerosis, thrombosis, emboli, low flow, and inadequate collateral circulation frequently seem to perform in concert to produce strokes or TIAs. It is often difficult to decide which is the prime cause of the cerebral infarct.

Emboli strike like a bolt out of the blue. They originate in more proximal atherosclerotic lesions, primarily the internal carotid artery, or in the heart. If an embolus is suspected because of sudden onset and the absence of atherogenesis accelerators, search the heart for atrial fibrillation, mitral stenosis, mitral prolapse, recent myocardial infarction, and infective endocarditis. The site of lodgment of the embolus varies with the size of the embolus and determines the neurologic picture. A large embolus may land in the internal carotid artery, a smaller one strike the middle cerebral, and one as small as 2 mm end in a tiny artery and result only in a TIA.

TIAs are common. They probably result from microemboli composed of fibrin and platelets; these are formed on the ragged intima of stenotic carotid arteries. The transient neurologic picture they cause depends on where they land. TIAs recurring in the same area of the brain are probably the precursors of a cerebral thrombosis at an atheroma site. If the TIAs occur in different parts of the brain they are almost certainly caused by multiple emboli originating outside the brain. This makes sense!

Be aware that TIAs herald strokes. But the incidence of subsequent stroke is not so high as you might think. A single TIA may not recur, or it may recur infrequently or frequently. The stroke rate is 4 to 8%/year, perhaps higher.

Lacunar infarcts are tiny localized areas

of infarction resulting from the occlusion (thrombosis or embolus) of small perforating arteries. These produce specific neurologic pictures that reveal the location of the lacuna. These may also be preceded by TIAs.

DATA The patient is digitalized to slow the ventricular rate. Antihypertensive medication is altered. Supportive treatment is given and the diabetes is controlled. By day 3, the patient is able to move her big toe and seems to have improved slightly.

LOGIC Her slight improvement is gratifying. But there are still one or two doubts in your mind that were planted by the radiographic reports.

DATA A repeat CT scan again shows no evidence of a mass lesion or hemorrhage, but it does show an area of decreased density approximating the location of the internal capsule in the right cerebral hemisphere. This area is enhanced by dye and has the appearance of an infarct. The distinction between thrombosis and embolus cannot be made. Furthermore, the small questionable lucent area noted on the left side is no longer evident.

The chest x-ray is also repeated, and this time the patient is more cooperative. Hilar nodes are not enlarged.

After detailed instructions to the family, the patient is sent home to recover.

LOGIC You are completely satisfied with the diagnosis of cerebral thrombosis—your first and most likely consideration. Note that a CT scan may show nothing for 48 hours; thereafter it becomes positive for infarction. Nuclear magnetic resonance and positron emission tomography show the infarct much earlier, but these procedures are not yet widely available. Note how the CT scan made it possible to be certain, exclude other possibilities, omit other studies, decrease hospital stay, and cut overall costs. The two questionable radiographic abnormalities were somewhat counterproductive in this regard; they were misleading bits of false positive information.

DATA At home, over the next 10 days, gradual improvement is noted. Ambulation and physiotherapy have been started. You impress your patient with the need to give up cigarettes, adhere to her diet, and continue with her antihypertensive medication. Though you do not suspect an embolus, you are not absolutely certain, so the patient is advised to take dipyridamole too.

LOGIC Your reservations arise from the presence of atrial fibrillation. If a cervical bruit were present too, there would be yet more concern for embolization. The entire romance of bruits, carotid stenosis, emboli, and their treatment with medication or surgery has not yet been written.

It is a fascinating story about which much has recently been published. A bruit in the area of the carotid bifurcation, especially if accompanied by a palpable thrill, indicates significant (50 to 90%) diametric narrowing. If this is an asymptomatic physical finding, treatment is not necessary. If it is found in association with a TIA, a problem exists.

Numerous questions would arise. Is the carotid artery the source of an embolus? How much occlusion exists? What is the risk of subsequent stroke? Can platelet-aggregation inhibitors prevent emboli? Does a surgical endarterectomy prevent stroke? And at what risk? Does stenosis recur?

Most of these questions are still unanswered, though many multi-institutional cooperative studies are in progress. The data bank still has insufficient data. But the degree of stenosis and the impairment of cerebral blood flow can be measured. Noninvasive techniques offer only limited resolution; these include ophthalmodynamometry, oculoplethysmography, quantitative phonoangiography, Doppler studies, and ultrasound. Invasive studies are more accurate and give better definition; these include digital subtraction angiography and aortic arch arteriography. The latter procedure is still considered to be the gold standard test that clearly defines the carotid artery defect, pictures the circle of Willis, and assesses the cerebral circulation.

If emboli are suspected, yet the carotid arteries are normal, ultrasound may detect silent mitral stenosis, mitral valve prolapse, or clots adherent to the valves or endocardium. You can see that an individualized diagnostic protocol and a unique decision tree must be constructed for each patient.

Problem List

1. Cerebral thrombosis
2. Essential hypertension
3. Diabetes mellitus
4. Chronic suppurative otitis media
5. Chronic bronchitis
6. Hypertensive cardiovascular disease
7. Atrial fibrillation
8. Status postmastectomy
9. Cigarette abuse.

QUESTIONS

1. Suppose the patient in this case study was noted to be still sick on day 5. The neurologic picture is the same, her sensorium is clouded, the temperature is 38.7 C, and respirations are 28/minute. You should:
   (a) start antibiotics
   (b) request cerebral arteriography
   (c) examine the chest and repeat the chest x-ray
   (d) request blood and urine cultures.
2. On Thursday, 5 days after the big football game, the star halfback develops a gradually worsening, persistent headache in the left hemicranium. Neurologic examination is negative. The best thing to do is:
   (a) watch him carefully
   (b) lumbar puncture
   (c) arteriography
   (d) CT.
3. A 62-year-old man is admitted to the hospital with the sudden onset of paralysis of the right arm and leg. Reflexes confirm a corticospinal tract lesion. But he also has paralysis of the entire left side of his face (cannot wrinkle his forehead or blow out his left cheek, and the left corner of his mouth droops). There are no other abnormalities noted. The diagnosis is:
   (a) cortical infarction on both sides
   (b) pontine infarction on the left side
   (c) internal capsule infarction on the left side
   (d) internal capsule infarction on the left side plus an old facial palsy on the right side.
4. A 28-year-old patient complains of sudden paralysis of both legs. There are no other symptoms. Neurologic examination is normal. Reflexes are equal, there are no patho-

logic reflexes, and sensation is intact, but the legs are limp. The patient has:
(a) infectious polyneuritis
(b) thrombosis of an artery supplying the spinal cord
(c) multiple sclerosis
(d) hysteria.

ANSWERS

1. **(c) and (d) are correct.** Pneumonia or urinary tract infection is likely in sick bedridden patients such as this. Depending on the probable site of infection, the immediate institution of appropriate antibiotics might be considered a correct action too. Arteriography would be worthless.
2. **(d) is correct.** It has the highest specificity and sensitivity for a suspected subdural hematoma. To watch him might be dangerous since brain damage can result. A lumbar puncture is neither specific nor sensitive for this diagnosis, and it may be harmful. Arteriography is an excellent test, but it is invasive, bears risk, and is costly. Though expensive, tomography will tell you what you need to know at little risk and it will be less costly in the long run.
3. **(b) and (d) are correct.** Bicortical infarcts are statistically unlikely; moreover, both sides of the face would be involved. (c) would affect the right lower two-thirds of the face. An infarct in the pons could catch the uncrossed corticospinal tract and the emerging fibers of the seventh cranial nerve (crossed paralysis). Also, be aware that the facial palsy may be old and the thrombosis new. Note how (b) locates the lesion by noting where the longitudinal disease site crosses the vertical disease site—a fine example of topical diagnosis.
4. **(d) is correct.** (a) tends not to appear so abruptly, often has accompanying sensory symptoms, and has diminished-to-absent reflexes. The blood supply to the spinal cord is not such as to selectively affect only the upper motor neurons to the legs; even if it were, the reflexes would be hyperactive, and Babinski signs would be present. Multiple sclerosis can concurrently involve any areas of the nervous system, but if the nerve supply to both legs were involved in the spinal cord, hyperreflexia would exist. Inquiry into the psychodynamics is indicated.

   It is important to remember that true paralysis or weakness can result from lesions in the long motor pathway, lower motor neuron, nerve root, peripheral nerve, myoneural junction, or muscle.

COMMENT   This patient started with what looked like a common type of stroke and ended by being diagnosed so. But there were many distracting clues which turned out to be unrelated to the diagnosis, even though they might well have been connected. The running ear, breast cancer, chronic bronchitis, slow onset of symptoms, and atrial fibrillation were all irrelevant but this had to be proven. Bayes is your consultant, and he tells you that cerebral thrombosis is the most likely cause of hemiplegia in a bruitless elderly person who has diabetes and hypertension—atrial fibrillation notwithstanding. (*P. C.*)

Suggested Readings

1. Harrison MJJ, Dyken ML (eds): *Cerebral Vascular Disease.* London, Butterworth, 1983.
    This textbook is totally devoted to the subject of this case. It has the following very relevant chapters:
    (a) Mitchell JRA: Hypertension and stroke, pp 46–66.
    (b) Dyken ML: Natural history of ischemic stroke, pp 139–170.
    (c) Harrison MJJ: Thromboembolism, pp 171–195.
    (d) Harrison MJJ: Angiography and CT scanning, pp 196–214.
    (e) Ginsberg MD, Cebul RD: Noninvasive diagnosis of carotid artery disease, pp 215–253.
2. Toole JF, Cole C: Ischemic cerebrovascular disease. In Baker AB, Baker LH (eds): *Clinical Neurology.* Philadelphia, Harper & Row, 1984.
    This huge very important subject is detailed in 51 pages.
3. Kistler JP, Ropper AH, Heros RC: Medical progress. The therapy of ischemic cerebral vascular disease due to atherothrombosis (2 parts). *N Engl J Med* 311:27–33, 100–105, 1984.
    These two articles in consecutive issues present the latest information on strokes of all kinds—risk factors, pathophysiology, anatomy, embolism, diagnostic techniques, TIAs, carotid bruits, etc.
4. Plum F: What causes infarction in ischemic brain?

The Robert Wartenburg Lecture. *Neurology (NY)* 33:222–233, 1983.
    An excellent discussion of the mechanisms by a master in the field dispels some old ideas and projects new ones.
5. Masdeu JC: Infarct versus neoplasm on CT: four helpful signs. *AJNR* 4:522–524, 1983.
    An important differentiation between two often confused clinical and radiologic diagnoses.
6. Corston RN, Kendall BE, Marshall J: Prognosis in middle cerebral artery stenosis. *Stroke* 15:237–241, 1984.
    The incidence of subsequent serious strokes is high.
7. Grotta JC, Bigelow RH, Hu H, et al: The significance of carotid stenosis ulceration. *Neurology (NY)* 34:437–442, 1984.
    Depicts the difficulties in predicting what will happen.
8. Strother CM, Crummy AB: Cervical arteriosclerosis—diagnostic advances in need of a clinical answer. *Stroke* 13:551–556, 1982.
9. Wood GW, Lukin RR, Tomsick TA, et al: Digital subtraction angiography with intravenous injection: assessment of 1000 carotid bifurcations: *AJR* 140:855–859, 1983.
    Good correlation is achieved with concomitant arterial injection.
10. Thompson JE: Carotid endarterectomy, 1982—the state of the art. *Br J Surg* 70:371–376, 1983.
    Asymptomatic bruits, risk factors, and diagnosis are included.
11. Garth KE, Carroll BA, Sommer FG, et al: Duplex ultrasound scanning of the carotid arteries with velocity spectrum analysis. *Radiology* 147:823–827, 1983.
    Compares degree of stenosis with velocity ratios and turbulence.
12. Murie JA, Quin RO, Forrest MB, et al: Pulsed Doppler imaging and spectral analysis for detection of carotid artery disease. *Angiology* 35:215–221, 1984.
    The ability to diagnose exceeds the ability to decide on treatment.

Chapter 24

Multisystem Problems

Until now, each chapter has dealt with problems in its own field, and there has been only little overlap whereby a particular presentation could be caused by diseases in several systems. This chapter will deal with symptoms or clusters whose diagnosis can lie in any one of many systems, whose diagnosis can be a single multisystem disease, or whose diagnoses may be multiple.

Recall, for instance, that hypertension can be caused by vascular malformations, renal disease, or endocrine disease. Furthermore, hypertension affects many organ systems: the heart, kidney, blood vessels, and eyes. And it is common to see hypertension in patients who also have diabetes, arthritis, or duodenal ulcer—a concurrence of high-incidence diseases.

Multisystem problems are usually solved by collecting a complete data base and then selecting relevant clues. But the entire range of problem-solving techniques may be called upon: Clusters can be formed, key clues are sought, and clues pointing to a specific organ system are helpful. Once you have found a leading clue, you may branch into a subset of data. For example, if your patient complains of a swollen abdomen, and you elicit a history of heavy alcohol intake, look directly for signs of cirrhosis. A single question to the patient with long-standing fever—"Did you drink any goat's milk while you were in Mexico?"—may lead you directly to the solution. Undulant fever may then be confirmed by additional tests; the complete data base can be sidestepped.

However, the multisystem problems which follow almost always require the initial formation of a differential diagnosis. Each case presentation can be caused by a wide variety of diseases originating in different body systems. The mechanics of forming the differential was discussed in Chapter 9 and should now be reread.

Unless a key clue is uncovered in the history or physical examination, extensive tests and procedures are usually needed to exclude most possibilities and prove one. Here is your opportunity to exercise restraint and use thoughtful selectivity in ordering diagnostic procedures. (*P. C.*)

Case 59
Weakness, Weight Loss, Anorexia

PAUL CUTLER, M.D.

DATA You see a 62-year-old man who has had weakness, weight loss, and loss of appetite for 5 months. Prior to this he was perfectly well.

LOGIC This common triad is always ominous, especially in the patient's age group. It usually indicates serious organic disease or a depressive reaction. The symptoms are not specific and point to no particular organ or illness. By culling the various modules of pathophysiology stored in your brain, you compose a list of common problems to consider:

1. cancer (stomach, lung, colon, pancreas, prostate, kidney)
2. tuberculosis (pulmonary or generalized)
3. depression
4. uremia
5. hematologic disease (chronic anemia, leukemia, myeloma, lymphoma).

Less common causes, such as the malabsorption syndrome, a connective tissue disorder, or Addison's disease, must also be considered while sifting the clues which follow.

As you approach the patient for additional information, the signs and symptoms of the various diagnostic possibilities are whirling through your mind. Each positive or negative clue will give more or less credence to a diagnosis, and you hope to harvest a combination of findings that will fit the template for one of the listed possibilities.

DATA The patient has been working hard at his printing job and had taken on additional responsibilities as a church elder and Sunday school teacher. He attributed his symptoms to too much pressure but nevertheless continued in these activities because he enjoyed them. However, during the past

month his anorexia got worse and he noticed his clothes felt loose; a scale revealed a 30-lb weight loss in 5 months. In the week prior to coming to your office, he began to have severe, constant backache unrelated to activity or motion and unrelieved by heat and aspirin.

LOGIC It now appears that the backache is what really drove him to your office. He seems to deny the importance of the other symptoms. Severe weight loss, lack of evidence for depression, and the recent unrelenting backache cast an aura of organicity upon the situation. Remember the possibility that the backache may be unrelated to the other symptoms.

DATA A review of systems is negative. In particular, he has had no polyuria, polydipsia, nocturia, urgency, thin stream, or dysuria. There has been no indigestion, early satiety, abdominal pain, change in bowel habit, or black stools. He has had no fever, chills, night sweats, cough, chest pain, hemoptysis, or dyspnea; no pain, stiffness, or swelling of joints; no heat intolerance, insomnia, palpitations, or tremor. He is not aware of family, financial, or emotional problems and is not depressed, though he admits to being a bit worried about not feeling well.

LOGIC This long series of pertinent negative historical data leads you away from diabetes mellitus, prostatic obstruction, carcinoma of the stomach and bowel, tuberculosis, carcinoma of the lung, connective tissue disease, thyroid disease, and depression—in that order.

Diabetes as a cause of weight loss is unlikely anyway, since polyphagia rather than anorexia would be expected. Carcinoma of the prostate could metastasize body-wide, yet not be large enough or located so as to cause urethral obstruction. The absence of frequent greasy stools and the presence of anorexia are against malabsorption. Since there are no gastrointestinal (GI) symptoms, cancer along this tract is less likely though certainly not ruled out. Cancer of the stomach, pancreas, or colon could each present with a downhill course from generalized spread before giving localized symptoms. The absence of pulmonary symptoms is strong evidence against pulmonary tuberculosis or cancer; there, a lesion producing such a rapid, relentless course would probably cause local symptoms too. Depression seems even more remote.

DATA Examination discloses a chronically ill patient who is emaciated and shows signs of severe weight loss. He is 70 inches tall, weighs 138 lb, and has normal vital signs. There is no jaundice, cyanosis, or clubbing, but the conjunctivae, mucous membranes, and nailbeds are pale. The rest of the complete physical examination is normal. There are no palpable lymph nodes and no palpable abdominal masses or organs. A satisfactory rectal examination cannot be done because the rectum is filled with hard feces. No reason for the back pain is found on orthopaedic and neurologic examination.

LOGIC Weight loss is confirmed by the emaciation (loss of subcutaneous fat—i.e. sunken cheeks, hollowed temples, and deeply wrinkled, loose skin over the arms and abdomen). The patient is anemic and you clearly have a serious organic problem to manage. The absence of large nodes and spleen is against most forms of leukemia. The absence of jaundice, large liver, and supraclavicular nodes whispers against metastatic cancer. An enema must be given and the rectal examination redone. Uremia is virtually excluded by normal fundi, normal breath odor, and absence of hypertension. Pernicious anemia merits little further consideration because of the normal tongue and the absence of neurologic and GI symptoms and signs; also, this disease is not usually

characterized by weight loss. Further help is needed.

DATA Studies are done. The complete blood count shows 3 million red blood cells/mm^3, hemoglobin 9 g/dl, hematocrit 27%; white blood cell count, platelets, and blood smear normal. The urinalysis, chest x-ray, ECG, and purified protein derivative skin test are normal or negative. Stool examination is negative for excessive fat ('Sudan stain), ova, parasites, and occult blood. Tests of blood chemistry (glucose, blood urea nitrogen, creatinine, electrolytes, protein electrophoresis, calcium, phosphorus) are normal. X-rays of the lumbosacral spine and pelvis show numerous osteolytic and osteoblastic lesions.

LOGIC The solution is at hand. In the presence of a normochromic normocytic anemia, you are not surprised to find the stool negative for excessive fat and occult blood. Steatorrhea and chronic GI bleeding usually cause macrocytic and microcytic anemias, respectively. Malabsorption and a bleeding mucosal GI lesion are now most unlikely. Normal proteins and urinalysis virtually exclude multiple myeloma; also, myeloma causes osteolytic, not osteoblastic lesions. Leukemia, lymphoma, tuberculosis, and uremia are now very unlikely.

The x-rays indicate bone metastases. Cancer probably explains the backache, the anemia, and the entire picture. The primary source of the cancer must still be located. Since osteoblastic bone lesions are usually caused by prostatic cancer, your suspicion is strong and you aim directly for this target.

DATA Repeated enemas eventually clear the rectum, and a stony-hard nodular prostate is palpated. Acid and alkaline phosphatases are both ten times normal. Bone marrow aspiration shows sheets of small malignant cells.

LOGIC Had a proper rectal examination been possible at the start, this problem would have been quickly and easily solved.

The alkaline phosphatase is elevated because new bone is being laid down concomitant with bone destruction. Elevation of the acid phosphatase is highly specific for prostatic cancer. The anemia is at least partly caused by marrow infiltration and replacement by cancer cells. Treatment and patient education can now begin.

QUESTIONS

1. Assume this patient showed no evidence of cancer of the prostate and repeated stool examinations were positive for occult blood. You would then have suspected cancer in the GI tract. All except one of the following might be true:
   (a) Barium enema demonstrates cancer of the cecum.
   (b) The anemia is hypochromic.
   (c) The alkaline phosphatase is elevated.
   (d) A bleeding duodenal ulcer is the cause of the patient's problem.
2. Had there been no evidence for cancer of the prostate, no anemia, and had the stool been repeatedly negative for occult blood, you might have given serious consideration to cancer of the pancreas. If the latter disease were present, only one of the following statements would be false:
   (a) GI x-rays are usually of no help.
   (b) Jaundice may be present.
   (c) Pancreatic function tests are the diagnostic procedure of choice.
   (d) A left pleural effusion may be present.
3. In a patient with weakness and weight loss, yet a good appetite and no other symptoms, consider:
   (a) diabetes mellitus
   (b) hyperthyroidism
   (c) malabsorption
   (d) all of the above.
4. You have a 60-year-old woman with weakness, anorexia, and weight loss. She lost her husband 1 year ago, seldom sees her children, and has no hobbies or friends. The complete data base is otherwise normal. Advise her to:
   (a) take mood elevators
   (b) return in 3 months for reevaluation
   (c) see a psychiatrist
   (d) have superficial psychotherapy and return frequently for reevaluation.

ANSWERS

1. **(d) is correct.** It is the only unlikely answer. Even though a duodenal ulcer could be present too, it would hardly cause anorexia and weight loss. Cancer of the cecum often presents in

this way. A hypochromic iron deficiency type anemia results from chronic GI blood loss. The alkaline phosphatase could be elevated from liver or bone metastases originating in any primary GI cancer.
2. **(c) is correct since it is false.** Such studies are neither sensitive nor specific. The choice procedure today is the computed tomographic scan, though some prefer ultrasound, endoscopic retrograde pancreatography, and an eventual guided biopsy. Ordinary GI x-rays are not helpful unless the lesion is large and located in the head of the pancreas. Under these circumstances, jaundice from common bile duct obstruction is usually present too. A left pleural effusion may be the only hint for cancer in the pancreatic tail just under the left hemidiaphragm.
3. **(b) is correct.** There may be no other symptoms but plenty of signs. For diabetes to cause this cluster, polyuria and polydipsia would have to be present too. Malabsorption fits the cluster, but if weight loss were present, there would be considerable loss of fat in the stool resulting in frequent greasy stools—not present here.
4. **(d) is correct.** Depression is probably the principal issue. If so, patience, understanding, mild medication, and revisits should suffice. Furthermore, revisits are indicated to detect new clues should they appear. Cancer and depression are frequently confused. Do not be lulled into complacency. Have your patient make a serious conscious effort to eat well and gain weight. (a) is satisfactory but not without psychotherapy. Three months is too long a time between visits, either for depression or should something else be wrong. If she does not improve, psychiatric consultation would be indicated, along with a complete medical reevaluation.

COMMENT Nonspecific presentations of this sort must often be solved by the traditional method of gathering a complete data base and sifting through the clues. Many diseases in numerous organ systems can present as this one did. But even here, shortcuts are possible.

While weakness, weight loss, and anorexia are each nonspecific, the triad is ominous and conjures up a distinct differential diagnosis. Then added bits of information in the history and physical examination narrow the list by eliminating most possibilities (proof by exclusion) and suggesting very few. Noteworthy is the use of the pertinent negative clue. During the data-gathering process, anemia and backache are added to the cluster and augur the presence of a malignant disease.

In this case, the problem solver could have

thrown out a huge fishnet to see what he could catch, or he could have been more selective in his approach. The entire workup was done on an outpatient basis. Had the rectal examination been immediately achievable, the diagnosis would have been quickly evident. Had an alkaline phosphatase been included in the initial chemical battery, the final diagnosis might have been more readily apparent; the test result would have prompted a search for bone or liver metastases. In this instance, the value of battery screening is clearly seen.

GI x-rays and high-technology tests were not needed. But if the prostate gland and spine x-rays had been normal, a search for GI cancer or lymphoma would have necessitated such x-rays and at least a computed tomographic scan.

The absence of lower urinary obstructive symptoms in the presence of a large hard prostate gland is somewhat of a surprise and represents a false negative historical clue that was initially misleading. But carcinoma of the prostate gland is common in men past 60, and the laws of probability are thereby obeyed. (*P. C.*)

PROBLEM-BASED LEARNING Cases that present in this way may be solved simply, or may require that the problem solver have a large information base. You should know all about:

1. the array of diseases that may present similarly in this manner
2. the common carcinomas of men—lung, prostate, and GI tract—and their clinical features
3. carcinoma of the prostate in particular—its metastatic features and serum markers
4. the reliability of testing modes for prostatic cancer—acid phosphatase and biopsy
5. how to best test for the occult pancreatic cancer, e.g. the relative values of ultrasound, computed tomographic scan, guided biopsy, endoscopic retrograde cholangiopancreatography, etc
6. why cancer causes general symptoms of weight loss and anorexia.

Suggested Readings

1. Cello JP: Carcinoma of the pancreas. In Sleisenger MH, Fordtran JS (eds): *Gastrointestinal Disease,* ed 3. Philadelphia, Saunders, 1983, pp 1514–1527.
   A textbook description of all aspects of the disease.
2. Jones GW: Diagnosis and management of prostatic cancer. *Cancer* 51:2456–2459, 1983.
3. Hosking DH, Paraskivas M, Hellsten OR, et al: The cytologic diagnosis of prostatic cancer by transrectal fine needle aspiration. *J Urol* 129:998–1000, 1983.
   Describes an easy outpatient method for diagnosis.
4. Fair WR: Cancer of the prostate: current thoughts on diagnosis and staging. *Surg Clin North Am* 62:1085–1099,1982.
5. Jacobs SC: Spread of prostatic cancer to bone. *Urology* 21:337–344, 1983.
6. Goldenberg SL, Silver HKB, Sullivan LD, et al: A critical evaluation of a specific radioimmunoassay for prostatic acid phosphatase. *Cancer* 50:1847–1851, 1982.
   Compares radioimmunoassay method with standard enzyme assay.
7. Paulson DF, Perez CA, Anderson T: Genitourinary malignancies. In DeVita VT Jr, Hellman S, Rosenberg SA (eds): *Cancer—Principles and Practice of Oncology.* Philadelphia, Lippincott, 1982.
   pp 753–769 cover cancer of the prostate.
8. Warren KW, Christophi C, Armendariz R, et al: Current trends in the diagnosis and treatment of carcinoma of the pancreas. *Am J Surg* 145:813–818, 1983.
   Covers the clinical picture, diagnostic methods, and causes for diagnostic delay.
9. DiMagno EP, Malagelada JR, Taylor WF, et al: A prospective comparison of current diagnostic tests for pancreatic cancer. *N Engl J Med* 297:737–742, 1977.
   The reliability and specificity of ultrasound, pancreatic function tests, retrograde pancreatography, scan, arteriography, and thermography in the diagnosis of pancreatic lesions are verified at surgery.
10. Cutler SJ, Myers MH, White PL: Who are we missing and why? *Cancer* 37:421–425, 1976.
    Deals with the statistics of numerous cancers not diagnosed when they are still localized.
11. Hosoki T: Dynamic CT of pancreatic tumors. *AJR* 140:959–965, 1983.
12. Wesdorp RI: Cancer cachexia and its nutritional implications. *Br J Surg* 70:352–355, 1983.
    Why cancer patients become cachectic.

Case 60
Swelling of the Abdomen
H. LEONARD BENTCH, M.D.

DATA Dr. Jones, an obstetrician, refers you a 32-year-old married woman who sought his advice because she missed two menstrual periods and noticed mild abdominal swelling. She thought she was pregnant. Dr. Jones thought she was not because the uterus was normal in size and the pregnancy test was negative. He further commented that she would not have noticeable abdominal swelling so early even if she were pregnant. But then he gave you a little more to worry about by saying, "the right adnexa was normal, but I couldn't feel the left; and the blood count was normal except for a hemoglobin of 10 g/dl and a hematocrit of 33%."

LOGIC It was appropriate for the patient to consult her obstetrician. Not only did she think she was pregnant, but she, like many women, looks to her obstetrician-gynecologist for primary care. During the childbearing years, secondary amenorrhea is most commonly due to pregnancy. However, there are many other causes including inflammatory, metabolic, endocrine, infectious, and psychogenic disorders.

Mild anemia is not unusual in menstruating women who lose 5 to 10 mg of iron with each period and do not quite replace it in their diet. However, in conjunction with a large abdomen and amenorrhea it causes you some concern.

DATA The patient's comment that she has been unable to close her skirt for the past month plus a quick look and feel convince you that her abdomen is enlarged.

LOGIC Before going further, you think of the many causes of abdominal distention. Localized enlargement can result from large cysts (ovary, pancreas, mesentery), tumors (uterus, ovary), or a huge liver or spleen. Diffuse abdominal swelling can be caused by one of the traditional five—fat, feces, flatus, fluid, and fetus. Occasionally an ovarian cyst will be so large as to give diffuse swelling. Also, two or more items may coexist, such as hepatosplenomegaly and ascites.

It is common for patients to complain of abdominal distention for simple reasons like recently acquired obesity, severe constipation, or the presence of much gastrointestinal gas. This may need little problem solving: a few questions, then feel and tap the abdomen. For obesity—a pinch! For constipation—a history! And for gas—tympany on percussion. If still in doubt, an x-ray of the abdomen will help distinguish between the five "f's," but an x-ray is ill-advised if pregnancy is suspected. Remember that gaseous distention plus abdominal cramps can augur intestinal obstruction.

DATA The patient is the head nurse in the dialysis unit at your hospital. In addition to her two chief complaints, she noted mild fatigue, soreness of the wrist and hand joints, and a nonpruritic rash on her face and arms. These were attributed to a combination of overwork and the irritating scrub soap used in the unit. She had gained 15 lb despite dieting, and had taken a diuretic for the swelling. She had been depressed by the recent death of a favorite dialysis patient. Her appetite was good, and she had no abdominal pain or indigestion. She neither smokes nor drinks alcohol. Past history is negative except for an appendectomy and allergy to penicillin.

Vital signs are normal except for a temperature of 37.7 C. A large 1 × 2-cm dark nevus seems particularly stark on her back compared to her sallow complexion. No spider angiomas are seen, though there is a slightly scaling urticarial rash on the face and hands. The abdomen is generally protuberant and dull to percussion except for tympany about the umbilicus, from which numerous distended veins flow. Shifting dullness, fluid wave, and the puddle sign cannot be elicited, and there is no bulging in the flanks. No masses are felt; the spleen is not palpable, though the liver has 14 cm of vertical height and reaches 3 cm below the costal margin in the midclavicular line. It is slightly enlarged and ballottable. The liver edge is firm and blunt. The lungs are clear, there is a grade 2/6 systolic ejection murmur at the base, two-plus ankle edema is present. Dr. Jones' findings on pelvic examination are confirmed, and the rest of the examination is normal.

LOGIC The case is a complex one, has many ramifications, and you realize that invasive diagnostic techniques will be needed, so you admit the patient to the hospital. Ascites is the key clue about which your investigation will center. Fever, rash, heart murmur, and mild hepatomegaly are found on physical examination and augment the laboratory finding of anemia.

Much related and unrelated information is now available and must be sorted out. As a dialysis unit nurse, your patient is exposed to hepatitis, tuberculosis, bacteria and viruses of all sorts, drug availability, and depression. Fever is worrisome and suggests infection, inflammation, or neoplasia. The nevus is probably a false clue, since most patients have several such lesions. But malignant melanoma with liver and peritoneal implants cannot be dismissed.

Slight liver enlargement and a caput medusae imply liver disease with portal hypertension. The absence of spider angiomas does not rule out liver disease, especially in the nonalcoholic, but no other stigmata are present. Even though you are reasonably certain of ascites, the textbook signs of fluid wave and shifting dullness have poor sensitivity and specificity except in severe cases. Ballottement of an organ is a more accurate sign of ascites. The firm blunt liver edge suggests liver disease.

Another concern is for infective endocarditis superimposed upon another disease.

The fever, anemia, and heart murmur suggest this possibility. Nor have you yet settled the issue of the impalpable left adnexa. A huge ovarian cyst can fill the abdomen and mimic ascites yet not be felt in the pelvis.

DATA On the way up to the hospital room, the patient had an x-ray of the abdomen and chest, and blood is taken for studies. The chest film shows a normal-sized heart, no pulmonary infiltrates, and a small right pleural effusion. The abdominal x-ray shows normal air distribution and an overall ground-glass hazy appearance characteristic of ascites.

LOGIC You review the common causes of ascites:

1. cirrhosis of the liver
2. congestive heart failure
3. metastatic cancer
4. tuberculous peritonitis

as well as some of the less common ones:

5. nephrotic syndrome
6. constrictive pericarditis
7. inferior vena cava, hepatic vein, or portal vein thrombosis
8. myxedema
9. pancreatic carcinoma, cyst, or inflammation
10. malnutrition.

The first four cause more than 90% of cases of ascites. Age and geography are factors. Possibilities 2, 3, and 8 are unlikely at age 32. Diagnoses 4 and 10 are much more common in underdeveloped, primitive, or impoverished areas.

DATA Abdominal paracentesis is performed and 50 ml of clear straw-colored fluid are removed. By the next day, the blood and ascitic fluid studies return: hematocrit 31%; white blood cell count 4,200/mm^3, normal differential; platelets 80,000/mm^3; SGOT 550 U/liter (normal 5 to 41); alkaline phosphatase 200 U/liter (normal 30 to 115); bilirubin 1.7 mg/dl (normal 0.1 to 1.2). The urinalysis and the rest of the blood chemistry determinations are normal.

The ascitic fluid shows 20 cells/mm^3, no red blood cells, 75 mg glucose, 1.5 g protein, and 4 units amylase/dl. The Gram stain exhibits no organisms, the culture reveals no growth, and no malignant cells are seen on cytologic study.

Two blood cultures are negative. Protein electrophoresis discloses only 2.5 g albumin, but 4.1 g globulin/dl; marked β-γ bridging is noted. A liver-spleen scan shows patchy hepatic uptake, no lucent areas, and an enlarged spleen with increased radioactive material in the spleen and bone marrow.

LOGIC The clinical problem is becoming clear. She has ascites and the fluid is a transudate. Infection, inflammation, and neoplasia appear most unlikely. Had you accidentally tapped a pancreatic or ovarian cyst, the glucose content would have been almost nil in both, and the amylase would be high in the former. Furthermore, these cysts would have been accompanied by an abnormal gas pattern seen in a radiograph of the abdomen since the intestines would have been displaced. Tuberculosis would have shown a lymphocytic exudate. The scan, her age, and the absence of tumor cells are against cancer.

Endocarditis is unlikely since blood cultures are negative and no embolic phenomena are noted. Heart failure and constrictive pericarditis are ruled out by the normal (except for murmur) heart examination, absence of rales, and absence of distended neck veins. Nephrotic syndrome is excluded by the normal urinalysis. Myxedema can be discarded by a single glance at the face.

On the other hand, physical examination, liver function tests, protein electrophoresis, and liver-spleen scan point directly to a diffuse disease of the liver.

Some findings are now explainable. The ankle edema and small pleural effusion are probably caused by hypoproteinemia and secondary hyperaldosteronism. The diseased liver cannot detoxify aldosterone or manufacture albumin. Secondary hyperaldosteronism and low serum albumin will retain and sequester water and salt. This decreases renal blood flow and invokes the renin-an-giotensin-aldosterone mechanism which completes the vicious circle. Fever may be related to the disease process in the liver. Anemia occurs for many reasons in liver disease; these include hemolysis, bleeding, and depressed marrow function. The heart murmur remains incompletely explained, though it may result from the anemia or fever. Low platelets, and anemia too, can be caused by hypersplenism secondary to portal hypertension. Amenorrhea probably results from an alteration in the metabolism of hormones upon which normal ovulation and menstruation depend.

Severe liver disease causes ascites in many ways: portal hypertension, low serum protein, intrahepatic lymphatic obstruction, and inability to detoxify fluid- and salt-retaining hormones.

The type of diffuse liver disease remains to be determined. It is not alcoholic cirrhosis: she does not drink alcohol. α_1-Antitrypsin deficiency is excluded by the presence of α_1-globulin on electrophoresis. Other inborn errors like hemachromatosis and Wilson's disease are uncommon and have associated clinical findings which are not present here, but appropriate tests must be done since these conditions are treatable. Secondary biliary cirrhosis has obvious clinical features. It is caused by extrahepatic biliary tract obstruction, usually stone or stricture, and is characterized by obstructive jaundice, elevated serum cholesterol, and an alkaline phosphatase that is elevated disproportionately to the SGOT. Primary biliary cirrhosis is a rare disease, especially in women under 50, and it is notable for the connective tissue and immunologic disorders associated with the manifestations of liver disease.

All considered, chronic active hepatitis, perhaps even consequent cirrhosis, is probably present. Only one study—liver biopsy—will provide an indisputable answer. At this point, the determination of the causative virus is mostly academic. But since a biopsy will require several days and since, for epidemiologic and intellectual reasons, you are anxious to verify the possible source of her disease (should it be chronic active hepatitis), a "hepatitis profile" that is suitable for late-stage disease is requested.

You already know that hepatitis A virus rarely if ever causes chronic active hepatitis. Also, hepatitis B virus and hepatitis non-A non-B virus do; furthermore, these are the varieties contracted by medical personnel, especially those working in dialysis units.

DATA The prothrombin time is normal and platelets are diminished though adequate on recheck. Directed needle liver biopsy is performed with the aid of a laparoscope. A macronodular liver with the classic histologic changes of chronic active hepatitis is found.

The results of the immunologic studies are as follows: (*a*) hepatitis A virus *antibodies* of the immunoglobulin M and G types are negative (IgM anti-HAV and IgG anti-HAV); (*b*) hepatitis B surface and core *antigens* (HBsAg and HBcAg) are negative; and (*c*) hepatitis B surface and core *antibodies* (anti-HBs and anti-HBc) are also negative.

LOGIC This establishes the exact diagnosis and explains all the findings. Her original episode of hepatitis must have been subclinical and progressed into this severe stage. It was probably contracted in the dialysis unit. The rash and joint pains are caused by altered immune mechanisms with resultant antigen-antibody complexes—a common manifestation of this type of liver disease. As testimony to this fact, the antinuclear antibody test is often positive.

Since the antigen and antibody tests are all negative, you may infer by exclusion that the causative virus in this patient was of the non-A non-B variety. There are as yet no known immunologic markers for this virus or group of viruses.

DATA Salt restriction, a mild diuretic, and steroids are begun. After a week, improvement is noted in many respects.

COMMENT Age and geography altered diagnostic likelihoods as we considered the common causes of ascites—the key clue. The absence of historical and physical evidence eliminated most possibilities. The presence of some clues supported others. Misleading features such as depression, overwork, no alcohol intake, use of scrub soap, and a large nevus clouded the issues and had to be suppressed. Fever, anemia, and heart murmur clustered to falsely suggest the presence of an additional disease. The sensitivity and specificity of classical clues for ascites were considered, and the importance of abdominal paracentesis in weeding out the causes of ascites was evident. However, the result of the liver biopsy was the decisive clue. (*P. C.*)

Suggested Readings

1. Bender MD, Ockner RK: Ascites. In Sleisenger MH, Fordtran JS (eds): *Gastrointestinal Disease*, ed 3. Philadelphia, Saunders,1983, pp 335–351.
   The causes, types, diagnosis, and treatment are detailed.
2. Sherlock S: *Diseases of the Liver and Biliary System*, ed 6. London, Blackwell, 1981, pp 270–294.
   Details the types of chronic hepatitis and their varied implications.
3. Shear L, Ching S, Gabuzda GJ: Compartmentalization of ascites and edema in patients with hepatic cirrhosis. *N Engl J Med* 282:1391–1396, 1970.
   This is the classic description of the hydrodynamics of ascites formation in cirrhosis.
4. Wands JR, Koff RS, Isselbacher KJ: Chronic active hepatitis. In Petersdorf RG, Adams RD, Braunwald E, et al (eds): *Harrison's Principles of Internal Medicine*, ed 10. New York, McGraw-Hill, 1983, pp 1801–1804.
5. Arthur MJ, Hall AJ, Wright R: Hepatitis B, hepatocellular carcinoma, and strategies for prevention. *Lancet* 1:607–610, 1984.
6. Francis DD, Hadler SC, Prendergast TF, et al: Occurrence of hepatitis A, B, and non-A/non-B in the United States. *Am J Med* 76:69–74, 1984.
   Throws the three types into epidemiologic perspective.
7. Oxman MN: Hepatitis B vaccination of high-risk hospital personnel. *Anesthesiology* 60:1–3, 1984.
   A sensible approach to a complex issue.
8. Krugman S: Hepatitis virus vaccines: present status. *Yale J Biol Med* 55:375–381, 1982.
   A chronological review and recommendations from a leading authority.
9. Dienstag JL: Non-A, non-B hepatitis. *Gastroenterology* 85:439–462, 1983.
   Recognition, epidemiology, and clinical features of the third type—in detail.
10. Cozzolino G, Lonardo A, Francica G, et al: Differential diagnosis between hepatic cirrhosis and chronic active hepatitis. *Am J Gastroenterol* 78:442–445, 1983.
    Describes sensitivity and specificity of physical and laboratory findings.

Case 61
High Blood Pressure
TIMOTHY N. CARIS, M.D.

DATA   A 43-year-old essentially asymptomatic black man comes to you for care. He is a self-employed gardner, and several weeks ago he had his blood pressure checked by a screening group in a shopping center. He was told it was 210/122. Subsequent daily recordings at a neighborhood clinic were 180/110, 192/108, 200/114, and 182/106.

LOGIC   At the onset, you recall that the prevalence of hypertension in this country approaches 20% of the adult population. High blood pressure is a major risk factor for stroke, congestive heart failure, renal failure, and coronary heart disease. You recall also that the ravages of hypertension are more likely to occur in blacks than in whites, and in men than in women. Your patient, then, is in a high-jeopardy category. Eighty-nine per cent of patients with high blood pressure suffer essential or primary hypertension, 6% have secondary causes for the elevation such as chronic renal parenchymal disease, and a final 5% have potentially surgically correctable secondary causes such as renal ischemic disease, coarctation of the aorta, pheochromocytoma, Cushing's syndrome, or primary aldosteronism. You therefore proceed with the remainder of your evaluation keeping appropriate categorization in mind.

DATA   The patient has been in excellent health and, as a consequence, has not undergone medical examination in years. When he was discharged from the army at age 20, he was asked to lie down for 3 hours and his blood pressure was checked every 30 minutes. He was told the pressure was high initially but returned to normal with rest. The patient was raised by a nonrelative, so family history is not obtainable. He has occasional occipital headaches late in the day which get worse as evening approaches; they usually respond to aspirin. He has not had exertional dyspnea, orthopnea, paroxysmal nocturnal dyspnea, palpitations, easy fatigability, chest discomfort, or chest pain. There have been no episodes of unsteady gait, memory defects, muscle weakness, sensory loss, difficulty in coordination, or visual disturbances. The remainder of the past history and history by systems was not contributory.

LOGIC   The natural development of essential hypertension (EH) includes lability of blood pressure during the second and third decades. Fixed hypertension usually appears in the thirties. Your patient fits this facet of the clinical picture. EH tends to occur in families but this fact is of no help in this situation.

EH is an insidious, painless disorder for many years—until target organs (heart, brain, kidneys) are significantly involved. Symptoms such as headaches, tinnitus, dizziness, fainting, and epistaxis that commonly have been ascribed to high blood pressure are nonspecific, and their incidence is found to be the same in normotensives as in hypertensives. Also, headaches occurring in the hypertensive patient are not temporally related to the height of the blood pressure. A pounding occipital headache which is present in the morning and which wears off as the day progresses does occur in some people with hypertension. This patient is describing a "tension" headache that may occur in anyone.

By history, he has no suggestion of left ventricular decompensation, myocardial ischemia, or cerebral ischemia. Pheochromocytoma is not likely since there is no history of paroxysmal headaches, sweating, racing of the heart, palpitations, tremulous sensations, or lightheadedness after arising abruptly from a seated or lying position.

DATA   The physical examination reveals a well-developed, moderately obese black male (72 inches tall, 224 lb). The pulse rate is 76/minute and regular, there are no bruits in the neck, and all the peripheral pulses are present, equal, and strong bilaterally. The remainder of the physical and neurologic examinations is completely normal except for the fundi which show narrowing of the arterioles and arteriovenous crossing defects. Blood pressure is 204/116 in the right arm and 200/114 in the left with the patient lying down. Blood pressure in the left arm is 200/116 when the patient is sitting and 194/118 when standing. Auscultation reveals a fourth heart sound at the apex and no bruits over the abdomen.

LOGIC   The ophthalmoscopic changes indicate long-standing hypertensive vascular disease. Patients with pheochromocytoma are likely to be hypermetabolic with tremor, tachycardia, and lean habitus; the lack of orthostatic drop in blood pressure also helps exclude this possibility. The absence of bruits in the neck is a point against significant carotid or vertebral atherosclerosis. Less than 20 mm Hg disparity between the blood pressures in the arms excludes the complications of aortic arch disorders such as occlusive atherosclerosis, dissecting aneurysm, or atypical coarctation. The diagnosis of ordinary coarctation of the aorta depends in part on diminished femoral pulses compared to the carotids. You can dismiss this possibility in your patient. The fourth heart sound indicates that concentric hypertrophy of the left ventricle has already begun—target organ involvement.

The absence of an abdominal bruit is important. In individuals less than 50 years old, a bruit is the most discriminatory clinical finding for renovascular ischemic disease causing secondary hypertension. Although abdominal bruits may be heard in up to 5% of patients with EH they are present in 50 to 60% of patients with renovascular hypertension in this age group.

To distinguish the bruit of renovascular stenosis from the innocent bruits commonly heard over the aorta, the nature of the bruit, its location, and the technique of auscultation are important. Aortic bruits in older people and in those with EH are soft, low-pitched, purely systolic, and heard in the epigastrium. The bruit caused by renal artery stenosis is high-pitched, continuous or systolic and diastolic, and is best heard in the subcostal margin and laterally into the flank; moderate pressure must be applied to the diaphragm of the stethoscope.

The characteristic central fat distribution of Cushing's disease or syndrome is not present in this patient. If you further consider the absence of ecchymoses, plethora, purple abdominal striae, and muscle weakness, this endocrine disease can be excluded.

DATA   Selected laboratory data needed to solve this problem are: urinalysis normal; hematocrit 44; serum creatinine 0.8 mg/dl, serum potassium 4.2 mEq/liter, fasting blood glucose 80 mg/dl; normal chest x-ray; and ECG shows early left ventricular hypertrophy.

LOGIC   A normal urinalysis helps exclude renal parenchymal disease as a source of secondary hypertension, while a normal serum creatinine speaks for good renal function. Primary aldosteronism is unlikely in the presence of a normal serum potassium. Neither history nor physical examination leads to the suspicion that coarctation of the aorta, pheochromocytoma, or Cushing's syndrome is the cause of the blood pressure elevation in this man. The normal blood glucose is another point against the last two.

Renal artery disease producing renal ischemia is the most common correctable cause for secondary hypertension. In this event, the elevated blood pressure tends to occur earlier in life and is of greater severity, and the course is more rapidly progressive than in the patient under discussion. But renal ischemic disease may closely mimic EH.

The absence of abdominal bruits is helpful but does not absolutely exclude renal artery disease. Some feel that despite the lack of clinical clues of renal artery stenosis, all patients should undergo a rapid infusion, rapid sequence intravenous pyelogram. Unequal size of kidneys, delay in visualization, or hyperconcentration of the contrast material on one side is considered indicative of renal vascular disease. Although still controversial, the present consensus is not to include intravenous pyelography in the initial evaluation of a hypertensive patient.

On the other hand, one must always consider and exclude renal artery disease if the patient has sustained hypertension and is less than 30 years old, if the patient is elderly and has severe elevation of blood pressure (i.e. sustained diastolic pressures of 130 mm Hg or greater), or if the patient has the documented sudden onset of fixed hypertension, rapidly worsening hypertension, or hypertension with an abdominal bruit.

There is no assurance that all patients with secondary hypertension will be identified; a very small number will slip through. If patients fail to respond to appropriate treatment for EH, these few should be reassessed. A more exhaustive diagnostic approach including renal arteriogram, renal vein renin measurements, urinary metanephrines and vanillylmandelic acid (VMA), plasma aldosterone and plasma renin activity determinations, angiotensin blocking agents, and dexamethasone suppression test might be undertaken at this point despite lack of clinical clues.

Recall that when first facing a patient with hypertension your main task is to decide whether this is garden variety EH or hypertension resulting from an endocrine disorder, renovascular disease, or renal disease. Doing so is most important because treatment is based primarily on this differentiation. EH is controllable, but not curable, and requires treatment for life. The hypertension caused by renal disease is only partially controllable and needs treatment during a curtailed life. But hypertension resulting from endocrine disorders and renovascular ischemia offers a good chance for cure.

Also, note that in deciding on the type of hypertension your patient may have, you are using both a multivariate analysis and an algorithmic technique that include critical factors such as age, gender, race, family history, rapidity of onset and severity of hypertension, and response to drug treatment.

The 90% with EH usually have a positive family history; their hypertension begins in the thirties and forties and becomes progressively worse. However, this type usually responds to diligent resourceful treatment.

Endocrine diseases associated with hypertension can be excluded by the clinical picture and a few well-selected tests.

Renovascular ischemic hypertension results mainly from either an atherosclerotic plaque causing 50% or more obstruction of a renal artery or fibromuscular dysplasia of one or both renal arteries. The former occurs mostly in males past 50 and the latter in females under 35. The common denominator is a marked decrease in perfusion pressure in the afferent arteriole of the glomerulus; this causes a release in renin which in turn invokes the renin-angiotensin-aldosterone mechanism. Hypertension results from the pressor action of angiotensin II abetted by the volume expansion caused by aldosterone. Somewhere between 1 and 5% of hypertensives have renovascular ischemic disease. Therefore, the following diagnostic pursuit applies only to a small minority of all hypertensive patients.

Once you suspect the presence of this problem, it must be proven—for surgery is the treatment of choice. There are many diagnostic procedures but each has its limitations.

The *saralasin test* causes a drop in blood pressure but this test is only 75% sensitive and the false positive rate of 15% that occurs mainly in high-renin essential hypertensives is unacceptable.

Inevitably you must come to the rapid sequence intravenous pyelogram. The criteria for test positivity result in 75% sensitivity and 89% specificity (11% false positives). While this is a fairly good distinguishing test since it is performed on a patient who is already highly suspect of having renovascular hypertension—P(D) = .50 or more—it is not reliable enough to hang your surgical gloves on.

If your suspicion is still high, two additional procedures must be done. First comes renal arteriography, invasive though productive in the detection of a stenotic lesion. But stenosis may exist yet not be the cause of the hypertension. Therefore the definitive test is done by sampling the blood in both renal veins via a catheter introduced into the femoral vein. Plasma renin activity (PRA) is measured in both renal veins. The PRA in the vein coming from the ischemic kidney should be much higher than the PRA coming from the nonischemic kidney. This difference is accentuated by the fact that the excessive secretion from the affected kidney suppresses the secretion from the normal one.

The presence of bilateral renal ischemia complicates the situation, though one side is usually more ischemic than the other. In effect, the arteriogram decides if stenosis exists, and venous sampling decides if the stenosis is the cause of the hypertension. These two studies will identify the 90% of those whose hypertension will be cured by surgery.

DATA Over the next 8 years, the patient was treated medically for EH. Since he felt well, he failed to take his medication regularly and visited his physician only rarely for acute minor problems. The blood pressure remained high, his heart got larger, albumin appeared in his urine, and hemorrhages were noted in his fundi.

At age 51, he suddenly developed severe chest, back, and abdominal pain requiring hospitalization. The ECG and enzymes remained normal, but he continued to be critically ill. Both legs became cold and pulseless, urine formation ceased, and he developed an aortic diastolic murmur and abruptly died.

LOGIC Poor patient compliance is common. Target organ involvement was becom-

ing more noticeable (heart, kidneys, fundi). His terminal event was a dissecting aortic aneurysm, not uncommon in hypertensives or patients with disorders like Marfan's syndrome and cystic medial necrosis. The dissection was extensive, involved and occluded the circulation to the legs and kidneys, then dissected retrograde to include the aortic valve and cause regurgitation. Probably dissection into the pericardial sac with tamponade caused sudden death.

QUESTIONS

1. Your patient is an asymptomatic 26-year-old woman whom you are examining for the first time. You note arteriovenous nicking on ophthalmoscopic examination and the BP is 220/132. She is hospitalized for an in-depth evaluation, to include renal arteriography, because you also find:
   (a) family history of hypertension
   (b) four to five white blood cells/high-power field on urinalysis
   (c) she is not using any oral contraceptives
   (d) a faint bruit in the left subcostal area that has short systolic and diastolic components.

2. The urinalysis shows 4+ glucosuria and a subsequent fasting blood glucose is 200 mg/dl. Which of the following is not causally related to hyperglycemia in a hypertensive patient?
   (a) diabetes mellitus
   (b) fibromuscular dysplasia of the renal artery
   (c) pheochromocytoma
   (d) Cushing's syndrome.

3. A patient with fixed hypertension has serum potassium levels of 2.8 mEq/liter. Which one of the following would have no bearing on this electrolyte disorder?
   (a) Patient is a chronic daily user of laxatives.
   (b) Patient is taking hydrochlorothiazide daily.
   (c) Patient may have primary aldosteronism.
   (d) Patient jogs 3 miles daily.

4. An 80-year-old asymptomatic man is referred to you because repeated blood pressure determinations in a neighborhood screening clinic have ranged from 180 to 200/70 to 80. Except for this finding, your physical examination reveals no abnormalities. The most likely explanation is:
   (a) beginning EH
   (b) aortic insufficiency
   (c) renal artery occlusive disease
   (d) atherosclerosis of aorta.

ANSWERS

1. **(d) is correct.** A young woman with severe hypertension and an epigastric bruit must be regarded as having hypertension secondary to renovascular ischemic disease until proven otherwise. Positive family history of hypertension does not relate to renal artery occlusive disease. Pyuria may suggest infection, but not renal artery disease. (c) merely excludes estrogen-containing pills as the cause of her hypertension.

2. **(b) is correct.** There is no relationship between hyperglycemia and fibromuscular dysplasia of the renal artery. The latter notably occurs in young women and may cause unilateral renal ischemia. Diabetes mellitus is a consideration. The incidence of this disorder is higher in hypertensives than in normotensives. Increased catecholamine levels result in transformation of glycogen stores in the liver to circulating blood glucose, and pheochromocytoma can be excluded if the catecholamine, metanephrine, and VMA levels in a 24-hour urine specimen are normal. Cushing's syndrome is related to adrenal hypercorticism, and hyperglycemia is a common manifestation of such a state because of excessive gluconeogenesis.

3. **(d) is correct.** There is no relationship between increased musculoskeletal activity and hypokalemia. Patients who are chronic daily laxative users deplete body potassium stores via the gastrointestinal tract. A 24-hour urine potassium determination would probably show less than 30 mEq, indicating the body is truly attempting to conserve potassium. Thiazides cause excess potassium excretion as well, particularly in the presence of the high-salt diet that is common in Americans. This drug should be discontinued for 4 weeks and the serum potassium levels reevaluated. The patient may well have primary aldosteronism. If so, the 24-hour urine potassium will be greater than 30 mEq despite hypokalemia, plasma renin activity will be low, and the aldosterone level will be high.

4. **(d) is correct.** The atherosclerotic aorta has lost its compliance. Absence of aortic distention with systolic expulsion of blood leads to high systolic pressure. The diastolic pressure remains normal. EH includes elevation of both systolic and diastolic pressures. There is no murmur to suggest aortic insufficiency. Renal ischemic disease that leads to hypertension includes diastolic pressure elevation as well.

COMMENT The high incidence of hypertension, the especially high incidence of the disease and its ravages in black men, and the fact that only 5% of hypertensives have possibly surgically correctable lesions influence your thoughts and management. The reliability of an abdominal bruit as a decision point is outlined.

An orderly stepwise approach in this case would be: (a) obtain family history for hypertension; (b) check BP in arm and leg; (c) seek evidence of target organ involvement; (d) study the urine, creatinine, potassium, VMA, ECG, and chest x-ray; (e) look for clues for renovascular hypertension; and (f) treat medically if none is present; do further studies if renal ischemia is suspected. The latter include an intravenous pyelogram, arteriogram, and PRA measurements from both renal veins. Each procedure has fairly well-established sensitivity and specificity, and the P(D) is altered by the results obtained by each one. If all are positive, you approach the 100% certainty that is desirable before surgery is performed. You have pinpointed the cause, evaluated the damage, and decided on treatment in six steps.

A decision tree, algorithm, or flow chart is ideally adaptable to the diagnostic process in this instance. (P. C.)

Suggested Readings

1. Kannel WB: Role of blood pressure in cardiovascular morbidity and mortality. *Prog Cardiovasc Dis* 17:5–24, 1974.
   An excellent overview of the significance of hypertension as determined by an 18-year longitudinal, prospective observation of a segment of the population in Framingham, MA.

2. Report of the Joint National Committee on Detection, Evaluation and Treatment of High Blood Pressure. *Arch Intern Med* 144:1045–1057, 1984.
   Here is the consensus of national authorities on the diagnostic and therapeutic approaches to patients with hypertension.

3. Caris TN: Initial evaluation of patients with hypertension—an office procedure. *South Med J* 71:403–407, 1978.
   Documents the rationale of relying on history, physical examination, and simple laboratory tests in the initial evaluation of a patient with high blood pressure.

4. Grim CE, Weinberger MH, Higgins JT, et al: Diagnosis of secondary forms of hypertension. *JAMA* 237:1331–1335, 1977.
   A comprehensive protocol for detection of correctable causes of high blood pressure.

5. Caris TN: *A Clinical Guide to Hypertension.* Littleton, MA, PSG Publishers, 1984.
   Chapter 4 in this comprehensive text details the secondary causes of hypertension with special attention to renovascular disease.

6. Ganguly A, Donohue JP: Primary aldosteronism; pathophysiology, diagnosis and treatment. *J Urol* 129:241–247, 1983.

7. Hansson L, Lundin S: Hypertension and coronary

heart disease: cause and consequence or associated diseases? *Am J Med* 76:41–44; 117–121, 1984.
8. Stamler J, Stamler R: Intervention for the prevention and control of hypertension and atherosclerotic diseases: United States and international experience. *Am J Med* 76:13–36, 1984.
    Shows a favorable decline in risk factors corre-

lating with decreased mortality.
9. Stringer DA, deBruyn R, Dillon MJ, et al: Comparison of aortography, renal vein renin sampling, radionuclide scans, ultrasound, and the IVU in the investigation of childhood renovascular hypertension. *Br J Radiol* 57:111–121, 1984.

Case 62
Sudden Coma

PAUL CUTLER, M.D.

It is 8:15 AM, July 3, and the attending physician is making rounds with two fledgling interns.

MD: I believe the patient we just saw with myocardial infarction is doing well. Whom shall we see next?

INTERN 1: We just got a call from the emergency room. A comatose patient is arriving by ambulance. He'll be on our service so we have to see him right away. Would you care to join us?

MD: Of course. Let's all go down and see what's wrong.

ER NURSE: Glad you got here so quickly, doctors! This man doesn't look too good.

INTERN 1: Does he have any family or friends with him?—And where is the ambulance driver?

NURSE: They're just leaving, but I'll get them.

MD: Good thinking. You can often find the answer from a relative or friend or the ambulance driver in a minute when it might take you all day to find out what's wrong by yourself. Suppose you, Jim (INTERN 2), get as much historical information as you can while Maria (INTERN 1) assesses the patient's vital signs and cardiorespiratory status. Maintenance of ventilation and circulation comes first.

INTERN 1: The patient is really comatose. I think he's about 50 years old. He doesn't respond to my voice or noxious painful stimuli. His pupils are equal, mid-dilated, and respond to light. The pulse is 110 but strong, the BP is 116/80, and the respirations are 18/minute with good depth. I don't see any cyanosis. The rectal temperature is 37.5 C.

MD: That's good. His circulation and respiration seem adequate, so he's not in shock and doesn't have cardiac or respiratory failure. What's more, the absence of fever is against meningitis. Now you can slow down a bit, but first do a Dextrostix test on a drop of capillary blood to rule out hypoglycemia. Draw some venous blood for determinations of glucose, creatinine, and toxic screen, and save a tube of blood in the icebox for possible future use. Before withdrawing the needle, inject 50 ml of 50% glucose to rule out hypoglycemia if the Dextrostix test is inconclusive. Also, inject 0.4 mg of naloxone hydrochloride intravenously; you should see a salutary effect in 2 minutes if he has taken an overdose of morphine, heroin, or opioids. Get some arterial blood for pH, pCO_2, and pO_2. Then get a urine sample, analyze it yourself, send a sample to the laboratory for further toxic screen, and leave the catheter in place. Don't forget a complete blood count, chest x-ray, and ECG.

As you can see, we're asking the laboratory to help eliminate acidosis, diabetes mellitus complications, hypoglycemia, drug intoxication, and uremia. Some advise against giving glucose routinely, but as far as I'm concerned it can't hurt, can help, and can give you the solution if the patient wakes up quickly.

The pupillary reactions tell us he hasn't had a massive cerebral or pontine hemorrhage; in that event one pupil would be unilaterally dilated and fixed or both would be constricted. Bilateral fixed dilatation would be alarming and might suggest extensive bilateral brain damage and impending death.

Suppose you proceed with your examination and ask the ER nurse to help you.

INTERN 2: We just got them in time—they were about to leave! The patient has no family and lives alone, but I got lots of information from his friend who lives in the next-door apartment. They're used to having breakfast together. He knocked on the door at 7 AM, found it open, and discovered the patient unconscious on the floor beside his bed. Last night while they were watching television together, he seemed perfectly well. They split two six-packs and said good night. The patient is 58 years old, a known diabetic for 15 years, takes pills for his diabetes, and his friend hinted that the patient sometimes "drinks a lot" to forget his divorced wife and children whom he never sees. He's never been known to have "fits" or "convulsions." The ambulance drivers had nothing to add; all they did was pick him up and bring him in. By the way, I asked the friend to check the apartment for any medicine bottles and let me know what he finds.

MD: That tells us a lot. The most common causes of coma are stroke, drug overdosage, diabetic complications, and trauma. If you review the various disease systems, you can appreciably lengthen this short list to include meningitis, encephalitis, myxedema coma, hysteria, the postictal state of epilepsy, brain tumor, brain abscess, uremia, hepatic coma, CO_2 narcosis, and shock from sepsis or massive myocardial infarction.

A "stroke" can be caused by thrombosis, hemorrhage, embolus, or subarachnoid hemorrhage. Trauma can result in a skull fracture, concussion, or subdural hematoma. Diabetes may be complicated by ketoacidotic coma, hyperosmolar coma, or hypoglycemia. Drug overdosage, in my experience, is usually caused by barbiturates, glu-

tethimide, diazepam, or heroin, although many other narcotics, sedatives, hypnotics, or mood changers can be the offending agents. Lately we've seen many patients who are unconscious from taking combinations of several drugs—anything they can get their hands on—including alcohol. We're not sure how "alcoholic" he is, but I'd be willing to bet that he drinks a lot, so we must be alert for alcoholic intoxication, hypoglycemia, and cranial trauma—the by-products of drinking. All those possibilities can be eliminated quickly with a multibranched but not necessarily thorough data base.

The fact that the patient had no preceding acute illness or gradual downhill course tells us the coma came on suddenly. This tends to rule out diabetic ketoacidosis, uremia, myxedema coma, brain tumor or abscess, hepatic coma, CO_2 narcosis (respiratory failure), and infectious disease. The absence of previous seizures is against epilepsy.

Where the patient is found may guide you. If he is picked up in an alley near a bar, foul play or acute alcoholic intoxication are suspect. Think of a stroke if he was known to be well earlier in the day and was later found unconscious at home. On the other hand, if he hasn't been feeling well and hasn't been seen for several days, gradual-onset diseases like diabetic coma, uremia, and meningitis are to be considered. So knowing when the patient was last seen well helps our logic too.

Don't get locked into a wrong hypothesis. Two common diseases often coexist and even relate to each other. An alcoholic patient may develop uremia. A comatose diabetic patient may have taken an overdose of drugs, suffered a stroke, or been mugged. Many a patient with alcohol on his breath has been jailed or sent home to die because the main illness was obscured.

Maria, tell us what you found.

INTERN 1: First we searched his pockets and found no medicine bottles or pills. His wallet contains a card saying he is diabetic and printed material suggestive of membership in Alcoholics Anonymous. So I don't know what his beer drinking really means. A catheterized urine sample showed nothing other than a trace of glucose. The Dextrostix test showed ample glucose, so I didn't give him any. I did give him the Narcan; it had no effect. He is well hydrated and has a laceration on the back of his head which is not bleeding. He isn't incontinent and hasn't bitten his tongue. There are no signs of meningeal irritation and no needle marks on his forearms. The fundi, heart, lungs, abdomen, extremities, genitalia, and rectum are normal, and the stool is negative for occult blood. In particular, there is no evidence of chronic liver disease or complications of diabetes. The neurologic examination is normal, but he has doll's-eye movements.

MD: He certainly doesn't have cirrhosis of the liver even though he does drink, but that's not surprising since only 20% of alcoholics get cirrhosis. You've pretty well ruled out meningitis and subarachnoid hemorrhage, so you can see there's no need to do a lumbar puncture routinely on every unconscious patient. One look at the patient tells you he doesn't have myxedema. He has neither Kussmaul nor Cheyne-Stokes respirations; this is against any type of acidosis or a large cerebral hemorrhage. Besides, he has no neurologic evidence of a stroke. And diabetic ketoacidosis is unlikely in the absence of dehydration and Kussmaul breathing. What do you think of the laceration on his scalp?

INTERN 1: Either he fell out of bed, or it represents inflicted trauma. I favor the fall because the trauma isn't great. And, oh, yes I forgot; his breath had no odor of alcohol or acetone, not did it resemble the breath of uremic or hepatic coma.

MD: Can you tell the difference?

INTERN 1: Yes. While in medical school, I smelled the breath of a patient with hepatic coma; I'll never forget it. The others are easy to identify.

MD: How can you tell that the unconscious patient didn't have a stroke?

INTERN 1: He doesn't have a hemiplegic posture, the reflexes and muscle tone are equal bilaterally, and there is no Babinski sign. Neither cheek blows out when he expires, and the face is symmetrical.

MD: Very good! What does the presence of doll's-eye movements mean?

INTERN 1: I'm not sure. Would you explain it?

MD: The eyes of a normal person whose head is slowly rocked side to side will move slightly in the opposite direction and then drift back slowly. In the patient who is stuporous or comatose from toxicity, metabolic disease, or cerebral disease, these movements are generally retained but exaggerated so that the eyes rotate more and return more slowly. If there is no movement at all, or only one eye moves, the lesion can be located in the pons, and the cause for unconsciousness is therefore more serious.

I'm a little concerned about the scalp laceration. It could have resulted from falling out of bed. On the other hand, somebody who has a stroke may fall and injure his head at the same time. The reverse is true too. The same incident which caused the laceration might have brought about a subdural hematoma. Foul play is always a consideration. Maybe we ought to do a lumbar puncture in this case in order to be sure.

INTERN 2: Do you think we should get a computed tomographic (CT) scan of the cranium and brain first?

MD: Not a bad idea! It *is* costly and I think we should be able to arrive at a diagnosis without it. But if cerebral thrombosis, cerebral hemorrhage, cerebral embolus, and subdural hematoma are viable possibilities, the CT scan may supersede other procedures and be of great help. These diagnostic possibilities seem unlikely to me, but in view of the laceration we'd better *do the scan before the lumbar puncture.* There's no telling what you might find. I've seen an occasional patient with a brain tumor that suddenly bled, a patient with cerebral metastases who was comatose, and a few with unsuspected subdural hematomas. In these cases a lumbar puncture might be dangerous and unnecessary.

Suppose Jim and I see some other patients. We'll return in an hour, Maria; the chemistries should be back by then too. Looks like you don't have any diabetes complications or stroke. Trauma and drugs are both possible.

(*It is 10:20 AM.*)

MD: Maria, we've just seen three patients: one with chronic obstructive lung disease, one with cirrhosis and bleeding, and a third for evaluation of hypertension. What have you found?

INTERN 1: The CT scan was normal so I did a lumbar puncture that revealed clear, colorless fluid under normal pressure; I sent the fluid to the laboratory for studies. There is no change in the physical examination. The ECG was normal. Tests have come back from the laboratory. The complete blood count, urinalysis, blood pH, pCO_2, pO_2, and creatinine are normal, the blood glucose is 164 mg/dl, and the toxic screen isn't back yet. The chest x-ray was normal.

MD: I suppose we can put diabetic complications and all causes for acidosis to rest. Subdural hematoma is essentially excluded now that the spinal fluid isn't xanthochromic and the CT scan is normal.

It's a bit late to mention it now, but while we were seeing the last three patients, it suddenly dawned on me that a lumbar puncture really wasn't necessary in this patient. The only reasons for doing it—possible meningitis and subarachnoid bleeding—would have already been ruled out by the clinical picture and the CT scan.

We now know what the diagnosis isn't, but we don't know what it is! Where do we go from here?

INTERN 2: Sir, I just got a telephone call from our patient's neighbor. He found two pill bottles in our patient's bathroom: one says, "Tolinase: take 1 tablet before breakfast and dinner" and the other says, "Seconal: take 1 capsule at bedtime for sleep." The first bottle has pills in it; the second is empty. I got the prescribing doctor's name and we're trying to get him on the phone now.

INTERN 1: The lab just called. The patient has a high barbiturate level in his blood. That clinches it. We'll start him on intravenous fluids, watch his blood gases carefully, and make sure he doesn't get into respiratory difficulty.

INTERN 2: The doctor was in his office. He says the patient saw him 3 days ago because he couldn't sleep, so he prescribed ten sleeping capsules. That means that the most he could have taken last night was seven or eight capsules, a sublethal dose. His physician then told me that the patient was depressed over his living pattern, missed his wife, and just heard she had remarried.

MD: Well, I guess I'll go back to my office. It's clear I'm not needed here. The patient should be well by tomorrow. Don't forget to have a psychiatrist see him.

COMMENT If this were June 3 instead of July 3, the seasoned intern would have preferred handling this case by himself. By June he would know the common causes for coma in the population with which he works. He would also know that the performance of life-maintaining maneuvers precedes diagnosis, and he would be familiar with the more unusual causes of coma too.

With no verbal information from the patient, the problem solvers had to flesh out the clinical picture from other important sources, such as the neighbor, ambulance driver, and treating physician.

Diabetes, alcoholism, and a scalp laceration were misleading false positive clues. Many pertinent negative clues were present too. The decisive clue related to the various circumstances surrounding barbiturate intoxication.

Although there are very many causes of coma, attention was given mainly to the common ones, as the less likely and easily recognizable ones were discarded almost by inspection alone. The laboratory took care of the rest.

Because drug overdose, stroke, and trauma are such common causes of coma, many emergency room protocols require intravenous Narcan, a toxic drug screen, and a CT scan for every unconscious patient—unless the cause for the clinical picture is obvious.

Many decision paths or flow charts have been made for the solution of coma, but they are of necessity very complicated, rigid, and incomplete. Especially in the comatose patient, a flexible, self-constructed flow chart should be utilized by the physician who must meet each somewhat varying problem of unconsciousness with a different "think as you go" approach. (*P. C.*)

Suggested Readings

1. Plum F, Posner JB: *The Diagnosis of Stupor and Coma*, ed 3. Philadelphia, Davis, 1980.
   A classic, short, excellent book on all the metabolic and structural causes of coma.

2. Ropper AM, Martin JB: Coma and other disturbances of consciousness. In Petersdorf RG, Adams RD, Braunwald E, et al (eds): *Harrison's Principles of Internal Medicine*, ed 10. New York, McGraw-Hill, 1983, pp 124–131.
   Alterations in consciousness are defined and the clinical approach to the unconscious patient is covered in a very few pages. Then the reader can look up the specific causes in detail.
3. Fitzgerald FT, Tierney LM Jr, Wall SD: The comatose patient. A systematic diagnostic approach for you to follow. *Postgrad Med* 74:207–215, 1983.
4. Hahn AL: Stupor and coma: a clinical approach. *Geriatrics* 38:65–67; 71–73, 1983.
5. Chang GY: Emergency evaluation of the comatose patient. *Hosp Pract (Off.)* 19: 182–183, 1984.
   Performed in an evacuation hospital in Korea.
6. Sananman ML: The use of EEG in the prognosis of coma. *Clin Electroencephalogr* 14:47–52, 1983.
7. Lundar T, James T, Lindegaard KF: Induced barbiturate coma; methods for evaluation of patients. *Crit Care Med* 11:559–562, 1983.

Case 63
Fainting Spells

PAUL CUTLER, M.D.

DATA   A 62-year-old priest is admitted to the hospital for study because of repeated episodes of fainting. During the last episode he fell and broke his nose; this prompted him to visit the doctor.

LOGIC   Fainting or syncope is a transient loss of consciousness which usually lasts no more than a minute or two. It must be differentiated from seizures, coma, and milder sensations such as giddiness, light-headedness, and "graying out" or presyncope. Seizures are episodes of loss of consciousness associated with convulsions. Coma is a prolonged period of unconsciousness. The other states may be milder, incomplete forms of syncope, or unrelated to any disorder associated with loss of consciousness.

DATA   The patient has had approximately 12 such episodes in the past 2 months. They come on quite suddenly without any premonitory symptoms; he faints and then "comes to" in about a minute or so. Others have observed several of the spells and tell him he lies motionless and quickly wakes up with no aftereffects. The episodes come at no particular time of day and do not seem to be related to any special event like eating, not eating, exercising, walking, urinating, coughing, suddenly standing up, shaving, or turning his head to the side. So far as he can recall, each episode occurred while he was sitting or standing, though he thinks one happened in bed.

A month ago he visited a physician who examined him and told him he could find nothing wrong. When advised to have further study, the patient said he was too occupied with his work but would consider it if the fainting recurred.

LOGIC   You are anxious to see if he has carotid sinus syncope but prefer to have him in a controlled environment before pressing on his carotid sinus. Because he is a priest and wears a high stiff collar, your first hypothesis is based more on a hunch than on logic and statistics. The history obtained so far has given you much to think about, and even more that you should not think about.

The causes of syncope range from benign emotional factors to malignant arrhythmias resulting in sudden death. A single fainting spell is commonly caused by a vasovagal reflex associated with fright, fear, or other passionate peaks. The relationship is obvious and these patients rarely reach the doctor. However, studies of large groups of patients with syncope reveal that one-third to one-half remain undiagnosed. In roughly half of those whose cause is found the origin is cardiovascular, and these have a more serious prognosis than the diagnosable non-cardiac cases or the undiagnosed cases.

The reasons for fainting are myriad, but they revolve mostly about five basic mechanisms: cerebral ischemia, decreased cardiac output, peripheral vasodilatation, reflexes, and altered composition of blood going to the brain, each alone or in combination. In these categories you must consider:

1. Transient ischemic attacks (vascular disease)
2. Heart disease: aortic stenosis, atrial myxoma or thrombosis, paroxysmal tachycardia, sinoatrial disease (sick sinus syndrome), atrioventricular (AV) block with Stokes-Adams attacks, angina pectoris, left ventricular failure; pulmonary embolus
3. Carotid sinus syncope
4. Orthostatic hypotension
5. Gastrointestinal hemorrhage
6. Hysteria
7. Decreased pO_2, pCO_2, glucose in blood
8. Syncope induced by cough, urination, or fluid removal from chest, celom, or bladder
9. Epilepsy (without seizures)
10. The common faint.

On the basis of the information thus far, many of the listed possibilities can be ruled out. Carotid sinus syncope and orthostatic hypotension occur only in the erect position. In the former instance, the patient stimulates a sensitive sinus by shaving, turning his head, wearing a stiff collar, or by unknown means; this lowers the blood pressure and often slows the pulse so that insufficient blood reaches the brain.

Orthostatic hypotension occurs in old, debilitated, or bedridden patients whose blood pressures drop and pulses slow when they stand up, resulting in cerebral ischemia. It is also seen in patients with diseases of the autonomic nervous system which preclude rapid adjustments by arterial constriction; included are some patients with diabetes, syphilis, amyloidosis, and generalized dysautonomia. These patients (especially the last group) often have other evidences of autonomic disturbance affecting sphincter control, pupils, potency, and so forth. In addition, marked orthostatic blood pressure changes causing syncope can occur when drugs are given to treat hypertension or when there is acute or chronic volume depletion.

Older people may already have modest decreases in cerebral blood flow because of hypertension, diabetes, and atherosclerosis. In addition, they often have inactive baroreceptors and sympathetic reflexes which impair mechanisms for homeostasis. These factors make them more susceptible to faint with postural change, carotid sinus sensitivity, inadvertent Valsalva maneuvers, and moderate drops in blood pressure seen in myocardial infarction, gastrointestinal hemorrhage, and paroxysmal tachyarrhythmias.

Healthy young soldiers may faint after prolonged motionless standing at attention during military displays—a dramatic yet benign form of syncope.

Gastrointestinal hemorrhages would not recur so frequently. Hypoglycemic syncope could occur from serious illness like insulinoma and severe liver disease; the episodes would come early in the morning or after a missed meal—not as in this case. Functional hypoglycemia which occurs 2 to 3 hours after a meal seldom, if ever, causes neurologic symptoms.

There is no demonstrable relation to any of the activities previously mentioned, so reflex syncope from cough, urination, and removed fluid can be discarded. Aortic stenosis is unlikely because exercise does not bring on an episode.

DATA Other than for mild diabetes which is well controlled by diet, he has been in good health. He has no chest pain, dyspnea, or orthopnea, but he occasionally feels a palpitation in his chest. His memory is good and he says he is still an effective capable priest; this is confirmed by his peers. He is obviously not emotional or disturbed and wants to return to work as soon as possible. The systems review is negative.

LOGIC   He has no symptoms of heart disease. The composite picture being formed of his personality would lead you to exclude hysteria as a viable cause of his problem. Also, the fact that he injured himself refutes hysteria.

As with attacks of any type, it is always good to examine a patient during an attack if possible. Checking the pulse, blood pressure, and ECG at these times is often helpful. Hysterical individuals have normal pulse and blood pressure. Those with cardiac causes do not.

Further points to consider are whether there are preceding symptoms. An aura suggests epilepsy. The common faint is induced by pain, an unpleasant sight, or an emotional disturbance and is preceded by sweating, pallor, tachycardia, and presyncopal "grayness." Transient ischemic attacks may be preceded by or accompanied by other neurologic symptoms like visual disturbances, sensory changes, aphasia, motor weakness, or vertigo, depending on the area involved. Numbness, tingling, and "difficulty in breathing" precede the giddiness and syncope of hyperventilation (alkalosis with low pCO_2). None of these factors is present here.

The occurrence of a single or many episodes is a key point. One faint can be caused by a gastrointestinal hemorrhage, a myocardial infarction, or a pulmonary embolus, but multiple episodes are not likely to have these causes. The rapidity of onset tells you much. Arrhythmias and cardiac arrest cause sudden syncope. Reflexes which induce vasodilatation and hypotension act slowly.

Overlap sometimes exists in that Stokes-Adams attacks and hypoglycemia may cause seizures too and may thus be confused with epilepsy. The length of time that the syncope lasts may be distinctive. For example, most cases of syncope recover in 1 or 2 minutes. But syncope caused by aortic stenosis, hypoglycemia, or hysteria lasts longer.

DATA   Finally, you examine the patient and go directly to the carotid sinuses and arteries. There are no bruits or thrills over the carotid, vertebral, or subclavian arteries, and pressure applied on each carotid sinus separately for 5 seconds causes a drop in blood pressure from 130/80 to 110/70, and a fall in pulse rate from 54 to 50. The patient is sitting up during the test, and he experiences no abnormal sensations.

LOGIC   The absence of bruits is against significant extracranial vascular disease, but this clue must be carefully weighed. Many older patients have bruits which are not clinically important. On the other hand, if stenosis exceeds 90%, there is not enough blood flow to cause a bruit. So this sign is neither sensitive nor specific.

Note that syncope resulting from extracranial cerebrovascular disease may result from disease of the vertebral as well as from the carotid arteries. So look for bruits in the subclavian triangle and suboccipital areas in addition to the site of the carotid bifurcations. Don't forget the special type of vertebrobasilar insufficiency caused by the subclavian steal syndrome.

As for carotid sinus pressure, many older people have sensitive sinuses and will exhibit circulatory changes but usually no syncope. This is especially true if there is associated heart disease. Even if you can induce syncope, it does not necessarily mean that this mechanism is the cause of the patient's syncope. The true cause may still be occult. However, if the carotid sinus is not sensitive and no symptoms are induced, then this mechanism is not the cause for syncope. It can be seen that this test needs careful, deliberate interpretation, for it has false positives but is not apt to have false negatives.

Hypothesis 1 is rejected. Now you proceed with the rest of the examination, having selected transient ischemic attacks or sudden decrease in cardiac output as your likely alternative possibilities.

DATA   Physical examination reveals the following vital signs: BP 130/80, P 54, R 14, T 37 C. The fundi, head and neck, heart, lungs, abdomen, rectum, genitalia, peripheral pulses, and neurologic examination are completely normal. In particular, there are no heart murmurs, thrills, or arrhythmias.

LOGIC   The mild bradycardia is the only abnormality noted. Aortic stenosis, already rendered unlikely by the absence of exertion-induced episodes, can be eliminated because there is no murmur, thrill, or abnormal apical and carotid impulse characteristic of this condition. He has no ventricular failure or angina by symptoms or signs. There is no reason why he should have a low pO_2 or pCO_2, since conditions causing such profound blood gas disturbances would be obvious to the naked eye. More studies are needed.

DATA   After lying flat for 15 minutes, he suddenly stands up. The BP hovers within 10 mm of his reclining BP for a full minute, so you discontinue this test. An electroencephalogram is normal and shows no epileptogenic focus. The chest and skull x-rays are normal. Fasting blood glucose, blood pH, pO_2, pCO_2, and urea nitrogen are normal. The 5-hour glucose tolerance test shows expectedly elevated levels at 1, 2, and 3 hours and no hypoglycemic phase. ECG shows a sinus bradycardia but is otherwise normal in all respects. Complete blood count and urinalysis are normal. An echocardiogram shows no mitral valve disease or evidence of a left atrial tumor or clot.

LOGIC   Orthostatic hypotension, epilepsy, hypoglycemia, and atrial myxoma are ruled out. Mild diabetes is confirmed. Blood gases are normal as predicted. The ECG offers no help except for the mild bradycardia which may be insignificant.

DATA   A 24-hour Holter monitor solves the problem. Three brief episodes of paroxysmal atrial tachycardia are noted; each is followed by a sinus pause of 5 to 6 seconds. One episode occurred while the patient slept; one occurred while he was sitting and he experienced no unusual sensations; but the third took place while he was walking about, and he almost blacked out. There was no evidence of altered AV conduction.

LOGIC   When testing for the causes of syncope, especially in the elderly, be wary of false negative and false positive results. Since arrhythmias are so common in this group, the detection of arrhythmias by the Holter monitor does not mean the arrhythmia is necessarily the cause of recurrent syncope. Furthermore, this procedure is not highly sensitive because nothing may happen during the 24 hours. But if syncope occurs *in conjunction with* a recorded arrhythmia, this is convincing evidence.

The patient no doubt has a sick sinus syndrome with paroxysms of tachycardia depressing his sinoatrial (SA) node so that it does not fire when called upon to do so. Had the asystole lasted a bit longer he would no doubt have fainted. Bradycardia and sinoatrial block are often present too.

Causes for this syndrome are not completely categorized. It may relate to myocardial disease in and around the SA node, disease of the artery to the SA node, coronary, hypertensive, or rheumatic heart disease, or unknown causes.

DATA   A transvenous pacemaker was passed. Very poor SA node recovery time was noted after atrial pacing. Also, a prolonged HV conduction time was detected on His bundle study. Therefore it was decided to implant a permanent state-of-the-art demand pacemaker. Antiarrhythmic drugs were considered since their use is safe with a pacemaker in place, but the decision was made to wait and see.

Since then, the patient has been free of syncope for 6 months, feels perfectly well, and is back at work. The precise cause of the disease in his SA node and ventricular conduction system remains obscure.

QUESTIONS

1. In the past 15 years, this patient's illness has been increasingly recognized and therefore apparently more common. Which of the following statements is incorrect?
   (a) Syncope results from the paroxysmal tachycardia.
   (b) Syncope results from the asystole following the tachycardia.

(c) The sick SA node may result in bradycardia and/or SA block.

(d) Carotid sinus sensitivity and AV conduction delays are common accompaniments.

2. "Low blood pressure" is falsely blamed for many symptoms. True orthostatic hypotension is associated with a profound drop in BP when the patient changes from a reclining to a standing position and may or may not be accompanied by syncope. It can occur in:

(a) hypertensive patients under treatment

(b) patients with blood volume depletion

(c) Addison's disease and pheochromocytoma

(d) patients with spinal cord diseases.

3. Stokes-Adams attacks are long-known causes of syncope or convulsions. Only one of the following statements about them is false:

(a) Complete heart block with episodes of asystole, ventricular tachycardia, or ventricular fibrillation is the usual mechanism.

(b) Coronary artery disease is the principal cause.

(c) Idiopathic disease of the conduction system is the principal cause.

(d) The ECG may not show complete heart block between attacks.

ANSWERS

1. **(a) is incorrect.** While tachycardia can cause syncope, in these cases it is usually the post-tachycardia asystole that results in transitory unconsciousness. (c) and (d) are true statements, though the causes are not perfectly clear. Generally it is difficult to speed such a patient's pulse with exercise or drugs. Drugs given to suppress the arrhythmias may make the SA disease worse, hence the need for permanent demand pacing.

2. **All are correct.** Drug therapy for hypertension may prevent the adequate vasoconstrictor action which adjusts for position change, allowing hypotension to develop. The tilt-table is used to detect volume depletion in hemorrhage or severe dehydration in like manner. In (c) both are known to be true by induction. In severe spinal cord disease, the autonomic control of vessels and sphincters may be lost.

3. **(b) is false.** Coronary disease is not the main cause. Degeneration of the conduction system (Lenègre's disease) is. (a) represents the usual mechanisms for attacks but, interestingly, (d) is also true, and the ECG may show lesser degrees of conduction system disease between attacks. Occasionally the interval ECG is normal.

COMMENT A crucial item of medical logic must be mastered here. Abnormalities that are found or induced may not necessarily be the cause of the patient's syncope. Modest orthostatic drops in blood pressure, arrhythmias noted by Holter monitor, and carotid sinus sensitivity may be *clinically relevant only if they induce syncope.* These aberrations are so common, especially in the aged, that their mere presence does not necessarily imply a cause and effect relationship. Other conditions may account for the fainting spells. The same logic holds true if you find a cardiac conduction disturbance or a cervical bruit. These too are so common that their presence may mislead you; other causes for syncope may be operative.

Most cases of diagnosed syncope can be solved by history and physical examination alone. When necessary, you can also do a blood count, serum glucose and electrolytes, arterial blood gases, and ECG. In unusual instances, you may need to do Holter monitoring, a ventilation-perfusion scan, an electroencephalogram, or programmed electrical stimulation of the heart. Brain scans are almost always fruitless.

This was a difficult presentation to solve. The author used at least 12 of the strategies and methods described in Chapters 3, 4, and 5 in order to reach a conclusion. Try your hand at identifying these techniques, and then compare your answers with the list printed at the end of the next case study (p. 549). Afterward, you should reread this case and see if you can detect where and how each of the listed strategies was used. (*P. C.*)

Suggested Readings

1. Weissler AM, Lewis RP, Boudoulas H, et al: Syncope. In Hurst JW (ed): *The Heart*, ed 5. New York, McGraw-Hill, 1982, pp 576–588.
   Cardiac and noncardiac causes of syncope are nicely discussed and made simple.

2. Noble JR: The patient with syncope. *JAMA* 237:1372–1376, 1977.
   A brief but worthwhile review of the causes of syncope as they relate to precipitating factors.

3. Kapoor WN, Karpf M, Wieand S, et al: A prospective evaluation and follow-up of patients with syncope. *N Engl J Med* 309:197–204, 1983.
   Shows that causes of syncope are often not found and offers proof of the frequency and serious nature of cardiac causes.

4. Lipsitz LA: Syncope in the elderly. *Ann Intern Med* 99:92–105, 1983.
   The serious aspects of syncope in the aged are discussed with special reference to the insensitivity and nonspecificity of many diagnostic procedures.

5. Boudoulas H, Weissler AM, Lewis RP, et al: The clinical diagnosis of syncope. *Curr Probl Cardiol* 7:1–40, 1982.

6. Madigan NP, Flaker GC, Curtis JJ, et al: Carotid sinus hypersensitivity. *Am J Cardiol* 53:1034–1040, 1984.
   Describes three types—cardioinhibitory, vasodepressor, and mixed.

7. Schatz I: Orthostatic hypotension: diagnosis and treatment. *Hosp Pract* 19:59–69, 1984.
   Reflex mechanisms, drugs, volume depletion, and neuropathy are included.
8. Klein GJ, Gulamhusein SS: Undiagnosed syncope: search for an arrhythmic etiology. *Stroke* 13:746–749, 1982.
   Concludes that the documented correlation of an arrhythmia with a syncopal attack is the only dependable diagnostic strategy.
9. Gibson TC, Heitzman MR: Diagnostic efficacy of 24-hour electrocardiographic monitoring for syn-cope. *Am J Cardiol* 53:1013–1017, 1984.
   Describes values and limitations.
10. Kaplan BM: The tachycardia-bradycardia syndrome. *Med Clin North AM* 60:81–97, 1976.
    An excellent analysis of the causes for syncope resulting from SA node disease, and the diseases which affect the SA node.
11. Gang ES, Reiffel JA, Livelli FD, et al: Sinus node recovery times following the spontaneous termination of supraventricular tachycardia. *Am Heart J* 105:210–215, 1983.
    This determines whether syncope will occur.

Case 64
Strange Behavior
PAUL CUTLER, M.D.

DATA   A woman of about 40 is brought to the emergency room by an employee of the YWCA because "she's been acting strange all day." Alcoholic intoxication is suspected because of the odor of her breath and the presence of several empty bourbon bottles in her room at the "Y." She is furtively alert and constantly changes her sitting position, does not seem to comprehend your questions, and seems to be listening intently for some sound.

LOGIC   You suspect an alcohol-related problem, but she does not seem to be merely drunk. Since alcohol has been recently ingested, you tend to minimize problems of the withdrawal syndrome and focus rather on the acute and chronic toxic effects. Chief among the possibilities from the available data are pathologic intoxication and acute alcoholic hallucinosis. The former is usually manifested by violent behavior following the consumption of even small amounts of alcohol, but is part of a spectrum which includes the possibility that this woman simply acts strangely whenever she drinks. Acute alcoholic hallucinosis typically comes several hours after a severe drinking bout but may develop during its course. It is thought that alcohol in this case allows the appearance of latent schizophrenic symptoms. In-deed, schizophrenia and alcoholism may co-exist, and the delineation and separation of the two must be determined by a longitudinal history. None of these conditions is likely to pose an immediate threat to life, although psychiatric hospitalization is often necessary for alcoholic hallucinosis.

DATA   You decide that further analysis of her problems is less urgent than that of the man with chest pain whom the nurse insists you see immediately. You ask the nurse to prepare the woman for an examination to be performed when you are able.

LOGIC   But while you listen to the heart of the patient with chest pain, your mind drifts back to the woman just seen. Could she be developing an alcohol withdrawal syndrome, even though she still has the odor of alcohol on her breath? Something doesn't seem to fit, so, having read about a similar case seen last week, you rethink the possibilities.

Patients who present with the seemingly sudden onset of strange behavior, delirium, or acute confusional states call to mind a wide assortment of disorders. These abnormal states are manifested by disturbances in perception, memory, thinking, concentration, orientation, insight, and mood, often coupled with bizarre movements and tremors.

A few, some, or many of these manifestations can be seen in any of the following clinical situations: (*a*) drug interaction or drug intoxication; (*b*) drug withdrawal, especially from sedatives; (*c*) alcohol intoxication; (*d*) alcohol withdrawal syndromes; (*e*) postsurgical states and acute severe medical illnesses, especially when complicated by fever or occurring in the elderly; (*f*) diseases specifically affecting the nervous system, such as encephalitis, meningitis, subdural hematoma, cerebral thrombosis, and brain tumor; postictal states; hypoglycemia; and trauma.

Medications well known to cause confusion in some patients include bromides, opiates, barbiturates, amphetamines, atropine, hyoscine, steroids, and antidepressants such as amitryptiline.

You recall that confusional states seeming to start suddenly may merely be *noticed* all at once. In retrospect, a family member may tell you that "Dad hasn't really been right" for several days, weeks, or months, but it suddenly became much worse. If the problem is therefore more long-standing, think of: hepatic encephalopathy or uremia; hyper- or hypo- osmolar, calcemic, natremic, or thyroid states; pernicious anemia; and chronic brain syndromes of the multiinfarct or Alzheimer's types.

DATA The nurse records the vital signs: oral temperature 38.5 C, blood pressure 144/85, radial pulse 105. She further notes that the patient is very restless and seems "startled" when her body is touched. The patient complains of headaches, which prompts the nurse to test for a stiff neck; this is absent. When informed of the temperature elevation and lack of nuchal rigidity, you request a complete blood count with white cell differential, clean-catch urinalysis, chest x-ray, serum glucose, serum calcium and sodium, and urea nitrogen. Had you not been so scholarly and selective, you would have simply ordered an 18-test blood chemistry profile. The results will be available in

about 45 minutes, at which time you expect to be seeing the patient again. You decline the nurse's suggestion of acetaminophen for the patient.

LOGIC Knowing that the patient is febrile raises additional diagnostic possibilities. In the present of altered mental status, infection of the central nervous system must be a consideration. An important factor is that the patient did not appear acutely ill; adults with bacterial meningitis are almost always toxic: they look sick. This feature accounted for the relatively slow pace of assessment. The white blood cell count is a good screen for bacterial infection in this age group, and a differential count showing a leftward shift could provide further diagnostic support. The urinalysis and chest film are screening tests for common sites of infection and are ordinarily indicated in the evaluation of infection without obvious source. The measurement of glucose, calcium, sodium, and urea nitrogen is routine in the evaluation of acutely altered function of the central nervous system. The symptom of headache is consistent with subdural hematoma, another problem associated with alcoholism, because such patients often get hurt after a fall or brawl.

DATA The samples are obtained. You have just assessed the cardiac patient when you receive a "stat" page to the x-ray department. You rush over and find that your "alcoholic" patient has had a grand mal seizure; the onset was not observed. Her blood pressure and pulse are about the same. She is awake and shows little or no postictal depression. There is a minor laceration on her tongue, but no evidence of sphincteric incompetence. You note that she has no sign of recent or remote cranial trauma, and the tympanic membranes and fundi are normal; the pupils are 3 mm in diameter, equal, and react directly and consensually to light. There is no nuchal rigidity and the Kernig and Brudzinski signs are absent. Movement of all extremities is forceful and the tendon reflexes are very brisk, although clonus is absent. You cannot assess the plantar reflexes because of withdrawal. If anything, she seems more in contact with her surroundings and she says she still has a terrible headache, which she knows "will only get better with some Fiorinal."

Limited general physical examination reveals: several spider angiomas on the upper trunk; normal thyroid, lungs, and heart; a smooth, soft, nontender liver felt 3 cm below the costal margin in the midclavicular line; no abdominal tenderness or masses; and stool negative for occult blood. Admission is planned and the patient is prepared for lumbar puncture.

LOGIC Note the form of the physical assessment. Since an acute neurologic event has just occurred, the immediate focus is on whether there is some intracranial process which needs instant action to save life. There is no evidence for this so the search then must focus on abnormalities of major organ systems that could have caused the seizure. With an acutely ill patient in the x-ray examining room, only the most basic physical assessment should be done.

The tentative hypothesis that the patient was simply suffering from the acute toxic effect of alcohol is now disproven with the occurrence of a seizure. The headache, fever, and seizure suggest intracranial infection or bleeding, but the patient's relatively good appearance and lack of meningeal signs are difficult to reconcile with these serious possibilities. Examination of the cerebrospinal fluid is nevertheless indicated since missing the diagnosis of bacterial meningitis could be a fatal error. The absence of ophthalmoscopic evidence for increased intracranial pressure permits removal of cerebrospinal fluid with relative safety. A lack of lateralizing signs serves to reduce the probability of a subdural hematoma, but is by no means definitive since the injury may have left few or no external traces and motor changes are usually late manifestations. The presence of symmetric hyperreflexia could be a valuable sign implying bilateral upper motor neuron lesions; however, the uncertainty about the plantar reflexes weakens this proposition.

In view of the chronic headaches followed by strange behavior, a computed tomographic scan might have been more discreet before doing a valorous lumbar puncture. But the time of night, the temporary unavailability of technical skill, the need for transport to the radiology department, and the anticipated lack of patient cooperation induce you to proceed with the lumbar puncture. This decision may have been made more on the basis of rationalization and prejudice than on wisdom and sound medical judgment.

In addition to structural lesions of the nervous system, hepatic or uremic encephalopathy may also cause hyperreflexia with extensor plantar reflexes. As yet, no data are available to rule out renal failure. Is there hepatic insufficiency? The liver is described as being 3 cm below the costal margin, but this is not necessarily abnormal, since the determinant of hepatomegaly is the total span. The qualitative features of the palpable liver were normal, arguing against acute hepatic enlargement, cirrhosis, or infiltrative disease. The lack of a palpable spleen is consistent with a lack of portal hypertension but is not decisive, since spleens are often difficult to palpate. Spider angiomas are a sign of major hepatic disease, but small numbers of them may be seen in normal individuals, more often in women.

Fever, tachycardia, altered mental status, and even seizures may be features of thyrotoxicosis, but the normal-sized thyroid and absence of other clinical features are against this. The normal auscultatory examination of the heart and lungs serves to minimize the possibility of infection of those sites, and of the heart as the source of a cerebral embolus.

DATA Lumbar puncture produces crystal-clear, colorless fluid at normal pressure, containing no microscopic abnormalities; it is sent for glucose and protein determination, and culture. The previously obtained laboratory data are available: hematocrit 40%; hemoglobin 13.3 g/dl; white blood cells (WBCs) 7800/mm^3 (differential not performed); the urine is negative for glucose and protein, ketones are 2+, and there are three to four WBCs/high-power field, no casts, and many vaginal epithelial cells. The urea nitrogen is 14 mg/dl, the glucose 88 mg/dl, the calcium 9.7 mg/dl, and the serum sodium 135 mEq/liter. The senior resident arrives in the emergency room and, after studying the available data and briefly examining the patient, proposes what in 48 hours proves to be the correct diagnosis.

LOGIC   The grossly normal cerebrospinal fluid rules out bacterial meningitis and minimizes the possibility of many other intracranial processes under consideration. The normal blood urea nitrogen, glucose, and calcium rule out encephalopathy due to uremia, hypo- or hyperglycemia, and parathyroid disorders. The normal WBC count minimizes the possibility of serious infection, and the lack of anemia reduces the likelihood of several categories of major systemic disease. The urine specimen was contaminated by vaginal secretions, but the lack of many WBCs is against the diagnosis of pyelonephritis. The ketonuria probability reflects the effects of fasting.

DATA   In seeking the patient's prior medical history, the resident learned that she had no local physician and was living at the YWCA because she had just come to this city. She stated that she drank liquor to help her headaches because her usual medicine had to be prescribed by a doctor. Usually she drank "only one shot at most three times a week." For about 6 months she had been taking self-increased doses of Fiorinal (contains aspirin, 200 mg; phenacetin, 130 mg; caffeine, 40 mg; butalbital, 50 mg), and most recently was using 16 to 20 tablets or capsules/day. She had been accustomed to getting prescriptions from each of five physicians, but had run out of the drug the day before.

LOGIC   Doses of butalbital in this range could produce physical dependence and an abstinence syndrome on sudden cessation. Hyperreflexia and seizures are common features of this syndrome. Bizarre mental states including frank psychosis may occur. Mild elevation of temperature is frequent.

DATA   The neurologic findings were further amplified by demonstrating a flexor plantar response upon stroking the foot appropriately after "spanking" the sole to reduce light tactile sensitivity, and by the finding of a glabellar reflex. The BP dropped to 90/78 when she stood up.

LOGIC   The glabella is just above the point where the eyebrows come closest together. A glabellar reflex, the nonextinguishing contraction of one or both orbicularis oculi muscles after tapping the glabella, is seen in virtually only sedative-hypnotic withdrawal and in some cases of parkinsonism. Orthostatic hypotension is another common feature of the barbiturate withdrawal syndrome. And a flexor plantar response is to be expected in the absence of long tract disease.

DATA   This woman's abstinence syndrome was treated by standard methods of gradual withdrawal. She was seen by an empathic house officer who is not content with the low probability estimate for an intracranial space-taking lesion and aims for certainty. So extensive studies, including a computed tomographic scan and electroencephalogram, were done and failed to yield a structural cause of her headaches. But strong evidence of psychoneurotic depression was elicited by additional interview. Tests of hepatic function were normal and there were no positive bacterial cultures. The patient participated briefly in a group psychotherapeutic process after discharge but was lost to follow-up.

LOGIC   We readily accept the danger of drugs but not of alcohol—which is just another drug. Alcoholic patients are prone to develop numerous complicating diseases. Some have already been mentioned. Aside from pathologic intoxication and various withdrawal syndromes, they may get nutritional diseases such as pellagra, beriberi, polyneuropathy, and Wernicke-Korsakoff syndrome. There is a high incidence of liver disease and alcoholic gastritis. During an episode of intoxication, the patient may develop a Mallory-Weiss syndrome from vomiting or a subdural hematoma from trauma, may suffocate from aspiration or a "café coronary," or may kill or be killed in an automobile accident. Severe hypoglycemia can result from a spree of drinking without eating. Alcohol may cause thrombocytopenia, acute pancreatitis, and acute muscle necrosis.

And as if all this were not enough, there are various brain diseases of uncertain pathogenesis associated with alcoholism: cerebellar degeneration, cerebral atrophy, and pontine myelinosis. And remember the marital discord, disturbed family relations, and altered work performance!

The alcoholic is damned if he does and damned if he doesn't. Withdrawal syndromes include severe tremulousness, hallucinosis, "rum fits" or withdrawal seizures, and, most serious, delirium tremens. The latter disorder usually occurs 2 to 4 days after enforced cessation of alcohol consumption. Characteristically, a patient is admitted to the hospital with pneumonia or to jail to dry out, seems to be doing well, and goes rapidly into a state of delirium combined with tremors—a picture well known to almost everybody. Such incidents are thought by some to be humorous and inspire many jokes. In fact, they are serious, may be fatal, and require urgent care.

COMMENT Physicians often behave as though they do not like to care for alcoholics, perhaps in part because of the failure of the conventional medical approach. Probably because of this bias and the fact that the patient did not look very sick, there was little initial effort at assessment. This is an example of how the diagnostic process may be clouded by a too obvious clue: the smell of alcohol. Many tales are told about drunkards who die in jail or are dismissed from the emergency room only to die at home. These persons all smell of alcohol but the real problem is overlooked. Always remember that devotees of Bacchus have a predilection for some diseases but are subject to all.

Assessment became more active with the report of fever, but the dramatic seizure really catalyzed vigorous and appropriate data gathering. It was not until these failed to yield solutions that a few questions and tests of a specific hypothesis gave the answer—drug withdrawal. Even so, additional studies were needed to pinpoint the reason for taking so much medication.

This case demonstrated the processing of abundant clues—true positives, pertinent true negatives, a misleading false positive, and several key clues. Cluster formation, differential diagnosis, hypothesis generation, and pruning the differential all took part in the evolution of a diagnosis. The problem solvers made decisions on the sequence of testing and alternate strategies were weighed.

In today's fast-moving emergency rooms this patient might have been managed with a brief history and a scant selective physical examination followed by a toxic screen, an 18-test blood chemistry profile, a blood alcohol level, a CT scan, and a lumbar puncture—all in a matter of a few hours. Economy, order, and thoroughness are thereby replaced by speed and accuracy. Even so, in spite of the use of high technology procedures and tests, additional history and examination data were needed. The procedures told you what the patient *did not* have. The history and physical examination told you what she *did* have. (*P. C.*)

Answers to Comment on Case 63

1. positive clues
2. pertinent negative clues
3. key clue
4. false clue
5. decisive clue
6. sensitivity and specificity of clues
7. early hypothesis generation
8. proof by exclusion
9. pinpointing the diseased organ
10. traditional method
11. hunch
12. varied cause and effect relationships.

Suggested Readings

1. Victor M, Adams RD: Alcohol. In Petersdorf RG, Adams RD, Braunwald E, et al (eds): *Harrison's Principles of Internal Medicine*, ed 10. New York, McGraw-Hill, 1983, pp 1285–1295.

   An excellent review of all the syndromes and diseases which may result from alcohol, and their management.

2. Complications of alcoholism. *Med Clin North Am* 68, Jan 1984.

   This entire issue deals in depth with the various effects of chronic alcoholism on the brain, heart, liver, blood, glucose metabolism, skeletal muscle, endocrine glands, etc. Each chapter is a trove of information.

3. Thomson AD: The consequences of alcohol abuse. *Practitioner* 227:1427–1439, 1983.
   A world-wide viewpoint of the chronic effects.
4. Landers DF: Alcoholic coma and some associated conditions. *Am Fam Physician* 28:219–222, 1983.
   Covers a variety of acute alcoholic syndromes.
5. Favazza AR: Alcoholism. *Am Fam Physician* 27:274–278, 1983.
   A fine short exposition of the definition and complications of alcoholism.
6. Sherlock S: Nutrition and the alcoholic. *Lancet* 1:436–439, 1984.
   Why alcoholics become malnourished.
7. Ayd FJ Jr: Benzodiazepine dependence and withdrawal. *Md State Med J* 32:22–24, 1983.
   Withdrawal syndrome is neatly described.
8. Levy AB: Delirium and seizures due to abrupt alprazolam withdrawal: case report. *J Clin Psychiatry* 45:38–39, 1984.
   Documents how withdrawal from a sedative or anxiolytic can cause problems—only 2 pages.
9. Multry JT: Chemical dependency: a unified illness. *Am Fam Physician* 29:285–290, 1984.
   A practical analysis of how dependence on any drug can lead to loss of control, social disaster, denial, and ethical deterioration.
10. Gay MH, Ryan GP, Boisse NR, et al: Phenobarbital tolerance and physical dependence: chronically equivalent dosing model. *Eur J Pharmacol* 95:21–29, 1983.
   Dependence and abstinence syndromes in rats that mimic human reactions.

Case 65
Prolonged Fever
PAUL CUTLER, M.D.

INTERN: We need some help on a difficult problem. The patient is a 48-year-old construction worker who has had documented fever for 2 to 3 weeks. Many temperature readings are between 38.3 and 39 C. He has had no previous illnesses or operations and complains only of fever, malaise, and fatigue. We've checked him in the hospital for a week and don't have a diagnosis yet.

MD: You've just defined the Petersdorf and Beeson criteria for a fever of undetermined origin (FUO). It features are (*a*) illness of more than 3 weeks, (*b*) fever higher than 38.3 C on several occasions, and (*c*) diagnosis uncertain after 1 week of hospital study. I think these criteria are good but not explicit enough. Fever should be the principal symptom and, while there may be nonspecific associated symptoms like malaise, fatigue, weight loss, or even chills, there should be no symptoms present that point to an organ or system—for example, arthralgia, abdominal pain, and so forth.

Former criteria for FUO definition are now obsolete because new technology permits more studies in 1 week than were conceivable 10 years ago. You may have already done ultrasound, computed tomography, and gallium scans of the abdomen, followed by needle aspiration, catheter drainage, biopsy, or exploratory laparotomy. Often less than a week is required to transform an FUO into an FKO (fever of known origin). The time needed for study will vary with the aggressiveness of the physician and the complexity of the case.

How did the illness begin?

INTERN: He was seen in the emergency room several times and was thought to have nothing more than a viral infection. We're seeing a lot of that. So he was sent home on aspirin. When he returned after a total of 10 days' fever, we hospitalized him. It took us a few days to get a bed.

During the past week, his fever has been well documented. The temperature rises to 38.5 to 39 C every day and there are no new symptoms. The physical examination has remained normal; we check him carefully every day. Normal or negative studies include a complete blood count, urinalysis, six blood cultures, two urine cultures, chest and abdomen x-rays, ECG, and complete blood chemistries except for the alkaline phosphatase, which is twice the upper normal value.

The sedimentation rate is elevated: 26 mm/hour, and the intermediate strength purified protein derivative (PPD) test is positive.

MD: I assume you've already asked all the appropriate questions and sought the physical findings that go with febrile disease?

INTERN: Yes. There's no dyspnea, cough, expectoration, disorientation, stiff neck, sore throat, joint pains, frequent or painful urination, nausea, vomiting, diarrhea, or abdominal pain. The patient has had no unpasteurized cow's or goat's milk products and no recent dental work or urethral instrumentation. While he has had no recent contact with tuberculosis, his sister died of that disease 25 years ago. He has no evidence of meningeal irritation, no heart murmur, rash, jaundice, arthritis, enlarged liver, spleen, or nodes.

MD: You just rattled off a lot of negative information. Can you tell me why you mentioned these items and what their absence or negativity means?

INTERN: I've listed what I feel are pertinent negatives. That is, they tend to exclude certain possibilities. The absence of dyspnea, cough, and expectoration is against advanced fibrocaseous pulmonary tuberculosis being a cause of fever. Meningitis is unlikely in the absence of disorientation, stiff neck, sore throat, and signs of meningeal irritation. No joint pains, arthritis, or rash are against an autoimmune collagen disorder. Infective endocarditis is less likely if there has been no dental work or urethral instrumentation. The other negative findings are against brucellosis, enteric fevers, and leukemias or lymphomas.

MD: That's good reasoning! Well, the patient doesn't look sick nor does he look like he's lost weight. He should be weighed daily. He has no other serious disease and is not immunosuppressed, so we're not in any great hurry to make a diagnosis. No need rushing in with invasive procedures just yet. Time may be better than tests. Few syndromes give rise to more abuse and ineffective use of diagnostic procedures than do prolonged fevers.

We've got to consider the anxiety of the patient and the yield, risk, and cost of each procedure against the morbidity, risk, and cost of the illness. It might be wiser from the economic and patient morale standpoints to proceed rapidly. But remember that many FUOs will diagnose themselves by the appearance of a new symptom or sign as we observe the patient. Still other patients (5 to 8%) get well without a diagnosis ever having been made.

The rapid erythrocyte sedimentation rate and elevated alkaline phosphatase are nonspecific markers for disease, but the latter suggests liver or bone involvement. An absence of leukocytosis and chills is against an occult abscess; the absence of a heart murmur and negative blood cultures are against endocarditis. The positive PPD skin test is a bit confusing. His sister had tuberculosis 25 years ago, so he may have become positive then. I don't know what to make of it. If negative, it would have been more helpful since anergy is uncommon even in miliary tuberculosis. Has he received any antibiotics or is he taking medication?

INTERN: Before he came into the hospital he was given penicillin and tetracycline by a physician, but he's taking no medication whatsoever now.

MD: Previous antibiotics may make it difficult to get a positive blood culture even if endocarditis exists; and it's interesting to note how often medications of any kind can cause fever. Antibiotics, barbiturates, iodides, Dilantin, propylthiouracil, allopurinol, methyldopa, procainamide, and quinidine are common offenders.

Well-defined FUOs are caused mainly by "the big three": infection in 40% of cases, malignancy in 20%, and collagen-vascular disease in 15%. Infections include tuberculosis, infective endocarditis, and localized but hidden infection such as perinephric, subphrenic, prostatic, tubo-ovarian, and hepatic abscesses. Less common infections are cytomegalovirus disease, histoplasmosis, coccidioidomycosis, typhoid, paratyphoid, and undulant fever, chronic meningococcemia, and gonococcemia.

As for malignancies and tumors, the most

common types that cause fever are lymphomas, Hodgkin's disease, and leukemias, though renal cell carcinoma, hepatoma, atrial myxoma, and metastastic cancer in the liver may also present with fever as the sole manifestation for some time.

The likelihoods depend on the subset with whom you work too. In my experience, malignancy is the most common cause of FUO, infection a close second, and collagen disorders a distant third.

I once saw an elderly male patient with widely spaced episodes of chills and fever recurring over a period of 6 months. Each time he got better with a "shot of penicillin" and asked me to give him the same thing. His regular physician was away. But by this time he already had constipation and red rectal bleeding too. Barium enema and subsequent surgery disclosed a carcinoma of the sigmoid colon in an area of diverticulitis with multiple microabscesses which were seeding his bloodstream. Who would think that cancer could cause chills and fever?

INTERN: That's a strange one! How about the third category?

MD: Collagen-vascular diseases are far more common in women, and include systemic lupus erythematosus, polymyalgia rheumatica, periarteritis nodosa, rheumatoid arthritis, and hypersensitivity angiitis; fever may sometimes be the sole symptom in these diseases long before other manifestations appear, but this is not usual. Better get some immunologic markers.

And don't forget a large miscellaneous group which makes up the remaining 20%! Each is most uncommon by itself but must be considered if one of the preceding triad is not found. In this list are factitious fever, habitual hyperthermia, drug fever, active cirrhosis or hepatitis, inflammatory bowel disease, malaria, periodic fever (familial Mediterranean fever—FMF), nonspecific granulomatous disease, Whipple's disease, atrial myxoma, and the undiagnosed cases. All can present as an FUO, though sooner or later additional signs appear.

Go after the common causes first, then consider the rare. Don't do anything highly invasive. I'll be back in a few days.

(Four days later)
INTERN: Glad you returned! The patient has been studied from top to bottom and we still don't have the answer.

MD: Tell me about it.

INTERN: Blood, urine, and stool cultures are all still negative and some have been incubating for as long as 10 days. Radioisotopic liver-spleen and liver-lung scans, abdominal sonogram, and computed tomography show no evidence of subphrenic, hepatic, or perinephric abscess. The scan and physical examination now suggest that the liver may be a little enlarged—14 cm on vertical percussion. A whole-body scan with gallium-67 detects no evidence of intraabdominal malignancy or infection. Prostatic examination is again normal. Serologic studies for fungi and cytomegalovirus are negative, and agglutination tests for enteric pathogens are negative. A Giemsa stain of a thick blood smear for malaria parasites is negative too.

The intravenous pyelogram and barium enema are normal. Rheumatoid factor, antinuclear antibody, and anti-DNA antibody are negative, and there is no eosinophilia. An echocardiogram shows no evidence of atrial myxoma and there's no mitral murmur.

While there have been no new symptoms or findings, the nurse reports a 4-lb weight loss in 2 weeks. I think we have to get to the bottom of this soon. We've pretty much ruled out the various possibilities you discussed. What about factitious fever, cyclic fever, and habitual fever?

MD: They're unusual. I'm sure you've already eliminated factitious fever by having the nurse continuously present while the temperature is being taken. But devious patients can fool the nurse by warming the mouth in advance. To get around this, you can take the temperature of a simultaneously voided urine sample or take the temperature by instantaneous probe. Also, factitious fever doesn't follow a diurnal pattern and drops suddenly without diaphoresis.

Cyclic fever (FMF) occurs in people who come from the Mediterranean basin, is usually accompanied by signs of serositis, and is cyclic and familial, as the name implies.

Habitual hyperthermia is a normal situation found mostly in young women in their twenties or thirties who have easily detectable psychoneurotic traits. They may have temperatures as high as 38 C daily, and though this is not pathologic, such patients often undergo extensive fruitless studies for FUO.

Drug-induced fevers are becoming more commonly recognized, but this patient is not taking medications and antibiotics were stopped a while ago, so that possibility may be excluded.

I would agree with you that more aggressive studies are indicated. Suppose we get biopsies of the liver, bone marrow, and gastrocnemius muscle. The liver is a good place to biopsy if diffuse visceral disease is expected, and the bone marrow gives essentially the same information. A muscle biopsy is for detecting vascular disease. Hold off on possible laparotomy or a therapeutic trial. Exploratory surgery is rarely necessary now that there are so many new diagnostic techniques.

(Three days later)

INTERN: We have the answer! The muscle and bone marrow biopsies were normal. But the liver biopsy showed multiple caseating granulomas typical of miliary tuberculosis. The pathologist even found tubercle bacilli in them. I was surprised at the normal chest x-ray, but, on reading, I found this to be common early in the disease.

MD: That's correct. You can begin treatment now and you should see some good results in 2 to 3 weeks. There's some difference of opinion on the value of liver biopsy in FUOs, but I don't think there can be any dispute here.

This case reemphasizes the need to "think common." There are several dozen causes of FUO, but tuberculosis, endocarditis, occult bacterial infection, lymphoma, cancer, and collagen disease head the list and are statistically far more common than the numerous but infrequent stragglers.

Fortunately, we did not have to consider the ponderous questions of exploratory laparotomy and therapeutic trials. These are "last resort" decisions, and often difficult to make. Therapeutic trials are especially risky, since you often do more harm than good when treating almost blindly with antibiotics or steroids. But sometimes your hand may be forced:

INTERN: This case bothers me. Don't you feel we should have had the answer sooner?

MD: Yes, I do. It bothers me too. I think we may have proceeded too slowly, and I must accept responsibility for that. The cluster of fever, a positive PPD, and an elevated alkaline phosphatase should have directed our inquiry more rapidly into a liver biopsy. Most of the studies could have been bypassed. There are indeed some diseases associated with fever where speedy diagnosis is essential to prevent rapid deterioration. This is especially true for miliary tuberculosis, infective endocarditis, and intraabdominal infection.

In the future, when confronted with diagnostic problems of this sort, try to form an early hypothesis by clustering a few clues. Then do a directed or selective study. For example, if your patient with fever just returned from an African safari, do a blood smear for malaria. If your patient with fever just had an appendectomy or complicated bowel surgery, look for intraabdominal suppuration with a computed tomographic scan, a gallium scan, or an ultrasound study. It would be senseless to request a PPD skin test or an antinuclear antibody titer. So rather than use a general checklist for all causes of FUO, evaluate the problem as it exists in a specific clinical setting. If your initial hypothesis is not supported by selected studies, you may have to formulate a new one.

In this regard, the key clue may often be found in the history—previous illnesses or surgery, drugs or alcohol, social and occupational history, hobbies, travel, and animal exposure.

If no hypothesis is feasible, then you must resort to an orderly battery of tests and studies for an FUO.

Hospitalized cases can be quite complicated. Often the clinical setting offers many possible causes for fever. Suppose you have a 60-year-old man who had a mitral valve replacement performed 5 days ago. He begins to have fever. Because of the surgery it is still difficult for him to cough and clear his chest. There is a catheter in his bladder because he is having trouble voiding, an intravenous catheter is in place for fluids and electrolytes, and he is being given two antibiotics either of which sometimes causes fever. On examination there are signs of a left pleural effusion.

Based on this information, you may postulate suppurative thrombophlebitis at the intracath site, infective endocarditis, infected incision, acute urinary tract infection, pneumonia, empyema, pulmonary embolus, and drug fever. With these presumptions, you would then order the appropriate confirmatory tests and actions. It would be farfetched to hunt for collagen disease or cancer under these circumstances.

By the way, recheck our patient's fundi for choroid tubercles.

INTERN: The next patient we'd like you to see has a problem which was very easy to solve. Just by looking at her, I could tell....

QUESTIONS

1. In general, therapeutic trials are frowned upon, but if the patient is deteriorating and no diagnosis has been made, you might try:
   (a) antibiotics if endocarditis is suspected
   (b) steroids if collagen-vascular disease is suspected
   (c) isoniazid and adjunctive therapy if miliary tuberculosis is suspected
   (d) antimetabolites if lymphoma is suspected.
2. In miliary tuberculosis, which of the following circumstances is excluded?
   (a) enlarged liver and spleen
   (b) signs of meningeal irritation
   (c) leukopenia and anemia
   (d) leukemia-like blood picture
   (e) normal chest x-ray
   (f) abnormal chest x-ray
   (g) positive PPD skin test
   (h) negative PPD skin test.
3. Which of the following questions is important in trying to determine the cause of an FUO?
   (a) Have you been bitten by a rat in the past 2 months?
   (b) Do any other members of your family suffer from recurrent fevers?

   (c) Do you have shaking chills?
   (d) Are you of Indian extraction?

ANSWERS

1. **(a) and (c) are correct.** For example, a young patient with a heart murmur and fever who appears ill may be given intelligent antibiotic treatment even if an etiologic agent is not identified and you are suspicious but not certain. There are definite risks. So too if miliary tuberculosis is suspected but not identified as such. But steroids are nonspecific in their action, may mask most diseases, and may make the patient susceptible to others. Their use is therefore inadvisable in almost all instances. Suspected lymphomas should not be treated without a tissue diagnosis, even if it necessitates laparotomy.

2. **None is correct because all are possible.** Widespread miliary involvement can enlarge the liver and spleen, cause meningitis, and involve the bone marrow. It may replace the marrow, causing leukopenia and anemia, or irritate the marrow, causing a leukemoid reaction. If miliary spread results from a caseous hilar node eroding a pulmonary vein, the chest x-ray may remain normal until miliary lesions in the lung coalesce and become radiologically visible. On the other hand, the chest x-ray may be abnormal from the start since it may show reinfection tuberculosis. The PPD skin test is usually positive, though it is sometimes negative if the patient is debilitated, anergic, or overwhelmed.

3. **(a), (b), and (c) are correct.** Rat-bite fever can be caused by either Spirillum minus or Streptobacillus moniliformis. Fever in another member of the family suggests FMF, especially if the extraction is Italian, Sephardic Jewish, or Arab. Shaking chills suggest malaria, sepsis, or abscess formation somewhere. Whether the patient is Asian or American Indian seems to have no bearing if he lives here.

COMMENT   The principal technique used here was the traditional exhaustive one. A complete data base was needed, and even then the problem remained unsolved. Fever was the key clue since other symptoms were too vague, and the conclusive clue resided in the liver biopsy. Bayes' mathematics again proved that common diseases deserve prime consideration, and that even uncommon manifestations of common diseases must be kept in mind before thinking of the rare.

Note the unreliability of statistics as demonstrated by the fact that causes for FUO will vary with its definition and with the vigor of diagnostic study during the first week. Further variability hinges on whether the patient is female, young, or old—and whether your population subset does or does not contain Mediterraneans who get FMF, underprivileged persons who are more susceptible to tuberculosis, addicts who are prone to endocarditis, or soldiers returning from the tropics who may harbor the malaria plasmodium.

The order, speed, urgency, cost, and danger of studies received careful consideration in a patient who was not desperately ill, and in whom tincture of time was an important ingredient in mandating that a definite diagnosis be made before giving treatment—usually a good idea. But in this case, a more rapid, hypothesis-driven approach would have been more advisable. The physician's zeal for teaching and the intern's thirst for learning and passion for thoroughness may not have been in the best interests of the patient and health care costs. (*P. C.*)

Suggested Readings

1. (a) Petersdorf RG, Beeson PB: Fever of unexplained origin: report on 100 cases. *Medicine* 40:1–30, 1961.
   (b) Larsen EB, Featherstone NJ, Petersdorf RG: Fever of undetermined origin: diagnosis and follow-up of 105 cases, 1970–1980. *Medicine* 61:269–292, 1982.
   These two articles compare the same subject two decades apart; both are partly authored by the original describer of FUO.

2. Vickery DM, Quinnell RK: Fever of unknown origin: an algorithmic approach. *JAMA* 238:2183–2188, 1977.
   The authors present a well-structured, step-by-step method of solving FUOs.

3. Hurley DL: Fever in adults. What to do when the cause is not obvious. *Postgrad Med* 74:232–244, 1983.
   Advocates scans as a replacement for laparotomy.

4. Kauffman CA, Jones PG: Diagnosing fever of unknown origin in older patients. *Geriatrics* 39:46–51, 1984.
   Covers the subject in only 6 pages—infections, neoplasms, drugs, etc.

5. Coon WW: Diagnostic celiotomy for fever of undetermined origin. *Surg Gynecol Obstet* 157:467–470, 1983.
   Cites the advantages of "diagnosis by looking in."

6. Williamson LM, Hull D, Mehta R, et al: Familial Hibernian fever. *Q J Med* 51:469–480, 1982.
   Reviews periodic fevers and gives the Irish equivalent of FMF.

7. Calamia KT, Hunder GG: Giant cell arteritis (temporal arteritis) presenting as FUO. *Arthritis Rheum* 24:1414–1418, 1981.

9. Mitchell DP, Hanes TE, Hoyumpa AM, et al: Fever of unknown origin: assessment of the value of liver biopsy. *Arch Intern Med* 187:1001–1004, 1977.
   A contrary view on the value of liver biopsy in FUO.

Section Four

Special Aspects of Problem Solving

Chapter 25. Information Retrieval

Chapter 26. Triage, Screening, Urgent Care

Chapter 27. Drug- and Doctor-Induced Disease

Chapter 28. The Psychiatric Patient

Chapter 29. The Pediatric Patient

Chapter 30. The Geriatric Patient

Section Four

Introduction

There are many population subsets in whom problem solving is somehow different. Special rules need to be observed, selected dictums must be followed, and varying techniques must be used.

Such groups of patients may consist of alcoholics, addicts, psychoneurotics or psychotics, the abused, the improperly treated, infants, children, adolescents, adults, the elderly, the poor, the rich, the underprivileged, the overprivileged, emergencies, and on and on. In each category there are distinctive features of data gathering, data evaluation, diagnostic possibilities, decision making, and problem solving.

The following chapters deal with some of these patient subsets. First and foremost, however, is the very important chapter on information retrieval—how to learn all about the patient's problems. This includes what you once knew and forgot, what you never knew, and what's new. (*P. C.*)

Chapter 25

Information Retrieval

DAVID A. KRONICK, PH.D.

The logic sessions in Section Three have required you to apply information to the solution of specific patient problems. This information is organized and stored in your personal memory and retrieved through a process of critical judgments about relevance to the particular case at hand. The extent to which your personal memory has stored the necessary information, and the extent to which you have been able to update, replenish and purge it of obsolete materials, will determine the degree to which you can bring it to bear on the solution of a problem.

Despite the extraordinary storage capacity of the brain, it is unlikely that your memory can acquire and store the information you will need to solve all medical problems. Because of the increased pace of medical innovation and the growth of medical literature it is no longer possible, as William Osler once said, to keep up "with half an hour's reading in bed as a steady practice" (1). Screening, digesting, synthesizing, and extracting the useful elements from the literature now comprise a task which must be shared with other individuals and agencies. If you are to function as an effective problem solver in clinical medicine, you must learn how to use these "external memory" and communications systems effectively.

There are two primary techniques for using information sources. The first is an anticipation of future needs, which is sometimes called *maintaining current awareness* or *knowledge of the state of the art.* It is also sometimes called "keeping up with the literature." This is a responsibility which must

be shared with your teachers, your colleagues, and other individuals through such mechanisms as hospital grand rounds, journal clubs, luncheon and dinner conversations, and other forms of continuing education. Each physician doubtlessly develops his own techniques or combination of techniques to maintain his current awareness.

Journal reading or systematically scanning a carefully selected number of clinical journals is a widely accepted strategy. Among the other techniques for current awareness are the review series which annually try to synthesize all the advances in clinical medicine for the previous year, such as the *Year Book of Medicine* and *Current Diagnosis.* Included also are all the forms of continuing education which are made available to physicians, as well as attendance at the various local, regional, and national meetings of general and special medical societies. Abstract journals such as the various sections of *Excerpta Medica* and the abstract sections of many clinical journals are also useful. Audiotape journals and seminar series make it possible to enhance your current awareness through a playback unit in your car or home.

The second primary technique for accessing information sources is in *response to a specific information need.* For example, you have a problem in diagnosis or treatment and wish to know if there have been any changes in the state of the art, or wish to supplement your knowledge about the subject. You must first specifically and precisely identify the type of information you need and articulate it in such a way that you can share it with another individual or information system. Not being aware that you may lack data or information is generally regarded as a greater intellectual misdemeanor than not having it. Obviously if you do not know you lack the information it is unlikely that you will acquire it. At this point it becomes important to know how to use external memory systems so you can plan your strategy for retrieving the information as effectively and efficiently as possible.

Many physicians and students collect and organize their own information files derived from journals, reprints, courses, and conferences. Several systems have been described for organizing personal information files (2, 3). One is simply to file notes and reprints under general subject terms which reflect your interests. Another is to keep reprints in accession order and maintain author and subject indexes. Since these are personal files they do not need to conform to any special procedure.

Standard subject heading lists such as the one used by *Index Medicus* can be helpful, since they help you maintain some consistency in your indexing vocabulary. Remember not to start a personal information system which will make more demands on your time than you can spare. Bear in mind that libraries are highly organized information files with a well-developed apparatus to provide access to them. Since they are not personal files you must know how they are organized in order to use them effectively.

One of the first places to look is in general medical texts which attempt to summarize the state of the art in a single work. Since these texts are so comprehensive they may omit some of the detail in which you are interested. In that case there will probably be one or more specialty texts covering your particular subject interest. The specialty texts as well as the general texts all provide references to document their discussions and to suggest sources of additional information. All textbooks, however, have experienced a certain amount of obsolescence by the time they are in print. The statement is some-

times made, although it is difficult to confirm or deny, that the "half-life" of medical information is 7 years. That is, at least half the information you possess today will be obsolete in 7 years. The standard general medical texts are usually issued in new editions every 3 to 5 years. The information included may be even older because of the inevitable lag between the time a manuscript for a book is completed and the time it is printed and sold.

Textbooks are supplemented by various handbooks and compendia, some of which supply key references to papers on a large number of clinical problems. Krupp's (Marcus A. Krupp et al (eds): *Current Medical Diagnosis and Treatment* (Los Altos, CA, Lange, 1985) is a good example; it is revised yearly.

Inevitably one must come, however, to the *Index Medicus* which is the major index to the international biomedical journal literature. *Index Medicus* is produced by the National Library of Medicine. Its present form dates from 1960 and its computer-based version from 1963. It indexes some 3,000 journals and is published monthly. An annual cumulation replaces the monthly issues and covers about 250,000 articles a year, half of which are in English.

If you are not familiar with the *Index Medicus*, a few minutes spent reading the preface to the most recent January issue and browsing through any issue will acquaint you with its construction. The most important fact to remember is that the index uses a special controlled vocabulary in which only approved terms are selected for indexing. These terms are listed in a compilation which is revised and issued each year under the title *Medical Subject Headings* (MeSH) as a part of the *Index Medicus*. This list will refer you from terms not used (but which may be your terms of reference) to terms which are used. It will also show you an array of related terms in its "Categorized Lists" which will suggest other appropriate terms for searching. The National Library of Medicine also publishes the *Abridged Index Medicus* which confines itself to 125

English-language journals. With this index and some knowledge of information services available through the developing national Biomedical Information Network no physician should lack access to the latest medical information no matter where he is located in this country.

This body of literature now numbering about 6 million articles is stored in computers, and access is provided on-line through an international communications system known as MEDLINE. On terminals located in more than 1,500 medical libraries, research institutions, and hospitals, the results of literature searches can be printed either directly at the site or, if the references are too numerous, off-line at the remote computer site. The same vocabulary is used for both the printed *Index Medicus* and the computer-based services. Most searches, if properly formulated with respect to the requirements of the search logic, can be completed in 5 to 15 minutes. Machine searches are especially helpful for inquiries in which you must coordinate a number of concepts. Examples of subjects which can be searched by MEDLINE are: Magnesium deficiency associated with lung function, and the relationship between hypoglycemia and alcoholism.

A computer terminal gives you access to 20 other specialized data bases stored with the National Library of Medicine. These are spinoff products of the *Index Medicus*. For example, Physician Data Query (PDQ) provides cancer information in an on-line interactive mode. The toxicology information program (TIP) and CHEMLINE tell you all about drugs, toxins, and chemicals. Anyone who writes a paper, does research, or wishes detailed information about any medical subject whatsoever must become familiar with these superb resources.

Medical information networks (MINET) that offer computer assistance from data bases on drugs, diseases, medical nomenclature, and poison control centers are available as a service of the American Medical Association. These services are being expanded.

Case 30 (in Chapter 18: Gastrointestinal

Problems) provides good examples of how some of the library information or "external memory" resources can be used. The problem concerns hematemesis which may be associated with a number of different conditions or causes. By consulting MeSH we learn that "hematemesis" is used as an indexing term in *Index Medicus*. If you look in the "Categorized Lists" (Fig. 25.1) at the back of MeSH you find that hematemesis is listed under the more general term "hemorrhage, gastrointestinal" along with "melena" and "peptic ulcer hemorrhage" which are also terms under which articles may be indexed. In the 1981 *Cumulated Index Medicus* we can find an article on actively bleeding Mallory-Weiss tears under "hematemesis" with the subheading "surgery." There are also several articles under the heading "hematemesis—etiology" which seem to be of interest.

Cancer of the stomach, on the other hand, is found under "stomach neoplasms" since the policy is to index articles on neoplasms either by name of the histologic type, "carcinoma," "melanoma," etc, or under the name of the site, "breast neoplasms," "kidney neoplasms," etc. There are about 40 articles in English in the 1981 *Cumulated Index Medicus* on "stomach neoplasms—diagnosis" and as many in other languages, but none of them seems to relate specifically to hematemesis.

"Osler's disease" provides an example of how several information sources may be consulted. We learn from a medical dictionary that the eponym is used in conjunction with polycythemia vera (Osler-Vaquez disease or Vaquez-Osler disease, de-

ESOPHAGITIS	C6.306.620
HERNIA, DIAPHRAGMATIC	C6.306.700
HERNIA, HIATAL ·	C6.306.700.490
GASTROESOPHAGEAL REFLUX	C6.306.780
GASTROINTESTINAL DISEASES	C6.405
GASTROENTERITIS	C6.405.236
GASTROINTESTINAL NEOPLASMS	C6.405.282
HEMORRHAGE, GASTROINTESTINAL	C6.405.348
HEMATEMESIS	C6.405.348.336
MELENA	C6.405.348.531
PEPTIC ULCER HEMORRHAGE	C6.405.348.718
HERNIA	C6.405.396
HERNIA, DIAPHRAGMATIC	C6.405.396.216

· INDICATES MINOR DESCRIPTOR

Fig. 25.1. Medical subject headings, "categorized list."

pending on your source) and hereditary hemorrhagic telangiectasia (Rendu-Osler-Weber disease, which is also found in several permutations). MeSH does not use either eponym but refers you from Osler-Vaquez disease and Osler-Rendu disease to the alternative terms.

Eponymic diseases are a good illustration of the use of another important index which is also computer-produced but quite different in technique than *Index Medicus*. The *Science Citation Index* is a multidisciplinary index to citations (references) found in journal articles published in any particular year. It enables you to discover who has cited a particular article published in any preceding year. In the case of Osler-Rendu or Rendu-Osler-Weber disease we must first find the references to the original articles. This is done quite easily by consulting such sources as Jablonski (Stanley Jablonski: *Illustrated Dictionary of Eponymic Syndromes and Diseases and Their Syndromes*. Philadelphia, Saunders, 1969) or Magalini (Sergio Magalini and Euclide Scrasia: *Dictionary of Medical Syndromes*, ed 2. Philadelphia, Lippincott, 1981) or that encyclopedic compendium of medical historical conferences which is referred to as Garrison-Morton (Leslie T. Morton: *A Medical Bibliography (Garrison and Morton)*, ed 3. Philadelphia, Lippincott, 1970). In any of these sources we will find references to both Rendu's and Osler's original articles. If we look in the "Citation Index" section of the *Science Citation Index* for 1982 under the citation for Osler's article which appeared in the *Johns Hopkins Hospital Bulletin* in 1901 we find that five authors have cited this paper in articles they published in 1981 and 1982 (Fig. 25.2). We must then look up each of these articles in the "Source Index," which will provide us with their full titles, to determine whether they may be relevant to our particular information needs.

Mallory-Weiss syndrome, on the other hand, although not listed in some medical dictionaries, is used as an indexable term in *Index Medicus*. The Mallory-Weiss article can also be found in Jablonski and in Ma-

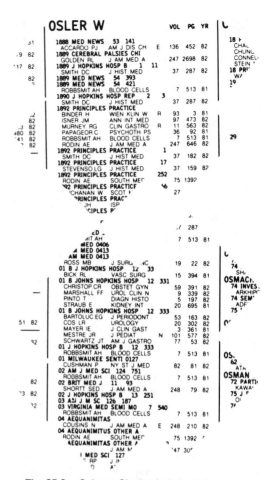

Fig. 25.2. *Science Citation Index,* citation index.

galini and can be used as the basis for the same approach in the *Science Citation Index*. The *Science Citation Index* can, of course, also be used with noneponymic terms by beginning with a citation to any earlier article on the subject of our interest.

This logic session on hematemesis also presents a likely opportunity for a MEDLINE search, since there are several concepts we may wish to coordinate. We learn from an outline inquiry at the terminal that there are 128 articles in the MEDLINE data base which have been assigned "hematemesis" as a subject heading along with any number of other subject headings and subheadings. When we coordinate "hematemesis" with some of the other suggested headings—"duodenal ulcer," "stomach neoplasms."

"Mallory-Weiss syndrome," etc—we find there are about 50 articles which have both the heading "hematemesis" and at least one of the others. When we instruct the system that we are interested only in English language aticles and only those dealing with humans, the number is reduced by half. A number of this magnitude can be printed directly on the terminal and screened for relevance. If the number had been much larger we could have asked for an off-line print and received it from the central computer site in about 3 days.

Practicing physicans, who labor under a chronic shortage of time and who may not be fully aware of their library's increasing resources, can easily lose the habit of reinforcing and acquiring medical information. You can practice medicine for years without visiting a library, researching a subject, or reading a journal.

But the good physician does otherwise. He is familiar with the library's facilities and the librarian's potential, and he may even know how to use the library independently by searching the card catalog, the periodical indexes, the *Index Medicus*, and the on-line computer.

One of the attractive aspects of medicine as a profession is that it forces the physician to be a lifelong student. The process is considerably facilitated by developing good scholarly habits and techniques and by learning how to use the available information resources and services.

Afterword

Confessions of an Information Seeker. The author of this chapter has just given you a simplified flow pattern for obtaining information about a patient's problems. Those who work in libraries are trained in library sciences. You aren't. And so as you, the novice, enter the library portals, you encounter many hurdles, sandtraps, and obstacles in your quest for medical data.

Things are not so simple as they tell you. And while we urge students and house officers to read and learn in a problem-based mode, we usually do not give these learners the 10 or more hours of education and training that are needed to utilize the library's facilities intelligently and speedily. Under these circumstances, consult your librarian who can channel you in the right direction.

If you seek elementary information about a set of diseases, any one of which may exist in a patient, the task may be easy. Just scan a general textbook, first noting the pages in the index. But if you wish to find out all there is to know at the intersection of three situations—e.g. rheumatoid arthritis, gold therapy, and at which degree of renal damage to stop treatment—the task becomes more difficult. And if you are preparing a case for presentation at chief's rounds or at grand rounds, if there is an unsolved diagnostic problem, or if you seek the best recent references about a case (as was done for each case in Section Three), the search becomes yet more laborious.

It is advantageous to know the physical structure and arrangement of your library— where indexed files, textbooks, current journals, and older journals are to be found and how they are categorized. A guided tour of the library accomplishes this. Remember that textbooks are filed by author and by subject, and books noted to be on the "reserve list" or "not to be taken outside of the library" are most frequently used and therefore probably the most valuable.

A good general rule to follow is that you must always *transcribe information and numbers correctly to your search list.* It may seem puerile to encourage the reader to copy correctly the name of the journal, exact title, authors, date, volume number, and book file number. But I give this advice only after having made the same mistakes dozens of times.

Now we get to the search for recent good literature. First, find out the exact manner in which your subject material is titled and numbered by consulting MeSH and Categorized Lists. This allows you to deal with the controlled vocabulary used by *Index Medicus* and MEDLINE. You may now look up articles under accepted known

MeSH headings. Bear in mind that there is a monthly edition of *Index Medicus* for the current year, but annual cumulations for previous years. You may search back in time as far as you wish.

Once you have selected and formed a list of journal articles you wish to peruse, then you must seek them out in their respective locations. Look them over, decide which are worth reading, and make note of what you have learned. You may have to deal with difficulties like journals being bound and therefore unavailable, journals being used by others or signed out, or journals not stored in your library. In the latter instance, interlibrary loan facilities may be employed.

Last, but not least, you may decide to perform a computer search using MED-LINE and the National Library of Medicine's huge stored data base. Information must be requested by carefully selecting MeSH headings; this usually requires the librarian's help. Within 24 hours you should have a computer print-out of all the reference sources you wish. Many references have brief abstracts attached. At this point you must again go to the stacks and seek out the actual articles.

For example, you may request all articles published in English and French between 1980 and the present on the subject of ventricular tachycardia and its various treatments. Or you may ask for all articles in the past decade on the diagnosis and treatment of hyponatremic states—perhaps only hyponatremic states associated with congestive heart failure. The subject may often be broadened or narrowed by adding or subtracting related MeSH headings.

The proper use of the library is like any other acquired skill. Students must first be taught, then they must perform several times under supervision, and finally they can be turned loose among the files, sources, and stacks. User-friendly expert librarians are always available and eager to help should a problem be encountered. Don't be easily discouraged. You learn only by doing.

(*P. C.*)

References

1. Osler W: The medical library in post-graduate work. In McGovern JP, Roland CG (eds): *Wm. Osler: The Continuing Education*, Springfield IL, Charles C Thomas, 1969, pp 209–223. Reprinted from *Br Med J* 2:925–928, 1909.
2. Alarcon RD: A personal medical reference index. *Lancet* 1:301–305, 1969.
3. Fuller EA: A system for filing medical literature. *Ann Intern Med* 68:684–693, 1968.

Suggested Readings

1. Warren KS (ed): *Coping with the Biomedical Literature: A Primer for the Scientist and the Clinician.* New York, Praeger, 1981.
   An overview of problems and procedures in dealing with the literature.
2. Morton LT, Godbolt S (eds): *Information Sources in the Medical Sciences*, ed 3. London, Butterworths, 1984.
   An excellent introduction to the medical library.

Chapter 26

Triage, Screening, Urgent Care

PAUL CUTLER, M.D.

Triage is a rapid method of separating patients with various illnesses into sets which need different types and speeds of care. As such, it is a method of problem solving used in the initial encounter with the patient. Based on the chief complaint, the patient is quickly channeled into the proper division of the health care system by a few well-selected questions or observations. This is the ultimate in speedy problem solving.

The word "triage" is a derivation of the French word, *trier*, which means to sort, sift, or select, and it is defined in *Webster's Third International Dictionary* as "the sorting of and allocation of treatment to patients and especially battle and disaster victims according to a system of priorities designed to maximize the number of survivors."

In the practice of medicine, problems must often be solved rapidly. An extreme example of such a situation, as in the Webster definition, is the management of mass casualties at the scene of a disaster or in war. In fact, the entire system of triage as we know it had its origins on the battlefields of recent wars, where rapid screening was crucial. Because available medical care facilities may be overwhelmed, quick assessments must be made as to who will benefit from the resources on hand. The *casualties are triaged into three groups:* no benefit because injury is minor, no benefit because death is likely despite care, and major benefit because emergent intervention may be lifesaving. Fortunately, decisions of such dramatic proportions are rare—but the process of triage is not.

Such sorting can be done by properly trained physicians' assistants, "paramedics," nurses, or physicians. If done by someone who is well-trained in disease processes, no special format need be followed and medical common sense may be used. Those who are less trained in medicine can be guided by printed algorithms especially designed for each complaint. Some less-trained individuals can perform intelligent triage because they know the patient populations, have common sense, and have acquired much experience.

Some Common Examples. The physician's assistant performs triage when making an appointment. What sounds urgent gets an immediate appointment, while routine revisits and unprompted complete examinations can wait a while. The diabetic patient who is seen every 3 months and now has an infected foot must be seen immediately. Screening of telephone calls also requires instant triage. Must the physician speak right away, may he call back later since he's seeing a patient now, or can the assistant handle the call? Then too a patient who looks "awfully sick" may be spotted in the waiting room and you are told "I think you'd better see him right away." The emergency room (ER) nurse may tell you to stop what you are doing and go directly to room 4 because the patient in there is cyanotic and has chest pain.

If you should stop at the scene of an automobile accident, quick decisions must be made. Three people are sprawled on the ground. One is screaming and covered with blood, but pressure on a single head laceration stops the bleeding and he is otherwise well. A second is hysterical, but has a good pulse and no apparent injury. The third complains of abdominal pain and has no visible injury but is pale, cold, and clammy; his pulse is weak and thready. Triage is easy here. The last patient needs the most and quickest care.

Without conceptualizing it, the physician performs triage many times each day. In his office he can quickly spot the patient who needs sympathy, one who needs symptomatic or curative medication, and one who needs elective or instant hospitalization. If the problem is complicated but not urgent, the patient may be asked to return in 2 days when the physician will have more time to do a complete examination.

Actually, triage is the most difficult problem-solving exercise of all. The triageur is face to face with a patient. Rapid decisions must be made. Books, consultants, laboratory aids, and diagnostic procedures are not used. Here, judgment, intuition, experience, common sense, and hunch play important roles. A mistake at this level can be fatal, and urgent matters cannot be overlooked. Ideally, perhaps, the triageur should be the most capable member of the medical team—not a person who merely follows printed instructions.

Protocols and Algorithms. For the less experienced or less trained person, triage can be carried out, as previously mentioned, according to carefully devised rules, protocols, and algorithms.

Protocols are commonplace in medicine. The formal expression of an experimental cancer chemotherapeutic regimen is a protocol. The Jones criteria for the diagnosis of acute rheumatic fever and the Romhilt and Estes criteria for the electrocardiographic diagnosis of left ventricular hypertrophy are protocols. You can establish a protocol in your own intensive care unit for the management of acute myocardial infarction or gastrointestinal hemorrhage. These are all carefully written-down, explicit plans.

It often seems that the diagnostic process follows implicit rules when we hear the professorial attending physician say "this smells like perinephric abscess." Usually such seemingly inspired utterances are the result of informal, internalized, logical analyses. Efforts to pinpoint the essential features of these analyses, as they apply to the diagnostic impressions, have resulted in the development of screening protocols. These aids to triage, sometimes called algorithms, have enabled minimally trained individuals to assess large numbers of patients and are especially useful in an ambulatory setting. The publication of an excellent series of protocols of self-directed health care—including whether to see your physician and how urgently—is an attempt to achieve the ultimate, though perhaps dangerous.

The Rise of the Emergency Room. Over the past 20 years, hospital ERs have experienced great increases in the number of patient visits. There are numerous reasons for this, such as physician unavailability, patient habit patterns, and the realization that ERs are not only for emergencies but can be visited for minor illnesses too. This has resulted in ER personnel being confronted not only with ambulance emergencies but with all sorts of situations, ranging from minor to life-threatening. Different levels of resources and skills are needed. Add to this the gap between patient load and resources; then time becomes a factor and quick triage becomes urgent. Long waits in the ER waiting room are not only tiresome, boring, and frustrating—*they may be fatal.*

Thus the entire system of triage has gained acceptance since it is designed to rapidly screen, separate, and decide the seriousness of the problem and the level of care needed, and, finally, to assign the patient to a health care resource most appropriate to his need. The system aims to speed patient flow, release the physician for higher level activities, and provide quick, quality care.

Patient disposition may be to an outpatient clinic, a walk-in acute care clinic, the ER surgical room, the triage physician for guidance, or the chief resident for further evaluation and admission to the hospital, or the patient may be sent home.

Triage may be conducted by a trained

secretary, technician, nurse, or physician. The latter utilize their own logic, while the former may have to depend on the carefully designed algorithms that have been set down by physicians and educators.

Some military hospitals have as many as 70 algorithms for the numerous common complaints seen in the ER. Thus, in an area where meningococcal disease may become epidemic, a patient with a sore throat may be triaged with a very simple algorithm, depending on the presence of headache or nuchal rigidity. If the patient has headache and can touch his chin to his chest, he is sent to a medical assistant for definitive care. If he has a headache but cannot touch his chin to his chest, he is sent to major medicine immediately. Associated complaints such as sinus problems, allergy, runny/stuffy nose, fever, and muscle aches are noted but are not crucial to the disposition of this particular problem.

Much more detailed protocols exist for the management of upper respiratory infections and a large variety of other situations. The answer to each question leads either to another question, to another algorithm, or to a disposition. These protocols can get quite complex and may thus outgrow their usefulness.

The hospital ER of a typical urban hospital serves not only to save the near-dead through elaborate technology, but is often the only way of getting into the health care system, i.e., to the clinic, to a bed, or to a consultant.

Triage in Action. Several studies have shown that the need for acute care can be emergent, urgent, or nonurgent and the relative proportions of these categories in an urban setting are 5-30-65. In the first category, care is needed at once; in the second it can wait a few hours; and in the third there is no hurry at all.

Emergent cases are those in which there is an immediate threat to life. These instances are usually obvious. In the case of infants, however, it is more common for a parent to arrive with a swaddled child and no blare of sirens. The triageur must quickly look at the tiny new arrival: Is there stridor

or adequate ventilatory movement? There is nothing more tragic than a death which occurs while the patient is waiting to be seen.

Separating the urgent from the nonurgent case is the most important function of triage. A problem requiring urgent care may be defined as an acute disorder with the potential for serious effect if unattended within a period of hours. Usually several simple questions or mere inspection is sufficient to make the judgment. The four determinants for need of urgent care are:

1. Assurance of respiration
2. Maintenance of circulation
3. Prevention of sepsis or other complications of infection
4. Preservation of function of organs.

This is where mistakes are made. In some cases, to look at the patient is to know he needs urgent care. The unconscious or near-unconscious patient must be evaluated—a sometimes difficult task if no one observed the onset of the present state. Abnormal breathing may be due simply to an emotional reaction, but this should never be easily assumed. Evaluate rapid, laboring breaths with caution too. Beware of sleepy people who breathe slowly or irregularly. Gross hemorrhage from external injury is an obvious "red flag." The loss of even small amounts of blood is significant too if it comes from the mouth (coughing or vomiting), the anus, or especially the pregnant uterus.

The chief complaint, coupled with a confirmatory examination of the affected site, serves to identify other patients needing urgent evaluation. A patient with chest pain or severe pain at any site must be assessed. Even slight pain must be studied if it is in the eye; the same is true for a foreign body in the eye or the acute loss of visual acuity. Nausea and vomiting are usually not urgent in adults. But if accompanied by crampy pains and abdominal distention, be careful because obstruction may be present. Vomiting is never pleasurable, but for infants it can represent a potentially life-threatening loss of fluids. Severe diarrhea poses the same danger.

Fever is the most common abnormal sign, but when is it most important? The febrile patient who looks very sick needs care. Yet a patient with the same degree of fever who complains only of mild malaise can usually be sent home, especially if these symptoms are typical of the current virus. But while an acute febrile illness may not be serious, if the temperature is 40.6 C and the environment is hot and humid, heat stroke may rapidly ensue when the patient goes home. So watch him for awhile.

The presence of fever and pain in a specific site demands that a possible causal relationship be defined. Flank pain, abdominal pain, and pelvic pain suggest pyelonephritis, peritonitis, and pelvic inflammatory disease. Follow the algorithm into its various branches before deciding where to send the patient.

It can be seen that the matter of deciding whether a symptom is serious depends on associated symptoms and findings. However, this decision can usually be made with a few questions. When you see a large number of patients in a busy clinic or ER, this skill is essential. If language barriers exist and interpreters are needed, there is even greater need for *fewer but better selected questions.*

Suppose the patient complains of headache. If he has had them for 10 years, speedy diagnosis is not needed. But if he played football last week and now has a headache which started 24 hours ago, a red flag goes up for subdural hematoma. Headaches for years can be delayed or referred; a severe headache for 3 hours needs more attention. See if the neck is stiff.

Similarly, suppose a patient complains of abdominal pain. The duration, nature, and location of the pain, and the presence or absence of tenderness, distention, peristalsis, nausea, vomiting, or diarrhea channel your patient via a decision path to his home, the pharmacy, an observation area, or the operating room.

Experimental computer programs that help the ER physician decide on the disposition of patients with abdominal pain or chest pain are available. Their performances are "reasonably good" and when additional requested patient data are entered, the recommended diagnosis and management are alleged to compare favorably with a physician's accuracy in the same situation.

Newer technology has been imported into the ER setting and is available for the quick screening needed in urgent cases. Ultrasound may help diagnose a ruptured ectopic pregnancy. Rapid drug screens can be obtained for comatose patients. Computed tomographic scans of the cranium and brain may be performed in emergency situations by transporting the patient down the hall.

Some Difficulties and Pitfalls. Deciding on the speed of care that is needed is usually not difficult. But mistakes are unfortunately made in busy ERs or offices. In most cases, there is no question. If circulatory or respiratory failure is evident by shock, cyanosis, feeble slow respirations, or very rapid respiration, hospitalization is indicated. Vital signs are a good guide here; blood gases are better. Coma, drug overdose, stroke, hematemesis, and typical myocardial infarction present no problem. But beware the more subtle impending disasters—the patient who gets a "stitch in the side" after a long bus trip, the 48-year-old diabetic man with vague "indigestion" for 24 hours, the patient with neurologic disease who suddenly develops nasal speech (the respiratory center is a millimeter away), and the healthy young man who has generalized urticaria and then becomes hoarse. These critical situations—pulmonary embolus, myocardial infarction, impending respiratory paralysis, and laryngeal edema—may be easily overlooked.

Further difficulties are encountered in evaluating seemingly minor complaints in patients who are prone to express their diseases differently from the average healthy young adult. In the elderly and the very young, typical patterns are often absent or incomplete. Meningitis may not cause meningeal signs. Sepsis may not result in fever. Cardiac decompensation may be expressed as "senility" and the patient is said to have a chronic brain syndrome. Persons with major physiologic disabilities may not tolerate otherwise minor problems. A minor wound infection in a 55-year-old beach vacationer merits cursory first aid; if that person were diabetic or immunosuppressed, the same lesion would demand detailed attention and follow-up.

Unfortunately, an occasional patient is sent home from the ER and dies. The known cardiac patient who has an obvious severe gastroenteritis is sent home and dies of acute coronary insufficiency and ventricular fibrillation. Nobody paid attention to his dehydration, cyanosis, depleted blood volume, and diminished coronary and systemic blood flow. Then there is the man with the odor of alcochol on his breath whose symptoms are not regarded seriously and who dies in jail or after being sent home.

Health care facilities are too limited to evaluate everyone fully. Patients with minor problems should resent the major financial expenses of "defensive medicine." Someone who has multiple aches and pains after an auto accident need not be x-rayed from head to toe. Not all patients can or should be extensively evaluated. Those with limited homeostatic capacity (infants, aged, debilitated, chronically ill) need more attention. Those who live alone and cannot summon help if needed also require more attention. The affected site is important. Pain in the right leg will not lead to rapid, mortal consequences even if due to an osteosarcoma. On the other hand, the pudgy child with a croupy cough, who probably does not have inspiratory obstruction, could possibly have epiglottitis, a disorder which is potentially fatal within a few hours. The consequences of being wrong in this instance are great, so observation with available ventilatory assistance is necessary even though the child most likely has the croup.

If the triageur classifies a patient as a *nonurgent encounter*, patient disposition is made according to the hospital's specific health care system—i.e. refer elsewhere, schedule for clinic, examine and treat, call consultant, etc. It is often wise to look be-

neath the seeming cause for the encounter. Hospital facilities for unscheduled care do not usually have a charming ambiance: The patient who registers is not seeking entertainment. While he may be well aware of the physiologic insignificance of his complaint, this may be his penultimate way of reaching out for human contact because he is unable to articulate his need for psychologic care in any other way. This subtlety can easily be missed by even the most experienced triage person.

The ER offers neither the time nor the place for complete evaluations. A look, a few questions, examination of one or two areas, and a decision of disposition must be made. This type of problem solving—perhaps the most important of all—can usually be done in a minute or two.

Suggested Readings

1. Kelman RH, Lane DS: Use of the hospital emergency room in relation to use of private physicians. *Am J Public Health* 66:1189–1191, 1976.
2. Brook RH, Stenson RL: Effectiveness of patient care in an emergency room. *N Engl J Med* 283:904–907, 1970.
   These articles emphasize the need for ER triage.
3. Wilkins EW Jr (ed): *MGH Textbook of Emergency Medicine*, ed 2. Baltimore, Williams & Wilkins, 1983.
   Of particular interest are pp 1–68 on life support, pp 817–878 on the history of emergency medical services, and pp 879–890 on triage and screening.
4. Murphy GJ, Jacobson S: Assessing the quality of emergency care: the medical record versus patient outcome. *Ann Emerg Med* 13:158–165, 1984.
   A careful analysis of the way patients with asthma are triaged and managed in a Philadelphia emergency room setting.
5. Levy R, Goldstein B, Trott A: Approach to quality assurance in an emergency department: a one year review. *Ann Emerg Med* 13:166–169, 1984.
   Assesses the quality of care by an audit of 75,000 charts in a busy Cincinnati emergency room.
6. Eliaston M, Sternbach GL, Bressler MJ: *Manual of Emergency Medicine*, ed 4. Chicago, Year Book, 1983.
   This is an excellent 468-page pocket-size book that covers the entire field of emergency care.
7. Quick JD, Moorhead G, Quick JC, et al: Decision making among emergency room residents; preliminary observations and a decision model. *J Med Educ* 58:117–125, 1983.
   Observes the various patterns residents use to make quick decisions.

Chapter 27

Doctor- and Drug-Induced Diseases

DAVID W. HAWKINS, PHARM.D.

The amount of disease, morbidity, and mortality caused by physicians is unknown. This includes the effect of drugs, treatments, and surgery which are usually correctly but sometimes injudiciously administered. The right drug for the wrong diagnosis, the wrong drug for the right diagnosis, and even the right drug for the right diagnosis can cause troublesome effects.

Such inadvertent results can be audited in a hospital setting; in the private office they are unmeasurable. Physicians are often unaware of the problems they have created. But when you approach any new patient you must *always consider the possibility* of iatrogenic or drug-induced disease as you list the possible causes for the patient's presentation. To find out what is wrong with him, a careful analysis of past and present treatments and medications is necessary.

Too often, a drug causes unrecognized side effects, interactions with other medications, or even toxicity from outright overdose. The physician may not realize that the resulting signs and symptoms are related to the drug, since the clues are very often nonspecific, attributed to something else, or even considered to be part of the disease for which the patient is being treated.

Confusing situations involving a psychogenic overlay of clues can be created by a physician who uses an ill-selected word, who pauses too long while examining the heart, or who visibly raises his eyebrow, thus planting an unshakable lifelong neurosis. A med- ical diagnosis given when no disease exists can do the same thing.

Frequently the physician can set a chain of events in motion, whether the diagnosis and treatment are correct, incorrect, or partially so. For example, consider the patient with a ruptured Baker's cyst, who is mistakenly though understandably thought to have thrombophlebitis. Anticoagulants are given and hematuria develops (at abnormally high or therapeutic prothrombin times). This calls for an intravenous pyelogram from which the patient may suffer anaphylaxis and die or develop acute renal failure. Should this not occur, and the x-ray be normal, subsequent cystoscopy may cause acute pyelonephritis; gentamicin is appropriately given for an identified organism and can cause renal failure. You may have to enter into a problem-solving exercise at any link in this confounding chain.

While the medical literature is replete with problems caused by medications, the difficulties directly attributable to the doctor's actions are not so well publicized. Many result from surgery or diagnostic procedures. Who has not heard the whispers in the hospital corridor about the lady whose uterus was removed and who now has anuria because the ureters were damaged, tied, or cut—or some such other catastrophic event? These could well become diagnostic problems because postoperative anuria can have other causes too. And what about the duodenal fistulae, bile fistulae, and anal incontinence that sometimes result from surgery? Then there are the catheters lost in the pulmonary artery, lumbar punctures resulting in death, central venous lines that cause pneumothorax, barium enemas that result in radiopaque pulmonary arteries, and on and on. Fortunately, these complications are not common.

Needless surgery is on the decrease, but drug-induced diseases continued to grow in frequency and threaten to become *one of the worst epidemics* of recent times. The plethora of available drugs, many proprietary names for the same generic drug, flagrant polypharmacy, and the inability of the physician to keep abreast of the mushrooming subjects of pharmacokinetics and drug interactions are among the causes of this threat.

Epidemiologic surveys have shown that 2 to 5% of admissions to the medical and pediatric services of general hospitals are caused by drug-induced problems. Another 5 to 30% of patients experience adverse drug reactions during hospitalization for other reasons. These statistics, plus the fact that polypharmacy has become an integral part of modern medical practice, mandate the inclusion of drug-induced problems in almost every differential diagnosis list.

The causes of drug-induced problems include:

1. genetically determined alterations in drug metabolism
2. disease-induced alteration in a drug's pharmacokinetic properties
3. exaggerated pharmacologic action
4. allergic or hypersensitivity state
5. idiosyncratic reaction
6. drug interaction
7. drug overdose.

The problem arising from any one of these seven known causes may manifest itself as a disease, syndrome, physical sign, symptom, or abnormal clinical laboratory value, thus confusing the physician. Food-drug interactions, lack of drug stability, packaging problems, and errors perpetrated by the patient, the doctor, or the pharmacist may cause additional confusion.

Medical conditions that result from drugs can also be caused by diseases, and that's where the need for problem solving arises. You can easily see how hyponatremia, hypokalemia, renal failure, hepatic cell damage, arrhythmias, deafness, hematologic disorders, gastrointestinal bleeding, or strange behavior can each be caused by *a variety of diseases or a drug.* That's why a drug history is so important in the formulation of almost every differential diagnosis.

For example, a drug can induce a disease—e.g. aplastic anemia can result from chloramphenicol and a systemic lupus erythematosus-like syndrome can result from hydralazine. On the other hand, a drug may simply cause a rash, a headache, or an elevated transaminase. How confusing this can be in evaluating a clue! The changes associated with adverse drug reactions are usually nonspecific, seldom characteristic for any one particular drug, and indistinguishable from the changes caused by other etiologic agents. The types of tissue injuries due to drugs are the same as those of any other disease-producing agent (e.g. thermal, radiation, viral, bacterial, etc). Thus, an objective means of demonstrating a causal relationship between a drug and a reaction is usually lacking.

Despite this limitation you can attempt to reasonably identify drug-induced problems using a systematic approach* which involves six successive steps:

1. Obtain a complete drug history.
2. Check the drug list against the problem list.
3. Establish temporal eligibility of a drug.
4. Check for dose dependency.
5. Apply the differential.
6. Verify the diagnosis.

Obtain a Complete Drug History. A complete drug history consists of a patient's current use of prescribed and nonprescribed or over-the-counter (OTC) drugs, past medi-

---

* Irey provides a detailed diagnostic scheme of deductive reasoning for establishing the presence of drug-induced diseases.

cation history, recent exposure to radiopaque media, drug allergies, and compounds often not perceived as drugs (e.g.
birth control pills).

Drug histories obtained by physicians often fail to take into account a major source
of drug-induced problems: the frequent use
of nonprescribed drugs. The patient may not
consider the use of an OTC agent as a drug-
taking activity, and the importance of knowing what nonprescribed drugs the patient is
taking is illustrated by the following case.

A real estate broker with congestive heart
failure (CHF) had been hospitalized three
times during the past year for increasing
frequency and severity of paroxysmal nocturnal dyspnea (PND). On his first admission a drug history revealed that he was
taking 0.25 mg of digoxin and 40 mg of
furosemide daily. During his third hospital
stay he confessed that unsuccessful negotia-
tions on large pieces of real estate had occurred just prior to each admission. These
business failures resulted in an upset stomach for which he took frequent doses of
Alka-Seltzer. The most likely cause for this
patient's PND is a sudden increase in sodium ingestion. Each Alka-Seltzer tablet
contains 532 mg of sodium (23 mEq). A
patient with CHF may easily become sodium overloaded by taking two Alka-Seltzer
tablets two or three times daily.

Various techniques are used as memory
joggers in an attempt to ascertain a patient's
OTC drug use habits. One method is similar
to the review of systems component of the
medical history. Several common disorders
ranging from dandruff to athlete's foot are
often self-treated with nonprescribed drugs
(Table 27.1). A review of these disorders
with the patient may elicit additional drug
history.

Another method involves simply inquir-

Table 27.1.
Disorders Commonly Self-Treated

Constipation	Insomnia
Diarrhea	"Tired blood"
Colds	Upset stomach
Cough	Headaches

Table 27.2.
Commonly Used OTC Agents

Antacids	Cold preparations
Analgesics	Alka-Seltzer
Laxatives	Vitamins
Cough syrup	Topical agents

ing about self-administration of commonly
used OTC agents; these are listed in Table
27.2. By combining these two methods you
can probably acquire a meticulously complete OTC drug history.

The past medication history is important
for two reasons. First, some drugs have been
known to cause problems long after they
have been discontinued. For example, one
form of aplastic anemia associated with
chloramphenicol may occur 1 to 2 months
after stopping the drug. Second, you may
learn that the patient has previously experienced an adverse drug reaction. Patients
who have had one adverse reaction are predisposed to developing others.

Recent exposure to certain radiopaque
media is frequently overlooked. Organic io-
dine-containing contrast media may interfere with radioactive iodine uptake and
scans of the thyroid for as long as several
years. Such drug-induced modifications of
tests can cause misdiagnoses and complicate
disease assessment.

**Check the Drug List against the Problem
List.** A list of drugs obtained from the patient's present and past medication history
should be compared against all the patient's
known problems (diseases, syndromes,
signs, symptoms, and abnormal laboratory
findings) in search of a possible relationship.
On occasion, you will quickly be able to
match a drug with a problem. Instant analysis occurs, for example, when a patient
presents with hypoglycemia and is a known
diabetic on insulin. On most occasions, however, a causal relationship between a drug
and a problem will not be immediately apparent. One may need to consult one or
several references to verify a possible connection.

Establish Temporal Eligibility of a Drug.
The time lapse between starting a drug and

subsequent development of an adverse reaction varies considerably. Anaphylactic reactions may occur within a few minutes following the intravenous administration of radiologic contrast media. On the other hand, corticosteroid-induced cataract usually requires more than 2 years of continuous therapy. Some adverse drug reactions occur at random. Methyldopa-induced hepatotoxicity, for example, usually occurs within the first 2 months of treatment but may not develop until 3 years after initiating therapy. Other adverse drug reactions occur at a predictable time during the treatment cycle. The chronology of adverse effects associated with penicillamine therapy is remarkably reproducible among patients who receive the drug for the long-term treatment of rheumatoid arthritis. You can predict with certainty when rash, mouth ulcers, thrombocytopenia, and nephrotic syndrome will occur.

A patient with infective endocarditis was admitted to the hospital, cultures drawn, and tobramycin and ticarcillin started. Cultures grew a gram-negative bacillus. The patient's admitting blood chemical tests were all within normal limits except for a slightly elevated urea nitrogen and serum creatinine. On the second hospital day, the renal function decreased markedly and he developed hematuria and heavy albuminuria. Tobramycin was discontinued because an aminoglycoside-induced nephritis was suspected.

This case illustrates two points concerning the temporal eligibility of a drug for the induction of a clinical problem. The first point seems patently obvious but is one that is frequently ignored. That is, in order for a drug to cause a disease its initiation must precede the onset of disease. In this particular case, the decline in renal function started before therapy with tobramycin was begun. A more likely cause for the patient's sudden onset of renal disease is an immune-complex form of glomerulonephritis associated with infective endocarditis.

A second point worth emphasizing is that the onset of aminoglycoside nephrotoxicity usually begins after the fourth or fifth day of treatment. Thus, in this case, the duration of therapy and the onset of kidney disease do not correlate for two reasons.

Check for Dose Dependency. Drug-induced problems are attributable to either immunologic or pharmacologic mechanisms. Examples of antibody-mediated drug reactions include anaphylaxis, serum sickness, contact dermatitis, hemolytic anemia, drug fever, and thrombocytopenia. As a general rule, hypersensitivity reactions to drugs occur independent of the dose.

On the other hand, adverse reactions attributable to the pharmacologic action of a drug are dose-dependent. For example, amphotericin B produces a predictable, dose-related (total dosages in excess of 4 g) nephrotoxicity. If a patient with previously normal renal function develops acute renal failure after receiving a total dosage of 2 g of amphotericin, it is not likely that the amphotericin is responsible for the acute renal insufficiency. One should, of course, discontinue the antifungal agent and then search for some other cause of renal deterioration.

Because of individual differences in the way drugs are handled by the body, a dose tolerated by some patients may cause side effects in others. This is especially true in patients with pathophysiologic or genetic conditions which affect drug metabolism and excretion. For example, drugs eliminated primarily by hepatic metabolism will accumulate to toxic levels in patients with severe liver disease. Drugs and active drug metabolites that depend upon urinary excretion will accumulate rapidly in patients with renal insufficiency. Variations in drug metabolism as a result of inherited deficiencies or abnormal enzyme systems may also lead to abnormal drug responses or an increased risk of adverse reactions.

A hypertensive patient on hydrochlorothiazide 100 mg b.i.d., propranolol 80 mg b.i.d., and hydralazine 50 mg b.i.d. developed polyarthralgia, myalgias, fever, and a butterfly rash across the face. Blood studies revealed an elevated erythrocyte sedimentation rate, a positive lupus erythematosus cell preparation, and a positive antinuclear antibody test. A diagnosis of hydralazine-induced lupus-like syndrome is entertained, but not without some degree of skepticism since a daily dosage in excess of 400 mg is usually required to produce this adverse reaction.

This patient's past medical history revealed that he had a similar reaction while on isoniazid, a drug he received 10 years ago for pulmonary tuberculosis. Tests at that time indicated that he was a slow acetylator of isoniazid. Slow acetylation is inherited as an autosomal recessive trait. Hydralazine is believed to be inactivated by the same liver enzyme that metabolizes isoniazid. That being the case, it is conceivable that this patient's lupus-like reaction resulted from gradual accumulation of hydralazine due to slow inactivation of the drug, despite a daily dose of only 100 mg.

Apply the Differential. Before deciding that a problem is drug-induced, one should consider factors other than the suspected drug which may have been responsible or at least partly responsible for the adverse effect. These include another drug not initially considered, the primary disease or diseases, another therapeutic modality, and interactions of two or more drugs.

A 52-year-old well-controlled hypertensive and diabetic male patient on hydrochlorothiazide and chlorpropamide was admitted to a hospital with hyponatremia. Because the patient was hypertensive he had been instructed to refrain from adding any salt to his food. When he presented complaining of muscle cramps, lethargy, headache, nausea, and vomiting, and was found to have a serum sodium of 110 mEq/liter, the thiazide diuretic was promptly discontinued. He was cautiously given hypertonic saline, but this had no effect on his serum sodium. The patient's chlorpropamide therapy was discontinued because of a fasting blood sugar of 80 mg/dl reported on the fourth hospital day. Following discontinuation of chlorpropamide therapy, the serum sodium started gradually climbing and was back within normal limits by the eighth hospital day. During this time the patient's

blood pressure had steadily increased and hydrochlorothiazide was reinstituted. By the tenth hospital day the patient's blood pressure had normalized and his serum sodium remained within physiologic limits.

Chlorpropamide may cause a syndrome of inappropriate secretion of antidiuretic hormone (SIADH) characterized by hyponatremia, urine that is hypertonic to plasma, and renal sodium wasting. So although this patient's hyponatremia might have resulted from hydrochlorothiazide administration, one could not rule out the possibility that the chlorpropamide was responsible. Evidence in support of a chlorpropamide-induced dilutional hyponatremia in this patient derives from two facts: (*a*) the serum sodium returned to within normal limits following discontinuation of the chlorpropamide, and (*b*) the serum sodium did not drop with reinstitution of hydrochlorothiazide therapy. At first, this patient was thought to have simple salt depletion. Had the correct diagnosis been recognized, simple fluid restriction for 1 or 2 days and discontinuation of chlorpropamide would have sufficed. It is interesting to note that thiazides occasionally cause SIADH too, but the sequence of events proved that this was not the case here.

The possibility that a problem may arise as a consequence of the primary disease, and not from the drug received, was alluded to earlier in the case dealing with nephritis secondary to subacute bacterial endocarditis.

Verify the Diagnosis. The final step in solving drug-induced problems is to verify the causal relationship between the drug and the problem. This is done by one or several of four methods.

1. First, the responsible drug can sometimes be qualitatively identified or quantitatively measured in the blood or urine. For some drugs, the serum concentration at which toxic signs and symptoms ensue is well delineated. For example, digitalis-induced cardiac arrhythmias are more likely to be associated with serum digoxin concentrations above 2 ng/ml than below. Ataxia

in an epileptic patient on phenytoin is most likely drug-induced if the serum phenytoin concentration is above 30 μg/ml. Serum drug concentrations are also useful in verifying toxicity secondary to quinidine, procainamide, lidocaine, salicylates, aminoglycosides, theophylline, lithium, and tricyclic antidepressants.

2. The second method makes use of pattern diagnosis in which a constant relationship between a drug and a clinical picture has been documented. Application of this method is not foolproof because of the nonspecificity of drug-tissue reactions.

3. The exclusion method is often used when more than one drug may have been responsible. The application of this method calls for a disease indicator-time graph (Fig. 27.1). Note that this method establishes temporal eligibility and by itself does not prove causation. In the case represented in the figure, the patient experienced a rise in serum glutamic-oxaloacetic transaminase (SGOT) while on *four drugs known to sometimes be hepatotoxic.* You can see that α-methyldopa was the only drug eligible to initiate the liver cell damage and the rise in SGOT in this case. Furthermore, soon after this drug was stopped, the SGOT began to drop and kept declining in the face of treatment with isoniazid, hydrochlorothiazide, and rifampin, each of which is potentially hepatotoxic.

Such a clinical event may exist in a patient who is given Aldomet for hypertension and

whose SGOT subsequently begins to rise. The Aldomet is discontinued. In the meantime he is found to have a strongly positive purified protein derivative skin test, so isoniazid is started—another hepatotoxic drug. The test was done because the patient had a chronic cough and his daughter had recently contracted active pulmonary tuberculosis. The chest x-ray was normal and the sputum was negative for acid-fast bacilli. Hydrochlorothiazide, a common first-line treatment for hypertension, was substituted; only rarely does this drug cause liver damage. Six weeks after isoniazid had been started, the sputum culture was found to be positive for *Mycobacterium tuberculosis* and rifampin was added to the regimen. An apical lordotic chest x-ray showed a small infiltrate in the left apex. Note that the SGOT fell to normal levels.

Similar instances where one of several drugs may be responsible for an abnormality are common in medicine.

4. A final, seldom intentionally used method applies to situations where disease indicators are noted to come and go repeatedly, coincident with giving and withholding the drug. This would call for rechallenging the patient with the suspected drug, a practice generally considered unethical.

Beware the Elderly. Old folks are walking culture plates for the incubation of doctor- and drug-induced diseases. This is reasonable for more of them are sick, polypathic, and take a variety of medications. The stage is set.

Old people are more susceptible to drug reactions because of altered pharmacokinetics. With increasing age there is a decreased volume of distribution, increased half-life, diminished system clearance, altered receptor sensitivity, and less albumin binding for many drugs. These changes are variable, require dosage adjustments, and cause toxicity.

The symptoms of drug-induced illness often mimic the underlying disorder being treated or other diseases commonly associated with aging. For example, forgetfulness, weakness, confusion, tremor, anorexia, anx-

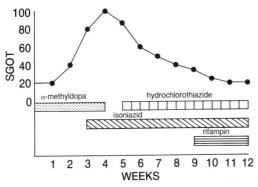

Fig. 27.1. Disease indicator-time graph showing temporal eligibility of α-methyldopa for the production of elevated SGOT.

iety, dry mouth, blurred vision, constipation, or urinary retention *can result from disease or drugs.* Many an old man has had a prostatectomy when cessation of anticholinergics would have sufficed. In other circumstances, prolonged searches for cancer and neurologic diseases have been instigated although a medication had caused the symptoms.

The Physician's Aids. *Plasma drug levels* not only help you decide on drug toxicity and tell you if drug-related illness is possible, but they also guide you in day-to-day treatment.

Drug information services that are readily available to the physician should help decrease toxicity, reactions, and interactions. These treasuries of instruction are accessible by letter, telephone, or computer communication with programs offered by the American Medical Association, the National Library of Medicine, private companies, and many hospitals.

Quinidine sulfate has been used for decades to *treat* arrhythmias; but it *causes* them too. So when a treated arrhythmia persists or worsens, is it the disease or the drug? Stop the drug and you may learn that it is often more knave than knight.

In any similar instance, before undertaking prolonged studies or symptomatic relief with yet more drugs, stop all medication for a few days. Very little harm can result, but much good may ensue.

Suggested Readings

1. Irey NS: When is a disease drug induced? In Riddel RH (ed): *Pathology of Drug-Induced and Toxic Diseases.* New York, Churchill Livingstone, 1982, pp 1–8.
   An excellent discussion on methods of analyzing and diagnosing cases of adverse drug reactions.
2. Rawlings MD, Thompson JW: Pathogenesis of adverse drug reactions. In Davies DM (ed): *Textbook of Adverse Drug Reactions,* ed. 2. New York, Oxford University Press, 1981, pp 11–34.
   Focuses attention on factors involved in the diagnosis, management, and prevention of adverse drug reactions, including drug interactions.
3. Ouslander JG: Drug therapy in the elderly. *Ann Intern Med* 95:711–722, 1981.
   Altered pharmacokinetics, polypharmacy, and poor compliance in the aged are well explained.

Chapter 28

Special Aspects of Problem Solving in the Psychiatric Patient

CHARLES L. BOWDEN, M.D,

Problem solving is especially difficult in the psychosomatic or psychiatric patient for three main reasons. Data gathering has its booby traps, psychiatric possibilities make incursions into every differential diagnosis, and there is the ever present issue of separating functional from organic illness.

Histories may be overly lengthy, unreliable, illogical, distorted, or difficult to obtain. The possibility that such patients may also have organic diseases probably constitutes the *single greatest difficulty* encountered in all of diagnosis. Many times each day the physician faces this dilemma as he questions himself: "Am I seeing the usual profusion of psychoneurotic symptoms in this patient? Is there an organic disease present this time? Am I missing something serious?"

Errors are common in either direction. The patient is often labeled "functional" or "neurotic" and bears this label for life. In this way, many cases of carcinoma of the pancreas, myxedema, and brain tumor are overlooked, and these patients may even be referred to psychiatrists or institutionalized because of persistence of unexplained symptoms. It is wise to remember that everyone eventually dies of organic disease.

On the other hand, many neurotic patients are unjustifiably given incorrect and unscientific diagnostic labels because of a borderline abnormality. Sometimes this is done because of the unwillingness or inability of the physician to take the time to explain the truth. It is easier to say that the patient has low blood pressure, anemia, menopause, sluggish glands, or nervous exhaustion than to explain the psychodynamics of functional disease.

This chapter tells you why and how psychologic factors influence and modify the problem-solving process. It also describes how psychologic issues present as physical symptoms and accompany physical illness.

Of primary importance is the fact that psychosomatic aspects of illness are very frequent. In a large outpatient clinic, 81% of new patients had psychologic factors as a basis for their presenting complaints. In 69%, no organic disease was present (1). While these statistics may not precisely fit each subset of the patient population, the implications are clear. Odds are that the next new patient you see *will not have organic disease.* Expressed differently, most patients have psychosomatic problems either as the prime reason for seeing a physician or as an overlay to their medical illnesses. You can see why some busy physicians tend erroneously to regard almost all patients as neurotic and thus may compromise the quality and quantity of their medical care.

A Venn diagram or Boolean notation can serve to indicate the overlap of people who have psychosomatic disease (PD), and those who have organic disease (OD). Roughly speaking, PD = .80, OD = .50, and PD ∩ OD = .30. Thus, patients with purely PD = .50, and purely OD = .20. These figures are percentage approximations based on estimates given by many primary care physicians (Fig. 28.1). The implications are obvious.

This broad and troublesome group of patients is most likely to be in lower socioeconomic classes and/or medically indigent. They tend to overutilize medical services and physician time, complain about their medical care, exhibit a lack of gratitude toward their physicians, migrate from one doctor to another, and are often passive-aggressive with physicians and others in authority.

Many factors incline patients toward psychosomatic dysfunction. Ignorance of the structure and functions of the body may cause a patient to misinterpret and/or exaggerate symptoms. Prescientific notions of causality result in patients attributing complaints to implausible or impossible sources. Fear or shame about the subjective meaning of a set of symptoms may make a patient unwilling to openly discuss the meaning or actual medical implications of a disorder. Secondary gain in the way of disability income, compensation for a job-related injury, or avoidance of an unpleasant job may cause a person to hang on to or exaggerate symptoms.

Factors within the medical care system may worsen such complaints. *Fragmentation of medical care* may result in each specific organ system complaint being assessed by a different doctor in a different clinic and being ruled out with a complex battery of tests. The patient is told there is nothing wrong, but continues to suffer. Doctor shopping often enters the picture, and resentment grows toward physicians who seem to dismiss the complaints out of hand or who are annoyed or bored by the patient. In part, these problems stem from our having too narrow a concept of disease. Environmental, psychologic, and interpersonal factors can significantly influence the patient's response to organic disease or may precipitate symptoms which the patient interprets as organic illness.

It is common to see a patient with a single symptom wander from one specialist to another. This is usually the result of the patient's idiosyncratic concept of the cause of his problem. It may result from advice given by well-meaning friends. Because of chronic headaches, he sees an ophthalmologist; new spectacles may or may not be prescribed, but the patient does not get better. So he consults an otolaryngologist who finds nothing wrong, may remove "diseased tonsils," or may treat his sinuses. Still no help, so he sees a neurologist who tells him he has no brain tumor. He then wends his weary way through a sequence of physicians, each of whom may or may not find an inconsequential problem. Eventually, he may stumble upon the right physician, who nails the complaint to the correct cause: trouble with his employer.

Psychosomatic aspects of illness can be grouped into useful categories with different diagnostic patterns and clues (2). The so-called classical psychosomatic disorders—peptic ulcer, bronchial asthma, etc—will not receive primary attention for several reasons. Foremost, they do not present major diagnostic dilemmas. Moreover, psychologic investigation and theorizing have not proven

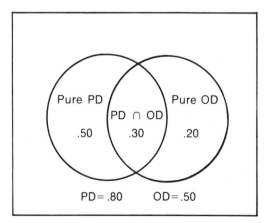

Fig. 28.1. Overlap of people who have psychosomatic disease (PD) and those who have organic disease (OD). Decimal equals percentage.

especially helpful in the management of these disorders, in contrast with others which will be discussed. It is not desirable that you memorize facts about a few so-called classical psychosomatic disorders. Instead, you should recognize the value of a psychosomatic perspective about a wide range of illnesses. This attitude reflects a move toward a systems view of disease causation, wherein circumstances or events stressful to the individual can cause, precipitate, or aggravate symptoms, and contribute to the development of anatomic or physiologic changes in one or more organ systems.

Categories of Psychosomatic Dysfunction

Psychologic Presentations of Organic Disease. Practically any organic disease can present solely as, or be accompanied by, psychologic symptoms (2). Subtle changes in personality function or behavior, especially an exaggeration of the person's usual personality style, or atypical behavior often observable only to family or close friends, can indicate an organic brain disorder. Conditions which often *present with depression* include cancer, anemias, and congestive heart failure. Some patients unconsciously deny or minimize the organic problem. They may even self-diagnose their condition as psychosomatic in an effort to conceal or distract the physician's attention from a physical illness they fear exists. Anxiety and depression may be aroused by subjective awareness of disturbed physical health. Disorders with major components of pain, especially if chronic, may result in personality alterations such that the patient superficially appears to have only a psychologic disturbance. The implications are clear. The physician must constantly be alert to the possibility of psychologic symptoms which *mask organic illnesses.*

Cancer is especially important because of the great similarity in early phases to pure depressive illness. Weight loss, anorexia, decreased interest and energy, as well as depressed mood, are common to both. Since depression is far more common than cancer, all such patients should be questioned in detail regarding previous depressions, family history of depressions, recent setbacks, and stresses. Symptoms indicative of primary unipolar depression, such as early morning awakening and morning fatigue and hopelessness, with gradual improvement as the day progresses, should be asked about. Have greater *concern about cancer* if cachexia and anorexia are profound, or if the depressive response is out of keeping with the patient's prior response to stresses. A screening medical history and physical examination are indicated in all severe depressions, and should be more thorough in older patients or those in whom symptoms develop suddenly, severely, and inexplicably. An inexplicable physical or laboratory abnormality should always be clarified by further examination or history.

Psychologic Complications of Organic Disease. Diseases which *impair brain oxygenation* are among the most common in this category. Arteriosclerosis, arrhythmias, emphysema, pulmonary fibrosis, and anemias are examples. Postsurgical effects of anesthesia and postoperative sequelae of open-heart surgery also may produce sensorial clouding which can interfere with effective management.

Complications *secondary to drugs* and other diagnostic and therapeutic measures require the physician's special alertness. Drugs with anticholinergic properties can produce mild to severe acute confusional states. Steroids, especially in larger doses, cause disturbances in mood and idiosyncratic, autistic thinking. Electrolyte imbalance, especially hyponatremia, can present as depression. Insulin overdose can cause a severe acute delirious state.

Hepatic and renal failure are associated with *organic brain syndromes.* Infections, both systemic and in the central nervous system, can also cause an organic brain syndrome. Space-occupying lesions, such as tumors and subdural hematomas, are causal factors too. The above listing, broadly representative though not exhaustive, emphasizes the reversible rather than irreversible organic brain syndromes for important reasons. Diagnosis is less difficult and treatment largely supportive for the latter group. By contrast, treatment of the underlying disorder in reversible organic brain syndromes can often be curative. Too, organic brain syndromes are often overlooked. This is especially the case when the physician is already busy treating a serious medical problem, such as renal failure, or managing the postoperative cardiac surgery patient. Although the circumstances accounting for such inattention to subtle signs of confusion and affective disturbance are understandable, they are also avoidable.

Psychologic Reactions to Organic Disease. The distinctions between psychologic presentations of organic diseases, psychologic components, and reactions is in part arbitrary. There is practical merit both for diagnosis and management in such separation. Psychologic reactions are influenced by the person's prior personality structure, the symbolic meaning to him of the disease and the impact of treatment, the kinds of support he has from friends, and cultural and socioeconomically related attitudes toward the illness in question. The degree of functional loss and physical distress caused by the disease and any prior experiences with it also contribute. A last important variable is the patient's relationship with his doctor and others on the health care team. In general, disorders which are especially stressful, traumatic, chronic, or which involve changes in body image are likely to evoke such reactions. Myocardial infarction is in ways paradigmatic of such conditions. Denial, sometimes coupled with efforts to prove that physical vigor and endurance are unimpaired, often complicates the diagnosis and management of such patients.

Somatic Presentation of Psychiatric Disorders. Only the more common and diagnostically difficult conditions will be described.

Depression. Among the most common of all disorders, depression is the psychiatric disorder most often presenting as an organic condition. Pain, impotence, insomnia, fatigue, anorexia and weight loss, and palpitations are among the most common complaints. Depression is the most common disorder among patients presenting with somatic complaints who do not have signs of organic disease; therefore one's index of suspicion in such cases should be high. The diagnosis, as for other psychiatric disorders, must be based on positive emotional, behavioral, and historical features of the specific illness.

Somatization Disorder and Conversion Disorder. The complex characteristics of these functionally caused presentations of physiologic dysfunction usually require physical and laboratory examination as well as psychiatric assessment to arrive at a reasonably clear diagnosis. Assessment over a period of time is often necessary for clarification. Suggestive supporting data are the presence of recent stress and a history of response to stress with somatic complaints. The complaints usually involve the special senses or the person's conceptualization of the anatomic location of organs and nerves. Rarely is this consistent with actual distribution and function. Pain is probably the most common of all conversion complaints. Easy to categorize is the patient who has pain in every part of the body at once—from head to toe—constantly, night and day, even when sleeping. Conversion symptoms are more common in patients who lack a sophisticated, scientific understanding of the structure and functions of the body. A symbolic meaning of the complaint and secondary gain are common, but may also be secondarily acquired with any organic illness.

Anxiety Disorder. Since anxiety can be a secondary accompaniment to practically any disorder, we are here limiting the term to the clinical syndrome. In this syndrome, anxiety with characteristic history, sense of apprehension, observable behavior, and physiologic concomitants dominates the picture. At times the patient may appear calm, and even deny subjective anxiety, but show the physiologic concomitants. Autonomic symptoms predominate. Somatic disturbances are always a part of the syndrome.

Among the most common disturbances are cardiorespiratory symptoms, in particular those which make up the *hyperventilation syndrome.* The patient reports palpitations, a subjective feeling of inability to inhale sufficient air, apprehension, lightheadedness, numbness and tingling of extremities and perioral areas, and (in severe cases) fainting. This is the most common cause of "shortness of breath" seen in the primary care physician's office, and enters into your differential logic when you consider heart disease, lung disease, or fainting spells. Many of the symptoms are caused by self-induced respiratory alkalosis.

Musculoskeletal complaints, including *tension headaches,* neck and shoulder pain, and low back pain are frequent. The concentration of tension-related musculoskeletal symptoms in the head, neck, and spinal column areas is characteristic and helpful diagnostically.

Irritable Colon Syndrome. Closely related to anxiety, this is by far the most common of stress-related gastrointestinal disturbances. Alternating diarrhea and constipation, cramping, flatulence and eructation, and occasional mucus in the stool are the common features of this reversible condition.

Hypochondriasis. These patients are characterized by the diffuse and varied nature of their complaints (3). They appear intensely worried by their symptoms, which they present in an overly detailed manner, often including specific dates and medical jargon which they have learned. Their symptoms arise from heightened awareness of normal body function. An occasional peristaltic movement of bowel is interpreted as an ulcer. Feeling the xiphisternum for the first time, the patient assumes it is a cancerous growth. The patient is preoccupied with all bodily functions and passes a lifetime in what may be called illness-claiming behavior. As such, he has spent an excessive amount of time seeing many physicians. His symptoms become worse rather than better when he is reassured that a particular complaint does not indicate major disease. Many patients may have reactive or transient hypochondriacal responses secondary to major stressful illnesses. It is the chronic, ingrained hypochondriac, whose entire life revolves around his symptoms, who needs to be specifically recognized so that appropriate management can be initiated.

The psychoneurotic or hypochondriacal patient may often be recognized by the multiplicity of unrelated complaints which have no pathophysiologic unity. Also suspect are the patient with a long list of written problems ("*maladie du petit papier*") and the patient with multiple operations or numerous hospitalizations. It is common to see a patient with long-standing abdominal pain and six abdominal scars. First a "chronic gallbladder" was removed, then two or three operations for postoperative "adhesions," followed by "chronic appendicitis," and, last, the removal of the uterus, both ovaries, and tubes. Probably none was indicated; the pain continues. And, finally, be alerted by the patient who has been to many physicians, some of known repute, and "nothing wrong could be found."

Schizophrenia. The schizophrenic's somatic symptoms are characterized by their bizarreness and their basis in a disturbed body image. Such patients often have delusional beliefs about the cause or explanation of a symptom. Most commonly, the complaints are neuromuscular (tension states), genital, or involve special senses (strange tastes or odd hearing complaints, often related to delusions or hallucinations). These patients are often incorrectly diagnosed as hypochondriasis or conversion neurosis. In addition to the presence of the specific clinical features of schizophrenia, the bizarreness of the symptom and the fixity with which the patient holds on to it, or to his conviction of the kind of treatment intervention he requires, help to establish the diagnosis.

Clarifying the Diagnostic Process

As can be seen from the above clinical examples, a major problem posed by psychosomatic complaints is the confounding of the medical problem-solving process. The physician needs to *avoid the dual errors* of, on one hand, overlooking occult ominous organic disease and, on the other, diagnosing as physically ill a patient who actually has no organic disorder. Once a patient is labeled psychoneurotic, the physician tends to regard this as the cause for each subsequent visit. He is usually correct. But this is where errors often occur. The chronic complainer can develop abdominal cancer with only a slight variation of his usual symptom complex. Each new symptom should be regarded with respect, since it may augur organic disease. The following principles can facilitate accurate diagnosis—and management—of patients with psychosomatic aspects to their problems.

Do not accept the patient's definition of the problem. The patient whose chief complaint is anxiety may be hyperthyroid. The patient concerned that he has cancer may have a severe depressive illness. Therefore, always have the patient explain what he means by a word, rather than assume that you and he are giving it the same definition.

Be alert to historical consistency of a patient's complaints. A patient with prior severe depressions or prior blood-loss anemia can, in a Bayes' theorem fashion, be assumed likely to have a recurrence of the previous conditions. Conversely, the patient with new, not readily explainable symptoms, regardless of how characteristic of a psychosomatic disorder they may be, should be treated with great concern for possible cancer or other organic disease.

Avoid using medical terminology or jargon with such patients. The anxiety level or excessive bodily concern of the patient may result in his indelibly latching on to your passing reference to "slightly depressed T waves" or a "funny shadow in the left apex of the chest" with a personalized, maladaptive interpretation of the remark. The same advice holds for the physical examination. The patient may infer from your listening to the aortic area for a few extra moments that you have uncovered serious pathology. If you recognize the patient's overconcern, an accompanying statement that "your heart is

in good condition and is functioning very well" can short-circuit misunderstanding.

Laboratory tests and medications also need to be ordered with circumspection. Whereas you may be ordering a test to ensure the absence of an unlikely possibility, the patient may infer that the test per se means the presence of disease in the organ system. Again, an accompanying explanation of the rationale for your particular testing or mode of intervention can reduce misunderstanding. When interpreting results of diagnostic tests to the patient, explain clearly the psychosomatic nature of the complaint if in fact no organic disease is found. To the degree that we brush off the patient with a prescription, when attention to the meaning of his illness or complaint is called for, we perpetuate and worsen this patient's responses.

Do follow such patients regularly and frequently, carefully documenting your observations in the medical record. Often an unequivocal diagnosis cannot be made at one visit. Establishing a baseline for the patient's behavior, appearance, and physical findings can in due time help to clarify the problem.

Avoid diagnosing "nondisease." The marginally low hemoglobin should not result in the diagnosis of anemia in the absence of other corroborative findings. A single positive latex fixation test should not lead to a diagnosis of rheumatoid arthritis in a patient with only mild subjective complaints of joint pain.

Do not prematurely initiate treatment which would mask occult disease. Tricyclic antidepressants may improve mood and overall function in patients with cancer, by virtue of both placebo and specific neuropharmacologic effects. Such treatment could delay recognition of the underlying disorder.

The patient who responds affirmatively to every question poses even more problems. You must suppress some of the information and try to form a reasonable cluster if you suspect organic disease. But though these usually tend to be hypochondriacal patients, they may be persons with primary problems of anxiety, conversion, or major organic illnesses. The first major concern posed by such patients is to avoid overtesting; the second is to convince the patient that there is no organic disease. It may be useful to say, "Mr. Jones, the examination I have done makes me reasonably certain that your heart is in good condition. It is wise that we get one additional test to ensure that your heart is fine. Though I expect the test to come back normal, I will discuss it with you as soon as we have the results." These patients often feel that physicians are avoiding them, and that symptoms which to them are serious are not being so treated by the physician. This can result in the patient becoming more firmly convinced of or fearful of his "disease."

Deal with these fears by performing at least a cursory examination of those parts of the person's body about which he is concerned. Even when you are certain that the patient's heart is functioning normally, your statement to him will be much more effective if you have listened to his heart with your stethoscope. Encourage questions from such patients. Failure to correct erroneous conclusions and associations can lead to a hardening of hypochondriacal beliefs.

Following a negative normal examination, do not proclaim that nothing is wrong with the patient. Rather, indicate that the organ system in question is in good condition—that the patient's very real symptoms reflect his body's way of responding to stress. Indicate that though rest or a drug may be helpful, the primary need is to help him identify and deal with the stresses.

References

1. Kaufman RM, Bernstein S: A psychiatric evaluation of the problem patient. *JAMA* 163:108–111, 1957.
2. Hall RCW: *Psychiatric Presentations of Medical Illness.* New York, Spectrum, 1980.
3. Kenyon FE: Hypochondriacal states. *Br J Psychiatry* 129:1–14, 1976.

Suggested Readings

1. Tumulty PA: The patient with a functional disorder. In *The Effective Clinician.* Philadelphia, Saunders, 1973, pp 125–135.
   A general approach to problem solving in patients with psychosomatic complaints.
2. Bowden CL: Coping with common patient reactions. In Bowden CL, Burstein AG (eds): *Psychosocial Basis of Health Care*, ed 3. Baltimore, Wilkins & Wilkins, 1983, pp 269–275.
   Practical guidelines both for preventing hypochondriacal responses from becoming ingrained, and for managing those which are ingrained.

Chapter 29

Special Aspects of Problem Solving in the Pediatric Patient

ALEXANDER W. PIERCE, JR., M.D.

Finding out what is wrong with the pediatric patient involves five special considerations:

1. Different techniques for data collection
2. Use of unique data
3. Different diagnostic probabilities
4. Increased likelihood of a single diagnosis
5. Diagnostic entities unique to pediatrics.

Obtaining a history from and doing a physical examination on an adult offer many difficulties, but in children these difficulties are often compounded and the physician must interact differently. The gestational, birth, and perinatal history, infant feeding practices, and the assessment of growth and development are data sets unique to problem solving in the pediatric patient; growth and development will be detailed to illustrate the use of unique data.

As for diagnostic probabilities, the spectrum is shifted in the child. For example, there is more infection and less malignancy than in the adult. The differential diagnosis of the pain syndromes of childhood will be used to exemplify pediatric probability sets. Disease incidences generally increase with age, and it is no surprise that old people are often polypathic, while children are far more apt to have a single disease. And the fact that there are diagnostic entities unique to pediatrics is a self-evident truth and needs no further discussion. The first four considerations, however, will be discussed in detail.

Different Techniques for Data Collection. Although the pediatric history is frequently obtained from relatives or guardians in addition to or instead of the patient, it is still the most important part of the data base. Often the history is obtained from *multiple informants* simultaneously; this requires unique interview skills. Failure to direct a multiple informant interview properly is a common cause for ineffective performance or poor time utilization. Maintenance of *interview control* and *directive interviewing* are necessary skills in obtaining a data base from a reactive adolescent and his parent, or from the preadolescent with an excessively dominating parent. Too often, when there is difficulty in maintaining interview control, the most direct source of information is neglected—the patient himself.

Patient compliance is critical to obtaining valid reproducible data by physical examination. The older child and adult understand and respect the expectation of compliance. The nonverbal infant and "terrible" 2-year-old, beset by stranger anxiety, do not understand this expectation. Evaluation of the patient's personal-social development (his level of maturity) is established at the beginning of the patient encounter. Compliance is facilitated by relating to a child in a manner commensurate with his level of development (his personal-social age) rather than his chronologic age or physical size.

The child who is "spoiled" or "immature" may be considered retarded in his personal-social development; he does not relate to peers, parents, or health care professionals on a level of sophistication commensurate with his chronologic age. The spoiled 4-year-old must be approached with the same firm, understanding, consistent patience required to examine the terrible, negative, normal 2-year-old. The adolescent who refuses to disrobe, or giggles and squirms during the examination, requires the structured, authoritarian, directive approach more commonly employed with the preadolescent.

In the infant and preschool child, *the physical examination is intentionally disordered.* The greater value of compliance justifies the possibility of introducing errors of omission which result from a disordered physical examination. Procedures which produce discomfort, or may be perceived by the child as producing discomfort, must be deferred to the terminal portions of the examination.

Similarly, because compliance may not be sustained, examine those areas most relevant to the presenting problem during the earlier portion of the examination. In the child who presents with respiratory symptoms, auscultate the chest prior to examining the upper respiratory tract. With the child who presents with acute abdominal pain, the rectal examination may be deferred to late in the course of events, but careful observation, auscultation, and palpation of the abdomen are done early.

Use of Unique Data. The assessment of growth and development, both by history and by observation, is to the pediatric data base what the review of systems is to the data base of the adult patient. It is a screening device to assess the patient's general health and detect unsuspected health problems. Deficits in the child's physical health or physical or social environment are reflected by deficits in growth or development. In childhood, growth and development normally proceed pari passu, and they are usually taught concurrently. As a consequence, students frequently fail to discriminate between the two processes. Growth refers to increments of physical size; development refers to increase in complexity of function.

In the evaluation of development, care must be taken to differentiate categories of development which are retarded or disordered. Gross motor development, fine motor-adaptive development, language development, and personal-social development must each be evaluated.

Parameters used to monitor growth are divergent in infancy and in the older child. Because length or height measurements are difficult to reproduce in the infant, weight is used to monitor growth prior to the achievement of an erect posture. Disorders of growth in this age group are referred to as "failure to thrive." Once the child has learned to stand erect, height is a superior parameter for gauging growth. Disorders of growth in this age group are referred to as "short stature."

Data useful in evaluating growth include not only the height and weight at a single visit, but, more importantly, changes in physical measurements with time (growth rate). When growth is suspect, the height of parents, grandparents, and siblings is elicited. If physical measurements are incongruous with genetic expectations or the growth rate slowed ("falling off the curve"), determination of skeletal maturation ("bone age") is indicated.

It is important to differentiate disordered from retarded growth or development. Disordered growth or development is that which occurs in an abnormal fashion or in an abnormal sequence, as opposed to being delayed or advanced. For example, while isolated language retardation may be due to environmental deprivation, diminished auditory acuity, or developmental aphasia, these diagnostic considerations are not appropriate to the child with disordered language development such as a lisp or stutter. Similarly, premature breast development (premature thelarche) in the absence of other evidence of sexual precocity may be considered disordered growth and development of the reproductive system. Acromegaly and hemihypertrophy are examples of disordered growth.

Different Diagnostic Probabilities. The

probabilities in pediatrics are different from those encountered in the adult patient. The child with acute chest pain, independent of its localization or radiation, does not have coronary insufficiency. Acute chest pain in children is usually the result of inflammatory disease (pneumonitis or pleuritis). If the pain is localized to the precordial region and radiates to the left shoulder, it may represent pericarditis. Chronic chest pain in the pediatric patient is most commonly psychophysiologic or "functional" in origin.

A disorder of the digestive system is improbable in the child with chronic recurrent abdominal pain; the cholecystogram and gastrointestinal series will be unrewarding. Again, the pain is most likely psychophysiologic. If chronic abdominal pain in a child has an organic basis, it usually involves the urinary tract.

There are *three principal recurrent pain syndromes* in childhood. Recurrent abdominal pain is found in 11%, recurrent head pain in 10%, and recurrent multiple extremity pain in 4% of pediatric patients. The incidence of major organic disease in children with the recurrent pain syndromes ranges from 3 to 6%. The incidence of a positive history of psychosocial environmental stress and a family history of related symptoms ranges from 50 to 75% in each of these three groups.

The pediatric patient who presents with *retarded or disordered growth or development* offers unique diagnostic considerations. Students are frequently too quick to seek consultative help. The most common diagnosis in patients referred for evaluation of retarded or disordered language development is mental retardation. The physician has responded to a complaint of "can't talk" or "isn't talking right" with referral for speech and language evaluation without prior evaluation of other development categories. On the other hand, the child of 18 months to 2 or 3 years of age who presents with retarded language development, but otherwise normal developmental parameters, probably has a congenital sensory-neural hearing deficit.

Similarly, the 1- to 2-year-old child with isolated retardation of gross motor development without associated retardation of other developmental categories most likely has a neuromuscular or musculoskeletal disorder. Congenital dislocation of the hip may present as "can't walk" in an otherwise bright child.

Retardation of fine motor-adaptive development in infancy is the best correlate or predictor of ultimate cognitive function. It is not usually impaired without involvement of other developmental parameters. Isolated retardation of fine motor-adaptive development is usually associated with disorders of the extrapyramidal motor tract.

The infant with retarded growth (failure to thrive) is most likely suffering from caloric deprivation. If a measured caloric intake fails to result in growth, major organ system failure must be considered. If both growth and development are retarded, a disorder of the central nervous system is probable. If development is normal and growth retarded, the system most frequently involved is cardiovascular (Table 29.1). Neurologic or cardiovascular disorders are usually easily detected by physical examination. If major organ system involvement is not readily apparent on physical examination of the child with growth failure and adequate caloric intake, the most common system to be involved is genitourinary.

The older child with growth failure (short stature) and adequate caloric intake must be considered in light of his genetic background. While racial differences in height are largely a reflection of environmental differences, the height of relatives must never-

Table 29.1.
Growth Retardation Due to Major Organ System Failure: Order of Probability

1. Central nervous system
2. Cardiovascular system
3. Genitourinary system
4. Respiratory system
5. Gastrointestinal system
6. Endocrine system
7. Hematopoietic system
8. Skeletal system

theless be used to determine growth potential for the individual patient. The hallmarks of genetically determined short stature are a normal growth rate and a normal bone age. The second common cause of short stature, constitutional delayed growth, is associated with a normal growth rate, a modestly delayed bone age, and delayed pubescence. Thus, in constitutional delayed growth, the height age and bone age are concordant and the ultimate statural height is compatible with genetic expectations.

Increased Likelihood of a Single Diagnosis. An inherent assumption in the initial approach to the pediatric patient is *"one patient, one diagnosis."* This principle is equally applicable to the child presenting to the emergency room with an unexpected finding unrelated to the presenting complaint and to the electively admitted patient with multiple complaints. Careful consideration of all possibilities for a common etiologic or pathophysiologic basis for multiple problems precedes consideration of multiple diagnoses.

In the infant with chronic progressive lower airway obstructive disease and easy bruisability, there is a high probability for the diagnosis of mucoviscidosis with associated hypoprothrombinemia resulting from malabsorption of fat-soluble vitamin K. Chronic lung disease and an unrelated primary coagulation defect are unlikely. Similarly, the older child with muscle weakness and dark urine is more apt to have myoglobinuria associated with a primary myopathy than renal disease with hematuria and a musculoskeletal disorder.

Suggested Readings

1. Homer C, Ludwig S: Categorization of etiology of failure to thrive. *Am J Dis Child* 135:848–851, 1981.
2. McGrath PJ, Goodman JT, Firestone P, et al: Recurrent abdominal pain: a psychogenic disorder? *Arch Dis Child* 58:888–890, 1983.
3. Barnes N: Excessive growth. *Arch Dis Child* 58:845–846, 1983.
4. Buckler JM: How to make the most of bone ages. *Arch Dis Child* 58:761–763, 1983.
5. Goldbloom RB: Failure to thrive. *Pediatr Clin North Am* 29:151–166, 1982.

Chapter 30

Special Aspects of Problem Solving in the Geriatric Patient

PAUL CUTLER, M.D.

Perhaps the most stirring description of old age to be found anywhere is in the Book of Ecclesiastes (1). The coming of "the evil days when thou shalt say 'I have no pleasure in them' " is beautifully and poetically portrayed. And the problems of old age, such as blindness, dreariness, tremors, bowed back, loss of teeth, lack of opportunity, light sleep, deafness, fear of heights, and fear of stumbling are depicted in allegoric verse:

"Before the sun, and the light, and
the moon,
And the stars, are darkened,
And the clouds return after
the rain;
In the days when the keepers of the
house shall tremble,
And the strong men shall bow themselves,
And the grinders cease because they
are few . . . ."

Read—where it is written.

Who He Is. The definition of a geriatric patient is "one who is 10 or more years older than the one who does the defining." Until recently, 65 marked the onset of the geriatric age, but many now regard it as upward of 70. A century ago, one was "old" at 50, but with the advent of means of preserving the abilities to see, hear, chew, and locomote, even people of 70 are no longer "old."

To the patient who sadly tells you: "Doctor, it's terrible to get old," you can honestly respond: "It's worse *not* to!"

The fact that a separate chapter of this book is devoted to the geriatric patient implies that *problem solving is somehow different in the elderly.* And so it is. Getting the history is more difficult and presents certain obstacles peculiar to this age. The physical examination and laboratory data must be interpreted differently because some findings that are abnormal in middle age are considered normal in an older person. Furthermore, disease incidences and likelihoods shift since certain conditions become much more common with advancing years. And last, elderly patients often react differently and less vigorously to an illness, thus making the presenting picture less recognizable.

Getting the History. There are many reasons why history taking can be very difficult in a geriatric patient. So too are there ways to make it easier. Try to take time to make friends with the patient. Treat him or her courteously, with respect and dignity; at the same time, be warm, kind, and considerate. For example, it often helps to ask about the family and former jobs and to talk about "old times."

Most older people retain their intelligence, compensate for a slower rate of learning by their greater store of well-learned long-term knowledge and experience, maintain their problem-solving skills, lead active independent lives, and are more flexible than people think.

Do not ever underestimate the intelligence of the patient. A person is not feeble-minded because he is old. On the contrary, most often, old patients are wise and should not be treated like "old Granny" or "Gramps." It might help to remember that the world is run mostly by people of geriatric age, and that Tennyson, Shaw, Goethe, Chagall, Schweitzer, Picasso, and Churchill, among others, did their best work after 60, and even after 80. But, on the other hand, many old folks do have waning mental faculties and altered mental mechanisms, so that it is necessary to assess the patient's intelligence, memory, and verbal powers at the same time that you take the history, and try to detect dramatization, distortion, and confabulation.

It is important to make sure the patient hears and understands you, and that you understand the meaning of his terminology.

Thus, a number of factors may make history taking difficult and the history itself distorted or untrue. The patient may not hear you correctly and may answer not what you asked, but what he thinks you asked. He may pretend to understand you and confabulate the answer, or he may even deliberately fabricate. His memory may be poor, or his answers may be twisted or false because of fear or denial. Often the elderly patient suffers with a chronic illness of insidious onset and he is unable to delineate a distinct beginning and a clear sequence of events because of a poor sense of time span.

Sometimes it is advisable to *consult other members* of the patient's family, especially for items relative to indications of mental deterioration, forgetfulness, personality changes, deafness, nutritional intake, or weight loss—items which may be more noticeable to the family than to the patient. Then too the history is often more accurate if retaken 1 or 2 days later when the patient is more lucid, less ill, and not under the effects of a calmative or analgesic drug. Indirect questions (discussed in Chapter 2) may be especially helpful in the elderly, who may have subconsciously learned how to eliminate or modify symptoms by altering their behavior.

Prominent Symptoms. Some symptoms are particularly common in old people; only a few will be discussed. For example, when the patient complains of "dizziness," you must know exactly what he means and you must get an accurate description of the symptom. He may not have true vertigo, but may merely feel weak, lightheaded, "funny," or have other similar, even less distinct symptoms. But if true vertigo exists, you sweep your diagnostic pointer in a different direction to include cerebral arteriosclerosis, Ménière's disease, labyrinthine disease, etc.

Constipation can be a vexing problem. If this symptom is recent and especially if it is accompanied by cramps and rectal bleeding, think of cancer. But far more often it is the result of improper diet, inadequate fluids, and poor habit patterns. Do not forget to do a rectal examination in all such cases. Frequently old people develop fixations on their bowels, and happiness is having a good bowel movement. So daily laxatives or enemas are in common usage.

Insomnia is a common complaint of old age. Older patients seem to need less sleep. Furthermore, they often nap in the daytime, thus making a full night's sleep more difficult. Then too they are consciously aware only of the numerous waking moments during the night and it seems to them that they have been awake all night. In Ecclesiastes (1), Koheleth says, " . . . and one shall start up at the voice of a bird," implying that the old sleep lightly and are easily and early awakened—also generally true.

A worrisome but common complaint is loss of appetite. It may mean many things, but think first of depression and cancer.

Often, the patient will complain of falling—once or frequently. This can be a Chinese puzzle. What caused the fall? Was there a transient episode of weakness, cerebral ischemia, cerebral thrombosis, or a cardiac arrhythmia? Or was it simply because of slow reflexes and lack of coordination, disabling arthritis of the knees, slipping on a loose rug, or tripping on a piece of furniture? The patient usually cannot furnish the answer. If there is a fracture present, did the patient fall because of a pathologic hip fracture, or did he sustain a fracture because of the fall? If he is unconscious after the fall, is it because the unconsciousness preceded or caused the fall, or was it the result of the fall?

Syncope is common in the elderly. There are many known causes (see Case 63) but the source is often never found. Cardiovascular origins tend to be serious and have a high annual mortality.

Note how many symptoms are *"can't symptoms,"* such as "can't sleep, can't eat, can't urinate, can't move bowels, can't see, can't hear, can't walk, and can't breathe."

Under the heading of "things that don't work anymore," the eyes and ears are very important. Failing vision is most common because of simple presbyopia, cataracts, glaucoma, and retinal degeneration; some of these can be helped. Deafness usually results from nerve degeneration, though conductive deafness may be present too, and hearing aids may be indicated.

Nocturnal leg *cramps* and leg *pains* occur with surprising frequency. If there is no detectable neurologic disease, the former have no known cause and are treated symptomatically. The latter may result from diabetic neuropathy or vascular disease.

Numerous more specific symptoms which clearly relate to organ disease (heart, gastrointestinal tract, urinary tract) may be present too, but these need no elaboration. Their causes are usually easily traceable.

The "Normal" Examination. There are a number of physical findings which are so common in the elderly that they may be regarded as "normal," even though such findings in younger people would indicate disease.

The purplish spots on the dorsum of the hands or on the arms are nothing more than "senile purpura" and do not indicate disease of the capillaries or coagulation mechanism. Brown spots on the dorsum of the hands are not "liver spots"; they mean nothing. Arcus senilis is nothing more than its name implies, and is significant only in younger patients. Tremor of the hands and a slow shuffling gait are so common that they are considered to be signs of old age, though they probably relate to degeneration of certain cerebellar and extrapyramidal centers.

Partial nerve deafness and ripening cata-racts are ubiquitous. Heart murmurs are more often heard than not. As the aortic valve scleroses and the aorta stretches and uncurls, basal murmurs become frequent. Not uncommonly the costovertebral articulations become fixed, the neck becomes rigid due to osteoarthritic changes, and the chest becomes barrel-shaped. This may interfere with the mechanics of respiration and may even be associated with senile emphysema. The neck contour makes it difficult to lie down without two pillows.

Blood pressure may be "alarmingly low," e.g. 87/60, though in reality normal; yet it is often considered high when it is found to be 180/80 mm Hg. The latter figure is probably normal and represents slight systolic elevation only, perhaps a mechanism to compensate for the loss of aortic elastic recoil and the relatively low diastolic pressure. Other cardiovascular findings such as premature atrial contractions and atrial fibrillation are commonly present; the former probably has no significance, whereas the latter may signify a well-tolerated mild cardiac disorder. The aorta which is fixed at either end can become tortuous with the continual pounding of time. This tortuosity may be falsely perceived as an abdominal aneurysm.

Abdominal reflexes are lost in a high percentage of geriatric persons (20 to 50%). Sometimes there is a normal loss of the Achilles reflex too. And loss of vibration sense in the legs is extremely common. These are important facts to keep in mind in persons who are prone to diseases like pernicious anemia and cerebrovascular accidents which affect these nerve tracts.

Certain laboratory test variations must also be kept in mind. The upper normal limit for blood glucose is higher and the criteria for an abnormal glucose tolerance test are at higher levels. This must be remembered before labeling the patient with diabetes. Also increased are the upper normal levels for blood urea nitrogen, creatinine, and cholesterol. Anemia must never be regarded lightly, but the lower limits of normal are 10.11 g/dl among presumably healthy, elderly men and 10.38 g/dl in women. These values are lower than in younger adults. Investigation is clearly indicated if the hemoglobin is below 10 g/dl, and possibly even if below 11 g/dl. As in interpreting other tests, it is helpful to know a previous value.

Especially Common Diseases. Since heart disease, stroke, and cancer are the three leading causes of death, you can expect them to be the most common diseases of the aged. This simple truth must always weight your logic. No matter what the clinical presentation, one of these illnesses must always be seriously considered, since they often hide behind what seems to be another disease.

Neuropsychiatric disorders commonly seen include anxiety, depression, melancholia, chronic brain syndrome, senile psychosis, effects of cerebral arteriosclerosis, stroke, acute confusional states, Parkinson's disease, dizziness, and loneliness.

In the special senses, you see cataracts, glaucoma, retinal arteriosclerosis, macular degeneration, presbyopia, deafness, and vertigo. Continuing into the gastrointestinal tract, the aged person suffers from inability to chew because of lost teeth; cancer from the mouth to the anus but mainly in the stomach, pancreas, colon, and rectum; cholelithiasis, diverticulosis, and diverticulitis; and last, but not least, hemorrhoids.

Cardiovascular diseases include mainly ischemic heart disease, congestive heart failure from many causes, arrhythmias, and peripheral vascular disease. In the lung, chronic obstructive lung disease, chronic bronchitis, and cancer head the list. As for hematology, anemias of all sorts, especially those of chronic disease and chronic blood loss from the gastrointestinal tract, are rampant. Leukemia, lymphoma, and multiple myeloma are not uncommon.

And in the bones and joints, arthritis, osteopenia, and Paget's disease are all frequent. Fractures can occur from seemingly atraumatic events like raising a window, moving a chair, or getting hugged. The genitourinary tract is notable for cancer (kidney, bladder, prostate, uterus, breast), benign prostatic hypertrophy, urinary incontinence, and atrophic vaginitis.

Endocrine diseases are very common, especially diabetes mellitus. While juvenile diabetics die young, and the peak incidence of onset of diabetes is in the forties and fifties, the percentage of people with diabetes rises with each decade. This confronts us with the enigma that diabetics die younger but live longer. In old age, all the endocrine glands remain very much alive except for the ovaries, but changes do occur in the responsiveness of neuroendocrine control circuits and feedback axes. As many as 30% of all cases of thyrotoxicosis are seen after 60; most are classical, but many pose diagnostic difficulty in that they are phlegmatic, apathetic, without goiter, and are obscured by the presence of concomitant disease. Hypothyroidism is common but often overlooked because its manifestations overlap with and are mistaken for those features which indicate that the patient is "getting older."

Points to Remember. Some additional items which make diagnosis difficult in the elderly are: Typical signs and symptoms of disease such as fever and pain are attenuated or absent; the effect of drugs is greater and so is the potential for confusing adverse reactions and interactions; physical disease often presents as a mental disorder as just stated; homeostatic mechanisms are not rapidly reactive; immunologic responses are altered; and last, the old patient tends to have a multiplicity of problems (medical, social, economic, etc). These are all pitfalls which stand in the way of correct diagnosis (2).

Thus, the older person may have pneumonia, sepsis, or pyelonephritis without fever; myocardial infarction or acute abdomen with little pain; easily induced hyponatremia, silent terminal bronchopneumonia, and congestive failure, infection, or anemia presenting as confusion. In fact, acute myocardial infarction may be classic in only one-third of cases; it presents primarily with confusion and restlessness in one-third, and with dyspnea, palpitations, and sweating in many of the rest.

Suppose that an anemia gradually develops. The symptoms of which the patient complains may not be from the anemia but from the unmasking of another latent disorder whose symptom threshold is surpassed because of the anemia. For example, subclinical coronary heart disease, barely compensated congestive failure, and asymptomatic cerebral arteriosclerosis may develop symptoms when anoxemia is superimposed.

A further point to remember is that many lanthanic problems exist in the aged. These usually give no symptoms and their mere presence is not necessarily the explanation for a presenting cluster. Since hiatal hernias, cholelithiasis, gastric mucosal atrophy, degenerative joint disease, and diverticulosis are so commonly present, they do not explain all instances of indigestion, abdominal pain and back pain which the patient may have. It is easy to fall into this type of diagnostic booby trap. On the other hand, since gallstones are so common (10 to 25%), and since perhaps 40% of these will eventually become symptomatic, it might be wiser to include a gallbladder study rather than a chest x-ray as part of an annual examination.

It is important to recall that old patients are highly *prone to adverse drug reactions* and that these may be the cause for or may modify the presenting symptoms, thus confusing the physician. In fact, adverse drug reactions and interactions are among the most common problems in this age group. Often, tolerance for a drug is lower because of associated renal or liver disease, deficiency of detoxifying mechanisms, or alterations in serum protein-binding capacity. Drugs may act differently. Barbiturates may cause stimulation or delirium, and hypotensives can cause syncope and symptoms of decreased cerebral perfusion. It is common for the patient to tell you, "That new medicine is making me sick!" He is probably correct. Remember too that these patients have multiple diseases, take many medications, and take them at ill-conceived intervals—a perfect background for confusion and mistakes, even if the patient were young.

In an excellent study (2) of 500 patients over the age of 65 who were admitted to the hospital, 193 developed complications and 44 developed intercurrent disease. Of the complications, 54 were drug reactions, 31 were procedure reactions, 61 resulted from accidents and trauma, 19 developed major psychologic decompensation, and 17 got hospital-acquired infections. Intercurrent diseases consisted mainly of pulmonary embolus and aspiration pneumonia, but also included fecal impaction, decubitus ulcer, parotitis, and urinary retention. One may conclude that hospitals are not completely safe—especially for the aged.

One last point! It would seem that Weed's problem-oriented medical records are of greatest value in geriatric medicine. These older patients have and have had multiple illnesses, take many medications, have had numerous consultations, have additional psychosocial problems, have isolated unclassifiable abnormal symptoms, physical findings, and paraclinical studies, and their records are therefore voluminous (2). How difficult it would be to track such a patient without a problem list to serve as a table of contents!

The Dementia Riddle. The problem of *senile dementia* has reached huge proportions and patients with this disease threaten to fill our nursing homes and institutions. Many public dollars will be saved if some dementias can be reversed.

The first thing to remember is that many cases of *seeming* dementia are temporary or reversible and are improved or remain static if treated. Numerous diseases masquerade as senile dementia. If undiagnosed, the patient may be institutionalized for life with no cure subsequently possible.

Commonly, concerned relatives bring you an old person who is acting strangely, is incoherent, disoriented, forgetful, and cannot manage his or her clothing and hygiene. This is the description of full-blown senile dementia. Only some of these features may be present. The picture may have existed for days, weeks, or months, and the patient may be coming from home or a nursing home where the family or staff can no longer cope.

"Senility" is assumed. But too often an organic illness is the cause. Just as in the thyroid disorders already discussed, many other situations may cause confusion, restlessness, and behavioral changes which, on the surface, are indistinguishable from senility. Treatable illness can easily be overlooked and the question to consider is: *Is this patient senile or sick?*

The history (obtained from somebody else), physical examination, and a "dementia profile" should successfully exclude most causes of organic dementia. *Medications are in a class by themselves since they are such common offenders.* Even the "correct dose" of digoxin, chlorpropamide, indomethacin, steroids, cimetidine, phenothiazines, or barbiturates may cause mental abnormalities, especially in the presence of polypharmacy and drug-drug interactions. *Depression* is another important cause of symptoms resembling senility. Your study must also exclude endocrine disorders, uremia, primary and metastatic brain tumors, subdural hematoma, cirrhosis of the liver, chronic alcoholism, pernicious anemia, cerebral anoxia from any cause (anemia, lung or heart diseases), normal-pressure hydrocephalus, nutritional deficiencies (vitamin B_1, riboflavin), collagen diseases, and those conditions associated with serum *sodium*, *calcium*, and *glucose* levels which are high enough or low enough to cause cerebral manifestations.

In addition to the various chemical tests needed to exclude most of these possibilities, intracranial lesions may require imaging techniques and electroencephalography.

Having eliminated all these possible abnormalities as a cause for the patient's dementia, there remain the two causes of most senile dementias—*multiinfarct dementia* and *senile dementia of the Alzheimer's type.* The former results from repeat cerebral infarcts, is episodic, and tends to occur in patients with hypertension, diabetes, and cardiovascular disease. The latter—Alzheimer's disease—is insidious, progresses slowly, and is inexorable. Once thought to be presenile since it was first described in people in the sixth decade of life, it presents the same clinical picture in older people. This consists of loss of memory and judgment, disorientation, and then loss of cognitive functions. Neurofibrillary tangles and plaques are seen throughout the brain in both age groups.

To Solve or Not. Inevitably, the issue of whether or not to pursue a diagnosis, and how vigorously to pursue it, arises in the elderly patient. There is no simple "yes" or "no" answer. An 80-year-old patient may have right upper quadrant pain, easily withstand a cholecystectomy, and live on for another 10 fruitful and enjoyable years.

On the other hand, an 80-year-old man with metastatic cancer should not have a coronary arteriogram for the investigation of chest pain. Nor should an 80-year-old with proven advanced triple vessel coronary artery disease have an extensive survey for suspected cancer. No matter what the results of such studies, you would do nothing anyway.

Do not push too hard with diagnostic studies in the very old, because their tolerance for such study is limited. The illness you are pursuing has probably already made the patient frail. If he has occult gastrointestinal bleeding which has already stopped, and the proctosigmoidoscopy and gastrointestinal x-rays are normal, it might be both more discreet and valorous to give iron for anemia rather than do visceral angiography. Often the diagnostic procedure causes more distress than the illness, and you should not gamble with the vitality of the patient by subjecting him to more tests than he can tolerate with reasonable safety (3).

Such attitudes may come more naturally to those who have practiced medicine for many years and have seen much of life and death. But such ideas may be heretical to today's intern or resident who, with a plethora of diagnostic tools, has not yet learned that he is not omnipotent and that Nature may often take its course in spite of him (4).

Some Final Reflections. Look deeply and carefully at your old patient, and you will usually see a compassionate, gentle, tolerant, and kind person. These are not the attributes of youth—or of middle age. Remember that every wizened old person once had youth, vigor, and dreams—as you do now. He still has those whom he loves and who love him. Though dignified and calm, he is fearful, for he knows each illness, each day, may be his last.

When he consults you, the thoughts of illness and death are always on his mind, for often "last night he heard the owl calling his name"—or so he thinks. He knows very well that the only condition with a 100% mortality is life itself—and he has had life. At this point, he needs your kindness and caring even more than your diagnostic skills, your science, and your medicine.

If, indeed, he is ill and is dying, the greatest fear is dying alone. And that is a fear we can treat and a problem we can solve without even knowing what is wrong with the patient. A perfunctory visit to the room of a dying man does more harm than good. But, just once, sit at the bedside, hold the dying man's hand, stroke his brow, smile to him, and help him to die—before, during, and after the event. Be there "as the silver cord is snapped asunder, as man goeth to his long home, and the dust returneth to the earth as it was" (1).

You will feel more like a "real physician" than ever, for helping your patient die can be a greater feat than helping him live.

References

1. Ecclesiastes 12:1–8.
   The classical features of old age are magnificently portrayed in this timeless writing.
2. Reichel W: Multiple problems in the elderly. *Hosp Prac* 11:103–108, 1976.
   This article is packed with wisdom concerning the management of geriatric patients, outlines the need for good record keeping, decries the diagnosis of "old age," and reveals what may

happen to old patients who are hospitalized.
3. Seegal D: The principle of minimal interference in the management of the elderly patient. *J Chronic Dis* 17:299–300, 1964.
4. Kampmeier R: Editorial: death and aging. *South Med J* 67:3–4, 1974.

Suggested Readings

1. Reichel W: *Clinical Aspects of Aging*, ed. 2. Baltimore, Williams & Wilkins, 1983.
   This comprehensive textbook was prepared under the direction of The American Geriatrics Society; it contains everything you might want to know about the geriatric patient.
2. Hodkinson HM: *An Outline of Geriatrics*, ed 2. London, Academic Press, 1981.
   In only 166 pages, this typically crisp British book covers the entire subject.
3. Charcot JM: *Clinical Lectures on the Diseases of Old Age* (translated). New York, W Wood & Co, 1881.
   This fascinating century-old book, written by a famous clinician, presents an array of diseases then attributed to old age.
4. Johnson JE III: Preparation in undergraduate medical education for improved geriatric care. *J Med Educ* 58:503–526, 1983.
   A superb discussion of the biologic mechanisms and pathophysiologic effects of aging that almost equals a textbook in only 24 pages.
5. Sivertson SE: Editorial: a framework for problem solving in geriatrics. *Postgrad Med* 57:129–131, 1975.
   A statistical analysis of the various causes for which 8181 geriatric patients visited a physician.
6. Beck CJ, Benson DF, Scheibel AB, et al: Dementia in the elderly: the silent epidemic. *Ann Intern Med* 97:231–241, 1982.
   The numerous causes of reversible dementia are discussed; special attention is given to Alzheimer's disease.
7. Cummings J, Benson DF, LoVerne S Jr: Reversible dementia: illustrative cases, definition, and review. *JAMA* 243:2434–2439, 1980.
   Elaborates on dementia mimics and their diagnosis.
8. Kokmen E: Dementia—Alzheimer type. *Mayo Clin Proc* 59:35–42, 1984.
   Recent understandings of histopathology and biochemical abnormalities—a solid review and update.

Index

Because this book consists principally of logic and ideas rather than facts, the index is scant. Diseases and their clinical features are not discussed in depth and are often only mentioned. Should the reader wish to seek out a subject, the table of contents may serve as a better guide.

Abdomen, swelling of, 527–530
  causes, 527
Abdominal pain, 387–392
  acute, 377–378
    causes, 378, 379, 380
    varying features of, 378
Abetalipoproteinemia, 385
Achalasia, 367
Alcohol
  harmful effects of, 548, 549
  intoxication syndromes, 545
  withdrawal syndromes, 408,
    545, 548, 549
Aldosteronism, primary, 451
Aldosteronoma, 285, 531
Algorithms, 161–163
  how to construct, 162, 163
  principal values of, 162
Alveolar hypoventilation, 26
Alzheimer's disease, 593
Amebic liver abscess, 401, 402
Amenorrhea, 467–470
  causes, 467
    minor, 467
    psychogenic, 468
  contraception, 467
  diagnostic protocol, 470
  drug related, 467
  galactorrhea associated, 468
  primary, 469
  secondary, 467, 470
American Rheumatism Associa-
    tion criteria, 491, 492
Amylase, in pancreatitis, 381
Analgesic nephropathy, 426, 445
Anatomic approach, 157
  examples of, 157, 158
Anemia
  aplastic, 256
  hemolytic, 245–248
    causes, 247
  iron deficiency, 228, 229, 230,
    231
  megaloblastic, 237–240, 256–
    257
  of chronic disorders, 229, 230,
    265

pernicious, 236–239
  sideroblastic, 229
Angina pectoris, 307
  pathophysiology, 307
  worsening, 309
Angiotensin converting enzyme,
    361
Ankylosing spondylitis, 498, 499
Anovulatory bleeding, 476
Antidiuretic hormone, 460
  inappropriate secretion of (see
    SIADH)
Antinuclear antibody test, 83–84,
    493
Antithrombin III deficiency, 234,
    235
Anxiety disorder, 580, 581
Aortic regurgitation, 298–301
  causes, 298
  physical findings in, 299, 300
Aortic stenosis, 299, 310–315
  causes, 312
  causes of aortic systolic mur-
    murs, 310, 311
  complications, 312, 313
  symptoms and signs, 311, 312
Appendiceal abscess, 388, 389
  sonography for, 390
Appendicitis, acute, 387–392
  atypical presentations, 389, 390
  character of pain, 388
  classical, 389
  differential diagnosis, 389, 390,
    391
  physical examination, 388
  radiographic features, 389
Arrhenoblastoma, 284
Arrhythmias, 315–318
  paroxysmal atrial fibrillation,
    316
  paroxysmal atrial flutter, 316
  paroxysmal atrial tachycardia,
    316, 317
  paroxysmal ventricular tachy-
    cardia, 316, 317
Arthritis
  acute monarticular, 481–485

diagnostic protocol, 484, 485
  value of arthrocentesis, 482,
    483
  polyarticular, 490–495
    causes, 490
    systemic lupus erythematosus
      vs rheumatoid arthritis,
      491–494
  septic, 481–485
    bacterial causes, 481
Ascaris lumbricoides, 152
Ascites, 527–530
  causes, 528
  role of liver, 529
  study of ascitic fluid, 529
Asterixis, 409
Atelectasis, 354
Atrial fibrillation, 320
Atrial septal defect, 313
Auer rods, 258
Augenblick, 55
Austin Flint murmur, 313

B_{12} binding capacity, 253, 255,
    361
Backache, 495–499
  causes, 495
  epidemiology, 495
Baker's cyst, 481, 570
Band keratopathy, 416, 455, 456
Barbiturate intoxication, 536–540
Barlow's syndrome, 317
Bartter's syndrome, 451, 452
Bayes' theorems, 67, 71, 81–88
  description of, 81–82
  limitations of, 88–89
  practical applications of, 83–84,
    94, 95
Behavior disorder, 545–550
Ben Gurion University of the
    Negev, xxvi
Bence-Jones protein, 242, 244
Benefit-cost analysis, 140
Bernstein test, 325, 368
Betz cells, viii
Bicipital tendonitis, 480
Biliary cirrhosis, 529

Biopsies, 118
  newer aspects of, 122–123
Blind loop syndrome, 385
Blood urea nitrogen: creatinine
      ratio, 417, 419, 439, 441
Boolean algebra, 67, 70–71
Bronchiectasis, 357
Bronchitis, chronic, 353, 354
Brudzinski's signs, 207
Bruit, abdominal, 532, 533

Cabot, Richard, 52
Calcitonin, 271
Calculi, renal, 416, 427–431 (*see
      also* Hematuria)
  causes and chemical composi-
      tion, 427, 428, 429
  oxalate, 430, 431
  pathophysiology, 430
  radiographic features, 430, 431
  symptoms, 427
  uric acid, 430
Camelot, 167
Carboxyhemoglobinemia, 253,
      255
Carcinoid, 279
Carcinoma
  of bladder, 418, 419
  of colon, 395
  of endometrium, 475, 476
  of kidney, 416, 417, 418, 419
      diagnosis, 417
  of lung, 329–334, 353–357
      bronchial obstruction, 354
      chronic bronchitis, 353, 354
      diagnosis, 355, 356
      endocrine abnormalities, 355
      hemoptysis, 353
      oat cell, 356
      operability, 355, 356
      physical signs, 354
      resectability, 355, 356
  of pancreas, 401, 402
  of prostate, 417, 418, 523–526
      anemia, 524, 525
      differential diagnosis, 523
      phosphatases, 524, 525
      symptoms, 523
  of thyroid, 272
      medullary, 271
Cardiomyopathy, 299
Cardiovascular problems, 295–
      326
  common presentations, 295
  technology in diagnosis, 296,
      297
Carey-Coombs murmur, 321, 322
Carotid sinus syncope (*see* Syn-
      cope)
Carpal tunnel syndrome, 486,
      487, 492
Case presentation, 199–204 (*see
      also* Skills)
  examples of, 201–204
  methods of, 199–201
      problem oriented, 200
      traditional, 199

Cause and effect, 61–62
Cavernous sinus syndrome, 153
Celiac sprue, 385
Cerebral embolus, 518
Cerebral thrombosis, 516–521
  clinical picture, 516, 517
  complications, 520
  diagnostic studies, 518, 519
  embolus vs thrombosis, 519
  pathophysiology, 518, 519
  role of computed tomographic
      scan, 517
  stroke mimics, 516, 517, 523
Chance node, 131
Chemistry profile
  6-test, 28
  12-test, 28
  18-test, 28
Chenodeoxycholic acid, 375
Chest pain, 323–326
  causes, 323
Cheyne-Stokes respiration, 538
Chlamydia trachomatis, 472
Cholecystitis, acute, 379
Cholelithiasis, 373, 375
  ultrasound in diagnosis of, 374,
      375, 382
Cholestasis, 397 (*see also* Jaun-
      dice)
  diagnostic protocol, 400, 402,
      403
  diagnostic techniques, 400, 402,
      403
  extrahepatic, 397, 398
  intrahepatic, 397, 398
  medical vs surgical, 399, 401
  physical signs, 399
  role of liver biopsy, 400, 402
Chymotrypsin test, 384
Cirrhosis of liver, 408–412
  cerebral manifestations, 408
  complications, 410, 411
  laboratory studies, 409
  peritonitis in, 410
  physical signs, 408, 409
  varied presentations of, 411
Classic cases, 92, 93
Clinical pictures, why they differ,
      62
Clinical reasoning, 12
Clubbing of fingers, 354, 355, 357
Clues, 40–48
  clustering, 33
  combinations of, 83
  contrary, 43
  decisive, 42
  definition of, 40
  false, 46, 48
  intersection of, 44
  key, 44, 48 (*see also* Problem-
      solving methods)
  negative, 33, 41
  pertinent negative, 41, 48
  positive, 41
  primary, 42
  quantitation of, 47

relation between, 43
relationship to disease
  demonstration by stick dia-
      grams, 78
  demonstration by Venn dia-
      grams, 77–78
  100% sensitive, 77
  100% sensitive and 100%
      specific, 78
  100% specific, 77
  overlap, 78
  varied and complex, 77
relative importance of, 45
relevance of, 32, 33
secondary, 42
sensitivity of, 45
sequence of, 46, 48
specificity of, 45
vanishing, 46
Coagulopathies, 232–236
Coarctation of aorta, 532
Coccidioidomycosis, 42
Cohort, 131
Coin test, 26
Coma, 536–540
  causes, 536, 537
  diagnostic logic, 536, 537, 538,
      539
  emergency management, 536,
      539
  role of computed tomographic
      scan, 538
  role of lumbar puncture, 538
Combination testing, 89, 91, 92,
      93 (*see also* Product of
      probabilities)
Computed tomography, 118,
      121–122
  benefits of, 121–122
  disadvantages of, 121
  uses of, 121
Computers, 165–167
  acronymic applications, 166
  pros and cons of, 165
  role of, 165–167
  specific mini-programs, 165
Confusional state, acute, 545–550
  causes, 546
  lumbar puncture, 547
Congestive heart failure, 302–306
  acute pulmonary edema, 302
  anasarca, 304
  causes for worsening, 305
  clinical picture, 302
  hyponatremia in, 303, 304
Contraceptives, 467, 468, 471,
      477
  complications of, 469
Convulsion, 507–511
  cardiovascular sources, 508
  causes, 507, 511
  hypoglycemia related, 509
  role of computed tomographic
      scan, 510
  toxic substance related, 508
  tumor related, 509

COPD (*see* Obstructive pulmo-
    nary disease, chronic)
Core curriculum, xxiv
Core of knowledge, 222, 223
Core of presentations, 222
Cori cycle, 5
Cost effectiveness analysis, 140
Creatine kinase, 308, 309
CREST syndrome, 492
Crighton, 57
Criteriology, 148
    for diagnosis, 88–89
Crohn's disease, 383
Crystal-induced arthropathies,
    482
CT (*see* Computed tomography)
Culdocentesis, 471
Cushing's disease, 87, 283 (*see*
    also Cushing's syndrome)
    clinical features, 284
    laboratory diagnosis, 285
Cushing's syndrome, 283 (*see*
    also Cushing's disease)
    causes, 283
Cutoff point, 79, 81, 94
Cystitis, acute, 422–426
    cystitis vs pyelonephritis, 424,
        426
    organisms, 423
    relation of gender and age, 423
    symptoms, 422
    urine studies in, 424

Data base
    complete, examples of, 188–
        192, 193–197
    components, 12, 50
    importance of history in, 13
Data clustering, 11 (*see also* Data
    resolution skills)
Data collection, 12–30
Data evaluation, 11 (*see also*
    Data resolution skills)
Data processing, 9, 11, 30–34,
    187, 198
Data resolution skills, 205–209
    (*see also* Skills)
    relevance determination, 209–
        217
    patient with anemia, 210,
        212, 213
    patient with chest pain, 210,
        214–216
    patient with jaundice, 211,
        216–217
    selection of data subsets, 205–
        209
    abdominal mass, 206–207
    cough and expectoration,
        207–208
    diminished vision, 208–209
    lump in groin, 209
    nipple discharge, 209
    single seizure, 207
    swollen legs, 206
    thyromegaly, 208

DEALE, 130
Decision analysis, 2
    for a specific case, 141–144
    case in point, 141
    foliate and prune, 142
    judgment, 142
    probabilities, 142
    selecting the optimal option,
        144
    test, 146
    tree, 143
    utilities, 144
    pros and cons, 144–147
Decision-making process, 58
    practical examples of, 58
Decision node, 131
Decision path, 160–161
Decision theory, 129
Decision tree, 130–135
    averaging out and folding back,
        134–135
    foliation of, 134
    outcomes of, 134
    structuring of, 130–131
    utilities of, 137–138
Decisions, 128
    based on mathematical preci-
        sion, 128, 129
Defensive medicine, 569
Dementia, 592–593
    Alzheimer's disease, 593
    causes, 593
    multiinfarct dementia, 593
Dendrograms, 159–160 (*see also*
    Problem-solving methods)
Depression, 579, 580
Devil's pinches, 233
Diabetes insipidus, 290–294
    clinical features, 290, 291
    diagnosis, 291, 292, 293
    differential diagnosis, 290, 291
    nephrogenic, 291
    psychogenic, 292
Diabetes mellitus, 273–277
    complications, 276, 277
    glycosuria, 273
    insulin reaction, 275
    pregnancy and, 275
Diagnosis, xxi, xxii
Diagnostic certainty, 7, 59–60, 92
    degree of, 149
    wrong labels, 60
Diagnostic hypothesis, 4 (*see also*
    Problem-solving methods)
Diarrhea, 382
    causes, 383
Dichotomous tests, 78
Differential diagnosis, (*see also*
    Problem-solving methods)
    formation of, 154, 155, 156
    pruning of, 41
    system for, 155
Digital subtraction angiography,
    118, 123
Digitalis intoxication, 66, 93
Digoxin serum assay, 66, 85, 93

Diphyllobothrium latum, 239
Disease
    action and reaction, 63
    definition of, 62
        description of, 148
        textbook cases, 149
    inoculum, 63
    symptom threshold, 63
    unanswered questions, 63
DISIDA isotope scan, 381, 382
Disk, herniated intervertebral,
    495–499
    electromyography, 498
    history, 497
    myelography, 498, 499
    physical signs, 497
    radiography for, 497
    role of computed tomographic
        scan, 498
Dissecting aneurysm, 534
Disseminated intravascular coag-
    ulation, 233, 234
Diverticulitis, 390, 391
Dizziness, 512–516
    benign positional vertigo, 512
    causes, 512–513
    definition, 512
    disabling positional vertigo, 512
    labyrinthitis, acute, 512
    vestibular neuronitis, 512
Doctor-induced disease (*see* Iatro-
    genic disease)
Doll's-eye movements, 538
Doppler studies, 519
Drop attacks, 515
Drug-induced problems, 570–576
    causes, 571
    examples, 572, 573
    identification of, 571–575
    in the elderly, 575–576
    scope, 571
Drug information services, 576
Drug levels in plasma, 576
Drug withdrawal syndrome, 545–
    550
Dupuytren's contracture, 408
Dysphagia, 365–369
    causes, 365, 366
        extraesophageal, 366
    cervical, 365, 367
    constancy or intermittency, 365
    location of, 365
    studies for, 366, 367, 368
    types, 365
Dyspnea
    four different presentations of,
        183–186
    on exertion, 17–18

Early hypothesis generation, 3
    (*see also* Problem-solving
    methods)
Ecclesiastes, 588, 589, 594
Ectopic pregnancy (*see* Preg-
    nancy)
Ehlers-Danlos syndrome, 299

Electrocardiogram
  left ventricular hypertrophy
    pattern, 298
    causes, 298
Electrolyte problems, 447–464
  disguises for, 447
Embolus, peripheral, 320, 321,
  322
Endocarditis, marantic, 43
Endocrine adenomatosis, multi-
  ple, 281
Endocrine problems, 266–294
  clues, 266, 267
  new technology, 266, 267
  pattern recognition, 266
  radioimmunoassay, 267
  reasons for overlooking, 267
  relative incidences, 268
Endoscopic retrograde cholangio-
  pancreatography, 400
Endoscopy, fiberoptic, 118
Epilepsy, idiopathic (see Convul-
  sion)
Epistaxis, 241
Eponymic syndromes, books, 562
Erythropoietin, 250, 251, 254
Esophageal diverticuli, 366
Esophageal spasm, diffuse, 366
Esophagitis, peptic, 366, 368, 374
Estimating the likelihood, 91, 94
  (see also Likelihoods)
Ethical dilemmas exposed, 132,
  133, 134, 139, 140, 146
  informed consent, 147
Evoked brain potentials, 31, 118
Experience, 2, 60

Farmer's lung, 360
Felty's syndrome, 257
Fetor hepaticus, 408
Fever, unknown origin, 550–555
  clinical settings for, 553, 554
  diagnosis, 552, 553
  factitious, 552
  miliary tuberculosis, 553, 554
  pertinent negatives, 551
  Petersdorf-Beeson criteria for,
    550
  principal causes, 551–552
Flexner, vii
Flow charts, 163–165 (see also
  Problem-solving methods)
Functional problems, 20

Gastritis, acute, 393
Gastrointestinal problems, 363–
  412
  consultations for, 364
  frequency of various, 363, 364
  physical signs, 363
  symptoms, 363
  tests for, 363
Gaucher's disease, 32
Gaussian curve, 47, 48
Geriatric patient, problem solving
  in, 588–594

adverse drug reactions, 592
difficulties with history, 588–
  589
"normal" findings, 590
prominent symptoms, 589
Ghor, vii
Gilbert's disease, 104
Glabellar reflex, 548
Globus hystericus, 367
Glucose 6-phosphate dehydrogenase deficiency, 247, 248,
  249
Gonorrhea, 471, 473
Gout, 481–485
  history of, 483
  joint fluid in, 483
  nephropathy in, 484
  pathophysiology, 483
  precipitating causes, 483
  serum uric acid, 482
Graham Steell murmur, 320
Granulomas, 329, 330
Growth and development, 586
Growth retardation, 586
Gynecologic problems, 465–478
  common presentations, 465
  endocrine overlap, 465

Halban's syndrome, 468, 469
Hamartoma, 329, 330
Hashimoto's disease, 208
Headache, 502–507
  brain tumor, 504
  causes, 503
  cervical osteoarthritis, 504
  intracranial infection, 504
  psychogenic, 503
  vascular, 504, 505, 506
Heinz bodies, 247
Hemachromatosis, 529
Hematemesis, 369–372
  assessment of severity of, 369
  causes, 369, 370
  diagnosis, 370
    procedures for, 370, 371
Hematologic problems, 225–265
  common clusters in, 226
  common presentations of, 225–
    226
  drugs in etiology of, 225
  new aspects of, 226
Hematuria, 415–422
  algorithm for, 420
  causes, 415, 416, 418, 419
  diagnostic procedures, 417, 418
    renal cyst vs cancer, 418,
      420, 421
  gross vs microscopic, 415, 418,
    419
  value of urinalysis, 415
Hemianopsia, 208, 209
Hemoglobinopathy, 247, 248
Hemoglobinuria, 247
Hemophilia, 234, 235
Hemoptysis, 340, 353, 354, 357

Hemorrhage, gastrointestinal,
  392–397 (see also Hema-
  temesis)
  causes, 395
  color of stool in, 393
  decision tree for, 396
  diagnostic protocols, 394, 395,
    396
  gastric aspiration in, 393
Hepatitis, 397–403
  alcohol-induced, 398
  amebic, 398
  B prodromes, 398
  chronic active, 527–530
    clinical picture, 527, 530
    immunologic studies, 530
    liver biopsy, 530
    non-A non-B type, 530
  drug-induced, 398
  immunologic markers, 400
  laboratory tests, 399, 400
  viral types, 400, 401
Hereditary spherocytosis, 247,
  249
Hirsutism, 282–286
  causes, 282, 283
  ethnic, 283
  idiopathic, 283
Histoplasmosis, 42
History taking
  ad hoc inquiry, 15
  body language, 14
  closed-ended questions, 13
  critical questions, 18
  disordered inquiry, 15
  do's and don'ts, 13
  eliciting the truth, 14
  errors commonly made, 181
  exclude and confirm technique,
    18
  hypothesis evaluation, 16
  hypothesis verification method
    of inquiry, 15
  independent, 19
  inquiry patterns, 14
  oblique questions, 18
  open-ended questions, 13, 174
  rigid and flexible formats, 14
  scanning questions, 16
  searching questions, 16
  silence, 14
  template matching, 16
  traditional method of inquiry,
    15
HLA-B27 and ankylosing spondylitis, 83
Hodgkin's disease, 260–265
  pruritus, significance of, 264
  staging of, 262, 263, 265
Holter monitor, 317, 543
Homans' sign, 206, 349
Horner's syndrome, 153, 154,
  515
Horton's headache, 506
HPO (see Pulmonary osteoarthropathy, hypertrophic)

Hunch, 60
  and intuition, 156, 157 (*see also* Medical intuition)
Hurler's syndrome, 299
Hydatidiform mole, 477
Hypercalcemia, 454–459
  causes, 454
    food and drugs, 454
    hyperparathyroidism, 454
    malignancy, 454, 456
  familial hypocalciuric, 458
  vagaries of calcium measurement, 454
Hypercalciuria, idiopathic, 428
Hyperkalemia, 452, 453
Hyperparathyroidism
  in stone formation, 428, 429
  primary, 454
    band keratopathy, 455, 456
    complications, 455
    laboratory tests, 456, 457, 458
    need for surgery, 458
    radiographic findings, 457
    symptoms, 455
Hyperpolymenorrhea, 475
Hypersensitivity pneumonitis, 360
Hypertension, 531–536
  causes, 531
  demographics, 531
  diagnostic protocol, 535
  hyperglycemia in, 534
  hypokalemia in, 534
  natural history, 531
  physical findings, 532
  renovascular, 532, 533, 534, 535
  tests for, 533, 534
  target organ involvement, 534
Hyperthermia, habitual, 553
Hyperthyroidism, 274, 286–290, 454, 455
  apathetic, 289
  clinical features, 287
  differential diagnosis, 287
  factitious, 289
Hypertrophy, left ventricle
  causes, 298, 299, 300
  physical findings in, 298, 299
  problem solving in, 301
Hyperventilation, 451
Hyperventilation syndrome, 581
Hyperviscosity syndrome, 241, 242, 252
Hypervitaminosis D, 427
Hypochondriasis, 581
Hypoglycemia, 278–282
  alimentary, 280
  causes, 279, 280, 281
  diagnosis, 280, 281
  factitious, 280
  insulin caused, 280, 281
  mimics, 278
  reactive, 279–280
  symptoms, 278

Hypokalemia, 449–453
  causes, 450, 452
  electrocardiographic changes, 449
  potassium kinetics, 450
  schema for diagnosis, 451
  surreptitious drug use, 452
  symptoms, 449
Hyponatremia, 459–464
  algorithmic approach, 462
  causes, 460
  differential diagnosis of symptoms, 459
  drug related, 461, 463
  laboratory evaluation, 461
  physical signs, 460
  sodium distribution, 460
  symptoms, 459, 460
Hypoparathyroidism, 288, 289
Hypothesis generation, 5 (*see also* Problem-solving methods)
Hypothyroidism, 288–289

Iatrogenic disease, 570–576
Idiopathic cyclic edema, 432
Idiopathic hypertrophic subaortic stenosis, 314
Ileus, paralytic, 406, 407
Imperfect information, concept of, 78, 93
Index Medicus, xxix, xxxi, 224, 560
  cumulated, 561
Indigestion, 372–377
  cholecystogram and ultrasound in diagnosis of, 374, 375
  functional vs organic, 373–374
  symptoms and causes, 373, 374
Infective endocarditis, 313, 314
Information retrieval, 559–564
Initial concepts, 15, 16
Initial hypothesis, 15
Inspection, 55–56
Insulinoma, 280, 281 (*see also* Hypoglycemia)
Intelligence
  artificial, 32
  natural, 31, 165
Interstitial nephritis, acute, 440
Intestinal obstruction, 403–407
  causes, 404, 406, 407
  distal vs proximal, 404, 406
  physical signs, 404, 405
  radiologic features, 405
  symptoms, 403, 404
Intestinal perforation, 405
Intestinal strangulation, 405, 406
Intraocular pressure, 26
Intuition, 60
Intussusception, 404
Irritable colon syndrome, 581

Jaundice, 397–403
  differential diagnosis, 397, 398
Jejunal biopsy, peroral, 385
Judgment, 2, 60, 168

Kartagener's syndrome, 153
Kayser-Fleischer ring, 45, 83
Kernig's sign, 207
Key clue, 3 (*see also* Problem-solving methods)
Kipling, 20
Krupp, Marcus A., 560
Kussmaul respiration, 538
Kveim-Siltzback test, 361

Laboratory automation, 28
Lactose intolerance, 376
Lacunar infarct, 516, 518–519
La Fontaine, 106
Lanthanic method, 157
Lasègue's sign, 497
Laurence-Moon-Biedl syndrome, 5
Lead intoxication, 225, 229
Left ventricular failure, 444 (*see also* Congestive heart failure)
Leiomyoma of uterus, 477
Leiomyosarcoma, 207
Lenègre's disease, 544
Leukemia
  acute, 257, 258, 259
  chronic, 258, 259
  radiation related, 259
Likelihood ratios, 88–91, 93, 94, 95, 103
Likelihood revision, 85–86, 93, 94
  by a negative clue, 86
  by a positive clue, 85
  by combinations of clues, 91, 92
Likelihoods, 4
Logic, 3, 8, 50
  causes of an effect, 52
  effects of a cause, 52
  maxims, 51, 52
  on basis of age, 50
  on basis of disease incidence, 52
  on basis of gender, 51
  on basis of geography, 51
  on basis of natural history, 51
  on basis of race, 51
  reverse gear, 52
Lyme disease, 34, 492, 494
Lymphadenopathy, 260–265
  causes, 260, 261
Lymphangiectasia, intestinal, 383, 385

Macroglobulinemia, 244
Magnetic resonance, 118, 123
Mainland, 47
Malabsorption syndrome, 382–387
  causes, 383, 384
  character of stool, 383
  chemical studies, 384
  clinical picture, 382, 383
  pathophysiology, 384
  radiographic features, 384
  role of liver disease, 386
  role of pancreatic disease, 386

Mallory-Weiss syndrome, 47, 369, 371, 562
Mammography, 125
Maneuvers with clues, 158
  exclusion, 158
  pattern building, 158
  screening, 158
  template matching, 158
  weight of evidence, 158, 159
Marfan's syndrome, 23, 153, 299, 534
Mathematical operations, 159 (see also Bayes' theorems, Boolean algebra, Mathematics, Venn diagrams)
Mathematical precision in medicine, 127–128
Mathematics, need for knowledge of, 65–66
McBurney's point, 388, 391
Meckel's diverticulum, 395, 396
Medical information base, 8, 50
Medical intuition, 3, 93, 128, 148, 156 (see also Problem-solving methods)
Medical Subject Headings (MeSH), 560
Mediterranean anemia, 227 (see also Anemia)
Mediterranean fever, familial, 552
Medline, 561
Medspeak, 130
Megaloblastic madness, 239
Melena, 392–397
  causes, 393
  roles for arteriography, endoscopy, isotopes, 396
Ménière's disease, 513
Menopause, 467–468, 469
  FSH level in, 468
Mesenteric occlusion, 379
Migraine, 504–505 (see also Headache)
  classic, 505
  common, 505
Milk-alkali syndrome, 427
Minimal change disease, 435, 436
Mistakes students make, 181–183 (see also History taking, Physical examination, Problem lists)
Mitral regurgitation, 298, 313–314
Mitral stenosis, 320–321
  catheterization studies, 321
  complications, 321, 322
  hemoptysis, 342
Mucoviscidosis, 587
Multiple choice questions, xxvi
Multiple myeloma, 241–244
  pathophysiology, 242, 243
Multisystem problems, 522–555
Musculoskeletal problems, 479–499
  immunology in, 480
  new technology, 479
  rheumatology and orthopaedics, 479

Myasthenia gravis, 365
Mycoplasma pneumonia, 247, 248
Myelofibrosis, 254, 257
Myeloma kidney, 440
Myeloproliferative disorders, 252, 254
Myocardial infarction, acute, 306–310
  clinical picture, 306, 307
  complications, 308, 309
  risk factors, 307, 309, 324
  ventricular premature depolarizations, 307, 308
Myoglobinuria, 247, 440
Myxoma, right atrium, 320, 321

National Library of Medicine, 560
Nephrotic syndrome, xxiv–xxv, 432–437
  causes, 434, 435, 436
  of edema, 432
  diagnosis of cause for, 434
  diagnostic triad, 433, 434
  laboratory tests, 434
  pathophysiology, 432, 433, 434
  role of biopsy, 435
  urinalysis in, 433
Neurologic problems, 500–521
  common presentations, 500
  technologic aids, 500–501
  topical diagnosis, 500, 520
Nil lesion, 435, 436
Nocturnal cramps, 590
Nosocomial anemia, 106
Nutritional history, 225
Nystagmus, 513, 514

Obesity, 282–286
  causes, 282
Objectives of book, xxiii–xxiv
Obstructive pulmonary disease, chronic, 303, 305, 335, 336, 339, 353–357
Obstructive uropathy, 415, 425, 441
Obturator sign, 388
Operating characteristics 75, 76, 77, 139 (see also Sensitivity, Specificity)
  alteration of, 76, 79–80
    tradeoffs by causing, 81
  applications of, 76
  derivation of, 75
  test efficiency, 75, 80
Option, alternative, 130
Organic brain syndromes, 579
Osler, William, 559
Osler's disease, 561
Osteoarthritis, 483, 491
Ovarian cyst, 472, 473
Over the counter drugs, 571, 572

Pancoast tumor, 487
Pancreatitis
  acute, 377–382
    clinical picture, 377, 378
    differential diagnosis, 378

laboratory diagnosis, 379
pathophysiology, 380
radiologic diagnosis, 380
chronic, 383
Papillary muscle rupture, 308
Papillary necrosis, 440
Paraproteinemia, 242, 243
Patient management, 7
Patient Management Problem, xxvi
Pediatric patient, problem solving in, 584–587
  different diagnostic possibilities, 585–586
  different techniques, 584
  monopathy, 587
  unique data sets, 585
Pel-Ebstein fever, 264
Pelvic inflammatory disease, 471, 472, 473
Pelvic pain, acute, 471–473
  causes, 471, 472
  ultrasound in diagnosis of, 473
Peptic ulcer, perforated, 381
Percutaneous transhepatic cholangiography, 400
Peritonitis, 410 (see also Cirrhosis of liver)
Peroxidase reaction, 258
Petersdorf-Beeson criteria for fever of unknown origin, 550 (see also Fever, unknown origin)
Pheochromocytoma, 279, 531, 532
Physical examination
  ad hoc, 21
  aids in recording, 187–188
    chest examination, 187–188
    flow charts, 188
    murmur description, 188
    sketches, 187
  attention to one item, 24
  causes for poor performance of, 23
  clinical measurement in, 23, 24
  complete, 21
  errors in doing, 22, 23
    excusable errors, 22
  examples of, 177, 190–192, 195–196
  general inspection, importance of, 21
  inaccuracies of, 24
  orderliness, importance of, 24
  palpation, uses of, 21, 22
  pitfalls in doing, 21
  positions of patient, 25
  skills, dissected, 24–25
    apex beat, 25
    eye examination, 25
    many per system, 25
  specific, 21
Physician Data Query (PDQ), 561
Pica, 225, 229
Pickwickian syndrome, 322
Pitressin, 292, 293

Pivotal clue, 154
aggregation of findings to form, 154
Plasma renin activity (PRA), 534
Pleural effusion, 346, 348–353
causes, 350
diagnostic studies, 351, 352, 353
dyspnea of sudden onset, 349
causes, 349
physical signs, 349
pleural fluid analysis, 350, 352
transudate vs exudate, 351
Plummer-Vinson syndrome, 365, 366
Pneumonia, 245–246, 344–348
complications, 246, 346, 347
in immunosuppressed host, 348
isolation of organism, 347
Klebsiella, 347
Legionella, 348
management, 346
mycoplasma, 346, 348
organisms, 345
physical signs, 344, 345
pneumococcal lobar, 344–345
Polyarthritis, 34
Polycystic ovaries, 284, 285 (*see also* Stein-Leventhal syndrome)
Polycythemia vera, 250–255
causes, 250, 253, 255
Polydipsia (*see* Diabetes insipidus)
Polymyalgia rheumatica, 502, 504
Polyuria (*see* Diabetes insipidus)
Portal-systemic encephalopathy, 408, 409
Positron emission tomography, 118, 123–124
PPD skin test (*see* Purified protein derivative skin test)
Precision, 6
in measurement, 57
Predictive value, 72
negative, 73
positive, 73
Pregnancy
ectopic, 468, 471, 472, 473
signs of, 468
test, 467, 468
Prevalence, 72
of disease P(D), 149–150
Prinzmetal's angina, 326
Probability, 4, 72
incremental change in, 74
of disease, P(D), 131, 149–150
estimate by Delphi technique for, 137
revision of, 150
posttest P(D), 74
pretest P(D), 74
theory, 2
Problem-based learning, xxvi–xxx, 231, 272, 301, 334, 368, 419, 453, 470, 484, 506, 526
Problem lists
assessment of, 6, 9, 179, 180,

192, 197–198
errors made in, 182
benefits of, 36
composition of, 34, 35
derivation of, 35
errors in construction, 35, 182
examples, 35, 36, 179, 192, 197, 285, 356, 520
final, 7, 9, 36, 180
formation, 34–37
initial, 7, 9, 36, 50, 179
level of resolution of, 35
Problem-oriented medical records, 2
Problem solving, xxi, xxii
minimal, 149
shortcuts in, 11 (*see also* Problem-solving methods)
teaching, xxv
Problem-solving methods, xxii, 148–169
algorithms, 161–163
cluster formation, 151
triads and tetrads, 152
weight of evidence, 152
computers, role of, 165–167
dendrograms, 159–160
early hypothesis generation, 151
hypothetico-deductive method, 151
initial concept, 151
string-together technique, 151
key clue, 154
divide and conquer strategy, 154
pattern recognition, 152, 153
gestalt, examples, 152, 153
syndromes, 153–154
traditional, 150–151
Procedures (*see* Tests)
Product of probabilities, 87, 93, 114
with maximal interdependence, 87, 88
with no interdependence, 87
with varying degrees of interdependence, 88, 89, 93
Programmed electrical stimulation, 296
Prolactinoma, 209, 468
Proof by exclusion, 155, 158
Proof by fleshing out, 156
Prostatic hypertrophy, benign, 415, 445
Protein-losing enteropathy, 432
Provisional hypotheses, 3 (*see also* Problem-solving methods)
Pseudobulbar palsy, 367
Pseudocyesis, 469
Pseudogout, 482, 484, 491
Pseudohyponatremia, 460, 461, 463
Psoas sign, 388
Psychiatric patient, problem solving in, 577–583
coping with, 582
organic vs "functional," 577

relative frequency of, 577–578
Psychogenic polydipsia (*see* Diabetes insipidus)
Psychosomatic disorders, 20, 578, 579
common symptoms, 20, 21
Pulmonary edema, 26
Pulmonary embolus, 304, 305, 341, 343, 349, 351
Pulmonary fibrosis, 359, 361
Pulmonary hypertension
causes, 319
diagnosis, 319
primary, 321, 358
Pulmonary nodule, 329–334
causes, 329
diagnosis, 330, 331, 332
doubling time, 329
Pulmonary osteoarthropathy, hypertrophic, 43, 354, 355
Pulmonary problems, 327–362
diagnostic aids, 327
patient presentations, 328
physical findings in, 327
symptoms of, 327
Purified protein derivative skin test, 330, 331, 343, 351, 355
Purpura, thrombocytopenic, 232–234
antibody mediated, 234
drug related, 234
thrombotic, 233, 234
Pyelonephritis
acute, 424, 425
complications, 425
chronic, 425

QALYS, 130
Quantification of terms, 56–58

Radioisotope studies, 118, 122
Raynaud's phenomenon, 366
Reading (*see also* Problem-based learning and Supplementary reading)
compulsory, xxxi
recommended, xxxi
Receiver-operator characteristics curve, 80–81
Red blood cell indices, 228, 238, 265
Red cell mass, 253, 255
Reed-Sternberg cells, 262
Reiter's syndrome, 490
Relevance of a clue, 31
Renal failure
acute, 437–442
causes, 438, 439
chemistry, 437
definition, 438
muscle necrosis as cause, 440, 441
vs chronic, 437, 438
chronic, 442–446
blood chemistry, 444
clinical picture, 442, 443, 445

Renal failure, chronic–*continued*
    differential diagnosis, 442, 445
    hypertension in, 445
    modes of presentation, 446
    pathophysiology, 442, 443, 444
    renal size in diagnosis of, 445
    tetany in, 443
Renal problems, 413–446
    clinical presentations, 413, 414
    new technology for, 414
    physical signs of, 413
Reticulocyte index, 228
Retroperitoneal fibrosis, 426, 445
Rhabdomyolysis, 441
Rheumatic valvular heart disease, 298, 312, 320
Rheumatoid arthritis, 491
    American Rheumatism Association criteria, 491
    manifestations, 491, 493
Rheumatoid factor, 491, 493
Richter's hernia, 406, 407
Riedel's lobe, 23
Right ventricular failure, 318–322
Risks, costs, benefits, 139
Rotator cuff injury, 486
"Rule of ones," 72
"Rule out," 16

SIADH, 292, 461
    causes, 463
    cancer, 463
Saralasin test, 533
Sarcoidosis, 358–362, 454, 456, 457
    anergy, 360
    diagnostic studies, 359, 360, 361
    hilar adenopathy, 360
    physical signs, 358
    pulmonary function tests, 359
    pulmonary hypertension, 358
    serologic tests, 360
    special features, 362
    stone formation in, 428
    symptoms, 358
Savatthi, King, ix
Scenario, 130
Schatzki's ring, 367
Schilling test, 387
Schizophrenia, 581
Science Citation Index, 562
Scleroderma, as cause of dysphagia, 367, 368
Sclerosing cholangitis, 397
Secretin test, 384
Secretin-cholecystokinin test, 384
Seizure (*see* Convulsion)
Self-evaluation exercises, xxiii
Sensitivity, 14, 15, 16, 45, 48, 75
    false negative rate, 72
    false positive rate, 72
    true negative rate, 72
    true positive rate, 72
Sensitivity analysis, 135

Sentinel pile, 212
Sequential multiple analyzer, 101
Set theory, 67, 68, 69, 94
    overlapping sets, 68, 69
Sheehan's syndrome, 289, 469
Sherlock Holmes, 42
Shortcuts, 55–56
    coup d'oeil, 55
    examples, 56
    how inspection helps, 55
    zeroing in, 55
Shoulder pain, 485–490
    applied anatomy, 486
    arthrocentesis, 489
    causes, 486
        extraarticular, 487
    physical examination, 487, 488
    radiography, 488
Sick sinus syndrome, 543
    causes for syncope in, 543–544
Sjögren's syndrome, 492
Skills
    case presentation, 199–204
    data acquisition, 174–181
    data analysis, 174–181
    data management, 173
    data relevance, determination, 209–217 (*see also* Data resolution skills)
    data subset selection, 205–209
    data synthesis, 174–181
    interpersonal, 10
    oral communication, 10, 174–177 (*see also* History taking)
    reasoning, 10
    self-assessment, 10
    transforming interview to written history, 174–179
    written communication, 10
SLE (*see* Systemic lupus erythematosus)
Society for Medical Decision Making, vii
Socratic sessions, xxvi
South India monkey trap, 127
Specificity, 14, 15, 16, 75
Spider angioma, 45, 46
Staghorn stones, 429
Stain
    periodic acid-Schiff, 258
    Sudan III, 387
    Wright's-Giemsa, 258
    Ziehl-Neelson, 332, 355
Steatorrhea, 385
Stein-Leventhal syndrome, 284, 469
Stick diagrams, 73
Stokes-Adams attacks, 541, 544
Subdeltoid bursitis, 486
Subdural hematoma, 504, 520
Suggested readings, viii, xxvii, xxix, xxxi
Sulkowich test, 429
Supplementary reading, xxvii, xxviii (*see also* Suggested readings)

Suppression of information, 156
Sutton's law, 45
Syllogisms, 60
    deductive reasoning, 61
    inductive reasoning, 61
    negative, 60
    positive, 60
Symptoms
    normality of, 19
    unreported, 19–20
Syncope, 540–545
    carotid sinus, 540, 542
    causes, 541
    cervical bruits, 542
    diagnostic logic, 542, 543
    equivalents, 540
Système Internationale, 104
Systemic lupus erythematosus
    American Rheumatism Association criteria, 492
    drugs causing, 492
    immunologic markers, 493
    manifestations, 491, 492

Tamponade, 308
Teaching, 6
    disease oriented, 6
    faculty faults, 6
    problem oriented, 6
Technologic procedures, 118–126
    cost-benefit-risk factors, 119, 124–126
    effect of Diagnosis-Related Groups, 120
    selection of, 119, 125–126
Temporal arteritis, 502, 504
Tension headache (*see* Headache)
Tentative diagnosis, 3 (*see also* Problem-solving methods)
Tests, 98–117
    alteration of testing formats, 111, 112
    availability, 101
    choosing the best test, 116
    continuous variable results, 103
    deciding on, 30
    Diagnosis-Related Groups, effect on, 112
    dichotomous test results, 103
    economic consideration, 114
    errors in testing, causes, 105
    expense, 101
    imperfect, 104
    invasive procedures, 102
    misuse, 108–110
    normality, 103–105
        "decision level," 103
        referent values, 103, 104
    order of testing, 99–100
        sequential strategy, 100
        tandem strategy, 100
    overuse, reasons for, 108
    patterns for ordering, 98
    perfect, 103–104
    profiles, batteries, panels, 101
        for coronary risk, 101

Torch profile, 101
reasons for testing, 99
  monitoring, 99
  screening, 99
  targeted screening, 99
reporting techniques, 102
risks, 102
selectivity of, 29
special, 107–108
  acid-fast stain, 108
  Campylobacter, 107
  carcinoembryonic antigen, 108
  cardiac enzymes, 107
  treadmill, 108, 325
strategies for testing, 106–107
  batteries vs selectivity, 106, 107
  combination testing, 113–116
  profiles and subprofiles, 106–107
  series or parallel, 113
  specific clinical problems, 116
unexpected test results, 110
Textbook picture of disease, 32 (*see also* Disease, definition of)
Thallium scan, 325
Threshold determinations, 132, 136–137
Thyroid function tests, 270, 274, 288, 289
Thyroid nodule, 269–272
  aspiration cytology, 270
  clues for malignancy, 271, 272
  dendrogram in diagnosis of, 272
  evidence of toxicity, 270
  radioisotope scan, 271
  sonogram, 271
Tietze's syndrome, 324
Tilt test, 393
Tophi, 45, 484 (*see also* Gout)
Toxic megacolon, 386

Transient ischemic attacks, 517, 518, 541
  as cause of convulsions, 508
Treadmill test, 108, 325
Triage, 565–569
  decisions on urgency, 568
  definition, 565
  emergency room role, 566
  emergent, urgent, nonurgent, 567
  need for selective data inquiry, 568, 569
  pitfalls, 568, 569
  protocols and algorithms, 566
Tuberculosis, 328, 330, 332, 341, 343, 351, 355
  miliary, 553, 554 (*see also* Fever, unknown origin)
Tumor markers, 118
Two by two tables, 73, 78, 84, 85, 92

Ulcerative colitis, 385, 386
Ultrasound, 118, 120–121
  M mode, 120
  two-dimensional, 120
  uses, 120–121
Uremic frost, 443
Urinary tract infection, 422–426
  obstruction in the etiology of, 425

Vaginal bleeding, abnormal, 474–478
  causes, 474, 475, 476
  evaluation, 475, 477
  pelvic examination, 475
  terminology, 475
Vasopressin, 292
Venereal Disease Research Laboratory Test, 28, 261
Venn diagrams, 67, 70, 77, 78, 578

Ventilation-perfusion scan, 304, 351, 352
Vertebrobasilar ischemia, 513, 514, 515
Vertigo (*see* Dizziness)
Vestibular neuronitis, 512
Virchow node, 45, 370
Virilism, 283
Vitamin D intoxication, 457
Voltaire, 20
Volvulus, 404
Von Willebrand's disease, 234, 235

Wallenberg's syndrome, 514
Wassermann test, 28
Weakness, weight loss, anorexia, 523–526 (*see also* Carcinoma, of prostate)
Wernicke-Korsakoff encephalopathy, 408, 409
Whipple's disease, 383, 385, 552
Whipple's triad, 281
Whispered pectoriloquy, 26
Willebrand, E. A. von (*see* Von Willebrand's disease)
Wilson's disease, 411, 529
Wolff-Parkinson-White syndrome, 108
Workup, 53–55
  complete, who needs a, 54
  depth of study, 53
  maxi-workup, 53
  midi-workup, 53
  mini-workup, 53

d-Xylose absorption test, 384, 386

Yearbook of Medicine, 559

Zenker's diverticulum, 365, 366
Zollinger-Ellison syndrome, 371